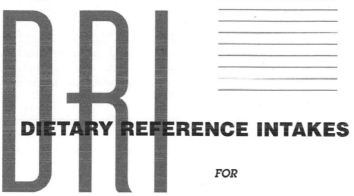

DIETARY REFERENCE INTAKES

FOR

Vitamin C,
Vitamin E,
Selenium, and
Carotenoids

A Report of the
Panel on Dietary Antioxidants and Related Compounds,
Subcommittees on Upper Reference Levels of Nutrients and
Interpretation and Uses of Dietary Reference Intakes, and the
Standing Committee on the Scientific Evaluation of
Dietary Reference Intakes

Food and Nutrition Board
Institute of Medicine

NATIONAL ACADEMY PRESS
Washington, D.C.

NATIONAL ACADEMY PRESS • 2101 Constitution Avenue, N.W. • Washington, DC 20418

NOTICE: The project that is the subject of this report was approved by the Governing Board of the National Research Council, whose members are drawn from the councils of the National Academy of Sciences, the National Academy of Engineering, and the Institute of Medicine. The members of the committee responsible for the report were chosen for their special competences and with regard for appropriate balance.

This project was funded by the U.S. Department of Health and Human Services Office of Disease Prevention and Health Promotion, Contract No. 282-96-0033; Health Canada; the Institute of Medicine; the Dietary Reference Intakes Private Foundation Fund, including the Dannon Institute and the International Life Sciences Institute; and the Dietary Reference Intakes Corporate Donors' Fund. Contributors to the Fund include Roche Vitamins Inc.; Mead Johnson Nutrition Group; Daiichi Fine Chemicals, Inc.; Kemin Foods, Inc.; M&M Mars; Weider Nutrition Group; Nabisco Foods Group; U.S. Borax; and Natural Source Vitamin E Association. The opinions or conclusions expressed herein do not necessarily reflect those of the funders.

Library of Congress Cataloging-in-Publication Data

Dietary reference intakes for vitamin C, vitamin E, selenium, and carotenoids : a report of the Panel on Dietary Antioxidants and Related Compounds, Subcommitties on Upper Reference Levels of Nutrients and of Interpretation and Use of Dietary Reference Intakes, and the Standing Committee on the Scientific Evaluation of Dietary Reference Intakes, Food and Nutrition Board, Institute of Medicine.
    p. ; cm.
Includes bibliographical references and index.
ISBN 0-309-06949-1 (case) – ISBN 0-309-06935-1 (paper)
  1. Antioxidants. 2. Reference values (Medicine). 3. Vitamin C. 4. Vitamin E. 5. Carotenoids. I. Institute of Medicine (U.S.). Panel on Dietary Antioxidants and Related Compounds.
  [DNLM: 1. Nutritional Requirements. 2. Ascorbic Acid. 3. Carotenoids. 4. Reference Values. 5. Selenium. 6. Vitamin E. QU 145 D56566 2000]
QP801.A66 D53 2000
612.3′9–dc21
00-035521

This report is available for sale from the National Academy Press, 2101 Constitution Avenue, N.W., Box 285, Washington, DC 20055; call (800) 624-6242 or (202) 334-3313 (in the Washington metropolitan area), or visit the NAP's on-line bookstore at **http://www.nap.edu**.

For more information about the Institute of Medicine or the Food and Nutrition Board, visit the IOM home page at **http://www.iom.edu**.

Printed in the United States of America

The serpent has been a symbol of long life, healing, and knowledge among almost all cultures and religions since the beginning of recorded history. The image adopted as a logotype by the Institute of Medicine is based on a relief carving from ancient Greece, now held by the Staatliche Museen in Berlin.

"Knowing is not enough; we must apply.
Willing is not enough; we must do."
—Goethe

INSTITUTE OF MEDICINE

Shaping the Future for Health

THE NATIONAL ACADEMIES

National Academy of Sciences
National Academy of Engineering
Institute of Medicine
National Research Council

The **National Academy of Sciences** is a private, nonprofit, self-perpetuating society of distinguished scholars engaged in scientific and engineering research, dedicated to the furtherance of science and technology and to their use for the general welfare. Upon the authority of the charter granted to it by the Congress in 1863, the Academy has a mandate that requires it to advise the federal government on scientific and technical matters. Dr. Bruce M. Alberts is president of the National Academy of Sciences.

The **National Academy of Engineering** was established in 1964, under the charter of the National Academy of Sciences, as a parallel organization of outstanding engineers. It is autonomous in its administration and in the selection of its members, sharing with the National Academy of Sciences the responsibility for advising the federal government. The National Academy of Engineering also sponsors engineering programs aimed at meeting national needs, encourages education and research, and recognizes the superior achievements of engineers. Dr. William A. Wulf is president of the National Academy of Engineering.

The **Institute of Medicine** was established in 1970 by the National Academy of Sciences to secure the services of eminent members of appropriate professions in the examination of policy matters pertaining to the health of the public. The Institute acts under the responsibility given to the National Academy of Sciences by its congressional charter to be an adviser to the federal government and, upon its own initiative, to identify issues of medical care, research, and education. Dr. Kenneth I. Shine is president of the Institute of Medicine.

The **National Research Council** was organized by the National Academy of Sciences in 1916 to associate the broad community of science and technology with the Academy's purposes of furthering knowledge and advising the federal government. Functioning in accordance with general policies determined by the Academy, the Council has become the principal operating agency of both the National Academy of Sciences and the National Academy of Engineering in providing services to the government, the public, and the scientific and engineering communities. The Council is administered jointly by both Academies and the Institute of Medicine. Dr. Bruce M. Alberts and Dr. William A. Wulf are chairman and vice chairman, respectively, of the National Research Council.

PANEL ON DIETARY ANTIOXIDANTS
AND RELATED COMPOUNDS

NORMAN I. KRINSKY *(Chair)*, Department of Biochemistry, Tufts University, Boston, Massachusetts

GARY R. BEECHER, U.S. Department of Agriculture Beltsville Human Nutrition Research Center, Beltsville, Maryland

RAYMOND F. BURK, Clinical Nutrition Unit, Vanderbilt University Medical Center, Nashville, Tennessee

ALVIN C. CHAN, Department of Biochemistry, Microbiology, and Immunology, University of Ottawa, Ontario, Canada

JOHN W. ERDMAN, JR., Division of Nutritional Sciences, College of Agricultural, Consumer and Environmental Sciences, University of Illinois at Urbana-Champaign

ROBERT A. JACOB, U.S. Department of Agriculture Western Human Nutrition Research Center, University of California, Davis

ISHWARLAL JIALAL, Department of Pathology and Internal Medicine, University of Texas Southwestern Medical Center, Dallas

LAURENCE N. KOLONEL, Cancer Research Center, University of Hawaii, Honolulu

JAMES R. MARSHALL, Cancer Prevention and Control, Arizona Cancer Center, University of Arizona, Tucson

SUSAN TAYLOR MAYNE, Department of Epidemiology and Public Health, Yale University School of Medicine, New Haven, Connecticut

ROSS L. PRENTICE, Division of Public Health Sciences, Fred Hutchinson Cancer Research Center, Seattle, Washington

KATHLEEN B. SCHWARZ, Division of Pediatric GI/Nutrition, Johns Hopkins Hospital, Baltimore, Maryland

DANIEL STEINBERG, Division of Endocrinology and Metabolism, University of California, San Diego

MARET G. TRABER, Department of Nutrition and Food Management, Oregon State University, Corvallis

Food and Nutrition Board Liaison
CHARLES H. HENNEKENS, Boca Raton, Florida

Federal Project Steering Committee Liaison
LTC KARL FRIEDL, U.S. Army Medical Research and Materiel Command, Ft. Detrick, Frederick, Maryland

Staff

SANDRA A. SCHLICKER, Study Director
ELISABETH A. REESE, Research Associate
ALICE L. VOROSMARTI, Research Associate
MICHELE R. RAMSEY, Senior Project Assistant

SUBCOMMITTEE ON UPPER REFERENCE
LEVELS OF NUTRIENTS

IAN C. MUNRO *(Chair)*, CanTox, Inc., Mississauga, Ontario, Canada
GEORGE C. BECKING, Phoenix OHC, Kingston, Ontario, Canada
RENATE D. KIMBROUGH, Independent Consultant, Washington, D.C.
RITA B. MESSING, Division of Environmental Health, Minnesota
   Department of Health, St. Paul
SANFORD A. MILLER, Graduate School of Biomedical Sciences,
   University of Texas Health Sciences Center, San Antonio
SUZANNE P. MURPHY, Cancer Research Center, University of Hawaii,
   Honolulu
HARRIS PASTIDES, School of Public Health, University of South
   Carolina, Columbia
JOSEPH V. RODRICKS, The Life Sciences Consultancy LLC,
   Washington, D.C.
IRWIN H. ROSENBERG, Jean Mayer U.S. Department of Agriculture
   Human Nutrition Research Center on Aging, Tufts University,
   Boston, Massachusetts
STEVE L. TAYLOR, Department of Food Science and Technology and
   Food Processing Center, University of Nebraska, Lincoln
JOHN A. THOMAS, Retired, San Antonio, Texas
GARY M. WILLIAMS, Department of Pathology, New York Medical
   College, Valhalla

Staff

SANDRA A. SCHLICKER, Study Director
ELISABETH A. REESE, Research Associate
MICHELE R. RAMSEY, Senior Project Assistant

SUBCOMMITTEE ON INTERPRETATION AND USES OF DIETARY REFERENCE INTAKES

SUZANNE P. MURPHY *(Chair)*, Cancer Research Center, University of Hawaii, Honolulu

LENORE ARAB, Departments of Epidemiology and Nutrition, University of North Carolina School of Public Health, Chapel Hill

SUSAN I. BARR, Department of Nutrition, University of British Columbia, Vancouver, Canada

SUSAN T. BORRA, International Food Information Council, Washington, D.C.

ALICIA L. CARRIQUIRY, Department of Statistics, Iowa State University, Ames

BARBARA L. DEVANEY, Mathematica Policy Research, Princeton, New Jersey

JOHANNA T. DWYER, Frances Stern Nutrition Center, New England Medical Center and Tufts University, Boston, Massachusetts

JEAN-PIERRE HABICHT, Division of Nutritional Sciences, Cornell University, Ithaca, New York

HARRIET V. KUHNLEIN, Centre for Indigenous Peoples' Nutrition and Environment, McGill University, Ste. Anne de Bellevue, Quebec, Canada

Consultant

GEORGE BEATON, GHB Consulting, Willowdale, Ontario, Canada

Staff

MARY I. POOS, Study Director
ALICE L. VOROSMARTI, Research Associate
MICHELE R. RAMSEY, Senior Project Assistant

STANDING COMMITTEE ON THE SCIENTIFIC EVALUATION OF DIETARY REFERENCE INTAKES

VERNON R. YOUNG *(Chair)*, Laboratory of Human Nutrition, School of Science, Massachusetts Institute of Technology, Cambridge

JOHN W. ERDMAN, JR. *(Vice-Chair)*, Division of Nutritional Sciences, College of Agricultural, Consumer and Environmental Sciences, University of Illinois at Urbana-Champaign

LINDSAY H. ALLEN, Department of Nutrition, University of California, Davis

STEPHANIE A. ATKINSON, Department of Pediatrics, McMaster University, Hamilton, Ontario, Canada

ROBERT J. COUSINS, Center for Nutritional Sciences, University of Florida, Gainesville

JOHANNA T. DWYER, Frances Stern Nutrition Center, New England Medical Center and Tufts University, Boston, Massachusetts

JOHN D. FERNSTROM, Western Psychiatric Institute and Clinic, University of Pittsburgh School of Medicine, Pittsburgh, Pennsylvania

SCOTT M. GRUNDY, Center for Human Nutrition, University of Texas Southwestern Medical Center, Dallas

CHARLES H. HENNEKENS, Boca Raton, Florida

SANFORD A. MILLER, Graduate School of Biomedical Sciences, University of Texas Health Sciences Center, San Antonio

WILLIAM M. RAND, Department of Family Medicine and Community Health, Tufts University School of Medicine, Boston, Massachusetts

U.S. Government Liaison

ELIZABETH CASTRO, Office of Disease Prevention and Health Promotion, U.S. Department of Health and Human Services, Washington, D.C.

Canadian Government Liaison

PETER W.F. FISCHER, Nutrition Research Division, Health Protection Branch, Health Canada, Ottawa, Ontario, Canada

Staff

ALLISON A. YATES, Study Director
GAIL E. SPEARS, Administrative Assistant

Preface

This report is one of a series that presents a comprehensive set of reference values for nutrient intakes for healthy U.S and Canadian populations. It is a product of the Food and Nutrition Board of the Institute of Medicine working in cooperation with scientists from Canada.

The report establishes a set of reference values for vitamin C, vitamin E, and selenium to replace previously published Recommended Dietary Allowances (RDAs) and Recommended Nutrient Intakes (RNIs) for the United States and Canada and examines data about β-carotene and the other carotenoids (α-carotene, β-cryptoxanthin, lutein, lycopene, and zeaxanthin). Evidence has been reviewed regarding the impact of these compounds on chronic disease along with their roles related to deficiency states. Although the reference values are based on data, the data were often scanty or drawn from studies that had limitations in addressing the various questions that needed to be dealt with in order to develop reference values for these nutrients and food components. Thus, scientific judgment was required in setting the reference values. The reasoning used is described for each nutrient in Chapters 5 through 8.

These compounds, vitamin C, vitamin E, selenium, β-carotene and other carotenoids, have been termed "dietary antioxidants" somewhat loosely by many. There has been intense interest by the public and the media in the possibility that increased intakes of dietary antioxidants protect against chronic disease. Many research programs are under way in this area.

Epidemiological evidence suggests that the consumption of fruits and vegetables reduces the risk of both cancer and cardiovascular disease, and it has been hypothesized that this is due in part to the presence of compounds with antioxidant properties found in these food groups. While dietary antioxidants is a convenient generic title, these compounds are multifunctional, and some of the actions observed in vivo may not represent an antioxidant function, even though the compounds have been frequently classified as antioxidant nutrients.

Although a definition of a dietary antioxidant is provided in this report at the specific request of the federal agencies, the above compounds were evaluated with respect to their role in human nutrition, without limiting the criteria to antioxidant properties or to only those compounds or nutrients which met the definition. Data were reviewed regarding the minimum amount of these compounds required to prevent deficiency diseases, as well as the amounts that might impact on chronic diseases regardless of whether or not the putatively protective mechanisms involved antioxidant properties. Thus, a major task of the Panel on Dietary Antioxidants and Related Compounds, the Subcommittee on Upper Reference Levels of Nutrients (UL Subcommittee), the Subcommittee on Interpretation and Uses of Dietary Reference Intakes (Uses Subcommittee), and the Standing Committee on the Scientific Evaluation of Dietary Reference Intakes (DRI Committee) was to analyze the evidence on beneficial and adverse effects of various intakes of vitamin C, vitamin E, selenium, and β-carotene in the context of setting Dietary Reference Intakes (DRIs) for these compounds.

Many of the questions raised about requirements for and recommended intakes of these nutrients cannot be answered fully because of inadequacies in the present database. Apart from studies of overt deficiency disease, there is a dearth of studies that address specific effects of inadequate intakes on specific indicators of health status. For these compounds, there is no direct information that permits estimating the amounts required by children, adolescents, lactating women, and the elderly. For β-carotene, data useful for the setting of Tolerable Upper Intake Levels (ULs) are inconsistent and for the other carotenoids data are sparse, precluding reliable estimates of the minimum intake above which there is the risk of adverse effects. For some of these nutrients, there are questions about how much is contained in the food North Americans eat. Thus, another major task of the report was to outline a research agenda to provide a basis for public policy decisions related to recommended intakes of vitamin C, vitamin E, selenium, and the carotenoids and ways to achieve those intakes.

The process for establishing DRIs is an iterative process and is thus evolving as the conceptual framework is applied to new nutrients and food components. With more experience, the proposed models for establishing reference intakes for use with nutrients and food components that play a role in health will be refined. Also, as new information or new methods of analysis are adopted, these reference values undoubtedly will be reassessed.

Because the project is ongoing as indicated above, many comments were solicited and have been received on the two reports previously published (*Dietary Reference Intakes for Calcium, Phosphorus, Magnesium, Vitamin D, and Fluoride* and *Dietary Reference Intakes for Thiamin, Riboflavin, Niacin, Vitamin B_6, Folate, Vitamin B_{12}, Pantothenic Acid, Biotin, and Choline*). Refinements have been included in the general discussion regarding approaches used (Chapters 1 through 4) and in the discussion of uses of DRIs (Chapter 9 in this report). For example, it is now clearly stated that animal data can be used as the critical adverse effect in setting a UL for a nutrient.

Among the comments received to date have been requests for additional guidance in the practical application of DRIs. The Uses Subcommittee, conceptually included since the beginning of the DRI process, was formed subsequent to the release of the first two reports. Although their activities will involve reports specifically addressing the rationale for using DRIs for assessing intake and planning, in this report Chapter 9 addresses some of the major issues that relate to the anticipated uses and applications of reference values.

This report reflects the work of the Food and Nutrition Board's DRI Committee, its expert Panel on Dietary Antioxidants and Related Compounds, UL Subcommittee, and Uses Subcommittee. It is important to acknowledge the support of the government of Canada and Canadian scientists in this initiative, which represents a pioneering first step in the standardization of nutrient reference intakes at least within a major part of one continent. A brief description of the overall project of the DRI Committee and of the panel's task are given in Appendix A. It is hoped that the critical, comprehensive analyses of available information and of knowledge gaps in this initial series of reports will greatly assist the private sector, foundations, universities, government laboratories, and other institutions with the development of a productive research agenda for the next decade.

The DRI Committee, the Panel on Dietary Antioxidants and Related Compounds, the UL Subcommittee, and the Uses Subcommittee wish to extend sincere thanks to the many experts who have assisted with this report by giving presentations, providing written materials, participating in discussions, analyzing data, and other means. Many, but far from all, of these people are named in Appendix B. Special thanks go to staff at the National Center for Health Statistics, the Food Surveys Research Group of the Agricultural Research Service, and the Department of Statistics at Iowa State University for extensive analyses of survey data.

The respective chairs and members of the panel and subcommittees have performed their work under great time pressure. Their dedication made the completion of this report possible. All gave of their time willingly and without financial reward; both the science and practice of nutrition are major beneficiaries.

This report has been reviewed in draft form by individuals chosen for their diverse perspectives and technical expertise, in accordance with procedures approved by the National Research Council's Report Review Committee. The purpose of this independent review is to provide candid and critical comments to assist the panel and subcommittee members and the Institute of Medicine in making the published report as sound as possible and to ensure that the report meets institutional standards for objectivity, evidence, and responsiveness to the study charge.

The content of the final report is the responsibility of the Institute of Medicine and the study panel and not the responsibility of the reviewers. The review comments and draft manuscript remain confidential to protect the integrity of the deliberative process. The panel wishes to thank the following individuals, who are neither officials nor employees of the Institute of Medicine, for their participation in the review of this report: Bruce N. Ames, Ph.D., University of California at Berkeley; Dennis M. Bier, M.D., Baylor College of Medicine; James R. Coughlin, Ph.D., Coughlin & Associates; Barry Halliwell, D.Sc., University of London, Kings College; John E. Halver, Ph.D., University of Washington; Richard J. Havel, M.D., University of California at San Francisco; Orville Levander, Ph.D., U.S. Department of Agriculture; Stanley D. Omaye, Ph.D., University of Nevada; Helmut Sies, M.D., Heinrich-Heine-Universität Düsseldorf; Thressa C. Stadtman, Ph.D., National Institutes of Health; and Walter Willett, M.D., Dr. P.H., Harvard School of Public Health.

The DRI Committee wishes to acknowledge, in particular, the commitment shown by Norman Krinsky, chair of the panel, who steered this difficult project through what at times seemed to some like "dangerous and uncharted waters." His ability to keep the effort and the various perspectives moving in a positive direction is very much appreciated. Thanks also are due to DRI Committee members Scott Grundy and John Fernstrom, in-depth internal reviewers for this report.

Special thanks go to the staff of the Food and Nutrition Board and foremost to Sandra Schlicker, who was the study director for the panel and without whose assistance, both intellectual and managerial, this report would neither have been as polished nor as timely in its release.

It is, of course, those at the Food and Nutrition Board who get much of the work completed and so the panel, subcommittees, and the Food and Nutrition Board wish to thank Allison Yates, Director of the Food and Nutrition Board, for constant assistance and it also recognizes, with appreciation, the contributions of Mary Poos, Elisabeth Reese, Alice Vorosmarti, Gail Spears, and Michele Ramsey. We also thank Florence Poillon and Sydne Newberry for editing the manuscript and Mike Edington and Claudia Carl for assistance with publication.

Vernon Young
Chair, Standing Committee on the Scientific
   Evaluation of Dietary Reference Intakes

Cutberto Garza
Chair, Food and Nutrition Board

Contents

SUMMARY   **1**

   What Are Dietary Reference Intakes?, 2
   Approach for Setting Dietary Reference Intakes, 6
   Nutrient Functions and the Indicators Used to Estimate
      Requirements for Vitamin C, Vitamin E, Selenium,
      and the Carotenoids, 12
   Criteria and Proposed Values for Tolerable Upper
      Intake Levels, 13
   Using Dietary Reference Intakes, 14
   Definition of a Dietary Antioxidant, 17
   Evidence of Oxidative Stress and the Risk of Chronic
      Degenerative Disease, 17
   Recommendations, 19

**1 INTRODUCTION TO DIETARY REFERENCE
   INTAKES**   **21**

   What Are Dietary Reference Intakes?, 21
   Categories of Dietary Reference Intakes, 22
   Parameters for Dietary Reference Intakes, 27
   Summary, 33
   References, 33

2   **VITAMIN C, VITAMIN E, SELENIUM, AND
    β-CAROTENE AND OTHER CAROTENOIDS:
    OVERVIEW, ANTIOXIDANT DEFINITION, AND
    RELATIONSHIP TO CHRONIC DISEASE**   35
    Overview, 35
    Definition and Criteria for a Dietary Antioxidant, 42
    Oxidative Stress, Antioxidants, and Chronic Disease, 44
    Conclusions, 51
    References, 52

3   **VITAMIN C, VITAMIN E, SELENIUM, AND
    β-CAROTENE AND OTHER CAROTENOIDS:
    METHODS**   58
    Methodological Considerations, 58
    Estimates of Laboratory Values, 67
    Nutrient Intake Estimates, 67
    Dietary Intakes in the United States and Canada, 69
    Summary, 71
    References, 71

4   **A MODEL FOR THE DEVELOPMENT OF
    TOLERABLE UPPER INTAKE LEVELS FOR
    NUTRIENTS**   73
    Background, 73
    Model for Derivation of Tolerable Upper
        Intake Levels, 75
    Risk Assessment and Food Safety, 75
    Application of the Risk Assessment Model to
        Nutrients, 80
    Steps in the Development of Tolerable Upper
        Intake Levels, 84
    Intake Assessment, 92
    Risk Characterization, 92
    References, 94

5   **VITAMIN C**   95
    Summary, 95
    Background Information, 95
    Selection of Indicators for Estimating the
        Requirement for Vitamin C, 101
    Factors Affecting the Vitamin C Requirement, 128
    Findings by Life Stage and Gender Group, 134
    Intake of Vitamin C, 154

Tolerable Upper Intake Levels, 155
Research Recommendations for Vitamin C, 165
References, 167

6 **VITAMIN E**   186
Summary, 186
Background Information, 187
Selection of Indicators for Estimating the Requirement
    for α-Tocopherol, 203
Factors Affecting the Vitamin E Requirement, 224
Findings by Life Stage and Gender Group, 226
Intake of Vitamin E, 243
Tolerable Upper Intake Levels, 249
Research Recommendations for Vitamin E, 260
References, 262

7 **SELENIUM**   284
Summary, 284
Background Information, 284
Selection of Indicators for Estimating the
    Requirement for Selenium, 287
Factors Affecting the Selenium Requirement, 291
Findings by Life Stage and Gender Group, 292
Intake of Selenium, 308
Tolerable Upper Intake Levels, 311
Research Recommendations for Selenium, 318
References, 319

8 **β-CAROTENE AND OTHER CAROTENOIDS**   325
Summary, 325
Background Information, 326
Selection of Possible Indicators for Estimating the
    Requirement for β-Carotene and Other
    Carotenoids, 331
Factors Affecting Carotenoid Bioavailability, 354
Findings by Life Stage and Gender Group, 358
Intake of Carotenoids, 360
Tolerable Upper Intake Levels, 366
Research Recommendations for β-Carotene and
    Other Carotenoids, 371
References, 372

9   USES OF DIETARY REFERENCE INTAKES   **383**
Overview, 383
Assessing Nutrient Intakes of Individuals, 384
Assessing Nutrient Intakes of Groups, 387
Planning Nutrient Intakes of Individuals, 392
Planning Nutrient Intakes of Groups, 392
Nutrient-Specific Considerations, 393
Summary, 399
References, 399

10 A RESEARCH AGENDA   **401**
Approach, 401
Major Knowledge Gaps, 402
The Research Agenda, 406

APPENDIXES
A   Origin and Framework of the Development of Dietary
      Reference Intakes, 409
B   Acknowledgments, 413
C   Dietary Intake Data from the Third National Health
      and Nutrition Examination Survey (NHANES III),
      1988–1994, 416
D   Dietary Intake Data from the Continuing Survey of
      Food Intakes by Individuals (CSFII), 1994–1996, 432
E   Canadian Dietary Intake Data, 1993, 1995, 438
F   Serum Values from the Third National Health and
      Nutrition Examination Survey (NHANES III),
      1988–1994, 440
G   Options for Dealing with Uncertainties, 458
H   Glossary and Acronyms, 463
I   Biographical Sketches of Panel and Subcommittee
      Members, 469

INDEX   **483**

SUMMARY TABLE, Dietary Reference Intakes:
   Recommended Intakes for Individuals,   **507**

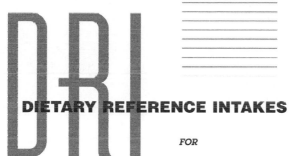

DIETARY REFERENCE INTAKES

FOR

Vitamin C,
Vitamin E,
Selenium, and
Carotenoids

Summary

This report provides quantitative recommendations for the intake of vitamin C, vitamin E, and selenium. It also discusses β-carotene and other carotenoids (α-carotene, β-cryptoxanthin, lutein, lycopene, and zeaxanthin) but does not provide quantitative recommendations for their intake. It is one volume in a series of reports that presents dietary reference values for the intake of nutrients by Americans and Canadians. The development of Dietary Reference Intakes (DRIs) expands and replaces the series of Recommended Dietary Allowances (RDAs) in the United States and Recommended Nutrient Intakes (RNIs) in Canada. The report includes current concepts about the roles vitamin C, vitamin E, selenium, and β carotene and the other carotenoids play in long-term health, going beyond a review of the roles they are known to play in traditional deficiency diseases. A major impetus for the expansion of this review is the growing recognition of the many uses to which RDAs and RNIs have been applied, and a growing awareness that many of these uses require the application of statistically valid methods that depend on reference values other than recommended nutrient intakes.

The overall project is a comprehensive effort undertaken by the Standing Committee on the Scientific Evaluation of Dietary Reference Intakes (DRI Committee) of the Food and Nutrition Board, Institute of Medicine, the National Academies, with active involvement of Health Canada. (See Appendix A for a description of the overall process and its origins.) This study was requested by the Federal Project Steering Committee for Dietary Reference Intakes (see Appendix B for membership), which is coordinated by the Office of Disease Prevention and Health Promotion of the U.S. Department of Health and Human Services, in collaboration with Health Canada.

Major new recommendations in this report include the following:

- A definition of a dietary antioxidant is provided.
- The Recommended Dietary Allowance (RDA) for vitamin E and selenium is the same for adult men and women regardless of age, representing the lack of specificity in data available.
- The Recommended Dietary Allowance (RDA) for vitamin C is different for adult men and women due to women's smaller lean body mass.
- α-Tocopherol alone is used for estimating vitamin E requirements and recommending daily vitamin E intake, since the other naturally occurring forms of vitamin E (β-, γ-, and δ-tocopherols and the tocotrienols) are not converted to α-tocopherol in the human and are recognized poorly by the α-tocopherol transfer protein in the liver.
- Tolerable Upper Intake Levels (ULs) for vitamin C, vitamin E, and selenium are established.
- Research recommendations for full-scale intervention trials to test the preventive potential of vitamin C, vitamin E, selenium, and β-carotene and other carotenoids for chronic disease are outlined. At the present time, there is no resolution of the possible impact of these nutrients or food components on chronic disease.

WHAT ARE DIETARY REFERENCE INTAKES?

Dietary Reference Intakes (DRIs) are reference values that are quantitative estimates of nutrient intakes to be used for planning and assessing diets for apparently healthy people. They include Recommended Dietary Allowances (RDAs) as well as three other types of reference values (see Box S-1). Although the reference values are based on published data, the data were often scanty or drawn from studies that had limitations in addressing the question. Thus, scientific judgment was required for evaluating the evidence and in setting the reference values and is delineated for each nutrient in Chapters 5 through 8.

Recommended Dietary Allowances

The process for setting the RDA depends on being able to set an *Estimated Average Requirement* (EAR). Before setting the EAR, a spe-

Box S-1 Dietary Reference Intakes

Recommended Dietary Allowance (RDA): the dietary intake level that is sufficient to meet the nutrient requirement of nearly all (97 to 98 percent) healthy individuals in a particular life stage and gender group.

Adequate Intake (AI): a recommended intake value based on observed or experimentally determined approximations or estimates of nutrient intake by a group (or groups) of healthy people that are assumed to be adequate—used when an RDA cannot be determined.

Tolerable Upper Intake Level (UL): the highest level of nutrient intake that is likely to pose no risk of adverse health effects for almost all individuals in the general population. As intake increases above the UL, the risk of adverse effects increases.

Estimated Average Requirement (EAR): a nutrient intake value that is estimated to meet the requirement of half the healthy individuals in a life stage and gender group.

cific criterion of adequacy is selected, based on a careful review of the literature. When selecting the criterion, reduction of disease risk is considered along with many other health parameters.

If the standard deviation (SD) of the EAR is available and the requirement for the nutrient is symmetrically distributed, the RDA is set at 2 SDs above the EAR:

$$RDA = EAR + 2\ SD_{EAR}.$$

If data about variability in requirements are insufficient to calculate an SD, a coefficient of variation (CV) for the EAR of 10 percent is ordinarily assumed, unless available data indicate a greater variation is probable.

If 10 percent is assumed to be the CV, then twice that amount added to the EAR is defined as equal to the RDA. The resulting equation for the RDA is then

$$RDA = 1.2 \times EAR.$$

If the distribution of the nutrient requirement is known to be skewed for a population, other approaches are used to find the ninety-seventh to ninety-eighth percentile to set the RDA. The RDA for a nutrient is a value to be used as a goal for dietary intake for the healthy individual. As discussed in Chapter 9 of this report, the

RDA is not intended to be used to assess the diets of either individuals or groups or to plan diets for groups.

Adequate Intakes

The *Adequate Intake (AI)* is set instead of an RDA if sufficient scientific evidence is not available to calculate an EAR. For example, the AI for young infants, for whom human milk is the recommended sole source of food for most nutrients up through the first 4 to 6 months, is based on the daily mean nutrient intake of apparently healthy, full-term infants who receive only human milk. The main intended use of the AI is as a goal for the nutrient intake of individuals. Other uses of AIs will be considered in future reports.

Comparison of RDAs and AIs

Although both the RDA and the AI are to be used as a goal for intake by individuals, the RDA differs from the AI. Intake of the RDA for a nutrient is expected to meet the needs of 97 to 98 percent of the individuals in a life stage and gender group. However, because no distribution of requirements is known for nutrients with an AI, it is not possible to know what percentage of individuals are covered by the AI. In determining the AI for a nutrient, it is expected to exceed the RDA for that nutrient, if it were known, and should cover the needs of more than 97 to 98 percent of the individuals (see Figure S-1). The degree to which an AI exceeds the RDA is likely to differ among nutrients and population groups, however.

For people with diseases that increase specific nutrient requirements or those who have other special health needs, the RDA and AI may each serve as the basis for adjusting individual recommendations; qualified health professionals should adapt the recommended intake to cover higher or lower needs.

Tables S-1 through S-3 give the recommended intake levels, whether RDAs or AIs, for vitamin C, vitamin E (α-tocopherol), and selenium by life stage and gender group. For these nutrients, AIs rather than RDAs are being proposed for infants to age 1 year.

Tolerable Upper Intake Levels

The *Tolerable Upper Intake Level* (UL) is the highest level of daily nutrient intake that is likely to pose no risk of adverse health effects for almost all individuals in the general population. As intake increases above the UL, the risk of adverse effects increases. The term

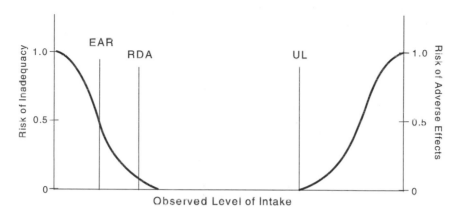

FIGURE S-1 Dietary reference intakes. This figure shows that the Estimated Average Requirement (EAR) is the intake at which the risk of inadequacy is 0.5 (50%) to an individual. The Recommended Dietary Allowance (RDA) is the intake at which the risk of inadequacy is very small—only 0.02 to 0.03 (2% to 3%). The Adequate Intake (AI) does not bear a consistent relationship to the EAR or the RDA because it is set without being able to estimate the average requirement. It is assumed that the AI is at or above the RDA if one could be calculated. At intakes between the RDA and the Tolerable Upper Intake Level (UL), the risks of inadequacy and of excess are both close to 0. At intakes above the UL, the risk of adverse effects may increase.

"tolerable intake" was chosen to avoid implying a possible beneficial effect. Instead, the term is intended to connote a level of intake that can, with high probability, be tolerated biologically. The UL is not intended to be a recommended level of intake. There is no established benefit for apparently healthy individuals if they consume nutrient intakes above the RDA or AI.

ULs are useful because of the increased interest in and availability of fortified foods and the increased use of dietary supplements. ULs are based on total intake of a nutrient from food, water, and supplements if adverse effects have been associated with total intake. However, if adverse effects have been associated with intake from supplements or food fortificants only, the UL is based on nutrient intake from these sources only, rather than on total intake. The UL applies to chronic daily use.

For some nutrients such as β-carotene and other carotenoids, there are insufficient data with which to develop a UL. This does

TABLE S-1 Criteria and Dietary Reference Intake Values for Vitamin C by Life Stage and Gender Group

Life Stage Group	Criterion
0 through 6 mo	Human milk content
7 through 12 mo	Human milk + solid food
1 through 3 y	Extrapolation from adult
4 through 8 y	Extrapolation from adult
9 through 13 y	Extrapolation from adult
14 through 18 y	Extrapolation from adult
19 through 30 y	Near-maximal neutrophil concentration
31 through 50 y	Extrapolation of near-maximal neutrophil concentration from 19 through 30 y
51 through 70 y	Extrapolation of near-maximal neutrophil concentration from 19 through 30 y
>70 y	Extrapolation of near-maximal neutrophil concentration from 19 through 30 y
Pregnancy	
≤18 y	Extrapolation of near-maximal neutrophil concentration plus transfer to the fetus
19 through 50 y	Extrapolation of near-maximal neutrophil concentration plus transfer to the fetus
Lactation	
≤18 y	Human milk content + age specific requirement
19 through 50 y	Human milk content + age specific requirement

[a] EAR = Estimated Average Requirement. The intake that meets the estimated nutrient needs of half of the individuals in a group.

[b] RDA = Recommended Dietary Allowance. The intake that meets the nutrient needs of almost all (97–98 percent) individuals in a group.

[c] AI = Adequate Intake. The observed average or experimentally set intake by a

not mean that there is no potential for adverse effects resulting from high intake. When data about adverse effects are extremely limited, extra caution may be warranted.

APPROACH FOR SETTING DIETARY REFERENCE INTAKES

The scientific data used to develop Dietary Reference Intakes (DRIs) have come from observational and experimental studies. Studies published in peer-reviewed journals were the principal

EAR (mg/d)[a]		RDA (mg/d)[b]		AI (mg/d)[c]	
Male	Female	Male	Female	Male	Female
				40	40
				50	50
13	13	15	15		
22	22	25	25		
39	39	45	45		
63	56	75	65		
75	60	90	75		
75	60	90	75		
75	60	90	75		
75	60	90	75		
	66		80		
	70		85		
	96		115		
	100		120		

defined population or subgroup that appears to sustain a defined nutritional status, such as growth rate, normal circulating nutrient values, or other functional indicators of health. An AI is used if sufficient scientific evidence is not available to derive an EAR. For healthy human milk-fed infants, the AI is the mean intake. **The AI is not equivalent to an RDA.**

source of data. Life stage and gender were considered to the extent possible, but the data did not provide a basis for proposing different requirements for men and for nonpregnant and nonlactating women in different age groups for any of the nutrients except vitamin C.

Three of the categories of reference values (Estimated Average Requirement [EAR], Recommended Dietary Allowance [RDA], and Adequate Intake [AI]) are defined by specific criteria of nutrient adequacy; the fourth (Tolerable Upper Intake Level [UL]) is defined by a specific endpoint of adverse effect, when one is avail-

TABLE S-2 Criteria and Dietary Reference Intake Values for α-Tocopherol[a] by Life Stage Group

Life Stage Group[b]	Criterion
0 through 6 mo	Human milk content
7 through 12 mo	Extrapolation from 0 to 6 mo
1 through 3 y	Extrapolation from adult
4 through 8 y	Extrapolation from adult
9 through 13 y	Extrapolation from adult
14 through 18 y	Extrapolation from adult
19 through 30 y	Prevention of hydrogen peroxide-induced hemolysis
31 through 50 y	Extrapolation of hydrogen peroxide-induced hemolysis from 19 through 30 y
51 through 70 y	Extrapolation of hydrogen peroxide-induced hemolysis from 19 through 30 y
>70 y	Extrapolation of hydrogen peroxide-induced hemolysis from 19 through 50 y
Pregnancy	
≤18 y	Plasma concentration
19 through 50 y	Plasma concentration
Lactation	
≤18 y	Human milk content + age specific requirement
19 through 50 y	Human milk content + age specific requirement

[a] α-Tocopherol includes *RRR*-α-tocopherol, the only form of α-tocopherol that occurs naturally in foods, and the 2*R*-stereoisomeric forms of α-tocopherol (*RRR*-, *RSR*-, *RRS*-, and *RSS*-α-tocopherol) that occur in fortified foods and supplements. Does not include the 2*S*-stereoisomeric forms of α-tocopherol (*SRR*-, *SSR*-, *SRS*-, and *SSS*-α-tocopherol), also found in fortified foods and supplements. The 2*R*-stereoisomeric forms of α-tocopherol, as defined in this report, are the only forms of Vitamin E that have been shown to meet human requirements.

[b] All groups except Pregnancy and Lactation are males and females.

[c] EAR = Estimated Average Requirement. The intake that meets the estimated nutrient needs of half of the individuals in a group, men and women combined.

able. In all cases, data were examined closely to determine whether an antioxidant function or a reduction of risk of a chronic degenerative disease could be used as a criterion of adequacy. The quality of studies was examined by considering study design; methods used for measuring intake and indicators of adequacy; and biases, interactions, and confounding factors.

Although the reference values are based on data, the data were often scanty or drawn from studies that had limitations in addressing the various questions that confronted the panel. Therefore,

EAR (mg/d)[c]	RDA (mg/d)[d]	AI (mg/d)[e]
		4
		6
5	6	
6	7	
9	11	
12	15	
12	15	
12	15	
12	15	
12	15	
12	15	
12	15	
16	19	
16	19	

[d] RDA = Recommended Dietary Allowance. The intake that meets the nutrient needs of almost all (97–98 percent) individuals in a group.

[e] AI = Adequate Intake. The observed average or experimentally set intake by a defined population or subgroup that appears to sustain a defined nutritional status, such as growth rate, normal circulating nutrient values, or other functional indicators of health. An AI is used if sufficient scientific evidence is not available to derive an EAR. For healthy human milk-fed infants, the AI is the mean intake. **The AI is not equivalent to an RDA.**

many of the questions raised about the requirements for and recommended intakes of these nutrients cannot be answered fully because of inadequacies in the present database. Apart from studies of overt deficiency diseases, there is a dearth of studies that address specific effects of inadequate intakes on specific indicators of health status. (A research agenda is proposed; see Chapter 10.) After careful review and analysis of the evidence, including examination of the extent of congruence of findings, scientific judgment was used to determine the basis for establishing the values. The reasoning

TABLE S-3 Criteria and Dietary Reference Intake Values for Selenium by Life Stage Group

Life Stage Group[a]	Criterion
0 through 6 mo	Human milk content
7 through 12 mo	Human milk + solid food
1 through 3 y	Extrapolation from adult
4 through 8 y	Extrapolation from adult
9 through 13 y	Extrapolation from adult
14 through 18 y	Extrapolation from adult
19 through 30 y	Maximizing plasma glutathione peroxidase activity
31 through 50 y	Extrapolation of plasma glutathione peroxidase activity from 19 through 30 y
51 through 70 y	Extrapolation of plasma glutathione peroxidase activity from 19 through 30 y
>70 y	Extrapolation of plasma glutathione peroxidase activity from 19 through 30 y
Pregnancy	
≤18 y	Saturation of fetal selenoprotein
19 through 50 y	Saturation of fetal selenoprotein
Lactation	
≤18 y	Human milk content + age specific requirement
19 through 50 y	Human milk content + age specific requirement

[a] All groups except Pregnancy and Lactation are males and females.

[b] EAR = Estimated Average Requirement. The intake that meets the estimated nutrient needs of half of the individuals in a group, men and women combined.

[c] RDA = Recommended Dietary Allowance. The intake that meets the nutrient needs of almost all (97–98 percent) individuals in a group.

[d] AI = Adequate Intake. The observed average or experimentally set intake by a

used is described for each nutrient in Chapters 5 through 8. While the various recommendations are provided as single rounded numbers for practical considerations, it is acknowledged that these values imply a precision not fully justified by the underlying data in the case of currently available human studies.

In this report, the scientific evidence related to the prevention of chronic degenerative disease was judged to be too nonspecific to be used as the basis for setting any of the recommended levels of intake. Furthermore, a quantitative relationship between the biomarkers of antioxidant function and the prevention of chronic

EAR (μg/d)[b]	RDA (μg/d)[c]	AI (μg/d)[d]
		15
		20
17	20	
23	30	
35	40	
45	55	
45	55	
45	55	
45	55	
45	55	
49	60	
49	60	
59	70	
59	70	

defined population or subgroup that appears to sustain a defined nutritional status, such as growth rate, normal circulating nutrient values, or other functional indicators of health. An AI is used if sufficient scientific evidence is not available to derive an EAR. For healthy human milk-fed infants, the AI is the mean intake. **The AI is not equivalent to an RDA.**

degenerative disease was lacking. Thus, for vitamin C, vitamin E, and selenium, EARs and RDAs are based on criteria specifically related to their general functions. For all of these nutrients, the EAR is higher than the amount needed to prevent overt deficiency diseases in essentially all individuals in the life stage group and is based on limited data indicating laboratory evidence of sufficiency. At this time, no DRIs have been set for any of the carotenoids. The indicators used in deriving the EARs and thus the RDAs are described below.

NUTRIENT FUNCTIONS AND THE INDICATORS USED TO ESTIMATE REQUIREMENTS FOR VITAMIN C, VITAMIN E, SELENIUM, AND THE CAROTENOIDS

Vitamin C (ascorbic acid) functions physiologically as a water-soluble antioxidant by virtue of its high reducing power. To provide antioxidant protection, the Recommended Dietary Allowance (RDA) for adults for vitamin C is set at 75 mg/day for females and 90 mg/day for males. This intake should maintain near maximal neutrophil ascorbate concentrations with little urinary excretion. Because smokers suffer increased oxidative stress and metabolic turnover of vitamin C, their recommended intake is increased by 35 mg/day.

Vitamin E is thought to function primarily as a chain-breaking antioxidant that prevents the propagation of lipid peroxidation. To estimate the requirement, data were examined on induced vitamin E deficiency in humans and the intake that correlated with in vitro hydrogen peroxide-induced hemolysis and plasma α-tocopherol concentrations. In addition, vitamin E acts as an in vivo antioxidant, maintaining normal physiological function in humans. The RDA for both men and women is 15 mg/day of α-tocopherol. Other naturally occurring forms of vitamin E (β-, γ-, δ-tocopherol and the tocotrienols) do not meet the vitamin E requirement because they are not converted to α–tocopherol in humans and are recognized poorly by the α-tocopherol transfer protein. In establishing recommended intakes α-tocopherol is defined as *RRR*-α-tocopherol, the only form of α-tocopherol that occurs naturally in food, and the 2*R*-stereoisomeric forms of α-tocopherol (*RRR*-, *RSR*-, *RRS*-, and *RSS*-α-tocopherol) that occur in fortified foods and supplements.

Selenium functions through selenoproteins, several of which are oxidant defense enzymes. The method used to estimate the requirement for selenium relates to the intake needed to maximize the activity of the plasma selenoprotein glutathione peroxidase, an oxidant defense enzyme. The RDA for both men and women is 55 µg/day. It is not clear if the diseases associated with selenium deficiencies, Keshan disease or Kashin-Beck disease, are due to oxidative stress. The selenium in several selenoproteins has a biochemical role in oxidant defense, and as such plays a role as a dietary antioxidant.

β-Carotene and other provitamin A carotenoids function as a source of vitamin A and, due to this provitamin A activity, can prevent vitamin A deficiency. Because specific functions beyond this role have not yet been sufficiently identified, no Dietary Reference Intakes (DRIs) have been established for any of the carotenoids including those which do not have provitamin A activity. In conjunction with the review of vitamin A, efforts are under way to establish ratios for the provitamin A carotenoids—β-carotene, α-carotene, and β-cryptoxanthin—based on their ability to be converted to vitamin A. A subsequent report will provide this analysis of the potential contributions of the carotenoids to the requirement for vitamin A.

CRITERIA AND PROPOSED VALUES FOR TOLERABLE UPPER INTAKE LEVELS

A risk assessment model is used to derive Tolerable Upper Intake Levels (ULs). The model consists of a systematic series of scientific considerations and judgments. The hallmark of the risk assessment model is the requirement to be explicit in all the evaluations and judgments made.

The ULs for adults for vitamin C (2,000 mg/day based on the adverse effect of osmotic diarrhea), vitamin E (1,000 mg/day of any form of supplemental α-tocopherol based on the adverse effect of increased tendency to hemorrhage), and selenium (400 μg/day based on the adverse effect of selenosis), shown in Table S-4, were set to protect the most sensitive individuals in the general population (e.g., those who might be below reference adult weight). Members of the general apparently healthy population should be advised not to exceed the UL routinely. However, intake above the UL may be appropriate for investigation within well-controlled clinical trials to ascertain if such intakes are of benefit to health. Clinical trials of doses above the UL should not be discouraged because it is expected that participation in these trials will require informed consent that will include discussion of the possibility of adverse effects and will employ appropriate safety monitoring of trial subjects.

The ULs for vitamin C and selenium are based on intake from diet and supplements. Vitamin E ULs are based on intake from supplements only.

A UL could not be established for β-carotene because of inconsistent data and could not be set for other carotenoids because of a lack of suitable data. In both cases, this signifies a need for additional information. It does not necessarily signify that people can tolerate chronic intakes of these substances at high levels. Like all chemical agents, nutrients and other food components can produce adverse effects if intakes are excessive. Therefore, when data are extremely limited, extra caution may be warranted. In particular, β-carotene supplementation is not advisable, other than for the

TABLE S-4 Tolerable Upper Intake Levels (UL[a]) by Life Stage Group

Life Stage Group	Vitamin C (mg/d)	α-Tocopherol (mg/d)[b]	Selenium (µg/d)
0 through 6 mo	ND[c]	ND	45
7 through 12 mo	ND	ND	60
1 through 3 y	400	200	90
4 through 8 y	650	300	150
9 through 13 y	1,200	600	280
14 through 18 y	1,800	800	400
19 through 70 y	2,000	1,000	400
>70 y	2,000	1,000	400
Pregnancy			
≤18 y	1,800	800	400
19 through 50 y	2,000	1,000	400
Lactation			
≤18 y	1,800	800	400
19 through 50 y	2,000	1,000	400

[a] The UL is the highest level of daily nutrient intake that is likely to pose no risk of adverse health effects to almost all individuals in the general population. As intake increases above the UL, the risk of adverse effects increases. Unless specified otherwise, the UL represents total nutrient intake from food, water, and supplements.

[b] The UL for α-tocopherol applies to any form of supplemental α-tocopherol.

[c] ND. Not determinable due to lack of data of adverse effects in this age group and concern with regard to lack of ability to handle excess amounts. Source of intake should be from food and formula in order to prevent high levels of intake.

prevention and control of vitamin A deficiency, in view of concerns about lung cancer and total mortality risk raised by recent randomized clinical trials in special at-risk populations.

USING DIETARY REFERENCE INTAKES

Suggested uses of Dietary Reference Intakes (DRIs) appear in Box S-2. The transition from using previously published Recommended Dietary Allowance (RDAs) and Reference Nutrient Intakes (RNIs) alone to using all DRIs appropriately will require time and effort by health professionals and others.

For statistical reasons that will be addressed in a future report and discussed briefly in Chapter 9, the Estimated Average Requirement (EAR) is the appropriate reference intake to use in assessing the nutrient intake of groups; the RDA is not appropriate. The prevalence of inadequacy may be estimated by determining the percentage of the population below the EAR as follows:

- Based on the Third National Health and Nutrition Examination Survey (NHANES III) data, about 11 percent of nonsmoking

---

Box S-2 Uses of Dietary Reference Intakes for Healthy Individuals and Groups

Type of Use	For the Individual	For a Group
Assessment	**EAR**[a]: use to examine the possibility of inadequacy of reported intake.	**EAR**[b]: use to estimate the prevalence of inadequate intakes within a group.
	AI[a]: intakes at this level have a low probability of inadequacy.	**AI**[b]: mean intake at this level implies a low prevalence of inadequate intakes.
	UL[a]: intake above this level has a risk of adverse effects.	**UL**[b]: use to estimate the prevalence of intakes that may be at risk of adverse effects.
Planning	**RDA**: aim for this intake.	**EAR**: use in conjunction with a measure of variability of the group's intake to set goals for the median intake of a specific population.
	AI: aim for this intake.	
	UL: use as a guide to limit intake; chronic intake of higher amounts may increase risk of adverse effects.	

EAR = Estimated Average Requirement
RDA = Recommended Dietary Allowance
AI = Adequate Intake
UL = Tolerable Upper Intake Level

[a] Requires accurate measure of usual intake. Evaluation of true status requires clinical, biochemical, and anthropometric data.
[b] Requires statistically valid approximation of usual intake.

adult women and 21 percent of nonsmoking adult men have dietary intakes of vitamin C that are less than the EAR for this nutrient.

• Although dietary intakes of selenium depend on the selenium content of the soil where a plant was grown, adults in North America are meeting their selenium needs, probably because food in the United States and Canada is so widely distributed beyond the region where it was grown.

• Only a small proportion of the adult men and women in the population reportedly has a vitamin E intake from food and supplements greater than the EAR. However, estimates of vitamin E intake are particularly difficult due to a propensity to underreport fat intake which results in its underestimation (dietary fat serves as the major carrier for vitamin E). In addition, the EARs for vitamin E are based on α-tocopherol only and do not include amounts obtained from the other seven naturally occurring forms of vitamin E (β-, γ-, δ-tocopherol and the four tocotrienols). Because the various forms of vitamin E cannot be interconverted in humans, EARs, RDAs, and AIs apply only to intake of the $2R$-stereoisomeric forms of α-tocopherol from food, fortified foods, and multivitamins. Currently, most nutrient databases, as well as nutrition labels, do not distinguish among the various tocopherols in food. They often present the data as α-tocopherol equivalents and include the contribution of all eight naturally occurring forms of vitamin E, after adjustment for bioavailability (e.g., γ-tocopherol is usually assumed to have only 10 percent of the availability of α-tocopherol). Because these other forms of vitamin E occur in foods (e.g., γ-tocopherol is present in widely consumed oils such as soybean and corn oils), the intake of α-tocopherol equivalents is greater than the intake of α-tocopherol alone. Based on NHANES III dietary intake data, approximately 80 percent of the α-tocopherol equivalents from food are from α-tocopherol, and thus can contribute to the body's requirement for vitamin E.

Data for intakes of vitamin C, vitamin E, and selenium from food and supplements in the United States are provided in this report. Data from Canada are available only for vitamin C from food. Detailed data for intakes of carotenoids from a recently released and expanded food composition database in the United States are presently being analyzed and are not available to be included in this report. Thus they will be included in the Appendix of a subsequent DRI report that will include vitamin A.

DEFINITION OF A DIETARY ANTIOXIDANT

A dietary antioxidant is a substance in foods that significantly decreases the adverse effects of reactive species, such as reactive oxygen and nitrogen species, on normal physiological function in humans. The definition is based on several criteria: the substance is found in human diets, the content of the substance has been measured in foods commonly consumed, and the substance decreases the adverse effects of reactive species in vivo in humans. Vitamin C, vitamin E, and selenium (in the form of selenocysteine or selenomethionine) are the food components reviewed in this report that meet this definition of a dietary antioxidant. The other food components covered in this report, β-carotene and the other carotenoids, do not meet the definition but influence biochemical reactions that involve the oxidative process.

EVIDENCE OF OXIDATIVE STRESS AND THE RISK OF CHRONIC DEGENERATIVE DISEASE

There is a considerable body of biological evidence that, at high levels, reactive oxygen and nitrogen species can be damaging to cells and thus may contribute to cellular dysfunction and disease. Hence, close attention has been given to evidence relating intake of vitamin C, vitamin E, selenium, and β-carotene and other carotenoids to reduction of the risk of chronic disease. Since the entire population is exposed to oxidative stresses through oxidative metabolism and only some develop a chronic disease, it is clear that more information is needed in order to understand how to evaluate the role of oxidative stress in the development of chronic disease. The potential role of oxidative stress in six chronic disease relationships is briefly described below.

Cancer

One theory holds that oxidative damage contributes to carcinogenesis. A great deal of epidemiological evidence indicates that diets rich in fruits and vegetables are associated with a lower risk of incurring a number of common cancers, especially cancers of the lung, oral cavity, pharynx, larynx, and cervix. However, these studies provide only limited support for a protective association of individual food components categorized as antioxidants. Data regarding the protection by individual food components against cancer in humans are not yet available.

Cardiovascular Disease

Of all the chronic diseases in which excess oxidative stress has been implicated, cardiovascular disease has the strongest supporting evidence. Oxidation of low-density lipoproteins may be a key step in the development of coronary atherosclerosis. Epidemiological studies indicate that diets rich in fruits and vegetables, vitamin C, vitamin E, and carotenoids are associated with a decreased risk of coronary heart disease. However, no randomized prospective studies have documented a favorable effect of vitamin C or carotenoids on cardiovascular morbidity and mortality. Four studies have examined the effects of vitamin E; only one reported a positive benefit while the other three were neutral. Thus available data do not adequately substantiate the premise that increasing the intake of vitamin C, vitamin E, or β-carotene and other carotenoids will reduce the risk of coronary heart disease. Ongoing randomized trials among high-risk, apparently healthy individuals and among patients with cardiovascular disease are expected to provide evidence useful in resolving this issue.

Cataracts

A number of observational epidemiological studies have examined the relationship between intakes of vitamin C, vitamin E, and carotenoids and the presence of cataracts in humans. Several studies indicate a lowered risk of cataracts associated with either an increased serum level of these dietary components or supplement use. These studies, since observational in nature, do not constitute at this time a sufficient basis for a conclusion that these dietary components can *prevent* cataracts in humans.

Age-Related Macular Degeneration

Epidemiological studies find a decreased likelihood of age-related macular degeneration (AMD) associated with higher intakes of fruits and vegetables, especially those that are rich in the carotenoids lutein and zeaxanthin. Protective effects of lutein and zeaxanthin are biologically plausible because these carotenoids selectively accumulate as the pigment of the macular region of the retina and account for the yellow color observed in this region. The association has also been observed in smokers, who have lower plasma levels of carotenoids and are also at an increased risk of developing AMD. However, all reports are associative in nature and have not established a causal relationship between intake or plasma concentrations of lutein and/or zeaxanthin and risk for AMD.

Central Neurodegenerative Diseases

Increasing evidence suggests that a number of common neurodegenerative diseases, such as Alzheimer's, Parkinson's, and amyotrophic lateral sclerosis, may reflect adverse responses to oxidative stress. Small intervention trials with either vitamin C or vitamin E have reported symptomatic improvement in those already afflicted with the disease. However, these preliminary findings do not constitute adequate proof of the usefulness of these antioxidants in decreasing the development or delaying the onset of these diseases.

Diabetes Mellitus

Although some evidence suggests that modifications observed in structural proteins in patients with diabetes mellitus may be attributable to either an oxidative stress or a stress due to reactive carbonyls, much of the research, with either single compounds or combinations of specific food components that may function as antioxidants, has been inconclusive. In addition, no clinical intervention trials have tested directly whether provision of antioxidants can defer the onset of the complications of diabetes.

RECOMMENDATIONS

Available Data on Food Composition

Because the various forms of vitamin E are not interconvertible and because plasma concentrations of α-tocopherol are dependent upon the affinity of the hepatic α-tocopherol transfer protein for the various forms, it is recommended that relative biological potencies of the various forms of vitamin E be reevaluated. Until this is done, the actual concentrations of each of the various vitamin E forms in food and biological samples should be reported separately, wherever possible.

Research

Five major types of information gaps were noted: (1) a dearth of studies designed specifically to estimate average requirements in apparently healthy humans; (2) a nearly complete lack of usable data on the nutrient needs of infants, children, adolescents, and pregnant and lactating women; (3) a lack of definitive studies to determine the role of these nutrients in lowering the risk of certain chronic diseases; (4) a lack of validated biomarkers to evaluate oxidative stress and the relationship between antioxidant intake and health and disease; and (5) a lack of studies designed to detect adverse effects of chronic high intakes of these nutrients.

Highest priority is thus given to research that has potential to prevent or retard human disease processes and to prevent deficiencies with functional consequences as follows:

• Studies to provide the basic data for constructing risk curves and benefit curves across the exposures to dietary and supplemental intakes of vitamin C, vitamin E, selenium, and β-carotene and other carotenoids. Studies should be designed to determine the relationship of nutrient intakes to validated biomarkers of oxidative stress. These studies should be followed by nested case-control studies to determine the relationship of the biomarkers of oxidative stress to chronic disease. Finally, full-scale intervention trials should be done to establish the preventive potential of a nutrient for chronic disease.

• Investigations of gender specificity of the metabolism and requirements for vitamin C, vitamin E, selenium, and β-carotene and other carotenoids.

• Studies to validate methods and possible models for estimating Dietary Reference Intakes (DRIs) in the absence of data for some life stage groups, such as children, pregnant and lactating women, and older adults.

• Research to determine the interactions and possible synergisms of vitamin C, vitamin E, selenium, and β-carotene with each other, with other nutrients and food components, and with endogenous antioxidants. Multifactorial studies are needed to demonstrate in vivo actions as well as synergisms that have been shown to occur in vitro.

• Studies to develop economical, sensitive, and specific methods to assess the associations of vitamin C, vitamin E, selenium, and β-carotene and other carotenoids with the causation, prevalence, prevention, and treatment of specific viral or other infections.

• Investigations of the magnitude and role of genetic polymorphisms in the mechanisms of actions of vitamin C, vitamin E, selenium, and β-carotene and other carotenoids.

1
Introduction to Dietary Reference Intakes

The term *Dietary Reference Intakes (DRIs)* refers to a set of at least four nutrient-based reference values, each of which has special uses. The development of DRIs expands on the periodic reports called *Recommended Dietary Allowances*, which have been published since 1941 by the National Academy of Sciences. This comprehensive effort is being undertaken by the Standing Committee on the Scientific Evaluation of Dietary Reference Intakes (DRI Committee) of the Food and Nutrition Board, Institute of Medicine, the National Academies, with the active involvement of Health Canada. See Appendix A for a description of the overall process and its origins.

WHAT ARE DIETARY REFERENCE INTAKES?

The reference values, collectively called the Dietary Reference Intakes (DRIs), include the Recommended Dietary Allowance (RDA), the Adequate Intake (AI), the Tolerable Upper Intake Level (UL), and the Estimated Average Requirement (EAR).

A requirement is defined as the lowest continuing intake level of a nutrient that, for a specified indicator of adequacy, will maintain a defined level of nutriture in an individual. The chosen criterion of nutritional adequacy is identified in each nutrient chapter; note that the criterion may differ for individuals at different life stages. Hence, particular attention is given throughout this report to the choice and justification of the criterion used to establish requirement values.

This approach differs somewhat from that used by the World Health Organization, Food and Agriculture Organization, and International Atomic Energy Agency (WHO/FAO/IAEA) Expert Consultation on *Trace Elements in Human Nutrition and Health* (WHO, 1996). That publication uses the term *basal requirement* to indicate the level of intake needed to prevent pathologically relevant and clinically detectable signs of a dietary inadequacy. The term *normative requirement* indicates the level of intake sufficient to maintain a desirable body store or reserve. In developing RDAs and AIs, emphasis is placed instead on the reasons underlying the choice of the criterion of nutritional adequacy used to establish the requirement. They have not been designated as basal or normative.

Unless otherwise stated, all values given for RDAs, AIs, and EARs represent the quantity of the nutrient or food component to be supplied by foods from a diet similar to those consumed in Canada and the United States. If the food source of a nutrient is very different (as in the diets of some ethnic groups) or if the source is supplements, adjustments may have to be made for differences in nutrient bioavailability. When this is an issue, it is discussed for the specific nutrient in the section "Special Considerations."

RDAs and AIs are levels of intake recommended for individuals. They should minimize the risk of developing a condition that is associated with the nutrient in question and that has a negative functional outcome. The DRIs apply to the apparently healthy general population. Meeting the recommended intakes for vitamin C, vitamin E, selenium, and carotenoids would not necessarily provide enough for individuals who are already malnourished, nor would they be adequate for certain disease states marked by increased requirements. Qualified medical and nutrition personnel must tailor recommendations for individuals who are known to have diseases that greatly increase requirements or who are at risk for developing adverse effects associated with higher intakes. Although the RDA or AI may serve as the basis for such guidance, qualified personnel should make necessary adaptations for specific situations.

CATEGORIES OF DIETARY REFERENCE INTAKES

Each type of Dietary Reference Intake (DRI) refers to average daily nutrient intake of individuals over time. In most cases, the amount taken from day to day may vary substantially without ill effect.

Recommended Dietary Allowance

The *Recommended Dietary Allowance* (RDA) is the average daily dietary intake level that is sufficient to meet the nutrient requirement of nearly all (97 to 98 percent) apparently healthy individuals in a particular life stage and gender group (see Figure 1-1). The RDA is intended to be used as a goal for daily intake by individuals. The process for setting the RDA is described below; it depends on being able to set an Estimated Average Requirement (EAR). That is, if an EAR cannot be set, no RDA will be set.

Estimated Average Requirement [1]

The *Estimated Average Requirement* (EAR) is the daily intake value that is estimated to meet the requirement, as defined by the specified indicator of adequacy, in half of the apparently healthy individuals in a life stage or gender group (see Figure 1-1). A normal or symmetrical distribution (median and mean similar) is usually assumed for nutrient requirements. At this level of intake, the other half of a specified group would not have its nutritional needs met. The general method used to set the EAR is the same for all of the nutrients in this report. The specific approaches, provided in Chapters 5 through 8, differ because of the different types of data available.

Method for Setting the RDA

The EAR is used in setting the RDA as follows. If the standard deviation (SD) of the EAR is available and the requirement for the nutrient is normally distributed, the RDA is defined as equal to the EAR plus 2 SDs of the EAR:

$$RDA = EAR + 2 \ SD_{EAR}.$$

---

[1] The definition of EAR implies a median as opposed to a mean, or average. The median and average would be the same if the distribution of requirements followed a symmetrical distribution and would diverge as a distribution became skewed. Three considerations prompted the choice of the term EAR: data are rarely adequate to determine the distribution of requirements, precedent has been set by other countries that have used EAR for reference values similarly derived (COMA, 1991), and the type of data evaluated makes the determination of a median impossible or inappropriate.

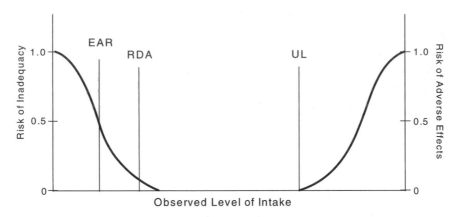

FIGURE 1-1 Dietary reference intakes. This figure shows that the Estimated Average Requirement (EAR) is the intake at which the risk of inadequacy is 0.5 (50%) to an individual. The Recommended Dietary Allowance (RDA) is the intake at which the risk of inadequacy is very small—only 0.02 to 0.03 (2% to 3%). The Adequate Intake (AI) does not bear a consistent relationship to the EAR or the RDA because it is set without being able to estimate the average requirement. It is assumed that the AI is at or above the RDA if one could be calculated. At intakes between the RDA and the Tolerable Upper Intake Level (UL), the risks of inadequacy and of excess are both close to 0. At intakes above the UL, the risk of adverse effects may increase.

If data about variability in requirements are insufficient to calculate an SD, a coefficient of variation (CV_{EAR}) of 10 percent will ordinarily be assumed and used in place of the SD. Because

$$CV_{EAR} = SD_{EAR}/EAR, \text{ and}$$
$$SD = (EAR \times CV_{EAR});$$

the resulting equation for the RDA is

$$RDA = EAR + 2 (0.1 \times EAR), \text{ or}$$
$$RDA = 1.2 \times EAR.$$

If the nutrient requirement is known to be skewed for a population, other approaches will be used to find the ninety-seventh to ninety-eighth percentile to set the RDA.

The assumption of a 10 percent CV is based on extensive data on the variation in basal metabolic rate (FAO/WHO/UNA, 1985; Garby and Lammert, 1984), which contributes about two-thirds of the daily energy expenditure of many individuals residing in Canada and the United States (Elia, 1992) and on the similar CV of 12.5 percent estimated for the protein requirements in adults (FAO/WHO/UNA, 1985). If there is evidence of greater variation, a larger CV will be assumed. In all cases, the method used to derive the RDA from the EAR is stated.

For vitamins C and E, and selenium, there are very few direct data on the requirements of children. Thus, EARs and RDAs for children are based on extrapolations from adult values. The method is described in Chapter 3.

Other Uses of the EAR

Together with an estimate of the variance of intake, the EAR may also be used in the assessment of the intake of groups or in planning for the intake of groups (Beaton, 1994) (see Chapter 9).

Adequate Intake

If sufficient scientific evidence is not available to calculate an EAR, a reference intake called an *Adequate Intake* (AI) is provided instead of an RDA. The AI is a value based on experimentally derived intake levels or approximations of observed mean nutrient intakes by a group (or groups) of apparently healthy people. In the judgment of the DRI Committee, the AI for children and adults is expected to meet or exceed the amount needed to maintain a defined nutritional state or criterion of adequacy in essentially all members of a specific, apparently healthy population, because it is set using presumably healthy populations. Examples of defined nutritional states include normal growth, maintenance of normal circulating nutrient values, or other aspects of nutritional well-being or general health.

The AI is set when data are considered to be insufficient or inadequate to establish an EAR on which an RDA would be based. For example, for young infants for whom human milk is the recommended sole food source for most nutrients in the first 4 to 6 months, the AI is based on the daily mean nutrient intake supplied by human milk for apparently healthy, full-term infants who are fed exclusively human milk.

Similarities Between the AI and the RDA

Both the AI and the RDA are to be used as a goal for individual intake. In general, the values are intended to cover the needs of nearly all persons in a life stage group. (For infants, the AI is the mean intake when infants in the age group are consuming human milk. Larger infants may have higher needs, which they meet by consuming more milk.) As with RDAs, AIs for children and adolescents may be extrapolated from adult values if no other usable data are available.

Differences Between the AI and the RDA

There is much less certainty about the AI value than about the RDA value. Because AIs depend on a greater degree of judgment than is applied in estimating the EAR and subsequently the RDA, the AI may deviate significantly from the RDA, if it could have been determined, and may be numerically higher than the RDA, if it were known. For this reason, AIs must be used with greater care than RDAs. Also, the RDA is always calculated from the EAR, using a formula that takes into account the expected variation in the requirement for the nutrient (see previous section "Estimated Average Requirement").

Tolerable Upper Intake Level

The *Tolerable Upper Intake Level* (UL) is the highest level of daily nutrient intake that is likely to pose no risk of adverse health effects in almost all individuals in the specified life stage group (see Figure 1-1). As intake increases above the UL, the risk of adverse effects increases. The term *tolerable intake* was chosen to avoid implying a possible beneficial effect. Instead, the term is intended to connote a level of intake that can, with high probability, be tolerated biologically. The UL is not intended to be a recommended level of intake, and there is no established benefit for healthy individuals if they consume a nutrient in amounts exceeding the recommended intake (the RDA or AI).

The UL is based on an evaluation conducted using the methodology for risk assessment of nutrients (see Chapter 4). The need for setting ULs grew out of the increased fortification of foods and the use of dietary supplements by more people and in larger doses. The UL applies to chronic daily use. As in the case of applying AIs, professionals should avoid very rigid application of ULs and first assess the characteristics of the individual or group of concern such as source of nutrient, physiological state of the individual, length of sustained high intakes, and so forth.

For vitamin C and selenium, the UL refers to total intakes—from food, fortified food, and nutrient supplements. In other instances (e.g., vitamin E), it may refer only to intakes from supplements, food fortificants, pharmacological agents, or a combination of the three. For some nutrients, such as β-carotene and other carotenoids, there may be inconsistent and insufficient data on which to develop ULs. This indicates the need for caution in consuming amounts greater than the recommended intakes; it does not mean that high intakes pose no risk of adverse effects.

The safety of routine, long-term intake above the UL is not well documented. Although members of the general population should be advised not to routinely exceed the UL, intake above the UL may be appropriate for investigation within well-controlled clinical trials. Clinical trials of doses above the UL should not be discouraged as long as subjects participating in these trials have signed informed consent documents regarding possible toxicity and as long as these trials employ appropriate safety monitoring of trial subjects.

Determination of Adequacy

In the derivation of the EAR or AI, close attention has been paid to the determination of the most appropriate indicators of adequacy. A key question is, Adequate for what? In many cases, a continuum of benefits may be ascribed to various levels of intake of the same nutrient. One indicator may be deemed the most appropriate to determine the risk that an individual will become deficient in the nutrient, while another may relate to reducing the risk of chronic degenerative disease such as common neurodegenerative diseases, cardiovascular disease, cancer, diabetes mellitus, cataracts, or age-related macular degeneration.

Each EAR or AI is described in terms of the selected criterion or outcome. The potential role of vitamin C, vitamin E, selenium, and β-carotene and other carotenoids in the reduction of disease risk was considered in developing the EARs for this group of nutrients. With the acquisition of additional data relating intake to chronic disease or disability, the choice of the criterion for setting the EAR may change. These nutrients, their role in health, and the types of evidence considered are discussed in Chapter 2.

PARAMETERS FOR DIETARY REFERENCE INTAKES

Life Stage Categories

The life stage categories described below were chosen by keeping in mind all the nutrients to be reviewed, not only those included in this report. Additional subdivisions within these groups may be added in later reports. If data are too sparse to distinguish differences in requirements by life stage or gender group, the analysis may be presented for a larger grouping.

Infancy

Infancy covers the period from birth through 12 months of age and is divided into two 6-month intervals. The first 6-month interval was not subdivided further because intake is relatively constant during this time. That is, as infants grow, they ingest more food; however, on a body weight basis their intake remains the same. During the second 6 months of life, growth velocity slows, and thus total daily nutrient needs on a body weight basis may be less than those during the first 6 months of life.

For a particular nutrient, average intake by full-term infants who are born to presumably healthy, well-nourished mothers and exclusively fed human milk has been adopted as the primary basis for deriving the Adequate Intake (AI) for most nutrients during the first 6 months of life. The value used is thus not an Estimated Average Requirement (EAR); the extent to which intake of human milk may result in exceeding the actual requirements of the infant is not known, and ethics of experimentation preclude testing the levels known to be potentially inadequate. Therefore, the AI is not an EAR in which only half of the group would be expected to have their needs met.

Using the infant fed human milk as a model is in keeping with the basis for estimating nutrient allowances for infants developed in the last Recommended Dietary Allowances (NRC, 1989) and Recommended Nutrient Intake (Health Canada, 1990) reports. It also supports the recommendation that exclusive human milk feeding is the preferred method of feeding for normal full-term infants for the first 4 to 6 months of life. This recommendation has also been made by the Canadian Paediatric Society (Health Canada, 1990), the American Academy of Pediatrics (AAP, 1997), and the Food and Nutrition Board report *Nutrition During Lactation* (IOM, 1991).

In general, for this report, special consideration was not given to possible variations in physiological need during the first month after birth or to the variations in intake of nutrients from human milk that result from differences in milk volume and nutrient concentration during early lactation. Specific Dietary Reference Intakes (DRIs) to meet the needs of formula-fed infants are not proposed in this report. The previously published RDAs and RNIs for infants have led to much misinterpretation of the adequacy of human milk because of a lack of understanding about the derivation of these values for young infants. Although they were based on the composition of human milk and the volume of intake, the previous RDA and RNI values allowed for lower bioavailability of nutrients from nonhuman milk.

Ages 0 through 6 Months. To derive the AI value for infants ages 0 through 6 months, the mean intake of a nutrient was calculated based on the average concentration of the nutrient from 2 to 6 months of lactation, using consensus values from several reported studies (Atkinson et al., 1995) and an average volume of milk intake of 0.78 L/day as reported from studies of full-term infants by test weighing, a procedure in which the infant is weighed before and after each feeding (Butte et al., 1984; Chandra, 1984; Hofvander et al., 1982; Neville et al., 1988). Because there is variation in both of these measures, the computed value represents the mean. It is expected that infants will consume increased volumes of human milk as they grow.

Ages 7 through 12 Months. There is no evidence for markedly different nutrient needs during the period of infants' growth acceleration and gradual weaning to a mixed diet of human milk and solid foods from ages 7 through 12 months. The basis of the AI values derived for this age category was the sum of the specific nutrient provided by 0.60 L/day of human milk, which is the average volume of milk reported from studies in this age category (Heinig et al., 1993), and that provided by the usual intakes of complementary weaning foods consumed by infants in this age category (Specker et al., 1997). This approach is in keeping with the current recommendations of the Canadian Paediatric Society (Health Canada, 1990), the American Academy of Pediatrics (AAP, 1997), and *Nutrition During Lactation* (IOM, 1991) for continued human milk feeding of infants through 9 to 12 months of age with appropriate introduction of solid foods.

One problem encountered in trying to derive intake data in infants was the lack of available data on total nutrient intake from a combination of human milk and solid foods in the second 6 months of life. Most intake survey data do not identify the milk source, but the published values indicate that cow milk and cow milk formula were most likely consumed.

Toddlers: Ages 1 through 3 Years

The greater velocity of growth in height during ages 1 through 3 compared with ages 4 through 5 provides a biological basis for dividing this period of life. Because children in the United States and

Canada from age 4 onwards begin to enter the public school system, ending this life stage prior to age 4 seemed appropriate. Data are sparse for indicators of nutrient adequacy on which to derive DRIs for these early years of life. In some cases, DRIs for this age group were derived from data extrapolated from studies of infants or of adults aged 19 years or older.

Early Childhood: Ages 4 through 8 Years

Because major physiological changes in velocity of growth and in endocrine status occur during ages 4 through 8 or 9 years (the latter depending on onset of puberty in each gender), the category of 4 through 8 years is appropriate. For many nutrients, a reasonable amount of data are available on nutrient intake and various criteria for adequacy (such as nutrient balance measured in young children aged 5 through 7 years) that can be used as the basis for the EARs for this life stage group.

Puberty/Adolescence: Ages 9 through 13 Years and 14 through 18 Years

Recognizing that current data support younger ages for pubertal development, it was determined that the adolescent age group should begin at 9 years. The mean age of onset of breast development (Tanner Stage 2) for white females in the United States is 10.0 ± 1.8 (standard deviation) years; this is a physical marker for the beginning of increased estrogen secretion (Herman-Giddens et al., 1997). In African-American females, onset of breast development is earlier (mean 8.9 years ± 1.9). The reason for the observed racial differences in the age at which girls enter puberty is unknown. The onset of the growth spurt in girls begins before the onset of breast development (Tanner, 1990). The age group of 9 through 13 years allows for this early growth spurt of females.

For males, the mean age of initiation of testicular development is 10.5 to 11 years, and their growth spurt begins 2 years later (Tanner, 1990). Thus, to begin the second age category at 14 years and to have different EARs for females and males for some nutrients at this age seems biologically appropriate. All children continue to grow to some extent until as late as age 20; therefore, having these two age categories span the period 9 through 18 years of age seems justified.

Young Adulthood and Middle Ages: Ages 19 through 30 Years and 31 through 50 Years

The recognition of the possible value of higher nutrient intakes during early adulthood on achieving optimal genetic potential for peak bone mass was the reason for dividing adulthood into ages 19 through 30 years and 31 through 50 years. Moreover, mean energy expenditure decreases during this 30-year period, and needs for nutrients related to energy metabolism may also decrease. For some nutrients, the DRIs may be the same for the two age groups. However, for other nutrients, especially those related to energy metabolism, EARs (and RDAs) are likely to differ.

Adulthood and Older Adults: Ages 51 through 70 Years and Greater than 70 Years

The age period of 51 through 70 years spans active work years for most adults. After age 70, people of the same age increasingly display variability in physiological functioning and physical activity. A comparison of people over age 70 who are the same chronological age may demonstrate as much as a 15- to 20-year age-related difference in level of reserve capacity and functioning. This is demonstrated by age-related declines in nutrient absorption and renal function. Because of the high variability in functional capacity of older adults, the EARs for this age group may reflect a greater variability in requirements for the older age categories. This variability may be most applicable to nutrients for which requirements are related to energy expenditure.

Pregnancy and Lactation

Recommendations for pregnancy and lactation may be subdivided because of the many physiological changes and changes in nutrient needs that occur during these life stages. In setting EARs for these life stages, however, consideration is given to adaptations to increased nutrient demand, such as increased absorption, and to greater conservation of many nutrients. Moreover, some nutrients may undergo net losses due to physiological mechanisms regardless of the nutrient intake. Thus, for some nutrients, there may not be a basis for EAR values that are different during these life stages than they are for other women of comparable age.

Reference Weights and Heights

The reference weights and heights selected for adults and children are shown in Table 1-1. The values are based on anthropometric data collected from 1988–1994 as part of the Third National Health and Nutrition Examination Survey (NHANES III) in the United States.

TABLE 1-1 Reference Heights and Weights for Children and Adults in the United States[a]

Gender	Age	Median Body Mass Index, kg/m²	Reference Height, cm (in)	Reference Weight,[b] kg (lb)
Male, female	2–6 mo	–	64 (25)	7 (16)
	7–12 mo	–	72 (28)	9 (20)
	1–3 y	–	91 (36)	13 (29)
	4–8 y	15.8	118 (46)	22 (48)
Male	9–13 y	18.5	147 (58)	40 (88)
	14–18 y	21.3	174 (68)	64 (142)
	19–30 y	24.4	176 (69)	76 (166)
Female	9–13 y	18.3	148 (58)	40 (88)
	14–18 y	21.3	163 (64)	57 (125)
	19–30 y	22.8	163 (64)	61 (133)

[a] Adapted from NHANES III, 1988–1994.
[b] Calculated from body mass index and height for ages 4 through 8 and older.

The median heights for the life stage and gender groups through age 30 were identified, and the median weights for these heights were based on reported median Body Mass Index (BMI) for the same individuals. Since there is no evidence that weight should change as adults age if activity is maintained, the reference weights for adults ages 19 through 30 years are applied to all adult age groups.

The most recent nationally representative data available for Canadians (from the 1970–1972 Nutrition Canada Survey [Demirjian, 1980]) were reviewed. In general, median heights of children from 1 year of age in the United States were greater by 3 to 8 cm (1 to 2 1/2 inches) than those of children of the same age in Canada measured two decades earlier (Demirjian, 1980). This could be explained partly by approximations necessary to compare the two data sets, but more likely by a continuation of the secular trend of increased heights for age noted in the Nutrition Canada Survey when it compared data from that survey with an earlier (1953) national Canadian survey (Pett and Ogilvie, 1956).

Similarly, median weights beyond age 1 year derived from the recent survey in the United States (NHANES III, 1988–1994) were also greater than those obtained from the older Canadian survey (Demirjian, 1980). Differences were greatest during adolescence— from 10 to 17 percent higher. The differences probably reflect the secular trend of earlier onset of puberty (Herman-Giddens et al., 1997), rather than differences in populations. Calculations of BMI for young adults (e.g., a median of 22.6 for Canadian women compared with 22.8 for U.S. women) resulted in similar values, indicating greater concordance between the two surveys by adulthood.

The reference weights chosen for this report were based on the most recent data set available from either country, recognizing that earlier surveys in Canada indicated shorter stature and lower weights during adolescence compared with those from surveys in the United States.

Reference weights are used primarily when setting the EAR or Tolerable Upper Level Intake (UL) for children or when relating the nutrient needs of adults to body weight. For the 4- to 8-year-old age group on an individual basis, a small 4-year-old child can be assumed to require less than the EAR and a large 8-year-old will require more than the EAR. However, the RDA or AI should meet the needs of both.

SUMMARY

Dietary Reference Intakes (DRIs) is a generic term for a set of nutrient reference values that includes the Recommended Dietary Allowance, Adequate Intake, Tolerable Upper Intake Level, and Estimated Average Requirement. These reference values are being developed for life stage and gender groups in a joint U.S. and Canadian activity. This report, one volume in a series, covers the DRIs for vitamin C, vitamin E, selenium, and β-carotene and the other carotenoids.

REFERENCES

AAP (American Academy of Pediatrics). 1997. Breastfeeding and the use of human milk. *Pediatrics* 100:1035–1039.

Atkinson SA, Alston-Mils BP, Lonnerdal B, Neville MC, Thompson MP. 1995. Major minerals and ionic constituents of human and bovine milk. In: Jensen RJ, ed. *Handbook of Milk Composition*. California: Academic Press. Pp. 593–619.

Beaton GH. 1994. Criteria of an adequate diet. In: Shils ME, Olson JA, Shike M, eds. *Modern Nutrition in Health and Disease, 8th edition*. Philadelphia: Lea & Febiger. Pp. 1491–1505.

Butte NF, Garza C, Smith EO, Nichols BL. 1984. Human milk intake and growth in exclusively breast-fed infants. *J Pediatr* 104:187–195.

Chandra RK. 1984. Physical growth of exclusively breast-fed infants. *Nutr Res* 2:275–276.

COMA (Committee on Medical Aspects of Food Policy). 1991. *Dietary Reference Values for Food Energy and Nutrients for the United Kingdom*. Report on Health and Social Subjects, No. 41. London: HMSO.

Demirjian A. 1980. *Anthropometry Report. Height, Weight, and Body Dimensions: A Report from Nutrition Canada.* Ottawa: Minister of National Health and Welfare, Health and Promotion Directorate, Health Services and Promotion Branch.

Elia M. 1992. Energy expenditure and the whole body. In: Kinney JM, Tucker HN, eds. *Energy Metabolism: Tissue Determinants and Cellular Corollaries.* New York: Raven Press. Pp. 19–59.

FAO/WHO/UNA (Food and Agriculture Organization of the United Nations/ World Health Organization/United Nations). 1985. *Energy and Protein Requirements Report of a Joint FAO/WHO/UNA Expert Consultation.* Technical Report Series, No. 724. Geneva: World Health Organization.

Garby L, Lammert O. 1984. Within-subjects between-days-and-weeks variation in energy expenditure at rest. *Hum Nutr Clin Nutr* 38:395–397.

Health Canada. 1990. *Nutrition Recommendations. The Report of the Scientific Review Committee 1990.* Ottawa: Canadian Government Publishing Centre.

Heinig MJ, Nommsen LA, Peerson JM, Lonnerdal B, Dewey KG. 1993. Energy and protein intakes of breast-fed and formula-fed infants during the first year of life and their association with growth velocity: The DARLING Study. *Am J Clin Nutr* 58:152–161.

Herman-Giddens ME, Slora EJ, Wasserman RC, Bourdony CJ, Bhapkar MV, Koch GG, Hasemeier CM. 1997. Secondary sexual characteristics and menses in young girls seen in office practice: A study from the Pediatric Research in Office Settings network. *Pediatrics* 99:505–512.

Hofvander Y, Hagman U, Hillervik C, Sjolin S. 1982. The amount of milk consumed by 1–3 months old breast- or bottle-fed infants. *Acta Paediatr Scand* 71:953–958.

IOM (Institute of Medicine). 1991. *Nutrition During Lactation.* Washington, DC: National Academy Press.

Neville MC, Keller R, Seacat J, Lutes V, Neifert M, Casey C, Allen J, Archer P. 1988. Studies in human lactation: Milk volumes in lactating women during the onset of lactation and full lactation. *Am J Clin Nutr* 48:1375–1386.

NRC (National Research Council). 1989. *Recommended Dietary Allowances,* 10th edition. Washington, DC: National Academy Press.

Pett LB, Ogilvie GH. 1956. The Canadian Weight-Height Survey. *Hum Biol* 28:177–188.

Specker BL, Beck A, Kalkwarf H, Ho M. 1997. Randomized trial of varying mineral intake on total body bone mineral accretion during the first year of life. *Pediatrics* 99:E12.

Tanner JM. 1990. *Growth at Adolescence.* Oxford: Oxford University Press.

WHO (World Health Organization). 1996. *Trace Elements in Human Nutrition and Health.* Geneva: World Health Organization.

2

Vitamin C, Vitamin E, Selenium, and β-Carotene and Other Carotenoids: Overview, Antioxidant Definition, and Relationship to Chronic Disease

OVERVIEW

This report focuses on vitamin C, vitamin E, selenium, and β-carotene and other carotenoids (α-carotene, β-cryptoxanthin, lutein, lycopene, and zeaxanthin). These compounds have frequently been called dietary antioxidants since in some cases they counteract oxidative damage to biomolecules (Halliwell, 1996), and the possibility exists that increased intakes of these compounds may protect against chronic disease. Although the term dietary antioxidants is a convenient description, these compounds are multifunctional, and some of the actions observed in vivo may not represent an antioxidant function, even though the compounds have been classified as antioxidant nutrients (Sies and Stahl, 1995).

Therefore, in this report the above compounds were evaluated with respect to their role in human nutrition, without limiting the investigation to antioxidant properties. Information was reviewed regarding the minimum amount of these nutrients required to prevent deficiency diseases, as well as the amounts that might impact on chronic diseases, regardless of whether the effect was an antioxidant effect or not. Resolution of any impact of these compounds on chronic disease will require evaluation of the many human intervention trials that are still under way (Table 2-1).

Four main tasks were assigned to the Dietary Reference Intakes Panel on Dietary Antioxidants and Related Compounds. The first task was to develop a definition of a dietary antioxidant; the second

TABLE 2-1 Intervention Trials: Antioxidants and Chronic Diseases

Study	Country	Study Type[a]	Study Population
Skin Cancer Prevention Study (Greenberg et al., 1990)	U.S.[c]	Secondary prevention; randomized, double-blind, placebo-controlled intervention	1,805 men and women with recent nonmelanoma skin cancer; aged 40–89 y
Linxian Cancer Prevention Study (Blot et al., 1993)	China	Primary prevention; randomized, double-blind, placebo-controlled intervention	29,584 poorly nourished men and women, aged 40–69 y
α-Tocopherol, β-Carotene Cancer Prevention Study (ATBC Cancer Prevention Group, 1994)	Finland	Primary prevention; randomized, double-blind, placebo-controlled intervention	29,133 male cigarette smokers, aged 50–69 y
Polyp Prevention Study (Greenberg et al., 1994)	U.S.	Secondary prevention; randomized, double-blind, placebo-controlled intervention	864 men and women with recent nonmelanoma skin cancer
The β-Carotene and Retinol Efficacy Trial (Omenn et al., 1996)	U.S.	Primary prevention; randomized, double-blind, placebo-controlled intervention	14,254 heavy smokers and 4,060 asbestos workers, aged 45–69 y
Cambridge Heart Antioxidant Study (Stephens et al., 1996)	U.K.[e]	Secondary prevention; randomized, double-blind, placebo-controlled intervention	2,002 patients with coronary atherosclerosis, mean age 62 y

Duration of Treatment (y)	Daily Dose	Primary Disease Outcome	Results[b]
5	50 mg β-carotene	Skin cancer	No effect on occurrence of new nonmelanoma skin cancers
5.25	15 mg β-carotene, 30 mg α-tocopherol, 50 mg selenium	Cancer	9% reduction in total mortality; 13% decrease in cancer mortality; 21% decrease in stomach cancer deaths; 10% decrease in cerebrovascular mortality (nonsignificant)
6	50 mg α-tocopherol and/or 20 mg β-carotene	Lung cancer	50% increase in hemorrhagic stroke deaths among vitamin E group; 11% increase in ischemic heart disease deaths among β-carotene group; 18% increase in lung cancer among β-carotene group; no effect of vitamin E on lung cancer
4	25 mg β-carotene, 1,000 mg vitamin C, 400 mg α-tocopherol	Colorectal cancer	No reduced incidence of adenomas
4	30 mg β-carotene, 25,000 IU retinol (as retinyl palmitate)	Lung cancer	28% increase in lung cancer; 26% increase in CVD[d] (nonsignificant); 17% increase in total mortality among treatment group
1.4	400 or 800 IU (268 or 537 mg) α-tocopherol	CVD death or nonfatal MI[f]	77% decrease in risk of subsequent nonfatal MI; no benefit on cardiovascular mortality

continued

TABLE 2-1 Continued

Study	Country	Study Type[a]	Study Population
Physicians' Health Study (Hennekens et al., 1996)	U.S.	Primary prevention; randomized, double-blind, placebo-controlled intervention	22,071 male physicians, aged 40–84 y
Nutritional Prevention of Cancer Study (Clark et al., 1996, 1998)	U.S.	Secondary prevention; randomized, double-blind, placebo-controlled intervention	1,312 men and women with history of basal or squamous cell carcinoma; aged 18–80 y
GISSI-Prevention Trial (GISSI-Prevenzione Investigators; 1999)	Italy	Secondary prevention; randomized, double-blind, placebo-controlled intervention	11,324 patients with recent MI
Women's Health Study (Lee et al., 1999)	U.S.	Primary prevention; randomized, double-blind, placebo-controlled intervention	39,876 healthy women, aged ≥45 y
Heart Outcomes Prevention Evaluation Study (HOPE Study Investigators, 2000)	Canada	Secondary prevention; randomized, double-blind, placebo-controlled intervention	9,541 high-risk men and women, aged ≥55 y

Studies In Progress

Study	Country	Study Type[a]	Study Population
MRC/BHF Heart Protection Study (MRC/BHF, 1999)	U.K.	Secondary prevention trial	20,536 high-risk men and women, aged 40–80 y

Duration of Treatment (y)	Daily Dose	Primary Disease Outcome	Results[b]
12	50 mg β-carotene (alternate days)	Cancer, CVD	No effects on CVD or cancer including among smokers
4.5	200 μg selenium	Skin cancer, prostate cancer	No effect on incidence of skin cancer; 63% reduction in prostate cancer incidence; reduction in total cancer mortality and total cancer incidence
3–5	300 mg α-tocopherol and/or 1 g ω-3 PUFA[g]	Total mortality	No benefit from vitamin E; 15% decrease in risk of death, nonfatal MI, and stroke from ω-3 PUFA
2.1	50 mg β-carotene (alternate days)	MI, stroke, or CVD death	No effect on incidence of cancer, CVD, or total mortality
4–6	400 IU (268 mg) α-tocopherol, ACE[h] inhibitor	MI, stroke, or CVD death	No benefit from vitamin E
≥5	20 mg β-carotene, 600 mg α-tocopherol, 250 mg vitamin C	Total mortality	No results yet

continued

TABLE 2-1 Continued

Study	Country	Study Type[a]	Study Population
Women's Antioxidant Cardiovascular Study (Manson et al., 1995)	U.S.	Secondary prevention; randomized, double-blind, placebo-controlled intervention	8,000 women with prior CVD event or ≥3 coronary risk factors, aged ≥40 y
Women's Health Study (Buring and Hennekens, 1992)	U.S.	Primary prevention; randomized, double-blind, placebo-controlled intervention	39,876 healthy women, aged ≥45 y
Physician's Health Study II (Hennekens, 1998)	U.S.	Primary prevention; randomized, double-blind, placebo-controlled intervention	15,000 healthy male physicians, aged ≥55 y
SUVIMAX (Hercberg et al., 1998)	France	Primary prevention; randomized, double-blind, placebo-controlled intervention	12,735 men and women, aged 35–60 y

[a] A primary prevention trial is one in which the study participants have no history of the disease outcome being investigated. Participants in a secondary prevention trial have had a prior occurrence of the outcome being investigated.

[b] Unless noted otherwise, results are statistically significant.

[c] U.S. = United States.

[d] CVD = cardiovascular disease.

task was to select, in addition to vitamin C, vitamin E, and β-carotene, other food components which might prove to be antioxidants and play a role in health; the third task was to assess the role of these compounds in health; and the fourth task was to develop Dietary Reference Intakes (DRIs) for the selected nutrients. The panel was asked to evaluate vitamin C, vitamin E, and β-carotene and other antioxidants. Since other dietary carotenoids share many,

Duration of Treatment (y)	Daily Dose	Primary Disease Outcome	Results[b]
4	50 mg β-carotene, 600 IU α-tocopherol, 500 mg vitamin C (alternate days)	CVD	No results yet
NR[i]	600 IU α-tocopherol, 100 mg aspirin (alternate days)	MI, stroke, or CVD death	No results yet
NR	50 mg β-carotene, 400 IU α-tocopherol (alternate days), 500 mg vitamin C, multivitamin (centrum silver)	CVD, cancer, eye diseases	No results yet
8	6 mg β-carotene, 30 mg α-tocopherol, 120 mg vitamin C, 100 µg selenium, 20 mg zinc	Cancer, ischemic heart disease	No results yet

[e] U.K. = United Kingdom.
[f] MI = myocardial infarction.
[g] PUFA = polyunsaturated fatty acid.
[h] ACE = angiotension-converting enzyme.
[i] NR = not reported.

although not all, of the properties of β-carotene, additional carotenoids (α-carotene, β-cryptoxanthin, lutein, lycopene, and zeaxanthin) were added as related nutrients that would be investigated. In addition, because of the important role that selenium plays as a cofactor for oxidant defense enzymes, it was also included as a related nutrient.

DEFINITION AND CRITERIA FOR A DIETARY ANTIOXIDANT

Definition of a Dietary Antioxidant

The definition was based on several criteria: (1) the substance is found in human diets; (2) the content of the substance has been measured in foods commonly consumed; and (3) in humans, the substance decreases the adverse effects of reactive species, such as reactive oxygen and nitrogen species in vivo. Thus, the definition of a dietary antioxidant is as follows:

> *A dietary antioxidant is a substance in foods that significantly decreases the adverse effects of reactive species, such as reactive oxygen and nitrogen species, on normal physiological function in humans.*

This stringent definition, with supporting information, was slightly modified from the proposed definition published earlier (IOM, 1998). The earlier report stated that the nutritional recommendations that will be presented in the final report for some of these dietary components may not be determined by or related to their possible action as antioxidants. The primary indicators for developing the Dietary Reference Intakes (DRIs) are based on specific actions and effects of the compounds that may or may not be attributed to their antioxidant activity. In particular, criteria chosen upon which to base EARs and thus RDAs for any of the compounds investigated are not related specifically to ameliorating chronic diseases because a scientific justification for such a requirement was not found.

The European Commission Concerted Action on Functional Food also adopted stringent criteria regarding the relationship between free-radical events and human disease, and whether antioxidants are capable of modulating these events and thus reducing the risk of disease (Diplock et al., 1998). The summary report concluded that, "there is at present insufficient evidence available on which to base a firm conclusion that antioxidants are capable of reducing risk of disease" (Diplock, 1998). Recommendations for the nutrients in this report are similar. However, it should be pointed out that a large number of human intervention studies are under way using the compounds discussed in this report, and the results of these studies may give rise to new conclusions.

Are Vitamin C, Vitamin E, Selenium, and β-Carotene and Other Carotenoids Dietary Antioxidants?

Vitamin C functions physiologically as a water-soluble antioxidant by virtue of its very strong reducing power (high redox potential) and facile regeneration via ubiquitous reductants such as glutathione, nicotinamide adenine dinucleotide, and nicotinamide adenine dinucleotide phosphate. The primary method used to estimate the requirement relates to the vitamin C intake needed to maintain near-maximal neutrophil ascorbate concentration with minimal urinary excretion. Because smokers suffer increased oxidative stress and metabolic turnover of vitamin C, their requirement is increased. Although there is ample evidence that vitamin C administration can result in decreases in markers of oxidative stress, a Recommended Dietary Allowance (RDA) derived from a direct antioxidant function of vitamin C could not be calculated because of the lack of a quantitative relationship between this antioxidant function and a health-related endpoint. Since vitamin C reduces markers of oxidative stress, it meets the definition of a dietary antioxidant.

Vitamin E functions as a chain-breaking antioxidant that prevents the propagation of lipid peroxidation. To estimate the requirement, data were examined on the intake of vitamin E that would prevent hydrogen peroxide-induced lysis of erythrocytes. Under these circumstances, vitamin E is acting as an ex vivo antioxidant, maintaining a normal physiological function in humans. Although it is not yet possible to relate vitamin E intake to a lowering of chronic disease risk, it still meets the definition of a dietary antioxidant.

Selenium functions through selenoproteins, several of which are oxidant defense enzymes. The criterion used to estimate the requirement for selenium relates to the intake needed to maximize the activity of the plasma selenoprotein glutathione peroxidase, an oxidant defense enzyme. It is not clear if the diseases associated with selenium deficiencies, Keshan disease or Kashin-Beck disease, are due to oxidative stress. The selenium in several selenoproteins has a biochemical role in oxidant defense, thus maintaining normal physiological function, and as such plays a role as a dietary antioxidant.

β-Carotene and other carotenoids function as sources of vitamin A and, due to this provitamin A activity, can prevent vitamin A deficiency. Because no other specific nutrient functions have been identified at this time, no requirements have been established for any of the carotenoids. β-Carotene and the other carotenoids display in vitro antioxidant activity, but the evidence that they act as in vivo antioxidants in humans is still controversial. Therefore, β-carotene does not meet the definition of a dietary antioxidant. Similar conclusions have been drawn for α-carotene, β-cryptoxanthin, lycopene, lutein, and zeaxanthin.

OXIDATIVE STRESS, ANTIOXIDANTS, AND CHRONIC DISEASE

Oxidative Stress

There have been many proposals as to how oxidative stress can be defined. Because all cells are exposed to oxidants, generated either endogenously from metabolism or exogenously from a variety of environmental insults, the problem arises as to what constitutes an oxidative stress. Furthermore, different cells can be exposed to the same level of oxidants, but depending on the level of antioxidants or protective mechanisms available to the cell, they may or may not experience an oxidative stress. Sies (1985) defined oxidative stress as "a disturbance in the prooxidant-antioxidant balance in favor of the former." Others have amplified this definition to include "short- and/or long-term disturbance of the prooxidant-antioxidant balance resulting in adverse effects that are due either to impaired antioxidation or to favored prooxidation" (Biesalski et al., 1997). Here, oxidative stress is defined as an *imbalance* between the production of various reactive species and the ability of the organism's natural protective mechanisms to cope with these reactive compounds and prevent adverse effects.

The primary reactive species include reactive oxygen species (ROS) and reactive nitrogen species (RNS). These in turn react in the body and generate radical intermediates of lipids, proteins, and nucleic acids that ultimately form the chemical end products of oxidative stress. The physiological consequences of these end products have been hypothesized to be the causes of many chronic diseases as well as the natural aging process (Ames, 1998; Halliwell, 1997). The protective mechanisms include protective enzymes, antioxidant or quenching compounds produced by the organism, and similar compounds made available in the diet. The evidence that chronic disease results from an imbalance between formation and removal of reactive species is discussed below.

The primary defensive compounds are antioxidants that can interact with and quench reactive radical species, and enzymes that can inactivate these species or their products. All of the compounds in this report—vitamin C, vitamin E, selenium in the form of selenoproteins, and β-carotene and other carotenoids—are in vitro antioxidants, and some evidence exists that they have in vivo antioxidant actions. The protective enzymes include, among others, superoxide dismutase, catalase, and selenium-containing glutathione peroxidases and thioredoxin reductase. Other antioxidant mechanisms include stimulation of the expression of antioxidant or repair enzymes, as well as chelation of transition metals. A recent review of the relationship between antioxidant supplementation and oxidative damage concludes that, with the exception of vitamin E and possibly vitamin C reducing markers of lipid peroxidation, the evidence is insufficient that antioxidant supplementation leads to a material reduction in oxidative damage in humans (McCall and Frei, 1999).

Biomarkers of Oxidative Stress

There have been numerous tests described to evaluate the level of markers of oxidative stress in living systems. Many of these markers represent oxidative breakdown products of normal tissue components and metabolites. Products derived from oxidized lipids include age pigments (lipofuscin), aldehydes, alkanes, and prostanoids such as the F_2-isoprostanes derived from unsaturated fatty acids. Oxidation of proteins produces protein carbonyls and amino acid derivatives such as methionine sulfoxide and nitrotyrosine, derived from the reaction of peroxynitrite ($ONOO^-$) with tyrosine. Purine and pyrimidine metabolites that are derived from oxidized nucleic acids can be detected in tissues and in urine. Since virtually all tissues are exposed to ROS and RNS, there will always be a baseline production of these biomarker molecules. What is important in evaluating the extent of oxidative stress is the *change* in the level of the biomarker compared to a baseline or steady-state level.

It is quite clear that dietary change can alter the levels of some of the biomarkers described above, and this phenomenon has been reported when the dietary intake of fruits and vegetables has been increased. Examples of such studies include reductions in biomarkers of deoxyribonucleic acid (DNA) damage (Pool-Zobel et al., 1997) or of lipid peroxidation (Miller et al., 1998), following consumption of diets rich in fruits and vegetables. Many of these studies have been reviewed recently (Halliwell, 1999).

A major problem with the use of biomarkers such as those described above is not knowing whether they reflect processes in the initiation of a disease state or whether they are products of a disease state. The validity of biomarkers, either intermediate or final, will not be settled until they are evaluated as part of intervention trials.

A causal relationship between the formation of a biomarker of oxidant stress and a chronic disease has not yet been validated.

Some attempts have been made to determine a more global measure of oxidative stress, such as TRAP (total radical-trapping antioxidant capability) (Wayner et al., 1985), ORAC (oxygen radical absorbance capacity) (Cao et al., 1993), TEAC (trolox equivalent antioxidant capacity) (Miller et al., 1993), and FOX (ferrous oxidation/xylenol orange) (Jiang et al., 1992) assays. However, because these markers do not measure the same oxidants or antioxidant defenses (Cao and Prior, 1998), it is difficult to validate them as useful markers of oxidant stress.

Evidence of Oxidative Stress and Chronic Disease

Aerobic metabolism produces energy, waste products such as carbon dioxide, and a small, but steady stream of radical by-products that are capable of reacting with all of the body's constituents to form oxidative damage products (Ames et al., 1993; Chance et al., 1979). Calculations have been made of the number of radical species formed per cell per day, but it is not at all clear how these numbers relate to diseases. Since the entire population is exposed to oxidative stresses and only a small fraction develops a chronic disease, it is clear that at this time, it is not understood how to evaluate the role of oxidative stress in the development of chronic disease. The potential role of oxidative stress in six chronic disease areas and aging is described briefly below.

Cancer

DNA is subject to damage, and either an exogenous or an endogenous mutagen can produce damage at a faster rate than the normal protective process of enzymatic repair (Ames et al., 1995). Under these circumstances, elevated levels of excision products will appear in the urine. The observation that 8-oxy-7,8-dihydro-2′-deoxyguanosine (8-oxodG) is a major urinary product of both oxidative damage to DNA and damage by ionizing radiation that produces ROS, has served as the basis for the hypothesis that oxidative DNA damage is carcinogenic (Ames et al., 1995). The presence of 8-oxodG in DNA would lead to a guanine-to-thymine transversion that would result in a DNA mutation and, depending on its location, an altered gene product. 8-OxodG is also produced by ionizing radiation, and since this process can be carcinogenic, it has been assumed that any condition that produces 8-oxodG will also be carcinogenic. However, a causal relationship between oxidative stress to DNA and cancer in humans has not yet been established (Poulsen et al., 1998).

A great deal of evidence based on epidemiological studies indicates that consuming diets rich in fruits and vegetables is associated with both a decrease in oxidative damage to DNA (Halliwell, 1998) and a lower risk of a number of common cancers. There are several mechanisms that could account for these observations, in addition to antioxidant components that scavenge radical intermediates. Other mechanisms include the modification of carcinogen activation by the inhibition of phase 1 enzymes, modification of carcinogen detoxification by phase 2 enzymes, and suppression of the abnormal proliferation associated with preneoplastic lesions (Wargovich, 1997).

Cardiovascular Disease

Of all the chronic diseases in which excess oxidative stress has been implicated, cardiovascular disease has the strongest supporting evidence. A coherent pathogenetic mechanism has been developed to account for the earliest stage in atherogenesis, namely, the development of the fatty streak lesion. Hypercholesterolemia and, particularly, increased concentrations of low-density lipoproteins (LDLs) cause the accumulation of cholesterol-loaded "foam cells" beneath the endothelial lining of major arteries, which in turn develop into a fatty streak. This lesion is clinically benign but is the precursor of later lesions (the fibrous plaque and the complex lesion) that ultimately give rise to clinical manifestations (angina pectoris and myocardial infarction) (Steinberg and Witztum, 1990).

An elevated LDL cholesterol level sufficiently increases the risk of cardiovascular disease. Brown and Goldstein (1986) demonstrated that the molecular defect in individuals with familial hypercholesterolemia was the absence of functional LDL receptors. The histological lesions in these patients cannot be differentiated from that of lesions in individuals who have normal LDL receptors. The implication therefore is that normal LDL taken up by way of the normal LDL receptor cannot be the basis for the formation of foam cells. In other words, the LDL must first be modified somehow and the modified form must be taken up into the monocytes or macrophages via one or more alternative receptors ultimately and develop into foam cells. One such modification, and the most extensively studied, is LDL oxidation, and several macrophage receptors have been shown to take up oxidatively modified LDL (oxLDL) and thus develop foam cells (Navab et al., 1995; Steinberg, 1997; Steinberg and Witztum, 1990; Steinberg et al., 1989; Steinbrecher, 1997).

In addition to its ability to cause foam cell formation, oxLDL can contribute to atherogenesis by virtue of a number of properties that differ from those of normal LDL (reviewed in Steinberg, 1997). The key question is whether these potentially proatherogenic properties of oxLDL are of sufficient importance that inhibition of the generation of oxLDL by antioxidants will have a significant impact on the rate of progression of atherosclerotic lesions.

The finding that a relationship existed between LDL levels and the incidence of cardiovascular disease was followed by the observation that oxLDL was associated with the development of atherosclerotic lesions in experimental animals. This association led to the hypothesis that oxLDL is the causative agent in the development of cardiovascular disease (Steinberg et al., 1989). This hypothesis has served as the basis for a number of human intervention trials, testing whether antioxidant agents capable of decreasing the extent of oxidation of LDL and thus decreasing oxLDL concentration might prove useful in decreasing the incidence of cardiovascular disease.

Several biomarkers of oxidative stress have been used to evaluate the extent of oxLDL formation and/or the extent of oxidative damage to lipids in general. OxLDL formation has been assessed after treating individuals with dietary antioxidants and evaluating the presence of oxLDL. In addition there have been reports of a potent effect of supplementary antioxidants in lowering the extent of ex vivo oxLDL formation. The results are not consistent, and as such, it is still not possible to conclude that dietary antioxidants prevent the formation of oxLDL in vivo. In addition, this modulation of LDL oxidation still must be validated as a marker of risk for cardiovascular disease (Zock and Katan, 1998).

The appearance of F_2-isoprostanes in urine has been suggested by a number of investigators as a reliable index of in vivo free radical generation and oxidative lipid formation. There is very strong evidence from animal studies that F_2-isoprostanes increase in plasma and urine as a result of oxidative stress, and in humans, these products are elevated in smokers (Morrow et al., 1995). Evidence is gradually accumulating that supplementary antioxidants, and vitamin E in particular, can both affect the level of F_2-isoprostanes in animal models of atherosclerosis and decrease the extent of arterial wall lesions (Pratico et al., 1998). Similar results have been obtained in humans (Hodis et al., 1995). Although some reviews point out that the protective role of antioxidants in animal models of atherosclerosis is only partially confirmed in human studies (Faggiotto et al.,

1998), others are much more supportive of a protective role for vitamin E in coronary heart disease (Pryor, 2000).

Cataracts

There have been a number of observational epidemiological studies of the risk of developing cataracts in humans. Many of these studies indicate that the risk of cataracts may be inversely proportional to the serum level of antioxidants (Knekt et al., 1992; Taylor et al., 1995) or may be reduced by supplement use (Jacques et al., 1997). These studies, however, have been considered to be inconclusive (Christen et al., 1996a; Leske et al., 1998). In the Alpha-Tocopherol, Beta-Carotene Cancer Prevention Study, 5 to 8 years of daily supplementation with either 50 mg of vitamin E or 20 mg of β-carotene or both resulted in no difference in the prevalence of cataracts in the men in this study (Tcikari et al., 1997).

Age-Related Macular Degeneration

This irreversible disease, which is the major form of blindness in the elderly in the United States, Canada, and Europe, has been related to antioxidants found in the diet. This is because the pigment in the macular region of the normal retina consists of the two xanthophyll carotenoids, lutein and zeaxanthin (Bone et al., 1988; Handelman et al., 1988). This observation, coupled with the epidemiological observations of an inverse relationship between the risk of age-related macular degeneration (AMD) and the ingestion of fruits and vegetables (Goldberg et al., 1988), led a number of groups to propose that the basis of this chronic disease was a nutritional deficiency of green, leafy vegetables and yellow and orange fruits and vegetables that were rich in lutein and zeaxanthin (EDCCSG, 1992; Seddon et al., 1994; Snodderly, 1995). Another association was the observation that smokers, who have lower plasma levels of carotenoids, also have a lower macular pigment (lutein and zeaxanthin) density (Hammond et al., 1996) and an increased risk of developing AMD (Christen et al., 1996b). However, all of these reports are associative in nature and do not demonstrate a causal relationship between deficiencies of lutein and zeaxanthin and development of AMD.

Central Neurodegenerative Diseases

There is increasing evidence that a number of common neurodegenerative diseases, such as Alzheimer's disease, Parkinson's disease, multiple sclerosis, and amyotrophic lateral sclerosis may include adverse responses to oxidative stress. Small intervention trials in patients with these diagnoses have reported some improvement with either vitamin E (Muller, 1994; Sano et al., 1997) or vitamin C (Morris et al., 1998; Riviere et al., 1998), but it is still too early to draw any conclusions as to the usefulness of these compounds in these diseases, or to their ability to delay onset of the disease.

Diabetes Mellitus

Cardiovascular complications are the major causes of death in diabetes. The incidence of coronary heart disease in type II diabetes is significantly higher than that in the general population (Kannel and McGee, 1979). In addition, individuals with diabetes experience microvascular complications (retinopathy, neuropathy, and nephropathy) secondary to their hyperglycemia. Thus, oxidative processes also may play an important role in the development or progression of diabetes mellitus.

In vitro oxidation of LDL from patients with diabetes mellitus proceeds at an accelerated rate, which suggests that they are more susceptible to the atherogenic process (Chisolm et al., 1992; Nishigaki et al., 1981; Reaven et al., 1995; Tsai et al., 1994). The several ways in which oxLDL is potentially more atherogenic than native LDL have been discussed above (see section "Cardiovascular Disease").

Diabetics tend to have smaller, denser LDL (associated with hypertriglyceridemia) and these LDLs are more susceptible to oxidative modification ex vivo (Feingold et al., 1992). The TRAP of plasma from patients with insulin-dependent diabetes is decreased (Tsai et al. 1994), which may account in part for the greater susceptibility of their LDL to oxidation.

Microvascular complications are believed to be the ultimate consequences of nonenzymatic glycosylation and the progressive accumulation of advanced glycosylation end products (AGEs). There is evidence that the formation of these complex carbohydrate-protein and carbohydrate-lipid complexes is accompanied and accelerated by oxidative processes, which may lead to diabetic complications (Brownlee et al., 1988; Dyer et al., 1993; Hunt et al., 1988; McCance et al., 1993; Mullarkey et al., 1990). The glycosylation process is associated with increased formation of free radicals, and the possibility that treatment with antioxidants might slow the development of AGEs is under investigation.

The issue of whether modifications observed in plasma and tissue proteins in patients with diabetes are due to an oxidative stress or a stress from reactive carbonyls has been discussed by Baynes and Thorpe (1999). A number of studies have tried altering the pathobiology of diabetes by treating patients with either single antioxidant-type compounds or combinations of compounds with antioxidant properties. The results have been inconclusive, which may reflect the fact that the underlying pathology is not caused exclusively by an oxidative stress, but by an inability to metabolize and inactivate reactive carbonyls appropriately. Under these circumstances, the oxidative damage may be exacerbated, resulting in an increase in many of the markers associated with oxidative stress but not caused directly by oxidative stress (Baynes and Thorpe, 1999).

Aging

Aging is not in itself a chronic disease, but rather is characterized by the active or passive presence of a chronic disease (cardiovascular disease, cancer, cataracts, Alzheimer's disease, etc.). It is not clear if an accumulation of chronic insults and weakened defenses renders the aging individual more susceptible to various diseases. Do antioxidants play a role in preventing aging or prolonging life? There is no direct evidence in humans for such an effect, although vitamin E supplementation appears to improve some immune responses in the elderly (Meydani et al., 1997). There have been suggestions that supplementing older animals with antioxidants may improve various physiological functions (Hagen et al., 1999), but the only experimental intervention that has resulted in prolongation of the life span of the animals has been the drastic reduction of food consumption (Pariza and Boutwell, 1987). Whether such a protocol would delay aging in humans has not yet been studied. Whether dietary antioxidants can lead to healthier aging remains to be proven.

CONCLUSIONS

There is little doubt that an imbalance in the production of free radicals and other reactive species and the natural protective systems available to organisms can lead to the production of oxidized products of lipids, nucleic acids, and proteins. These oxidation products, or biomarkers of this imbalance, may be related to early events in certain chronic diseases. However, they have not yet been adequately validated as markers of the onset, progression, or regression of any chronic diseases. Although vitamin C, vitamin E, and selenium have been shown to decrease the concentrations of some of the biomarkers associated with oxidative stress, the relationship between such observations and chronic disease remain to be elucidated. As a consequence, it has not been possible to establish that dietary antioxidants or other nutrients that can alter the levels of these biomarkers are themselves causally related to the development or prevention of chronic diseases.

REFERENCES

Ames BN. 1998. Micronutrients prevent cancer and delay aging. *Toxicol Lett* 102–103:5–18.

Ames BN, Shigenaga MK, Hagen TM. 1993. Oxidants, antioxidants, and the degenerative diseases of aging. *Proc Natl Acad Sci USA* 90:7915–7922.

Ames BN, Gold LS, Willett WC. 1995. The causes and prevention of cancer. *Proc Natl Acad Sci USA* 92:5258–5265.

ATBC (Alpha-Tocopherol, Beta Carotene) Cancer Prevention Study Group. 1994. The effect of vitamin E and beta carotene on the incidence of lung cancer and other cancers in male smokers. *N Engl J Med* 330:1029–1035.

Baynes JW, Thorpe SR. 1999. Role of oxidative stress in diabetic complications: A new perspective on an old paradigm. *Diabetes* 48:1–9.

Biesalski HK, Böhles H, Esterbauer H, Fürst P, Gey F, Hundsdörfer G, Kasper H, Sies H, Weisburger J. 1997. Antioxidant vitamins in prevention. *Clin Nutr* 16:151–155.

Blot WJ, Li J-Y, Taylor PR, Guo W, Dawsey S, Wang G-Q, Yang CS, Zheng S-F, Gail M, Li G-Y, Yu Y, Liu B-Q, Tangrea J, Sun Y-H, Liu F, Fraumeni JF Jr, Zhang Y-H, Li B. 1993. Nutrition intervention trials in Linxian, China: Supplementation with specific vitamin/mineral combinations, cancer incidence, and disease-specific mortality in the general population. *J Natl Cancer Inst* 85:1483–1492.

Bone RA, Landrum JT, Fernandez L, Tarsis SL. 1988. Analysis of the macular pigment by HPLC: Retinal distribution and age study. *Invest Ophthalmol Vis Sci* 29:843–849.

Brown MS, Goldstein JL. 1986. A receptor-mediated pathway for cholesterol homeostasis. *Science* 232:34–47.

Brownlee M, Cerami A, Vlassara H. 1988. Advanced glycosylation end products in tissue and the biochemical basis of diabetic complications. *N Engl J Med* 318:1315–1321.

Buring JE, Hennekens CH. 1992. The Women's Health Study: Summary of the study design. *J Myocard Isch* 4:27–29.

Cao G, Prior RL. 1998. Comparison of different analytical methods for assessing total antioxidant capacity of human serum. *Clin Chem* 44:1309–1315.

Cao G, Alessio HM, Cutler RG. 1993. Oxygen-radical absorbance capacity assay for antioxidants. *Free Radic Biol Med* 14:303–311.

Chance B, Sies H, Boveris A. 1979. Hydroperoxide metabolism in mammalian organs. *Physiol Rev* 59:527–605.

Chisolm GM, Irwin KC, Penn MS. 1992. Lipoprotein oxidation and lipoprotein-induced cell injury in diabetes. *Diabetes* 41:61–66.

Christen WG, Glynn RJ, Hennekens CH. 1996a. Antioxidants and age-related eye disease. Current and future perspectives. *Ann Epidemiol* 6:60–66.

Christen WG, Glynn RJ, Manson JE, Ajani UA, Buring JE. 1996b. A prospective study of cigarette smoking and risk of age-related macular degeneration in men. *J Am Med Assoc* 276:1147–1151.

Clark LC, Combs GF, Turnbull BW, Slate EH, Chalker DK, Chow J, Davis LS, Glover RA, Graham GF, Gross EG, Krongrad A, Lesher JL, Park HK, Sanders BB, Smith CL, Taylor JR. 1996. Effects of selenium supplementation for cancer prevention in patients with carcinoma of the skin. A randomized controlled trial. *J Am Med Assoc* 276:1957–1963.

Clark LC, Dalkin B, Krongrad A, Combs GF Jr, Turnbull BW, Slate EH, Witherington R, Herlong JH, Janosko E, Carpenter D, Borosso C, Falk S, Rounder J. 1998. Decreased incidence of prostate cancer with selenium supplementation: Results of a double-blind cancer prevention trial. *Br J Urol* 81:730–734.

Diplock AT. 1998. Defense against reactive oxygen species. *Free Rad Res* 29:463–467.

Diplock AT, Charleux JL, Crozier-Willi G, Kok FJ, Rice-Evans C, Roberfroid M, Stahl W, Vina-Ribes J. 1998. Functional food science and defense against reactive oxidative species. *Br J Nutr* 80:S77–S112.

Dyer DG, Dunn JA, Thorpe SR, Bailie KE, Lyons TJ, McCance DR, Baynes JW. 1993. Accumulation of Maillard reaction products in skin collagen in diabetes and aging. *J Clin Invest* 91:2463–2469.

EDCCSG (Eye Disease Case-Control Study Group). 1992. Risk factors for neovascular age-related macular degeneration. *Arch Ophthalmol* 110:1701–1708.

Faggiotto A, Poli A, Catapano AL. 1998. Antioxidants and coronary artery disease. *Curr Opin Lipidol* 9:541–549.

Feingold KR, Grunfeld C, Pang M, Doerrler W, Krauss RM. 1992. LDL subclass phenotypes and triglyceride metabolism in non-insulin-dependent diabetes. *Arterioscler Thromb* 12:1496–1502.

GISSI-Prevenzione Investigators. 1999. Dietary supplementation with n-3 polyunsaturated fatty acids and vitamin E after myocardial infarction: Results of the GISSI-Prevenzione Trial. *Lancet* 354:447–455.

Goldberg J, Flowerdew G, Smith E, Brody JA, Tso MO. 1988. Factors associated with age-related macular degeneration. *Am J Epidemiol* 128:700–710.

Greenberg ER, Baron JA, Stukel TA, Stevens MM, Mandel JS, Spencer SK, Elias PM, Lowe N, Nierenberg DW, Bayrd G, Vance JC, Freeman DH, Clendenning WE, Kwan. 1990. A clinical trial of beta carotene to prevent basal-cell and squamous-cell cancers of the skin. *N Engl J Med* 323:789–795.

Greenberg ER, Baron JA, Tosteson TD, Freeman DH, Beck GJ, Bond JH, Colacchio TA, Coller JA, Frankl HD, Haile RW, Mandel JS, Nierenberg DW, Rothstein R, Snover DC, Stevens MM, Summers RW, van Stolk RU. 1994. A clinical trial of antioxidant vitamins to prevent colorectal adenoma. *N Engl J Med* 331:141–147.

Hagen TM, Ingersoll RT, Lykkesfeldt J, Liu J, Wehr CM, Vinarsky V, Bartholomew JC, Ames AB. 1999. (R)-alpha-lipoic acid-supplemented old rats have improved mitochondrial function, decreased oxidative damage, and increased metabolic rate. *FASEB J* 13:411–418.

Halliwell B. 1996. Antioxidants in human health and disease. *Annu Rev Nutr* 16:33–50.

Halliwell B. 1997. Antioxidants and human disease: A general introduction. *Nutr Rev* 55:S44–S52.

Halliwell B. 1998. Can oxidative DNA damage be used as a biomarker for cancer risk in humans? Problems, resolutions and preliminary results from nutritional supplement studies. *Free Radic Res* 29:469-486.

Halliwell B. 1999. Antioxidant defence mechanisms: From the beginning to the end (of the beginning). *Free Radic Res* 31:261-272.

Hammond BR Jr, Wooten BR, Snodderly DM. 1996. Cigarette smoking and retinal carotenoids: Implications for age-related macular degeneration. *Vision Res* 36:3003–3009.

Handelman GJ, Dratz EA, Reay CC, Van Kuijk JG. 1988. Carotenoids in the human macula and whole retina. *Invest Ophthalmol Vis Sci* 29:850–855.

Hennekens CH. 1998. Antioxidant vitamins and cardiovascular disease: Current knowledge and future directions. *Nutrition* 14:50–51.

Hennekens CH, Buring JE, Manson JE, Stampfer M, Rosner B, Cook NR, Belanger C, LaMotte F, Gaziano JM, Ridker PM, Willett W, Peto R. 1996. Lack of effect of long-term supplementation with beta carotene on the incidence of malignant neoplasms and cardiovascular disease. *N Engl J Med* 334:1145–1149.

Hercberg S, Galan P, Preziosi P, Roussel AM, Arnaud J, Richard MJ, Malvy D, Paul-Dauphin A, Briancon S, Favier A. 1998. Background and rational behind the SU.VI.MAX Study, a prevention trial using nutritional doses of a combination of antioxidant vitamins and minerals to reduce cardiovascular diseases and cancers. SUpplementation en VItamines et Mineraux AntioXydants Study. *Int J Vitam Nutr Res* 68:3–20.

Hodis HN, Mack WJ, LaBree L, Cashin-Hemphill L, Sevanian A, Johnson R, Azen SP. 1995. Serial coronary angiographic evidence that antioxidant vitamin intake reduces progression of coronary artery atherosclerosis. *J Am Med Assoc* 21:1849–1854.

HOPE (Heart Outcomes Prevention Evalulation) Study Investigators. 2000. Vitamin E supplementation and cardiovascular events in high-risk patients. *N Engl J Med* 342:154–160.

Hunt JV, Dean RT, Wolff SP. 1988. Hydroxyl radical production and autoxidative glycosylation. Glucose autoxidation as the cause of protein damage in the experimental glycation model of diabetes mellitus and ageing. *Biochem J* 256: 205–212.

IOM (Institute of Medicine). 1998. *Dietary Reference Intakes. Proposed Definition and Plan for Review of Dietary Antioxidants and Related Compounds.* Washington, DC: National Academy Press.

Jacques PF, Taylor A, Hankinson SE, Willett WC, Mahnken B, Lee Y, Vaid K, Lahav M. 1997. Long-term vitamin C supplement use and prevalence of early age-related lens opacities. *Am J Clin Nutr* 66:911–916.

Jiang ZY, Hunt JV, Wolff SP. 1992. Ferrous ion oxidation in the presence of xylenol orange for detection of lipid hydroperoxide in low density lipoprotein. *Anal Biochem* 202:384–389.

Kannel WB, McGee DL. 1979. Diabetes and cardiovascular disease: The Framingham study. *J Am Med Assoc* 241:2035–2038.

Knekt P, Heliovaara M, Rissanen A, Aromaa A, Aaran RK. 1992. Serum antioxidant vitamins and risk of cataract. *Br Med J* 305:1392–1394.

Lee IM, Cook NR, Manson JE, Buring JE, Hennekens CH. 1999. β-Carotene supplementation and incidence of cancer and cardiovascular disease: The Women's Health Study. *J Natl Cancer Inst* 91:2102–2106.

Leske MC, Chylack LT Jr, He Q, Wu SY, Schoenfeld E, Friend J, Wolfe J. 1998. Antioxidant vitamins and nuclear opacities. The Longitudinal Study of Cataract. *Ophthalmol* 105:831–836.

Manson JE, Gaziano JM, Spelsberg A, Ridker PM, Cook NR, Buring JE, Willett WC, Hennekens CH. 1995. A secondary prevention trial of antioxidant vitamins and cardiovascular disease in women. Rationale, design, and methods. *Ann Epidemiol* 5:261–269.

McCall MR, Frei B. 1999. Can antioxidant vitamins maternally reduce oxidative damage in humans? *Free Radic Biol Med* 26:1034–1053.

McCance DR, Dyer DG, Dunn JA, Bailie KE, Thorpe SR, Baynes JW, Lyons TJ. 1993. Maillard reaction products and their relation to complications in insulin-dependent diabetes mellitus. *J Clin Invest* 91:2470–2478.

Meydani SN, Meydani M, Blumberg JB, Leka LS, Siber G, Loszewski R, Thompson C, Pedrosa MC, Diamond RD, Stollar BD. 1997. Vitamin E supplementation and in vivo immune response in healthy elderly subjects. A randomized controlled trial. *J Am Med Assoc* 277:1380–1386.

Miller ER III, Appel LJ, Risby TH. 1998. Effect of dietary patterns on measures of lipid peroxidation: Results from a randomized clinical trial. *Circulation* 98: 2390–2395.

Miller NJ, Rice-Evans C, Davies MJ, Gopinathan V, Milner A. 1993. A novel method for measuring antioxidant capacity and its application to monitoring the antioxidant status in premature neonates. *Clin Sci* 84:407–412.

Morris MC, Beckett LA, Scherr PA, Hebert LE, Bennett DA, Field TS, Evans DA. 1998. Vitamin E and vitamin C supplement use and risk of incident Alzheimer disease. *Alzheimer Dis Assoc Disord* 12:121–126.

Morrow JD, Frei B, Longmire AW, Gaziano JM, Lynch SM, Shyr Y, Strauss WE, Oates JA, Roberts LJ II. 1995. Increase in circulating products of lipid peroxidation (F_2-isoprostanes) in smokers. *N Engl J Med* 332:1198–1203.

MRC/BHF (Medical Research Council/British Heart Foundation). 1999. MRC/BHF Heart Protection Study of cholesterol-lowering therapy and of antioxidant vitamin supplementation in a wide range of patients at increased risk of coronary heart disease death: Early safety and efficacy experience. *Eur Heart J* 20:725–741.

Mullarkey CJ, Edelstein D, Brownlee M. 1990. Free radical generation by early glycation products. A mechanism for accelerated atherogenesis in diabetes. *Biochem Biophys Res Commun* 173:932–939.

Muller DP. 1994. Vitamin E and other antioxidants in neurological function and disease. In: Frei B, ed. *Natural Antioxidants in Human Health and Disease.* San Diego: Academic Press. Pp. 535–565.

Navab M, Fogelman AM, Berliner JA, Territo MC, Demer LL, Frank JS, Watson AD, Edwards PA, Lusis AJ. 1995. Pathogenesis of atherosclerosis. *Am J Cardiol* 76:18C–23C.

Nishigaki I, Hagihara M, Tsunekawa H, Maseki M, Yagi K. 1981. Lipid peroxide levels of serum lipoprotein fractions of diabetic patients. *Biochem Med* 25:373–378.

Omenn GS, Goodman GE, Thornquist MD, Balmes J, Cullen MR, Glass A, Keogh JP, Meyskens FL Jr, Valanis B, Williams JH Jr, Barnhart S, Cherniack MG, Brodkin CA, Hammar S. 1996. Risk factors for lung cancer and for intervention effects in CARET, the Beta-Carotene and Retinol Efficacy Trial. *J Natl Cancer Inst* 88:1550–1559.

Pariza MW, Boutwell RK. 1987. Historical perspective: Calories and energy expenditure in carcinogenesis. *Am J Clin Nutr* 45:151–156.

Pool-Zobel BL, Bub A, Muller H, Wollowski I, Rechkemmer G. 1997. Consumption of vegetables reduces genetic damage in humans: First results of a human intervention trial with carotenoid-rich foods. *Carcinogenesis* 18:1847–1850.

Poulsen HE, Prieme H, Loft S. 1998. Role of oxidative DNA damage in cancer initiation and promotion. *Eur J Cancer Prev* 7:9–16.

Pratico D, Tangirala RK, Rader DJ, Rokach J, FitzGerald GA. 1998. Vitamin E suppresses isoprostane generation in vivo and reduces atherosclerosis in ApoE-deficient mice. *Nat Med* 4:1189–1192.

Pryor WA. 2000. Vitamin E and heart disease: Basic science to clinical intervention trials. *Free Radic Biol Med* 28:141–164.

Reaven PD, Herold DA, Barnett J, Edelman S. 1995. Effects of vitamin E on susceptibility of low-density lipoprotein and low-density lipoprotein subfractions to oxidation and on protein glycation in NIDDM. *Diabetes Care* 18:807–816.

Riviere S, Birlouez-Aragon I, Nourhashemi F, Vellas B. 1998. Low plasma vitamin C in Alzheimer patients despite an adequate diet. *Int J Geriatr Psychiatry* 13:749–754.

Sano M, Ernesto C, Thomas RG, Klauber MR, Schafer K, Grundman M, Woodbury P, Growdon J, Cotman CW, Pfeiffer E, Schneider LS, Thal LJ. 1997. A controlled trial of selegiline, alpha-tocopherol, or both as treatment for Alzheimer's disease. The Alzheimer's Disease Cooperative Study. *N Engl J Med* 336:1216–1222.

Seddon JM, Ajani UA, Sperduto RD, Hiller R, Blair N, Burton TC, Farber MD, Gragoudas ES, Haller J, Miller DT, Yannuzzi LA, Willett W. 1994. Dietary carotenoids, vitamins A, C, and E, and advanced age-related macular degeneration. *J Am Med Assoc* 272:1413–1420.

Sies H. 1985. Oxidative stress. Introductory remarks. In: Sies H, ed. *Oxidative Stress.* London: Academic Press. Pp.1–8.

Sies H, Stahl W. 1995. Vitamins E and C, beta-carotene, and other carotenoids as antioxidants. *Am J Clin Nutr* 62:1315S–1321S.

Snodderly DM. 1995. Evidence for protection against age-related macular degeneration by carotenoids and antioxidant vitamins. *Am J Clin Nutr* 62:1448S–1461S.

Steinberg D. 1997. Low density lipoprotein oxidation and its pathobiological significance. *J Biol Chem* 272:20963–20966.

Steinberg D, Witztum JL. 1990. Lipoproteins and atherogenesis. Current concepts. *J Am Med Assoc* 264:3047–3052.

Steinberg D, Parthasarathy S, Carew TE, Khoo JC, Witztum JL. 1989. Beyond cholesterol. Modifications of low-density lipoprotein that increase its atherogenicity. *N Engl J Med* 320:915–924.

Steinbrecher UP. 1997. Dietary antioxidants and cardioprotein—Fact or fallacy? *Can J Physiol Pharmacol* 75:228–233.

Stephens NG, Parsons A, Schofield PM, Kelly F, Cheeseman K, Mitchinson MJ. 1996. Randomised controlled trial of vitamin E in patients with coronary disease: Cambridge Heart Antioxidant Study (CHAOS). *Lancet* 347:781–786.

Taylor A, Jacques PF, Epstein EM. 1995. Relations among aging, antioxidant status, and cataract. *Am J Clin Nutr* 62:1439S–1447S.

Teikari JM, Virtamo J, Rautalahti M, Palmgren J, Liesto K, Heinonen OP. 1997. Long-term supplementation with alpha-tocopherol and beta-carotene and age-related cataract. *Acta Ophthalmol Scand* 75:634–640.

Tsai EC, Hirsch IB, Brunzell JD, Chait A. 1994. Reduced plasma peroxyl radical trapping capacity and increased susceptibility of LDL to oxidation in poorly controlled IDDM. *Diabetes* 43:1010–1014.

Wargovich MJ. 1997. Experimental evidence for cancer preventive elements in foods. *Cancer Lett* 114:11–17.

Wayner DD, Burton GW, Ingold KU, Locke S. 1985. Quantitative measurement of the total, peroxyl radical-trapping antioxidant capability of human blood plasma by controlled peroxidation. The important contributions made by plasma proteins. *FEBS Lett* 187:33–37.

Zock PL, Katan MB. 1998. Diet, LDL oxidation, and coronary artery disease. *Am J Clin Nutr* 68:759–760.

3

Vitamin C, Vitamin E, Selenium, and β-Carotene and Other Carotenoids: Methods

METHODOLOGICAL CONSIDERATIONS

Types of Data Used

A number of disciplines have made key contributions to the evidence linking antioxidants to outcomes that may relate to human health (e.g., Hennekens and Buring, 1987). Basic biological research often involving animal models, provides crucial information on mechanisms that may link nutrient consumption to beneficial or adverse health outcomes. Clinical and epidemiological observational studies likewise play a valuable role in generating and testing hypotheses concerning the health risks and benefits of nutrient intake patterns. Randomized clinical trials in population groups of interest have the potential to provide definitive comparisons between selected nutrient intake patterns and subsequent health-related outcomes. Note, however, that randomized trials attempting to relate diet to disease states also have important limitations, which are elaborated below.

Animal Models

Basic research using experimental animals affords considerable advantage in terms of control of nutrient exposures, environmental factors, and even genetics. In contrast, the relevance to free-living humans may be unclear. In addition, dose levels and routes of administration that are practical and possible in animal experiments may differ greatly from those that are relevant to or possible with humans. Nevertheless, results from animal feeding experiments regarding vitamin C, vitamin E, selenium, and β-carotene and other carotenoids were included in the evidence reviewed in developing the decisions concerning the ability to specify the Dietary Reference Intakes (DRIs) for these nutrients.

Human Feeding Studies

Controlled feeding studies, usually in a confined setting such as a metabolic ward, can yield valuable information on the relationship between nutrient consumption and health-related biomarkers. Much of the understanding of human nutrient requirements to prevent deficiencies is based on studies of this type. Studies in which the subjects are confined allow for close control of both intake and activities. Complete collections of nutrient losses through urine and feces are possible, as is recurring sampling of biological materials such as blood. Nutrient balance studies measure nutrient status in relation to intake, whereas depletion-repletion studies measure nutrient status while subjects are maintained on diets containing marginally low or deficient levels of a nutrient, followed by correction of the deficit with measured amounts of the nutrient. However, these studies have several limitations: typically they are limited in time to a few days or weeks, so longer-term outcomes cannot be measured with the same level of accuracy. In addition, subjects may be confined, and therefore findings cannot be generalized to free-living individuals. Finally, the time and expense involved in such studies usually limit the number of subjects and the number of doses or intake levels that can be tested.

In spite of these limitations, feeding studies play an important role in understanding nutrient needs and metabolism. Such data were considered in the DRI process and were given particular attention in the absence of reliable data with which to directly relate nutrient intake to disease risk.

Observational Studies

In comparison, observational epidemiological studies are frequently of direct relevance to free-living humans but lack the controlled setting of human feeding studies. Hence they may be able to establish convincing evidence of an association between the consumption of a nutrient and disease risk, but they are limited in their ability to ascribe a causal relationship. A judgment of causality may be supported by a consistency of association among studies in diverse populations and may be strengthened by the use of laboratory-based tools to measure exposures and confounding factors, rather than other means of data collection such as personal interviews. In recent years, rapid advances in laboratory technology have made possible the increased use of biomarkers of exposure, susceptibility, and disease outcome in molecular epidemiological research. For example, one area of great potential in advancing current knowledge of the effects of diet on health is the study of genetic markers of disease susceptibility (especially polymorphisms in genes that encode metabolizing enzymes) in relation to dietary exposures. This development is expected to provide more accurate assessments of the risk associated with different levels of intake of both nutrients and nonnutritive food constituents.

While analytic epidemiological studies (studies that relate exposure to disease outcomes in individuals) have provided convincing evidence of an associative relationship between selected nondietary exposures and disease risk, there are a number of other factors that limit study reliability in research relating nutrient intakes to disease risks. First, the variation in nutrient intake may be rather limited in populations selected for study. This feature alone may yield modest relative risk trends across intake categories in the population, even if the nutrient is an important factor in explaining large disease rate variations among populations.

Second, the human diet is a complex mixture of foods and nutrients including many substances that may be highly correlated, which gives rise to particular concerns about confounding. Third, many cohort and case-control studies have relied on self-reports of diet, typically food records, 24-hour recalls, or diet history questionnaires. Repeated application of such instruments to the same individuals show considerable variation in nutrient consumption estimates from one time to another with correlations often in the 0.3 to 0.7 range (e.g., Willett et al., 1985). In addition, there may be systematic bias in nutrient consumption estimates from self-reports because the reporting of food intakes and portion sizes may depend on individual characteristics such as body mass, ethnicity, and age. For example, total energy consumption may tend to be substantially underreported (30 to 50 percent) among obese persons, with little or no underreporting among lean persons (Heitmann and Lissner, 1995). Such systematic bias, in conjunction with random measurement error and limited intake range, has the potential to greatly impact analytic epidemiological studies based on self-reported dietary habits. Note that cohort studies using objective (biomarker) measures of nutrient intake may have an important advantage concerning the avoidance of systematic bias, although important sources of bias (e.g., confounding) may remain.

Randomized Clinical Trials

By allocating subjects to the (nutrient) exposure of interest at random, clinical trials eliminate the confounding that may be introduced in observational studies by self-selection. The unique strength of randomized trials is that, if the sample is large enough, the study groups will be comparable with respect not only to those confounding variables known to the investigators, but also to any unknown factors that might be related to risk of the disease. Thus, randomized trials achieve a degree of control of confounding that is simply not possible with any observational design strategy and thus allow for the testing of small effects that are beyond the ability of observational studies to detect reliably.

Although randomized controlled trials represent the accepted standard for studies of nutrient consumption in relation to human health, they too possess important limitations. Specifically, persons agreeing to be randomized may be a select subset of the population of interest, which limits the generalization of trial results. For practical reasons, only a small number of nutrients or nutrient combinations at a single intake level are generally studied in a randomized trial (although a small number of intervention trials to compare specific dietary patterns have been initiated in recent years). In addition, the follow-up period will typically be short relative to the preceding period of nutrient consumption that may be relevant to the health outcomes under study particularly if chronic disease endpoints are sought. Also, dietary intervention or supplementation trials tend to be costly and logistically difficult, and the maintenance of intervention adherence can be a particular challenge.

Because of the many complexities in conducting studies among free-living human populations and the attendant potential for bias and confounding, it is the totality of the evidence from both observational and intervention studies, appropriately weighted, that must form the basis for conclusions regarding causal relationships between particular exposures and disease outcomes.

Weighing the Evidence

As a principle, only studies published in peer-reviewed journals have been used in this report. However, studies published in other scientific journals or readily available reports were considered if they appeared to provide important information not documented elsewhere. To the extent possible, original scientific studies have been used to derive the DRIs. Based on a thorough review of the scientific literature, clinical and functional indicators of nutritional adequacy and excess were identified for each nutrient.

The quality of the studies was considered in weighing the evidence. The characteristics examined included the study design and the representativeness of the study population; the validity, reliability, and precision of the methods used for measuring intake and indicators of adequacy or excess; the control of biases and confounding factors; and the power of the study to demonstrate a given difference or correlation. Publications solely expressing opinions were not used in setting DRIs. The assessment acknowledged the inherent reliability of each type of study design as described above and applied standard criteria concerning the strength, dose-response, and temporal pattern of estimated nutrient-disease or adverse effect associations; the consistency of associations among studies of various types; and the specificity and biological plausibility of the suggested relationships (Hill, 1971). For example, biological plausibility would not be sufficient in the presence of a weak association and lack of evidence that exposure preceded the effect.

Data were examined to determine whether similar estimates of the requirement resulted from the use of different indicators and different types of studies. For a single nutrient, the criterion for setting the Estimated Average Requirement (EAR) may differ from one life stage group to another because the critical function or the risk of disease may be different. When no or very poor data were available for a given life stage group, extrapolation was made from the EAR or Adequate Intake (AI) set for another group, by making explicit and logical assumptions about relative requirements. Because EARs can be used for multiple purposes, they were established whenever sufficient supporting data were available.

Data Limitations

Although the reference values are based on data, the data were often scanty or drawn from studies that had limitations in addressing the various questions that confronted the panel. Therefore, many of the questions raised about the requirements for and recommended intakes of these nutrients cannot be answered fully because of inadequacies in the present database. Apart from studies of overt deficiency diseases, there is a dearth of studies that address specific effects of inadequate intakes on specific indicators of health status, and thus a research agenda is proposed (see Chapter 10).

Thus, after careful review and analysis of the evidence, including examination of the extent of congruent findings, scientific judgment was used to determine the basis for establishing the values. The reasoning used is described for each nutrient in Chapters 5 through 8.

Pathways to Nutrient Requirements

The possible pathways that were considered in determining the requirement for each nutrient include the following:

1. The availability of a convincing totality of evidence, including randomized clinical trial data, that the nutrient reviewed reduces the risk of important health outcomes—demonstration that a biomarker of exposure influences a specific health outcome constitutes a key component of this body of evidence.

2. The availability of a convincing totality of evidence, including randomized clinical trial data, that the nutrient reviewed favorably affects a selected functional marker—this pathway was used with caution in view of the many examples where intervention effects on an intermediate outcome (biomarker) proved to be inconsistent with intervention effects on the chronic disease of interest.

3. The presence of a clinically important deficiency disease or nutritional syndrome that has been demonstrated to relate specifically to an inadequate intake of the nutrient reviewed—this pathway is facilitated by considering intakes needed to ensure adequate body stores or reserves of the nutrient or of pertinent compounds that the body produces in response to adequate intake of the nutrient.

Method to Determine the Adequate Intake for Infants

The AI for young infants is generally taken to be the average intake by full-term infants who are born to apparently healthy, well-nourished mothers and are exclusively fed human milk. The extent to which the intake of a nutrient from human milk may exceed the actual requirements of infants is not known, and the ethics of experimentation preclude testing the levels known to be potentially inadequate. Using the infant exclusively fed human milk as a model is in keeping with the basis for earlier recommendations for intake (e.g., Health Canada, 1990; IOM, 1991). It also supports the recommendation that exclusive intake of human milk is the preferred method of feeding for normal full-term infants for the first 4 to 6 months of life. This recommendation has been made by the Canadian Paediatric Society (Health Canada, 1990), the American Academy of Pediatrics (AAP, 1997), the Institute of Medicine (IOM, 1991), and many other expert groups, even though most U.S. babies no longer receive human milk by age 6 months.

In general, this report does not cover possible variations in physiological need during the first month after birth or the variations in intake of nutrients from human milk that result from differences in milk volume and nutrient concentration during early lactation.

In keeping with the decision made by the Standing Committee on the Scientific Evaluation of Dietary Reference Intakes, specific DRIs to meet the needs of formula-fed infants have not been proposed in this report. The use of formula introduces a large number of complex issues, one of which is the bioavailability of different forms of the nutrient in different formula types.

Ages 0 through 6 Months

To derive the AI value for infants ages 0 through 6 months, the mean intake of a nutrient was calculated based on (1) the average concentration of the nutrient from 2 to 6 months of lactation using consensus values from several reported studies, if possible, and (2) an average volume of milk intake of 0.78 L/day. This volume was reported from studies that used test weighing of full-term infants. In this procedure, the infant is weighed before and after each feeding (Allen et al., 1991; Butte et al., 1984; Chandra, 1984; Hofvander et al., 1982; Neville et al., 1988). Because there is variation in both the composition of milk and the volume consumed, the computed value represents the mean. It is expected that infants will consume increased volumes of human milk during growth spurts.

Ages 7 through 12 Months

During the period of infant growth and gradual weaning to a mixed diet of human milk and solid foods from ages 7 through 12 months, there is no evidence for markedly different nutrient needs for this group of nutrients. The basis of the AI values derived for this age category was the sum of (1) the content of the nutrient provided by 0.60 L/day of human milk, which is the average volume of milk reported from studies of infants who receive only human milk in this age category (Heinig et al., 1993), and (2) that provided by the usual intakes of complementary weaning foods consumed by infants in this age category. Such an approach is in keeping with current recommendations of the Canadian Paediatric

Society (Health Canada, 1990), the American Academy of Pediatrics (AAP, 1997), and the Institute of Medicine (IOM, 1991) for continued feeding of infants with human milk through 9 to 12 months of age, with appropriate introduction of solid foods. Selenium and vitamin C had published information about the intake from solid foods for infants aged 7 through 12 months, and thus followed this method.

For vitamin E, which did not have intake data from solid foods, the AI was calculated by extrapolating upward from the AI for infants ages 0 through 6 months, adjusting for metabolic body size and growth, and adding a factor for variability. The method is described below.

Method for Extrapolating Data from Adults to Children

Setting the EAR or AI

For vitamin C, vitamin E, and selenium, data were not available to set the EAR and RDA for children ages 1 year and older and adolescents. Because vitamin C is a water-soluble vitamin and boys have a larger lean body mass and total body water than girls, the adult EAR was adjusted for children and adolescents on the basis of differences in reference weights from Table 1-1. For vitamin E and selenium, the EAR has been extrapolated downward using an adjustment for metabolic body size and growth. The method relies on at least four assumptions:

1. Maintenance needs for vitamin E and selenium expressed with respect to body weight ($[\text{kilogram of body weight}]^{0.75}$) are the same for adults and children. Scaling requirements to the 0.75 power of body mass adjusts for metabolic differences demonstrated to be related to body weight, as described by Kleiber (1947) and explored further by West et al. (1997). By this scaling, a child weighing 22 kg would require 42 percent of what an adult weighing 70 kg would require—a higher percentage than if the requirement were based on body weight to a power of one.

2. The EAR for vitamin E and selenium for adults is an estimate of maintenance needs.

3. The percentage of extra vitamin E and selenium needed for growth is comparable with the percentage of extra protein needed for growth.

4. On average, total needs do not differ substantially for males compared to females until age 14, when reference weights differ.

The formula for the extrapolation is

$$\mathrm{EAR}_{child} = \mathrm{EAR}_{adult}\ (F),$$

where $F = (\mathrm{Weight}_{child}/\mathrm{Weight}_{adult})^{0.75}\ (1 + \text{growth factor})$. Reference weights from Table 1-1 are used. If the EAR differs for men and women, the reference weight used for adults in the equation differs by gender; otherwise, the average for men and women is used unless the value for women is derived from data on men. The approximate proportional increase in protein requirements for growth (FAO/WHO/UNA, 1985) is used as an estimate of the growth factor as shown in Table 3-1. If only an AI has been set for adults, it is substituted for the EAR in the above formula, and an AI is calculated; no RDA is set.

Setting the RDA for Children

To account for variability in requirements because of growth rates and other factors, a 10 percent coefficient of variation (CV) for the requirement is assumed unless data are available to support another value, as described in Chapter 1.

Method for Extrapolating Data from Young to Older Infants

This adjustment, the metabolic weight ratio method, involves metabolic scaling but does not adjust for growth because it is based on a value for a growing infant. To extrapolate from the AI for infants ages 0 through 6 months to an AI for infants ages 7 through 12 months, the following formula is used:

$$\mathrm{AI}_{7\text{--}12\ mo} = \mathrm{AI}_{0\text{--}6\ mo}\ (F),$$

where $F = (\mathrm{Weight}_{7\text{--}12\ mo}/\mathrm{Weight}_{0\text{--}6\ mo})^{0.75}$.

TABLE 3-1 Estimated Growth Factor by Age Group

Age Group	Growth Factor
7 mo–3 y	0.30
4–8 y	0.15
9–13 y	0.15
14–18 y	
Males	0.15
Females	0.0

SOURCE: Proportional increase in protein requirements for growth from FAO/WHO/UNA (1985) used to estimate the growth factor.

Methods for Determining Increased Needs for Pregnancy

It is known that the placenta actively transports vitamin C, vitamin E, and selenium from the mother to the fetus (Hytten and Leitch, 1971). However, for these three nutrients, experimental data that could be used to set an EAR and RDA for pregnancy are lacking. In these cases the potential of increased need for these nutrients during pregnancy is based on theoretical considerations, including obligatory fetal transfer, if data are available, and increased maternal needs related to increases in energy or protein metabolism, as applicable.

Methods to Determine Increased Needs for Lactation

For vitamin C, vitamin E, and selenium, it is assumed that the total requirement of lactating women equals the requirement for the nonpregnant, nonlactating woman of similar age plus an increment to cover the amount of the nutrient needed for milk production. To allow for inefficiencies in use of these nutrients, the increment may be somewhat greater than the amount of the nutrient contained in the milk produced. Details are provided in each nutrient chapter.

ESTIMATES OF LABORATORY VALUES

Substantial changes in analytical methods have occurred during the more than 40 years of studies considered in this report. Although the requirement for vitamin C is based on recent data, the studies that were utilized to determine the vitamin E requirement are 40 years old. Methodological problems have been documented for vitamin E intake assessment from food (see Chapter 6).

NUTRIENT INTAKE ESTIMATES

Reliable and valid methods of food composition analysis are crucial in determining the intake of a nutrient needed to meet a requirement. For vitamin E and selenium, analytic methods to determine the content of the nutrient in food have serious limitations, the specifics of which are discussed in Chapters 5 through 8.

Methodological Considerations

The quality of nutrient intake data varies widely across studies. The most valid intake data are those collected from metabolic study protocols in which all food is provided by the researchers, amounts consumed are measured accurately, and the nutrient composition of the food is determined by reliable and valid laboratory analyses. Such protocols are usually possible with only a small number of subjects. Thus, in many studies, intake data are self-reported (e.g., through 24-hour recalls of food intake, diet records, or food frequency questionnaires).

Potential sources of error in self-reported intake data include over- or underreporting of portion sizes and frequency of intake, omission of foods, and inaccuracies related to the use of food composition tables (Lichtman et al., 1992; Mertz et al., 1991). In addition, errors can occur due to a lack of information on how a food was manufactured, prepared, and served, because a high percentage of the food consumed in the United States and Canada is not prepared from scratch in the home. Therefore, the values reported by nationwide surveys or studies that rely on self-reporting may be somewhat inaccurate and possibly biased.

Four sources of measurement error are particularly important with regard to vitamin E intake: (1) energy intake is underreported in national surveys (Mertz et al., 1991), and fat intake (which serves as a major carrier for vitamin E) is likely to be more underreported than energy intake in the Third National Health and Nutrition Examination Survey (NHANES III) (Briefel et al., 1997); (2) the amount of fats and oils added during food preparation (and absorbed into the cooked product) is difficult to assess using diet recall methodologies, yet it contributes substantially to vitamin E intake; (3) uncertainties about the particular fats or oils consumed, particularly when food labels do not indicate the specific fat or oil in the product (e.g. "this product may contain partially hydrogenated soybean and/or cottonseed oil or vegetable oil") necessitate a reliance on default selections (and thus assumptions about the relative content of α- and γ-tocopherols; and (4) due to the small number of samples, the vitamin E content of food sources in the Continuing Survey of Food Intakes by Individuals (CSFII) and NHANES III databases is quite variable (J. Holden, Agricultural Research Service, USDA, personal communication, April 13, 1999).

Food composition databases that are used to calculate nutrient intake from self-reported and observed intake data introduce errors due to random variability, genetic variation in the nutrient content, analytical errors, and missing or imputed data. In general, when nutrient intakes for groups are estimated, the effect of errors in the composition data is probably considerably smaller than the effect of errors in the self-reported intake data (NRC, 1986). It is not known to what extent this is true for vitamin C, vitamin E, selenium, or β-

carotene and other carotenoids. However, adult men and women participating in NHANES III underreported energy intake by about 23 percent, as well as fat intake (which serves as a carrier for vitamin E) when expressed as a percentage of total energy intake (Briefel et al., 1997).

Adjusting for Day-to-Day Variation

Because of day-to-day variation in dietary intakes, the distribution of 1-day (or 2-day) intakes for a group is wider than the distribution of usual intakes even though the mean intake may be the same (for further elaboration, see Chapter 9). To reduce this problem, statistical adjustments have been developed (NRC, 1986; Nusser et al., 1996) that require at least 2 days of dietary data from a representative subsample of the population of interest. However, no accepted method is available to adjust for the underreporting of intake, which may average as much as 20 percent for energy (Mertz et al., 1991).

DIETARY INTAKES IN THE UNITED STATES AND CANADA

Sources of Dietary Intake Data

The major sources of current dietary intake data for the U.S. population are the Third National Health and Nutrition Examination Survey (NHANES III), which was conducted from 1988 to 1994 by the U.S. Department of Health and Human Services, and the Continuing Survey of Food Intakes by Individuals (CSFII), which was conducted from 1994 to 1996 by the U.S. Department of Agriculture (USDA). NHANES III examined 30,000 subjects aged 2 months and older. A single 24-hour diet recall was collected for all subjects. A second recall was collected for a 5 percent nonrandom subsample to allow adjustment of intake estimates for day-to-day variation. The 1994 to 1996 CSFII collected two nonconsecutive 24-hour recalls from approximately 16,000 subjects of all ages. Both surveys used the food composition database developed by USDA to calculate nutrient intakes (Perloff et al., 1990). National survey data for Canada are not currently available, but data for vitamin C have been collected in Québec and Nova Scotia. The extent to which these data are applicable nationwide is not known.

Appendix D gives the mean and the first through ninety-ninth percentiles of dietary intakes of vitamin C and vitamin E by age from the CSFII, adjusted for day-to-day variation by the method of Nusser et al. (1996). Appendix C provides comparable information for vitamin C, vitamin E, and selenium from NHANES III, adjusted by methods described by the National Research Council (NRC, 1986) and by Feinleib et al. (1993) for persons aged 6 years and older. Appendix E provides means and selected percentiles of dietary intakes of vitamin C for individuals in Québec and Nova Scotia.

Sources of Supplement Intake Data

Although subjects in the CSFII are asked about the use of dietary supplements, quantitative information is not collected. Data on supplement intake obtained from NHANES III were reported as a part of total nutrient intake (Appendix C). NHANES III data on overall prevalence of supplement use are also available (LSRO/FASEB, 1995). In 1986, the National Health Interview Survey queried 11,558 adults and 1,877 children on their intake of supplements during the previous 2 weeks (Moss et al., 1989). The composition of the supplement was obtained directly from the product label whenever possible. Table 3-2 shows the percentage of adults, by age, taking supplements of vitamin C, vitamin E, or selenium.

Food Sources of Vitamin C, Vitamin E, Selenium, and Carotenoids

For some nutrients in this report, two types of information are provided about food sources of nutrients: identification of the foods that are the major contributors of the nutrient to diets in the United States and food sources of the nutrient. The determination of foods that are major contributors depends on both the nutrient

TABLE 3-2 Percentage of Persons Taking Vitamin Supplements by Sex, Age, and Type of Vitamin Used: National Health Interview Survey, United States, 1986

Supplement Taken	Females All Adults 18+ y	18–44 y	45–64 y	65+ y	Males All Adults 18+ y	18–44 y	45–64 y	65+ y
Vitamin C	33.6	32.7	35.7	33.3	27.8	27.7	28.4	27.2
Vitamin E	28.9	28.5	30.3	27.9	23.1	22.4	24.4	23.9
Selenium	10.3	10.5	10.2	10.2	8.1	8.3	7.1	8.7

NOTE: The high use of supplements by pregnant women is not reflected in this table.
SOURCE: Moss et al. (1989).

content of a food and the total consumption of that food (amount and frequency). Therefore, a food that has a relatively low concentration of the nutrient might still be a large contributor to total intake if it is consumed in relatively large amounts. In contrast, the food sources listed are those with the highest concentration of the nutrient; no consideration is given to the amount consumed.

SUMMARY

General methods for examining and interpreting the evidence on requirements for vitamin C, vitamin E, and selenium, with special attention given to infants, children, and pregnant and lactating women; methodological problems; and dietary intake data are presented in this chapter. Relevant detail is provided in the nutrient chapters.

REFERENCES

AAP (American Academy of Pediatrics). 1997. Breastfeeding and the use of human milk. *Pediatrics* 100:1035–1039.

Allen JC, Keller RP, Archer P, Neville MC. 1991. Studies in human lactation: Milk composition and daily secretion rates of macronutrients in the first year of lactation. *Am J Clin Nutr* 54:69–80.

Briefel RR, Sempos CT, McDowell MA, Chien S, Alaimo K. 1997. Dietary methods research in the Third National Health and Nutrition Examination Survey: Underreporting of energy intake. *Am J Clin Nutr* 65:1203S–1209S.

Butte NF, Garza C, Smith EO, Nichols BL. 1984. Human milk intake and growth in exclusively breast-fed infants. *J Pediatr* 104:187–195.

Chandra RK. 1984. Physical growth of exclusively breast-fed infants. *Nutr Res* 2:275–276.

FAO/WHO/UNA (Food and Agriculture Organization of the United Nations/World Health Organization/United Nations). 1985. *Energy and Protein Requirements Report of a Joint FAO/WHO/UNA Expert Consultation.* Technical Report Series. No. 724. Geneva: World Health Organization.

Feinleib M, Rifkind B, Sempos C, Johnson C, Bachorik P, Lippel K, Carroll M, Ingster-Moore L, Murphy R. 1993. Methodological issues in the measurement of cardiovascular risk factors: Within-person variability in selected serum lipid measures—Results from the Third National Health and Nutrition Survey (NHANES III). *Can J Cardiol* 9:87D–88D.

Health Canada. 1990. *Nutrition Recommendations. The Report of the Scientific Review Committee 1990.* Ottawa: Canadian Government Publishing Centre.

Heinig MJ, Nommsen LA, Peerson JM, Lonnerdal B, Dewey KG. 1993. Energy and protein intakes of breast-fed and formula-fed infants during the first year of life and their association with growth velocity: The DARLING Study. *Am J Clin Nutr* 58:152–161.

Heitmann BL, Lissner L. 1995. Dietary underreporting by obese individuals—Is it specific or non-specific? *Br Med J* 311:986–989.

Hennekens C, Buring JE. 1987. Need for large sample sizes in randomized trials. *Pediatrics* 79:569–571.

Hill AB. 1971. *Principles of Medical Statistics,* 9th edition. New York: Oxford University Press.

Hofvander Y, Hagman U, Hillervik C, Sjolin S. 1982. The amount of milk consumed by 1–3 months old breast- or bottle-fed infants. *Acta Paediatr Scand* 71:953–958.

Hytten FE, Leitch I. 1971. *The Physiology of Human Pregnancy,* 2nd edition. Oxford: Blackwell Scientific Publications.

IOM (Institute of Medicine). 1991. *Nutrition During Lactation.* Washington, DC: National Academy Press.

Kleiber M. 1947. Body size and metabolic rate. *Physiol Rev* 27:511–541.

Lichtman SW, Pisarska K, Berman ER, Pestone M, Dowling H, Offenbacher E, Weisel H, Heshka S, Matthews DE, Heymsfield SB. 1992. Discrepancy between self-reported and actual caloric intake and exercise in obese subjects. *N Engl J Med* 327:1893–1898.

LSRO/FASEB (Life Sciences Research Office/Federation of American Societies for Experimental Biology). 1995. *Third Report on Nutrition Monitoring in the United States.* Washington DC: US Government Printing Office.

Mertz W, Tsui JC, Judd JT, Reiser S, Hallfrisch J, Morris ER, Steele PD, Lashley E. 1991. What are people really eating? The relation between energy intake derived from estimated diet records and intake determined to maintain body weight. *Am J Clin Nutr* 54:291–295.

Moss AJ, Levy AS, Kim I, Park YK. 1989. *Use of Vitamin and Mineral Supplements in the United States: Current Users, Types of Products, and Nutrients.* Advance Data, Vital and Health Statistics of the National Center for Health Statistics. Number 174. Hyattsville, MD: National Center for Health Statistics.

Neville MC, Keller R, Seacat J, Lutes V, Neifert M, Casey C, Allen J, Archer P. 1988. Studies in human lactation: Milk volumes in lactating women during the onset of lactation and full lactation. *Am J Clin Nutr* 48:1375–1386.

NRC (National Research Council). 1986. *Nutrient Adequacy. Assessment Using Food Consumption Surveys.* Washington, DC: National Academy Press.

Nusser SM, Carriquiry AL, Dodd KW, Fuller WA. 1996. A semiparametric transformation approach to estimating usual daily intake distributions. *J Am Stat Assoc* 91:1440–1449.

Perloff BP, Rizek RL, Haytowitz DB, Reid PR. 1990. Dietary intake methodology. II. USDA's Nutrient Data Base for Nationwide Dietary Intake Surveys. *J Nutr* 120:1530–1534.

West GB, Brown JH, Enquist BJ. 1997. A general model for the origin of allometric scaling laws in biology. *Science* 276:122–126.

Willett WC, Sampson L, Stampfer MJ, Rosner B, Bain C, Witschi J, Hennekens CH, Speizer FE. 1985. Reproducibility and validity of a semiquantitative food frequency questionnaire. *Am J Epidemiol* 122:51–65.

4

A Model for the Development of Tolerable Upper Intake Levels for Nutrients

BACKGROUND

The *Tolerable Upper Intake Level* (UL) is the highest level of daily nutrient intake that is likely to pose no risk of adverse health effects to almost all individuals in the general population. As intake increases above the UL, the risk of adverse effects increases. The term *tolerable* is chosen because it connotes a level of intake that can, with high probability, be tolerated biologically by individuals; it does not imply acceptability of this level in any other sense. The setting of a UL does not indicate that nutrient intakes greater than the Recommended Dietary Allowance (RDA) or Adequate Intake (AI) are recommended as being beneficial to an individual. Many individuals are self-medicating with nutrients for perceived prophylactic or curative purposes. It is beyond the scope of the model at this time to address whether there are benefits of higher nutrient intakes that may offset the risk of adverse effects. The UL is not meant to apply to individuals who are being treated with the nutrient or food component under medical supervision or to individuals with predisposing conditions that modify their sensitivity to the nutrient or food component. This chapter describes a model for developing ULs.

The term *adverse effect* is defined as any significant alteration in the structure or function of the human organism (Klaassen et al., 1986) or any impairment of a physiologically important function that could lead to a health effect that is adverse. This is in accordance with the definition set by the joint World Health Organization, Food and Agriculture Organization of the United Nations, and International Atomic Energy Agency Expert Consultation in *Trace Elements in Human Nutrition and Health* (WHO, 1996). In the case of nutrients, it is exceedingly important to consider the possibility that the excessive intake of one nutrient may alter in detrimental ways the health benefits conferred by another. Any such alteration (referred to as an adverse nutrient-nutrient interaction) is considered an adverse health effect. When evidence for such adverse interactions is available, it is considered in establishing a nutrient's UL.

ULs are useful because of the increased interest in and availability of fortified foods, the increased use of dietary supplements, and the growing recognition of the health consequences of excesses, as well as inadequacies of nutrient intakes. ULs are based on total intake of a nutrient from food, water, and supplements if adverse effects have been associated with total intake. However, if adverse effects have been associated with intake from supplements or food fortificants only, the UL is based on nutrient intake from these sources only, not on total intake. The UL applies to chronic daily use.

For many nutrients, there are insufficient data on which to develop a UL. This does not mean that there is no potential for adverse effects resulting from high intake. When data about adverse effects are extremely limited, extra caution may be warranted.

Like all chemical agents, nutrients can produce adverse health effects if intakes from any combination of food, water, nutrient supplements, and pharmacological agents are excessive. Some lower level of nutrient intake will ordinarily pose no likelihood (or risk) of adverse health effects in normal individuals even if the level is above that associated with any benefit. It is not possible to identify a single risk-free intake level for a nutrient that can be applied with certainty to all members of a population. However, it is possible to develop intake levels that are unlikely to pose risk of adverse health effects for most members of the general population, including sensitive individuals. For some nutrients or food components, these intake levels may however pose a risk for subpopulations with extreme or distinct vulnerabilities.

Whether routine, long-term intake above the UL is safe is not well documented. Although members of the general population should not routinely exceed the UL, intake above the UL may be appropriate for investigation within well-controlled clinical trials. Clinical trials of doses above the UL should not be discouraged, as long as subjects participating in these trials have signed informed consent documents regarding possible toxicity and as long as these trials employ appropriate safety monitoring of trial subjects.

MODEL FOR DERIVATION OF TOLERABLE UPPER INTAKE LEVELS

The possibility that the methodology used to derive Tolerable Upper Intake Levels (ULs) might be reduced to a mathematical model that could be generically applied to all nutrients was considered. Such a model might have several potential advantages, including ease of application and assurance of consistent treatment of all nutrients. It was concluded, however, that the current state of scientific understanding of toxic phenomena in general, and nutrient toxicity in particular, is insufficient to support the development of such a model. Scientific information regarding various adverse effects and their relationships to intake levels varies greatly among nutrients and depends on the nature, comprehensiveness, and quality of available data. The uncertainties associated with the unavoidable problem of extrapolating from the circumstances under which data are developed (e.g., the laboratory or clinic) to other circumstances (e.g., the apparently healthy population) adds to this complexity.

Given the current state of knowledge, any attempt to capture in a mathematical model all the information and scientific judgments that must be made to reach conclusions regarding ULs would not be consistent with contemporary risk assessment practices. Instead, the model for the derivation of ULs consists of a set of scientific factors that always should be considered explicitly. The framework under which these factors are organized is called *risk assessment*. Risk assessment (NRC, 1983, 1994) is a systematic means of evaluating the probability of occurrence of adverse health effects in humans from excess exposure to an environmental agent (in this case, a nutrient or food component) (FAO/WHO, 1995; Health Canada, 1993). The hallmark of risk assessment is the requirement to be explicit in all the evaluations and judgments that must be made to document conclusions.

RISK ASSESSMENT AND FOOD SAFETY

Basic Concepts

Risk assessment is a scientific undertaking having as its objective a characterization of the nature and likelihood of harm resulting from human exposure to agents in the environment. The characterization of risk typically contains both qualitative and quantitative information and includes a discussion of the scientific uncertainties in this information. In the present context, the agents of interest are nutrients, and the environmental media are food, water, and non-food sources such as nutrient supplements and pharmacological preparations.

Performing a risk assessment results in a characterization of the relationships between exposure to an agent and the likelihood that adverse health effects will occur in members of exposed populations. Scientific uncertainties are an inherent part of the risk assessment process and are discussed below. Deciding whether the magnitude of exposure is *acceptable* or *tolerable* in specific circumstances is not a component of risk assessment; this activity falls within the domain of *risk management*. Risk management decisions depend on the results of risk assessments but may also involve the public health significance of the risk, the technical feasibility of achieving various degrees of risk control, and the economic and social costs of this control. Because there is no single, scientifically definable distinction between safe and unsafe exposures, risk management necessarily incorporates components of sound, practical decision making that are not addressed by the risk assessment process (NRC, 1983, 1994).

A risk assessment requires that information be organized in rather specific ways but does not require any specific scientific evaluation methods. Rather, risk assessors must evaluate scientific information using what they judge to be appropriate methods and must make explicit the basis for their judgments, the uncertainties in risk estimates, and when appropriate, alternative scientifically plausible interpretations of the available data (NRC, 1994; OTA, 1993).

Risk assessment is subject to two types of scientific uncertainties: those related to data and those associated with inferences that are required when directly applicable data are not available (NRC, 1994). Data uncertainties arise during the evaluation of information obtained from the epidemiological and toxicological studies of nutrient intake levels that are the basis for risk assessments. Examples of inferences include the use of data from experimental animals to estimate responses in humans and the selection of uncertainty factors to estimate inter- and intraspecies variabilities in response to toxic substances. Uncertainties arise whenever estimates of adverse health effects in humans are based on extrapolations of data obtained under dissimilar conditions (e.g., from experimental animal studies). Options for dealing with uncertainties are discussed below and in detail in Appendix G.

Steps in the Risk Assessment Process

The organization of risk assessment is based on a model proposed by the National Research Council (1983, 1994) that is widely used in public health and regulatory decision making. The steps of risk assessment as applied to nutrients are as follows (see also Figure 4-1):

- Step 1. Hazard identification involves the collection, organization, and evaluation of all information pertaining to the adverse effects of a given nutrient. It concludes with a summary of the evidence concerning the capacity of the nutrient to cause one or more types of toxicity in humans.
- Step 2. Dose-response assessment determines the relationship between nutrient intake (dose) and adverse effect (in terms of incidence and severity). This step concludes with an estimate of the Tolerable Upper Intake Level (UL)—it identifies the highest level

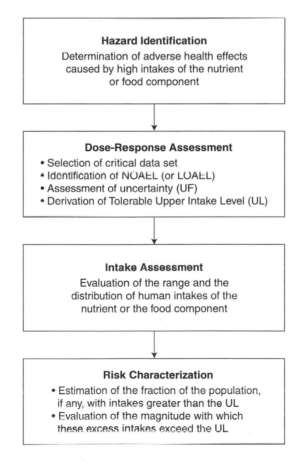

FIGURE 4-1 Risk assessment model for nutrient toxicity.

of daily nutrient intake that is likely to pose no risk of adverse health effects to almost all individuals in the general population. Different ULs may be developed for various life stage groups.

• Step 3. Intake assessment evaluates the distribution of usual total daily nutrient intakes among members of the general population. In cases where the UL pertains only to supplement use, and does not pertain to usual food intakes of the nutrient, the assessment is directed at supplement intakes only. It does not depend on step 1 or 2.

• Step 4. Risk characterization summarizes the conclusions from steps 1 and 2 with step 3 to determine the risk. The risk is generally expressed as the fraction of the exposed population, if any, having nutrient intakes (step 3) in excess of the estimated UL (steps 1 and 2). If possible, scientific characterization also covers the magnitude of any such excesses. Scientific uncertainties associated with both the UL and the intake estimates are described so that risk managers understand the degree of scientific confidence they can place in the risk assessment.

The risk assessment contains no discussion of recommendations for reducing risk; these are the focus of risk management.

Thresholds

A principal feature of the risk assessment process for noncarcinogens is the long-standing acceptance that no risk of adverse effects is expected unless a threshold dose (or intake) is exceeded. The adverse effects that may be caused by a nutrient or food component almost certainly occur only when the threshold dose is exceeded (NRC, 1994; WHO, 1996). The critical issues concern the methods used to identify the approximate threshold of toxicity for a large and diverse human population. Because most nutrients are not considered to be carcinogenic in humans, approaches used for carcinogenic risk assessment are not discussed here.

Thresholds vary among members of the general population (NRC, 1994). For any given adverse effect, if the distribution of thresholds in the population could be quantitatively identified, it would be possible to establish ULs by defining some point in the lower tail of the distribution of thresholds that would be protective for some specified fraction of the population. The method for identifying thresholds for a general population described here is designed to ensure that almost all members of the population will be protected, but it is not based on an analysis of the theoretical (but practically unattainable) distribution of thresholds. By using the model to derive the threshold, however, there is considerable confidence that the threshold, which becomes the UL for nutrients or food components, lies very near the low end of the theoretical distribution and is the end representing the most sensitive members of the population. For some nutrients, there may be subpopulations that are not included in the general distribution because of extreme or distinct vulnerabilities to toxicity. Data relating to effects observed in these groups are not used to derive ULs. Such distinct groups, whose conditions warrant medical supervision, may not be protected by the UL.

The joint Food and Agricultural Organization-World Health Organization (FAO/WHO) Expert Committee on Food Additives and various national regulatory bodies have identified factors (called *uncertainty factors* [UFs]) that account for interspecies and intraspecies differences in response to the hazardous effects of substances and for other uncertainties (WHO, 1987). Uncertainty factors are used to make inferences about the threshold dose of substances for members of a large and diverse human population from data on adverse effects obtained from epidemiological or experimental studies. These factors are applied consistently when data of specific types and quality are available. They are typically used to derive acceptable daily intakes for food additives and other substances for which data on adverse effects are considered sufficient to meet minimum standards of quality and completeness (FAO/WHO, 1982). These adopted or recognized UFs have sometimes been coupled with other factors to compensate for deficiencies in the available data and other uncertainties regarding data.

When possible, the UL is based on a no-observed-adverse-effect level (NOAEL), which is the highest intake (or experimental oral dose) of a nutrient at which no adverse effects have been observed in the individuals studied. This is identified for a specific circumstance in the hazard identification and dose-response assessment steps of the assessment of risk. If there are no adequate data demonstrating a NOAEL, then a lowest-observed-adverse-effect level (LOAEL) may be used. A LOAEL is the lowest intake (or experimental oral dose) at which an adverse effect has been identified. The derivation of a UL from a NOAEL (or LOAEL) involves a series of choices about what factors should be used to deal with uncertainties. Uncertainty factors are applied in an attempt to deal both with incomplete gaps in data and with incomplete knowledge regarding the inferences required (e.g., the expected variability in response within the human population). The problems of both data and inference uncertainties arise in all steps of the risk assessment. A discussion of options available for dealing with these uncertainties is presented below and in greater detail in Appendix G.

A UL is not, in itself, a description or estimate of human risk. It is derived by application of the hazard identification and dose-response evaluation steps (steps 1 and 2) of the risk assessment model. To determine whether populations are at risk requires an intake or exposure assessment (step 3, evaluation of intakes of the nutrient by the population) and a determination of the fractions of these populations, if any, whose intakes exceed the UL. In the intake assessment and risk characterization steps (steps 3 and 4), the distribution of actual intakes for the population is used as a basis for determining whether and to what extent the population is at risk (Figure 4-1). A discussion of other aspects of the risk characterization that may be useful in judging the public health significance of the risk and in risk management decisions is provided in the final section of this chapter "Risk Characterization."

APPLICATION OF THE RISK ASSESSMENT MODEL TO NUTRIENTS

This section provides guidance for applying the risk assessment framework (the model) to the derivation of Tolerable Upper Intake Levels (ULs) for nutrients.

Special Problems Associated with Substances Required for Human Nutrition

Although the risk assessment model outlined above can be applied to nutrients to derive ULs, it must be recognized that nutrients possess some properties that distinguish them from the types of agents for which the risk assessment model was originally developed (NRC, 1983). In the application of accepted standards for risk assessment of environmental chemicals to risk assessment of nutrients and food components, a fundamental difference between the two categories must be recognized: within a certain range of intakes, many nutrients are essential for human well-being and usually for life itself. Nonetheless, they may share with other chemicals the production of adverse effects at excessive exposures. Because the consumption of diets with variable levels of nutrients and food components is considered to be consistent with the development and survival of humankind over many millennia, there is generally less need for the large uncertainty factors that have been used in assessing risk of nonessential chemicals. In addition, if data on the adverse effects of nutrients are available primarily from studies in human populations, there will be less uncertainty than is associated with the types of data available on nonessential chemicals.

There is no evidence to suggest that nutrients consumed at the recommended intake (the Recommended Dietary Allowance [RDA] or Adequate Intake [AI]) present a risk of adverse effects to the general population.[1] It is clear, however, that the addition of nutrients to a diet through the ingestion of large amounts of highly fortified food, nonfood sources such as supplements, or both, may (at some level) pose a risk of adverse health effects. The UL is the highest level of daily nutrient intake that is likely to pose no risk of adverse health effects to almost all individuals in the general population. As intake increases above the UL, the risk of adverse effects increases.

If adverse effects have been associated with total intake, ULs are based on total intake of a nutrient from food, water, and supplements. For cases in which adverse effects have been associated with intake only from supplements and fortified food, the UL is based on intake from these sources only, rather than total intake. The effects of nutrients from fortified foods or supplements may differ from those of naturally occurring constituents of foods because of the chemical form of the nutrient, the timing of the intake and amount consumed in a single bolus dose, the matrix supplied by the food, and the relation of the nutrient to the other constituents of the diet. Nutrient requirements and food intake are related to the metabolizing body mass, which is also at least an indirect measure of the space in which the nutrients are distributed. This relation between food intake and space of distribution supports homeostasis, which maintains nutrient concentrations in this space within a range compatible with health. However, excessive intake of a single nutrient from supplements or fortificants may compromise this homeostatic mechanism. Such elevations alone may pose risks of adverse effects; imbalances among the vitamins or other nutrients may also be possible. These reasons and those discussed previously support the need to include the form and pattern of consumption in the assessment of risk from high nutrient or food component intake.

---

[1] It is recognized that possible exceptions to this generalization relate to specific geochemical areas with excessive environmental exposures to certain trace elements (e.g., selenium) and to rare case reports of adverse effects associated with highly eccentric consumption of specific foods. Data from such findings are generally not useful for setting ULs for the general North American population.

Consideration of Variability in Sensitivity

The risk assessment model outlined in this chapter is consistent with classical risk assessment approaches in that it must consider variability in the sensitivity of individuals to adverse effects of nutrients or food components. A discussion of how variability is dealt with in the context of nutritional risk assessment follows.

Physiological changes and common conditions associated with growth and maturation that occur during an individual's life span may influence sensitivity to nutrient toxicity. For example, sensitivity increases with declines in lean body mass and with declines in renal and liver function that occur with aging; sensitivity changes in direct relation to intestinal absorption or intestinal synthesis of nutrients; in the newborn infant, sensitivity is also increased because of rapid brain growth and limited ability to secrete or biotransform toxicants; and sensitivity increases with decreases in the rate of metabolism of nutrients. During pregnancy, the increase in total body water and glomerular filtration results in lower blood levels of water soluble vitamins for a given dose, such as vitamin C, and therefore reduces susceptibility to potential adverse effects. However, in the unborn fetus this may be offset by active placental transfer, accumulation of certain nutrients in the amniotic fluid, and rapid development of the brain. Examples of life stage groups that may differ in terms of nutritional needs and toxicological sensitivity include infants and children, the elderly, and women during pregnancy and lactation.

Even within relatively homogeneous life stage groups, there is a range of sensitivities to toxic effects. The model described below accounts for normally expected variability in sensitivity, but it excludes subpopulations with extreme and distinct vulnerabilities. Such subpopulations consist of individuals needing medical supervision; they are better served through the use of public health screening, product labeling, or other individualized health care strategies. (Such populations may not be at *negligible risk* when their intakes reach the UL developed for the apparently healthy population.) The decision to treat identifiable vulnerable subgroups as distinct (not protected by the UL) is a matter of judgment and is discussed in individual nutrient chapters, as applicable.

Bioavailability

In the context of toxicity, the bioavailability of an ingested nutrient can be defined as its accessibility to normal metabolic and physiological processes. Bioavailability influences a nutrient's beneficial effects at physiological levels of intake and also may affect the nature and severity of toxicity due to excessive intakes. Factors that affect bioavailability include the concentration and chemical form of the nutrient, the nutrition and health of the individual, and excretory losses. Bioavailability data for specific nutrients must be considered and incorporated by the risk assessment process.

Some nutrients may be less readily absorbed when they are part of a meal than when taken separately. Supplemental forms of some nutrients may require special consideration if they have higher bioavailability and therefore may present a greater risk of producing adverse effects than equivalent amounts from the natural form found in food.

Nutrient-Nutrient Interactions

A diverse array of adverse health effects can occur as a result of the interaction of nutrients. The potential risk of adverse nutrient-nutrient interactions increases when there is an imbalance in the intake of two or more nutrients. Excessive intake of one nutrient may interfere with absorption, excretion, transport, storage, function, or metabolism of a second nutrient. Possible adverse nutrient-nutrient interactions are considered as a part of setting a UL. Nutrient-nutrient interactions may be considered either as a critical endpoint on which to base a UL or as supportive evidence for a UL based on another endpoint.

Other Relevant Factors Affecting Bioavailability of Nutrients

In addition to nutrient interactions, other considerations have the potential to influence nutrient bioavailability, such as the nutritional status of an individual and the form of intake. These issues are considered in the risk assessment. With regard to the form of intake, fat-soluble vitamins such as vitamin E are more readily absorbed when they are part of a meal that is high in fat. ULs must therefore be based on nutrients as part of the total diet, including the contribution from water. Nutrient supplements that are taken separately from food require special consideration, because they are likely to have different bioavailabilities and therefore may represent a greater risk of producing adverse effects.

STEPS IN THE DEVELOPMENT OF TOLERABLE UPPER INTAKE LEVELS

Hazard Identification

Based on a thorough review of the scientific literature, the hazard identification step describes the adverse health effects that have been demonstrated to be caused by the nutrient or food component.

In vivo studies in humans and animals are the primary types of data used as background for identifying nutrient hazards in humans:

- *Human studies.* Human data provide the most relevant kind of information for hazard identification, and, when they are of sufficient quality and extent, are given greatest weight. However, the number of controlled human toxicity studies conducted in a clinical setting is very limited because of ethical reasons. Such studies are generally most useful for identifying very mild (and ordinarily reversible) adverse effects. Observational studies that focus on well-defined populations with clear exposures to a range of nutrient intake levels are useful for establishing a relationship between exposure and effect. Observational data in the form of case reports or anecdotal evidence are used for developing hypotheses that can lead to knowledge of causal associations. Sometimes a series of case reports, if it shows a clear and distinct pattern of effects, may be reasonably convincing on the question of causality.

- *Animal data.* Most of the available data used in risk assessments come from controlled laboratory experiments in animals, usually mammalian species other than humans (e.g., rodents). Such data are used in part because human data on nonessential chemicals are generally very limited. Moreover, there is a long-standing history of the use of animal studies to identify the toxic properties of chemical substances, and there is no inherent reason why animal data should not be relevant to the evaluation of nutrient toxicity. Animal studies offer several advantages over human studies. They can, for example, be readily controlled so that causal relationships can be recognized. It is possible to identify the full range of toxic effects produced by a chemical, over a wide range of exposures, and to establish dose-response relationships. The effects of chronic exposures can be identified in far less time than they can using epidemiological methods. All of these advantages of animal data, however, may not always overcome the fact that species differences in response to chemical substances can sometimes be profound, and any extrapolation of animal data to predict human response has to take into account this possibility.

Key issues that are addressed in the data evaluation of human and animal studies are listed in Box 4-1.

Evidence of Adverse Effects in Humans

The hazard identification step involves the examination of human, animal, and in vitro published evidence addressing the likelihood of a nutrient or food component eliciting an adverse effect in humans. Decisions regarding which observed effects are adverse are based on scientific judgments. Although toxicologists must consider the possibility that many demonstrable structural or functional alterations represent adverse effects with respect to nutrients, some alterations may be considered of little or self-limiting biological importance. As noted earlier, adverse nutrient-nutrient interactions are considered in the definition of an adverse effect.

Causality

The identification of a hazard is strengthened by evidence of causality. As explained in Chapter 3, the criteria of Hill (1971) are

---

BOX 4-1 Development of Tolerable Upper Intake Levels (ULs)

Components of Hazard Identification
- Evidence of adverse effects in humans
- Causality
- Relevance of experimental data
- Pharmacokinetic and metabolic data
- Mechanisms of toxic action
- Quality and completeness of the database
- Identification of distinct and highly sensitive subpopulations

Components of Dose-Response Assessment
- Data selection and identification of critical endpoints
- Identification of no-observed-adverse-effect level (NOAEL) (or lowest-observed-adverse-effect level [LOAEL])
- Assessment of uncertainty and data on variability in response
- Derivation of a UL
- Characterization of the estimate and special considerations

considered in judging the causal significance of an exposure-effect association indicated by epidemiological studies.

Relevance of Experimental Data on Nutrient Toxicity

Consideration of the following issues can be useful in assessing the relevance of experimental data.

Animal Data. Some animal data may be of limited utility in judging the toxicity of nutrients because of highly variable interspecies differences in nutrient requirements. Nevertheless, relevant animal data are considered in the hazard identification and dose-response assessment steps where applicable and, in general, are used for hazard identification unless there are data demonstrating they are not relevant to human beings or it is clear that the available human data are sufficient.

Route of Exposure.[2] Data derived from studies involving oral exposure (rather than parenteral, inhalation, or dermal exposure) are most useful for the evaluation of nutrients and food components. Data derived from studies involving parenteral, inhalation, or dermal routes of exposure may be considered relevant if the adverse effects are systemic and data are available to permit interroute extrapolation.

Duration of Exposure. Because the magnitude, duration, and frequency of exposure can vary considerably in different situations, consideration must be given to the relevance of the exposure scenario (e.g., chronic daily dietary exposure versus short-term bolus doses) to dietary intakes by human populations.

Pharmacokinetic and Metabolic Data

When available, data regarding the rates of nutrient absorption, distribution, metabolism, and excretion may be important in derivation of Tolerable Upper Intake Levels (ULs). Such data may provide significant information regarding interspecies differences and similarities in nutrient behavior, and so may assist in identifying

---

[2]The terms *route of exposure* and *route of intake* refer to how a substance enters the body (e.g., by ingestion, injection, or dermal absorption). These terms should not be confused with *form of intake*, which refers to the medium or vehicle used (e.g., supplements, food, or drinking water).

relevant animal data. They may also assist in identifying life stage differences in response to nutrient toxicity.

In some cases, there may be limited or even no significant data relating to nutrient toxicity. It is conceivable that in such cases, pharmacokinetic and metabolic data may provide valuable insights into the magnitude of the UL. Thus, if there are significant pharmacokinetic and metabolic data over the range of intakes that meet nutrient requirements, and if it is shown that this pattern of pharmacokinetic and metabolic data does not change in a range of intakes greater than those required for nutrition, it may be possible to infer the absence of toxic risk in this range. In contrast, an alteration of pharmacokinetics or metabolism may suggest the potential for adverse effects. There has been no case encountered thus far in which sufficient pharmacokinetic and metabolic data are available for establishing ULs in this fashion, but it is possible such situations may arise in the future.

Mechanisms of Toxic Action

Knowledge of molecular and cellular events underlying the production of toxicity can assist in dealing with the problems of extrapolation between species and from high to lower doses. It may also aid in understanding whether the mechanisms associated with toxicity are those associated with deficiency. In most cases, however, because knowledge of the biochemical sequence of events resulting from toxicity and deficiency is still incomplete, it is not yet possible to state with certainty whether or not these sequences share a common pathway.

Quality and Completeness of the Database

The scientific quality and quantity of the database are evaluated. Human or animal data are reviewed for suggestions that the substances have the potential to produce additional adverse health effects. If suggestions are found, additional studies may be recommended.

Identification of Distinct and Highly Sensitive Subpopulations

The ULs are based on protecting the most sensitive members of the general population from adverse effects of high nutrient or food component intake. Some highly sensitive subpopulations have responses (in terms of incidence, severity, or both) to the agent of interest that are clearly distinct from the responses expected for the presumably healthy population. The risk assessment process recognizes that there may be individuals within any life stage group who are more biologically sensitive than others, and thus their extreme sensitivities do not fall within the range of sensitivities expected for the general population. The UL for the general population may not be protective for these subgroups. As indicated earlier, the extent to which a distinct subpopulation will be included in the derivation of a UL for the general population is an area of judgment to be addressed on a case-by-case basis.

Dose-Response Assessment

The process for deriving the UL is described in this section and outlined in Box 4-1. It includes selection of the critical data set, identification of a critical endpoint with its no-observed-adverse-effect level (NOAEL) or lowest-observed-adverse-effect level (LOAEL), and assessment of uncertainty.

Data Selection and Identification of Critical Endpoints

The data evaluation process results in the selection of the most appropriate or critical data sets for deriving the UL. Selecting the critical data set includes the following considerations:

• Human data, when adequate to evaluate adverse effects, are preferable to animal data, although the latter may provide useful supportive information.
• In the absence of appropriate human data, information from an animal species whose biological responses are most like those of humans is most valuable. Pharmacokinetic, metabolic, and mechanistic data may be available to assist in the identification of relevant animal species.
• If it is not possible to identify such a species or to select such data, data from the most sensitive animal species, strain, or gender combination are given the greatest emphasis.
• The route of exposure that most resembles the route of expected human intake is preferable. This includes considering the digestive state (e.g., fed or fasted) of the subjects or experimental animals. Where this is not possible, the differences in route of exposure are noted as a source of uncertainty.
• The critical data set defines a dose-response relationship between intake and the extent of the toxic response known to be most

relevant to humans. Data on bioavailability are considered, and adjustments in expressions of dose-response are made to determine whether any apparent differences in response can be explained.

- The critical data set documents the route of exposure and the magnitude and duration of the intake. Furthermore, the critical data set documents the NOAEL (or LOAEL).

Identification of NOAEL (or LOAEL)

A nutrient can produce more than one toxic effect (or endpoint), even within the same species or in studies using the same or different exposure durations. The NOAELs and LOAELs for these effects will ordinarily differ. The critical endpoint used to establish a UL is the adverse biological effect exhibiting the lowest NOAEL (e.g., the most sensitive indicator of a nutrient's toxicity). Because the selection of uncertainty factors (UFs) depends in part upon the seriousness of the adverse effect, it is possible that lower ULs may result from the use of the most *serious* (rather than most *sensitive*) endpoint. Thus, it is often necessary to evaluate several endpoints independently to determine which leads to the lowest UL.

For some nutrients, there may be inadequate data on which to develop a UL. The lack of reports of adverse effects following excess intake of a nutrient does not mean that adverse effects do not occur. As the intake of any nutrient increases, a point (see Figure 4-2)

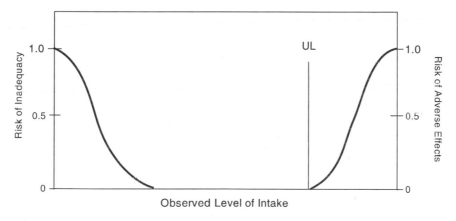

Observed Level of Intake

FIGURE 4-2 Theoretical description of health effects of a nutrient as a function of level of intake. The Tolerable Upper Intake Level (UL) is the highest level of daily nutrient intake that is likely to pose no risk of adverse health effects for almost all individuals in the general population. At intakes above the UL, the risk of adverse effects increases.

is reached at which intake begins to pose a risk. Above this point, increased intake increases the risk of adverse effects. For some nutrients, and for various reasons, there are inadequate data to identify this point, or even to make any estimate of its location.

Because adverse effects are almost certain to occur for any nutrient at some level of intake, it should be assumed that such effects may occur for nutrients for which a scientifically documented UL cannot now be derived. Until a UL is set or an alternative approach to identifying protective limits is developed, intakes greater than the Recommended Dietary Allowance (RDA) or Adequate Intake (AI) should be viewed with caution.

The absence of data sufficient to establish a UL points to the need for studies suitable for developing ULs.

Uncertainty Assessment

Several judgments must be made regarding the uncertainties and thus the uncertainty factor (UF) associated with extrapolating from the observed data to the general population (see Appendix G). Applying a UF to a NOAEL (or LOAEL) results in a value for the derived UL that is less than the experimentally derived NOAEL, unless the UF is 1.0. The greater the uncertainty, the larger the UF and the smaller the resulting UL. This is consistent with the ultimate goal of the risk assessment: to provide an estimate of a level of intake that will protect the health of virtually all members of the general population (Mertz et al., 1994).

Although several reports describe the underlying basis for UFs (Dourson and Stara, 1983; Zielhuis and van der Kreek, 1979), the strength of the evidence supporting the use of a specific UF will vary. Because the imprecision of the UFs is a major limitation of risk assessment approaches, considerable leeway must be allowed for the application of scientific judgment in making the final determination. Because data are generally available regarding intakes of nutrients and food components by human populations, the data on nutrient toxicity may not be subject to the same uncertainties as data on nonessential chemical agents, resulting in UFs for nutrients and food components typically less than the factors of 10 often applied to nonessential toxic substances. The UFs are lower with higher quality data and when the adverse effects are extremely mild and reversible.

In general, when determining an uncertainty factor, the following potential sources of uncertainty are considered and combined into the final UF:

- *Interindividual variation in sensitivity.* Small UFs (close to 1) are used to represent this source of uncertainty if it is judged that little population variability is expected for the adverse effect, and larger factors (close to 10) are used if variability is expected to be great (NRC, 1994).

- *Extrapolation from experimental animals to humans.* A UF to account for the uncertainty in extrapolating animal data to humans is generally applied to the NOAEL when animal data are the primary data set available. While a default UF of 10 is often used to extrapolate animal data to humans for nonessential chemicals, a lower UF may be used because of data showing some similarities between the animal and human responses (NRC, 1994). For example, in this report a UF of 3 was utilized to extrapolate from animal data to humans for vitamin E.

- *LOAEL instead of NOAEL.* If a NOAEL is not available, a UF may be applied to account for the uncertainty in deriving a UL from the LOAEL. The size of the UF applied involves scientific judgment based on the severity and incidence of the observed effect at the LOAEL and the steepness (slope) of the dose response.

- *Subchronic NOAEL to predict chronic NOAEL.* When data are lacking on chronic exposures, scientific judgment is necessary to determine whether chronic exposure is likely to lead to adverse effects at lower intakes than those producing effects after subchronic exposures (exposures of shorter duration).

Derivation of a UL

The UL is derived by dividing the NOAEL (or LOAEL) by a single UF that incorporates all relevant uncertainties. ULs, expressed as amount per day, are derived for various life stage groups using relevant databases, NOAELs and LOAELs, and UFs. In cases where no data exist with regard to NOAELs or LOAELs for the group under consideration, extrapolations from data in other age groups or animal data are made on the basis of known differences in body size, physiology, metabolism, absorption, and excretion of the nutrient.

Generally, age group adjustments are based solely on differences in body weight, unless there are data demonstrating age-related differences in nutrient pharmacokinetics, metabolism, or mechanism of action.

The derivation of a UL involves the use of scientific judgment to select the appropriate NOAEL (or LOAEL) and UF. The risk assessment requires explicit consideration and discussion of all choices made, regarding both the data used and the uncertainties accounted for. These considerations are discussed in the chapters on nutrients and food components. In this report, because of lack of consistency in the data, ULs could not be set for β-carotene. In addition, ULs could not be established for the other carotenoids due to a lack of suitable data.

Characterization of the Estimate and Special Considerations

If the data review reveals the existence of subpopulations having distinct and exceptional sensitivities to a nutrient's toxicity, these subpopulations are explicitly discussed and concerns related to adverse effects are noted; however, the use of the data is not included in the identification of the NOAEL or LOAEL, upon which the UL for the general population is based.

INTAKE ASSESSMENT

In order to assess the risk of adverse effects, information on the range of nutrient intakes in the general population is required. As noted earlier, in cases where the Tolerable Upper Intake Level (UL) pertains only to supplement use, and does not pertain to usual food intakes of the nutrient, the assessment is directed at supplement intakes only.

RISK CHARACTERIZATION

As described earlier, the question of whether nutrient intakes create a risk of adverse effects requires a comparison of the range of nutrient intakes (food, supplements, and other sources or supplements alone, depending upon the basis for the Tolerable Upper Level Intake [UL]) with the UL.

Figure 4-3 illustrates a distribution of chronic nutrient intakes in a population; the fraction of the population experiencing chronic intakes above the UL represents the potential at-risk group. A policy decision is needed to determine whether efforts should be made to reduce this risk. No precedents are available for such policy choices, although in the area of food additive or pesticide regulations, federal regulatory agencies have generally sought to ensure that the ninetieth or ninety-fifth percentile intakes fall below the UL (or its approximate equivalent measure of risk). If this goal is achieved, the fraction of the population remaining above the UL is likely to experience intakes only slightly greater than the UL and is likely to be at little or no risk.

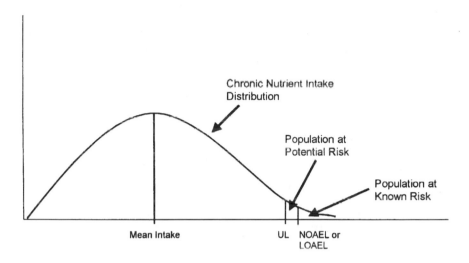

FIGURE 4-3 Illustration of the population at risk from excessive nutrient intakes. The fraction of the population consistently consuming a nutrient at intake levels in excess of the UL is potentially at risk of adverse health effects. See text for a discussion of additional factors necessary to judge the significance of the risk. LOAEL = lowest-observed-adverse-effect level, NOAEL = no-observed-adverse-effect level, UL= Tolerable Upper Intake Level.

For risk management decisions, it is useful to evaluate the public health significance of the risk, and information contained in the risk characterization is critical for this purpose.

Thus, the significance of the risk to a population consuming a nutrient in excess of the UL is determined by the following:

1. the fraction of the population consistently consuming the nutrient at intake levels in excess of the UL;

2. the seriousness of the adverse effects associated with the nutrient;

3. the extent to which the effect is reversible when intakes are reduced to levels less than the UL; and

4. the fraction of the population with consistent intakes above the NOAEL or even the LOAEL.

Thus, the significance of the risk of excessive nutrient intake cannot be judged only by reference to Figure 4-3, but requires careful consideration of all of the above factors. Information on these factors is contained in this report's sections describing the basis for each of the ULs.

REFERENCES

Dourson ML, Stara JF. 1983. Regulatory history and experimental support of uncertainty (safety) factors. *Regul Toxicol Pharmacol* 3:224–238.

FAO/WHO (Food and Agriculture Organization of the United Nations/World Health Organization). 1995. *The Application of Risk Analysis to Food Standard Issues.* Recommendations to the Codex Alimentarius Commission (ALINORM 95/9, Appendix 5). Geneva: World Health Organization.

FAO/WHO (Food and Agriculture Organization of the United Nations/World Health Organization). 1982. *Evaluation of Certain Food Additives and Contaminants.* Twenty-sixth report of the Joint FAO/WHO Expert Committee on Food Additives. WHO Technical Report Series No. 683. Geneva: World Health Organization.

Health Canada. 1993. *Health Risk Determination—The Challenge of Health Protection.* Ottawa: Health Canada, Health Protection Branch.

Hill AB. 1971. *Principles of Medical Statistics,* 9th edition. New York: Oxford University Press.

Klaassen CD, Amdur MO, Doull J. 1986. *Casarett and Doull's Toxicology: The Basic Science of Poisons,* 3rd edition. New York: Macmillan.

Mertz W, Abernathy CO, Olin SS. 1994. *Risk Assessment of Essential Elements.* Washington, DC: ILSI Press.

NRC (National Research Council). 1983. *Risk Assessment in the Federal Government: Managing the Process.* Washington, DC: National Academy Press.

NRC (National Research Council). 1994. *Science and Judgment in Risk Assessment.* Washington, DC: National Academy Press.

OTA (Office of Technology Assessment). 1993. *Researching Health Risks.* Washington, DC: Office of Technology Assessment.

WHO (World Health Organization). 1987. *Principles for the Safety Assessment of Food Additives and Contaminants in Food.* Environmental Health Criteria 70. Geneva: World Health Organization.

WHO (World Health Organization). 1996. *Trace Elements in Human Nutrition and Health.* Geneva: World Health Organization.

Zielhuis RL, van der Kreek FW. 1979. The use of a safety factor in setting health-based permissible levels for occupational exposure. *Int Arch Occup Environ Hth* 42:191–201.

5

Vitamin C

SUMMARY

Vitamin C functions physiologically as a water-soluble antioxidant by virtue of its high reducing power. It is a cofactor for enzymes involved in the biosynthesis of collagen, carnitine, and neurotransmitters in vitro, and it can quench a variety of reactive oxygen species and reactive nitrogen species in aqueous environments. Evidence for in vivo antioxidant functions of ascorbate include the scavenging of reactive oxidants in activated leukocytes, lung, and gastric mucosa, and diminished lipid peroxidation as measured by urinary isoprostane excretion. To provide antioxidant protection, a Recommended Dietary Allowance (RDA) of 90 mg/day for adult men and 75 mg/day for adult women is set based on the vitamin C intake to maintain near-maximal neutrophil concentration with minimal urinary excretion of ascorbate. Because smoking increases oxidative stress and metabolic turnover of vitamin C, the requirement for smokers is increased by 35 mg/day. Estimates of median dietary intakes of vitamin C for adults are 102 mg/day and 72 mg/day in the United States and Canada, respectively. The Tolerable Upper Intake Level (UL) for adults is set at 2 g/day; the adverse effects upon which the UL is based are osmotic diarrhea and gastrointestinal disturbances.

BACKGROUND INFORMATION

Vitamin C is a water-soluble vitamin that is essential for all humans and a few other mammals that lack the ability to biosynthesize the compound from glucose because they lack the enzyme gulonolactone oxidase. The term vitamin C refers to both ascorbic acid and dehydroascorbic acid (DHA), since both exhibit anti-scorbutic activity. Ascorbic acid, the functional and primary in vivo form of the vitamin, is the enolic form of an α-ketolactone (2,3-didehydro-L-threo-hexano-1,4-lactone). The two enolic hydrogen atoms give the compound its acidic character and provide electrons for its function as a reductant and antioxidant. Its one-electron oxidation product, the ascorbyl radical, readily dismutates to ascorbate and DHA, the two-electron oxidation products. Both the ascorbyl radical and DHA are readily reduced back to ascorbic acid in vivo. However, DHA can be hydrolyzed irreversibly to 2,3-diketogulonic acid. The molecular structure of ascorbic acid contains an asymmetric carbon atom that allows two enantiomeric forms, of which the L form is naturally occurring (the D-form, isoascorbic or erythorbic acid, provides antioxidant but little or no anti-scorbutic activity), as shown in Figure 5-1.

Function

The biological functions of ascorbic acid are based on its ability to provide reducing equivalents for a variety of biochemical reactions. Because of its reducing power, the vitamin can reduce most physiologically relevant reactive oxygen species (Buettner, 1993). As such, the vitamin functions primarily as a cofactor for reactions requiring a reduced iron or copper metalloenzyme and as a protective antioxidant that operates in the aqueous phase both intra- and extracellularly (Englard and Seifter, 1986; Halliwell and Whiteman, 1997; Tsao, 1997). Both the one- and the two-electron oxidation products of the vitamin are readily regenerated in vivo—chemically and enzymatically—by glutathione, nicotinamide adenine dinucleotide (NADH), and nicotinamide adenine dinucleotide phosphate (NADPH) dependent reductases (May et al., 1998; Park and Levine, 1996).

Vitamin C is known to be an electron donor for eight human enzymes. Three participate in collagen hydroxylation; two in carnitine biosynthesis; and three in hormone and amino acid biosynthesis. The three enzymes that participate in hormone and amino acid biosynthesis are dopamine-β-hydroxylase, necessary for the biosynthesis of the catecholamines norepinephrine and epinephrine; peptidyl-glycine monooxygenase, necessary for amidation of peptide hormones; and 4-hydroxyphenylpyruvatedioxygenase, involved in tyrosine metabolism. Ascorbate's action with these enzymes in-

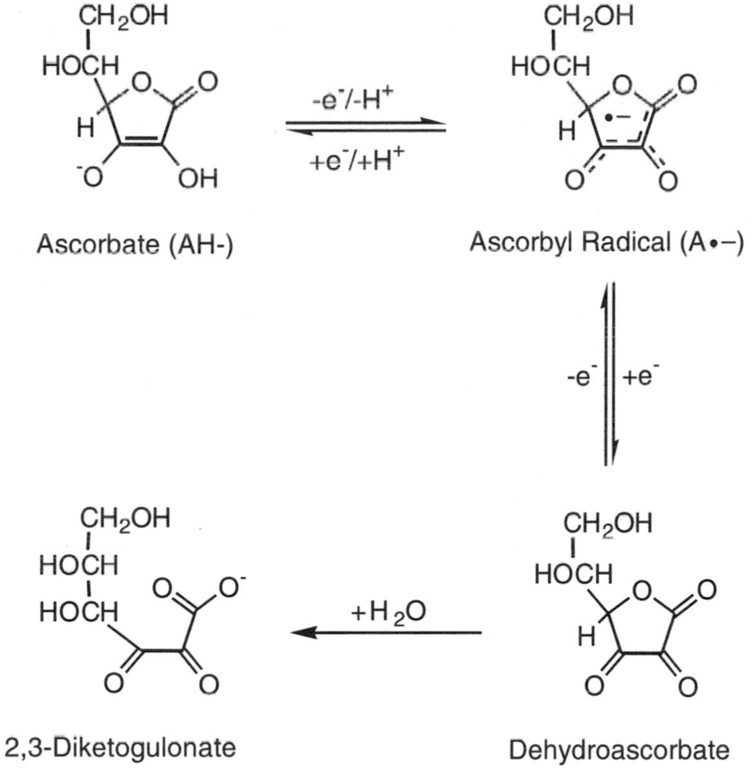

FIGURE 5-1 Chemical structure of ascorbic acid.

volves either monooxygenase or dioxygenase activities (Levine et al., 1996b).

As a cofactor for hydroxylase and oxygenase metalloenzymes, ascorbic acid is believed to work by reducing the active metal site, resulting in reactivation of the metal-enzyme complex, or by acting as a co-substrate involved in the reduction of molecular oxygen. The best known of these reactions is the posttranslational hydroxylation of peptide-bound proline and lysine residues during formation of mature collagen. In these reactions, ascorbate is believed to reactivate the enzymes by reducing the metal sites of prolyl (iron) and lysyl (copper) hydroxylases (Englard and Seifter, 1986; Tsao, 1997).

Evidence also suggests that ascorbate plays a role in or influences collagen gene expression, cellular procollagen secretion, and the biosynthesis of other connective tissue components besides collagen, including elastin, fibronectin, proteoglycans, bone matrix, and elastin-associated fibrillin (Ronchetti et al., 1996). The primary physical symptoms of ascorbic acid's clinical deficiency disease, scurvy, which involves deterioration of elastic tissue, illustrate the important role of ascorbate in connective tissue synthesis.

Ascorbic acid is involved in the synthesis and modulation of some hormonal components of the nervous system. The vitamin is a cofactor for dopamine-β-hydroxylase, which catalyzes hydroxylation of the side chain of dopamine to form norepinephrine, and α-amidating monooxygenase enzymes, involved in the biosynthesis of neuropeptides. Other nervous system components modulated by ascorbate concentrations include neurotransmitter receptors, the function of glutamatergic and dopaminergic neurons, and synthesis of glial cells and myelin (Englard and Seifter, 1986; Katsuki, 1996).

Because of its ability to donate electrons, ascorbic acid is an effective antioxidant. The vitamin readily scavenges reactive oxygen species (ROS) and reactive nitrogen species (RNS) (e.g., hydroxyl, peroxyl, superoxide, peroxynitrite, and nitroxide radicals) as well as singlet oxygen and hypochlorite (Frei et al., 1989; Halliwell and Whiteman, 1997; Sies and Stahl, 1995). The one- and two-electron oxidation products of ascorbate are relatively nontoxic and easily regenerated by the ubiquitous reductants glutathione and NADH or NAD-PH. The relatively high tissue levels of ascorbate provide substantial antioxidant protection: in the eye, against photolytically generated free-radical damage; in neutrophils, against ROS produced during phagocytosis; and in semen, against oxidative damage to sperm deoxyribonucleic acid (DNA) (Delamere, 1996; Fraga et al., 1991; Levine et al., 1994). Ascorbic acid protects against plasma and low-density lipoprotein (LDL) oxidation by scavenging ROS in the aqueous phase before they initiate lipid peroxidation (Frei et al., 1988; Jialal et al., 1990) and possibly by sparing or regenerating vitamin E (Halpner et al., 1998). Evidence suggests that ascorbate also provides antioxidant protection indirectly by regenerating other biological antioxidants such as glutathione and α tocopherol back to their active state (Jacob, 1995).

Ascorbic acid functions as a reducing agent for mixed-function oxidases in the microsomal drug-metabolizing system that inactivates a wide variety of substrates, such as endogenous hormones or xenobiotics (i.e., other chemical compounds such as drugs, pesticides, or carcinogens that are foreign to humans) (Tsao, 1997). The activity of both microsomal drug-metabolizing enzymes and cytochrome P-450 electron transport is lowered by ascorbate deficiency. The vitamin is involved in the biosynthesis of corticosteroids and aldosterone and in the microsomal hydroxylation of cholesterol in the conversion of cholesterol to bile acids. In reactions similar to the hydroxylation of proline for collagen synthesis, ascorbate is required along with iron at two steps in the pathway of carnitine biosynthesis. Ascorbic acid modulates iron absorption, transport, and storage (Gosiewska et al., 1996). Limited data suggest that ascorbate modulates prostaglandin synthesis and thus exerts bronchodilatory and vasodilatory as well as anticlotting effects (Horrobin, 1996).

Physiology of Absorption, Metabolism, and Excretion

Absorption and Transport

Intestinal absorption of ascorbic acid occurs through a sodium-dependent active transport process that is saturable and dose dependent (Rumsey and Levine, 1998; Tsao, 1997). At low gastrointestinal ascorbate concentrations, active transport predominates, while simple diffusion occurs at high concentrations. Some 70 to 90 percent of usual dietary intakes of ascorbic acid (30 to 180 mg/day) are absorbed; however, absorption falls to about 50 percent or less with increasing doses above 1 g/day (Kallner et al., 1979). The bioavailabilities of the vitamin from foods and supplements are not significantly different (Johnston and Luo, 1994; Mangels et al., 1993).

Cellular transport of ascorbic acid and DHA is mediated by transporters that vary by cell type (Jacob, 1999; Tsao, 1997). DHA is the form of the vitamin that primarily crosses the membranes of blood and intestinal cells, after which it is reduced intracellularly to ascorbic acid. Accumulation of ascorbate into neutrophils and lymphocytes is mediated by both high- and low-affinity transporters, and the vitamin is localized mostly in the cytosol. Intracellularly and in plasma, vitamin C exists predominately in the free reduced form as ascorbate monoanion, as shown in Figure 5-1 (Levine et al., 1994).

Metabolism and Excretion

Since the immediate oxidized forms of vitamin C are readily reduced back to ascorbic acid, relatively small amounts of the vitamin are lost through catabolism. The primary products of oxidation beyond DHA include oxalic and threonic acids, L-xylose, and ascorbate 2-sulfate (Jacob, 1999). With large intakes of the vitamin, unabsorbed ascorbate is degraded in the intestine, a process that may account for the diarrhea and intestinal discomfort sometimes reported by persons ingesting large doses (see section on "Adverse Effects").

Besides dose-dependent absorption, a second primary mechanism for regulation of body ascorbate content is renal action to conserve or excrete unmetabolized ascorbate. Recent studies have shown that little unmetabolized ascorbate is excreted with dietary intakes up to about 80 mg/day and that renal excretion of ascorbate increases proportionately with higher intakes (Blanchard et al., 1997; Melethil et al., 1986).

Body Stores

Dose-dependent absorption and renal regulation of ascorbate allow conservation of the vitamin by the body during low intakes and limitation of plasma levels at high intakes. Tissue-specific cellular transport systems allow for wide variation of tissue ascorbate concentrations. High levels are maintained in the pituitary and adrenal glands, leukocytes, eye tissues and humors, and the brain, while low levels are found in plasma and saliva (Hornig, 1975). Due to homeostatic regulation, the biological half-life of ascorbate varies widely from 8 to 40 days and is inversely related to the ascorbate body pool (Kallner et al., 1979). Similarly, catabolic turnover varies widely, about 10 to 45 mg/day, over a wide range of dietary intakes due to body pool size. A total body pool of less than 300 mg is associated with scurvy symptoms (Baker et al., 1971), while maximum body pools are limited to about 2 g (Kallner et al., 1979). At very low ascorbate intakes, essentially no ascorbate is excreted unchanged and a minimal loss occurs.

Clinical Effects of Inadequate Intake

Scurvy, the classic disease of severe vitamin C deficiency, is characterized by symptoms related to connective tissue defects. Scurvy usually occurs at a plasma concentration of less than 11 µmol/L (0.2 mg/dL). Clinical features of scurvy include follicular hyperkeratosis, petechiae, ecchymoses, coiled hairs, inflamed and bleeding gums, perifollicular hemorrhages, joint effusions, arthralgia, and impaired wound healing (Baker et al., 1971; Chazan and Mistilis, 1963; Levine et al., 1996b). Other symptoms include dyspnea, edema, Sjögren's syndrome (dry eyes and mouth), weakness, fatigue, and depression. In experimental subjects made vitamin C deficient but not frankly scorbutic, gingival inflammation (Leggott et al., 1986) and fatigue (Levine et al., 1996a) were among the most sensitive markers of deficiency. Vitamin C deficiency in infants may result in bone abnormalities such as impaired bone growth and disturbed ossification, hemorrhagic symptoms, and resultant anemia (Jacob, 1999).

Lack of ascorbate-related hydroxyproline and hydroxylysine formation needed for collagen cross-linking may explain many of the connective tissue and hemorrhagic manifestations of scurvy, however, the specific histologic defects have not been identified. Oxidative degradation of some blood coagulation factors due to low plasma ascorbate concentrations may contribute to hemorrhagic symptoms (Parkkinen et al., 1996).

Scurvy is rare in developed countries but is occasionally seen in individuals who consume few fruits and vegetables, peculiar or restricted diets, or in those who abuse alcohol or drugs. In the United States, low blood ascorbate concentrations are more prevalent in men, especially elderly men, than in women and are more prevalent in populations of lower socioeconomic status (LSRO/FASEB, 1989). Infantile scurvy is rarely seen, because human milk provides an adequate supply of vitamin C and infant formulas are fortified with the vitamin.

SELECTION OF INDICATORS FOR ESTIMATING THE REQUIREMENT FOR VITAMIN C

Antioxidant Functions

There is much support for the role of increased oxidative stress in the pathogenesis of cardiovascular disease (Jialal and Devaraj, 1996; Witztum and Steinberg, 1991). The most plausible and biologically relevant hypothesis is that the oxidative modification of low-density lipoprotein (LDL) and other lipoproteins promote atherogenesis (Berliner and Heinecke, 1996; Devaraj and Jialal, 1996; Witztum and Steinberg, 1991). Several lines of evidence suggest that oxidized LDL (oxLDL) is pro-atherogenic. Furthermore, data support the in vivo existence of oxLDL (Berliner and Heinecke, 1996; Witztum and Steinberg, 1991). In vitro studies have clearly shown that vitamin C at concentrations greater than 40 µmol/L (0.8 mg/dL) inhibits the oxidation of isolated LDL induced by transition metals, free-radical initiators, and activated human neutrophils and macrophages (Jialal and Grundy, 1991; Jialal et al., 1990; Scaccini and Jialal, 1994). This is because vitamin C effectively scavenges aqueous reactive oxygen species (ROS) and reactive nitrogen species (RNS), which prevents them from attacking LDL. Thus, in vitro vitamin C clearly functions as an antioxidant.

Studies shown in Table 5-1 examined the effect of vitamin C supplementation alone on biomarkers of lipid peroxidation. Of the 13 studies, 7 showed that vitamin C supplementation resulted in a significant decrease in lipid oxidation products in plasma, LDL, or urine. The vitamin C supplements that resulted in positive effects ranged from 500 to 2,000 mg/day. The most convincing evidence that vitamin C functions as an antioxidant in vivo is the study by Reilly et al. (1996) showing that supplementation of smokers with 2.0 g vitamin C for 5 days was associated with a significant reduction in urinary isoprostanes, an indicator of oxidative stress. In the remaining six studies in which vitamin C was supplemented in amounts ranging from 500 to 6,000 mg/day, there was no significant effect of vitamin C supplementation on lipid oxidation products in plasma, urine, or plasma LDL.

Carr and Frei (1999) examined the effect on LDL oxidation of supplementation with vitamin C in combination with vitamin E and β-carotene. Although these investigators have clearly shown that the supplements decrease LDL oxidation, it is difficult to assess the contribution of vitamin C alone.

Vitamin C supplementation (2,000 mg/day for 4 to 12 months) in 41 patients with non-atrophic gastritis decreased gastric mucosal nitrotyrosine, a measure of RNS activity (Table 5-2) (Mannick et al., 1996). Thus, from this study and the study by Reilly et al. (1996), it can be concluded that supplementation with vitamin C results in an antioxidant effect in vivo because it significantly reduces nitrotyrosine and urinary isoprostanes.

However, with respect to the effect of vitamin C on LDL oxidation, the data are inconclusive. This could be explained by the fact that, because vitamin C is water soluble, it does not partition into the LDL particle. Also, it must be pointed out that in one of the 13 studies summarized in Table 5-1, there was an increase in plasma thiobarbituric acid reactive substances (TBARS), an indicator of oxidative stress, with a 500-mg dose of ascorbic acid (Nyyssonen et al., 1997b).

Adhesion of mononuclear cells to endothelium is an early event in atherogenesis and may be triggered by oxidative stress. Smokers have low levels of vitamin C and increased oxidative stress. A recent study showed that monocytes of smokers display greater adhesion to endothelial cells than those of nonsmokers (Weber et al., 1996). When supplemented with 2,000 mg/day of vitamin C, the plasma ascorbate level of smokers increased, and adhesion of their monocytes to endothelium decreased to that seen in nonsmokers.

Impaired vascular function is crucial to the clinical manifestation of atherosclerosis. As depicted in Table 5-3, numerous investigators have reported a beneficial effect of high dose vitamin C administration, either orally or intraarterially, on vasodilation. This beneficial effect of vitamin C is most likely related to its antioxidant effect. Endothelium-derived relaxing factor, nitric oxide (NO), promotes vasodilation but is rapidly inactivated by superoxide. Vitamin C improves endothelial function and vasodilation, possibly by scavenging superoxide radicals, conserving intracellular glutathione, or potentiating intracellular NO synthesis. In human endothelial cells in culture, extracellular vitamin C at physiological concentrations increased cellular NO synthesis up to threefold, and the increase in NO synthesis followed a time course similar to ascorbate uptake into the cells (Heller et al., 1999).

Antioxidant Functions in Leukocytes

The content of vitamin C in leukocytes is especially important because the ROS generated during phagocytosis and neutrophil activation are associated with infectious and inflammatory stresses (Jariwalla and Harakeh, 1996; Levine et al., 1994). Along with pituitary and adrenal glands and eye lens, leukocytes contain the highest vitamin C concentrations of all body tissues (Moser, 1987). Studies with guinea pigs and monkeys show that the concentration of ascorbate in the leukocytes more accurately reflects liver and body pool ascorbate than does the concentration in plasma or erythrocytes (Omaye et al., 1987). The vitamin is transported into leukocytes by an energy-dependent transport system that concentrates the vitamin some twenty-five-, forty-, and eightyfold over plasma levels in neutro-

TABLE 5-1 Effect of Vitamin C Supplementation on
Biomarkers of Lipid Oxidation in Humans

Reference	Subjects	Vitamin C Dose[a] (mg/d)
Harats et al., 1990	17 smokers	1,000 1,500
Belcher et al., 1993	5 healthy men	1,000
Rifici and Khachadurian, 1993	4 healthy men and women	1,000
Cadenas et al., 1996	21 healthy men	1,000
Fuller et al., 1996	19 smokers (9 placebo)	1,000
Mulholland et al., 1996	16 female smokers (8 placebo)	1,000
Reilly et al., 1996	5 heavy smokers	2,000
Anderson et al., 1997	48 nonsmokers (24 females)	60 6,000
Nyyssonen et al., 1997b	59 male smokers (19 placebo)	500 (P[j]) 500 (SR[k])
Samman et al., 1997	8 male smokers	(40) 1,000
Wen et al., 1997	20 nonsmokers (9 placebo)	1,000
Harats et al., 1998	36 healthy men	(50) 500 (citrus fruit supplement)
Naidoo and Lux, 1998	9 healthy men, 6 healthy women	250, 500, 750 and 1,000

[a] Amount given in excess of variable amount consumed daily as part of the diet.
[b] LDL = low-density lipoprotein.
[c] TBARS = thiobarbituric acid reactive substances.
[d] LDL oxidizability is measured by the lag time and propagation rate of in vitro lipid peroxidation.
[e] VLDL = very low-density lipoprotein.
[f] CD = conjugated dienes.

Duration	Plasma Change	Findings
2 wk	2.0-fold	↓ Plasma and LDL[b] TBARS[c]
4 wk	2.3-fold	↓ Plasma and LDL TBARS
14 d	Not reported	LDL oxidation [d], no change
10 d	Not reported	↓ VLDL[e] and LDL oxidation (4 hour TBARS)
30 d	Not reported	Urine TBARS, no change
4 wk	3.9-fold	↓ LDL Oxidizability[d] (TBARS, CD[f])
14 d	3.0-fold	Serum TBARS, no change
5 d	Not reported	18 Urine 8-epi-PGF$_{2a}$
14 d	1.2-fold	Plasma MDA[g]/HNE,[h] no change ↑ TAC[i]
14 d	1.8-fold	Plasma MDA/HNE, no change ↑ TAC
2 mo	1.3-fold	LDL oxidizability, no change
2 mo	1.5-fold	Plasma ↑ TBARS with P Vit C No ↑ with SR Vit C
(2 wk)	(baseline)	LDL oxidizability (CD): no change
2 wk	2.0-fold	
4 wk	2.2-fold	↓ Plasma MDA (↑ erythrocyte Vit E and GSH[l]); no change LDL Vit E; no change in LDL oxidizability (TBARS and CD)
(1 mo)	(baseline)	↓ LDL oxidizability (CD)
2 mo	3.8-fold	
2 wk	1.5-fold (250) 2.0-fold (500) 2.0-fold (750 and 1,000)	↓ Plasma MDA and allantoin with 500, 750 and 1,000 mg/d

[g] MDA = malondialdehyde.
[h] HNE = hydroxynonenal.
[i] TAC = Total Antioxidant Capacity.
[j] P = plain.
[k] SR = slow release.
[l] GSH = reduced gluthione.

TABLE 5-2 Vitamin C Intake and Biomarkers of Gastric and Bladder Cancer

Reference	Subjects	Vitamin C Dose (mg/d)
Leaf et al., 1987	7 men	2–1,000
Young et al., 1990	18 healthy men	1,500
Dyke et al., 1994a	43 patients with gastritis	1,000
Dyke et al., 1994b	48 patients with gastritis	1,000
Drake et al., 1996	82 patients with dyspepsia	None
Mannick et al., 1996	84 patients with *Helicobacter pylori* infection	2,000
Satarug et al., 1996	31 healthy men, 80 men with liver fluke infection	300 with 300 mg/d proline

[a] DNA = deoxyribonucleic acid.
[b] ROS = Reactive Oxygen Species.
[c] RNS = Reactive Nitrogen Species.

TABLE 5-3 Vitamin C and Endothelium-Dependent Vasodilation in Humans

Reference	Subjects
Heitzer et al., 1996	10 chronic smokers 10 control subjects
Levine et al., 1996	46 coronary artery disease patients (20 placebo)
Ting et al., 1996	10 type II diabetic patients 10 control subjects
Motoyama et al., 1997	20 smokers 20 control subjects
Solzbach et al., 1997	22 hypertensive patients
Ting et al., 1997	11 hypercholesterolemic patients 12 healthy control subjects
Hornig et al., 1998	15 chronic heart failure patients 8 healthy control subjects
Taddei et al., 1998	14 hypertensive patients 14 healthy control subjects
Timimi et al., 1998	10 type I diabetic patients 10 control subjects

Duration	Findings
5–12 d	↓ In vivo nitrosation (N-nitrosoproline)
1 wk	↓ Urinary β-glucuronidase activity (linked to bladder cancer)
4 wk	↓ Gastric mucosa DNA[a] adduct formation
4 wk	↑ O^6-alkyltransferase DNA repair enzyme
—	Significant (p < .001) correlation between gastric mucosa ascorbyl radical concentration and ROS[b] activity
4–12 mo	↓ Nitrotyrosine in gastric mucosa (measure of RNS[c] activity)
1 d	↓ In vivo nitrosation by urinary nitrosoproline products

Vitamin C Dose	Findings
18 mg/min (infusion)	↑ Forearm blood flow 1.6-fold (measured after acetylcholine infusion)
2,000 mg (oral)	↑ Brachial artery dilation 3.2-fold (measured after 2 h)
24 mg/min (infusion)	↑ Forearm blood flow 1.4-fold (measured after methacholine infusion)
10 mg/min (infusion)	↑ Brachial artery dilation 1.7-fold (measured after 20 min)
3,000 mg (infusion)	↓ Coronary artery vasoconstriction 2.6-fold (measured after acetylcholine infusion)
24 mg/min (infusion)	↑ Forearm blood flow 1.3-fold (measured after methacholine infusion)
25 mg/min (infusion)	↑ Radial artery dilation 1.6-fold (measured after 10 min)
2,000 mg (oral)	↑ Radial artery dilation 1.5-fold (following 4 wk supplementation)
2.4 mg/min (infusion)	↑ Forearm blood flow 1.3-fold (acetycholine)
24 mg/min (infusion)	↑ Forearm blood flow 1.4-fold (measured after methacholine infusion)

phils, platelets, and lymphocytes, respectively (Evans et al., 1982; Jacob et al., 1992; Levine et al., 1996a). Metabolic priority for maintenance of intracellular lymphocyte ascorbate levels was demonstrated by its lower depletion rates compared to plasma and semen ascorbate levels during controlled vitamin C deficiency (intake of 5 mg/day) and faster recovery during vitamin repletion at 60 mg/day (Jacob et al., 1992). Intracellular ascorbate recycling (the intracellular regeneration of oxidized extracellular ascorbate) provides a cellular reservoir of reducing capacity (electrons) that can be transmitted both into and across the cell membrane (May et al., 1999).

The high intracellular concentration of ascorbate in leukocytes provides cellular protection against oxidant damage associated with the respiratory burst. In isolated neutrophils, ascorbate recycling is increased up to thirtyfold upon exposure of the cells to microbial pathogens (Wang et al., 1997b). Ascorbate effectively neutralizes phagocyte-derived oxidants without inhibiting the bactericidal activity of the phagosome (Anderson and Lukey, 1987). Evidence that ascorbate modulates leukocyte phagocytic action, blastogenesis, immunoglobulin production, chemotaxis, and adhesiveness has been reported in vitro, although evidence for the latter two functions has been mixed (Evans et al., 1982; Jariwalla and Harakeh, 1996).

Concentrations of ascorbate normally found in plasma (22 to 85 μmol/L [0.4 to 1.7 mg/dL]) were shown to neutralize hypochlorous acid (HOCl), one of many powerful oxidants generated by myeloperoxidase in activated neutrophils and monocytes (Halliwell et al., 1987; Heinecke, 1997). This action was hypothesized to protect α-1-antiprotease against inactivation by HOCl and thereby prevent proteolytic damage at inflamed sites such as the rheumatoid joint (Halliwell et al., 1987). Indeed, the ratio of oxidized to reduced ascorbate was found to be increased in the knee synovial fluid of active rheumatoid arthritis patients, which suggests that ascorbate is acting to scavenge phagocyte-derived oxidants in this locally inflamed area (Lunec and Blake, 1985). Similarly, increased ascorbate oxidation in the plasma of patients with adult respiratory distress syndrome (Cross et al., 1990) and in smokers (Lykkesfeldt et al., 1997) indicates protection against oxidant damage from activated neutrophils and other sources in the lung. Exposure of nine apparently healthy adults to 2,000 parts per billion (ppb) of ozone, an environmental pollutant, for 2 hours resulted in increased myeloperoxidase and decreased ascorbate concentrations in bronchoalveolar lavage fluid. These results imply that ascorbate protects against inflammatory oxidative stress induced by ozone (Mudway et al., 1999).

Ascorbate scavenging of myeloperoxidase-derived oxidants from phagocytic white cells may also be protective against in vivo LDL oxidation because HOCl-oxidized proteins have been identified in human atherosclerotic lesions (Hazell et al., 1996). In an in vitro system, ascorbate at a physiologically relevant concentration of 50 μmol/L (0.9 mg/dL) was the most effective antioxidant for preventing LDL oxidation due to myeloperoxidase-derived RNS (Byun et al., 1999).

Oxidative Deoxyribonucleic Acid and Chromosome Damage

Cellular Deoxyribonucleic Acid (DNA) Damage

Table 5-4 summarizes the results of five experimental human studies in which cellular markers of DNA damage were measured after various vitamin C intakes. Three of the studies varied vitamin C alone, while the other two studies varied vitamin C and other micronutrients.

Of the three studies that varied only vitamin C intake, one showed that 60 or 250 mg/day decreased sperm 8-hydroxy-7, 8-dihydro-2′-deoxyguanosine (8-oxodG), a measure of oxidative stress, but did not affect lymphocyte or urine 8-oxodG or DNA strand breaks (Fraga et al., 1991). In contrast, the second study showed no effect of either 60 or 6,000 mg/day vitamin C on lymphocyte DNA or chromosome damage as measured by comet assay (Anderson et al., 1997). The third study showed both decreases and increases in measures of lymphocyte DNA oxidative damage after vitamin C supplementation of 500 mg/day (Podmore et al., 1998). In a subsequent report of results from the study of Podmore et al. (1998), the investigators hypothesized that increases in serum and urine 8-oxodG following the decreases of lymphocyte 8-oxoguanine and 8-oxodG suggest a role for vitamin C in the repair of oxidant-damaged DNA (Cooke et al., 1998).

The two studies that co-supplemented with vitamin E and β-carotene (Duthie et al., 1996) or iron (Rehman et al., 1998) demonstrated mixed results in that both decreases and increases in lymphocyte DNA oxidant damage measures. Since the contribution of vitamin C alone to the results of these studies cannot be determined, these studies cannot be used to estimate a vitamin C requirement. Results of the latter study involving supplementation of apparently healthy individuals with both vitamin C and iron are discussed in the section "Tolerable Upper Intake Levels."

Inverse correlations of lymphocyte ascorbate and glutathione con-

TABLE 5-4 Vitamin C Intake and Biomarkers of Cellular
Oxidative DNA Damage in Humans

Reference	Subjects	Vitamin C Dose (mg/d)
Fraga et al., 1991	10 males	(250 baseline)[a] 5[a] 10 or 20[a] 60 or 250[a]
Duthie et al., 1996	50 male smokers	100 +280 mg/d vitamin E +25 mg/d β-carotene
	50 nonsmokers	100 +280 mg/d vitamin E +25 mg/d β-carotene
Anderson et al., 1997	48 nonsmokers (24 females)	60 6,000
Podmore et al., 1998; Cooke et al., 1998	30 healthy subjects (16 females and 14 males)	500
Rehman et al., 1998	10 healthy subjects	60 +14 mg/d Fe
	10 healthy subjects	260 +14 mg/d Fe

[a] Intake from controlled diet; no supplemental doses given.
[b] 8-oxodG = 8-oxo-7,8-dihydro-2'-deoxyguanosine.
[c] HPLC-EC = high-performance liquid chromatography-electrochemical detection
[d] DNA = deoxyribonucleic acid.

centrations with oxidized DNA bases in another study of 105 apparently healthy adults suggest that these two intracellular antioxidants protect human lymphocytes against oxidative damage (Lenton et al., 1999). In sum, the results of studies testing the effects of vitamin C on cellular DNA damage are mixed and cannot be used for estimating the vitamin C requirement.

Duration	Findings
(7–14 d)	
32 d	↑ Sperm 8-oxodG[b] (HPLC-EC[c])
28 d	↑ Sperm 8-oxodG (HPLC-EC)
28 d	↓ Sperm 8-oxodG (HPLC-EC)
	No changes in lymphocyte 8-oxodG or DNA[d] strand breaks
20 wk	↓ Lymphocyte DNA damage (comet assay)
20 wk	↓ Lymphocyte DNA damage (comet assay)
14 d	No change in lymphocyte DNA damage
14 d	(comet assay) or chromosome breakage
6 wk	↓ Lymphocyte 8-oxogua[e] and 8-oxodG (GC-MS[f])
	↑ Serum and urine 8-oxodG (GC-MS)
	↑ Lymphocyte 8-oxoade[g] (GC-MS)
12 wk	↓ Leukocyte 8-oxogua (GC-MS)
	↓ Leukocyte 8-oxoade (GC-MS)
12 wk	↓ Leukocyte 8-oxogua (GC-MS)
	↓ Leukocyte 8-oxoade (GC-MS)
	↑ Leukocyte 5-OH cytosine (GC-MS)
	↑ Leukocyte thymine glycol (GC-MS)
	↑ Total base damage at 6 wk, no change at 12 wk

[e] 8-oxogua = 8-oxoguanine.
[f] GC-MS = gas chromatography-mass spectroscopy.
[g] 8-oxoade = 8-oxoadenine.
SOURCE: Adapted from Carr and Frei (1999).

Urinary Markers of DNA Damage

Urinary excretion of DNA oxidant damage products, which is thought to represent the balance of total body DNA damage and repair has been measured in the studies shown in Table 5-5. This is a nonspecific measure used to assess changes due to micronutrient status. Except for the study by Cooke et al. (1998), no relationships between vitamin C intake and urinary markers of DNA damage were

TABLE 5-5 Vitamin C Intake and Urinary Excretion of Oxidative DNA Damage Products in Humans

Reference	Subjects	Vitamin C Dose (mg/d)
Fraga et al., 1991	10 males	(250 baseline)[a] 5[a] 10–20[a] 60–250[a]
Loft et al., 1992	83 subjects	72[d] 5.9 mg/d vitamin E[d] 1.1 mg/d vitamin A[d]
Witt et al., 1992	11 subjects	1000 +533 mg/d vitamin E +10 mg/d β-carotene
Prieme et al., 1997	18 male smokers 20 male smokers	500 500 (SR[e])
Cooke et al., 1998	14 males 16 females	500

[a] Intake from controlled diet; no supplemental doses given.
[b] 8-oxodG = 8-oxo-7,8 dihydro-2′-deoxyguanosine.
[c] HPLC-EC = high-performance liquid chromatography-electrochemical detection.
[d] Intake estimated from diet records; no supplemental doses given.

found. Thus, urinary markers of DNA damage cannot be used to determine vitamin C requirements.

Ex Vivo Damage

The five studies in Table 5-6 measured DNA and chromosome damage ex vivo after supplementing the subjects with vitamin C. Single large doses of vitamin C (1 g/day or more) provided protection against lymphocyte DNA strand break damage induced ex vivo by radiation or hydrogen peroxide (H_2O_2) as measured by the comet assay (Green et al., 1994; Panayiotidis and Collins, 1997). In contrast, Crott and Fenech (1999) reported that a single 2-g dose of vitamin C neither caused DNA damage nor protected cells against hydrogen peroxide-induced toxicity. The two other studies measured DNA chromosome damage after treatment of lymphocytes with bleomycin, a test for genetic instability. Following vitamin C supplementation for two weeks, Pohl and Reidy (1989) found de-

Duration	Findings
(7–14 d)	Urine 8-oxoG[b]: no changes (HPLC-EC[c])
32 d	
28 d	
28 d	
2 wk	Urine 8 oxodG: not correlated (HPLC-EC)
1 mo	Urine 8-oxoG: no changes (HPLC-EC)
2 mo	Urine 8-oxodG: no changes (HPLC-EC)
2 mo	Urine 8-oxodG: no changes (HPLC-EC)
6 wk	↑ Urine 8-oxodG (GC-MS[f])

[e] SR = slow release.
[f] GC-MS = gas chromatography-mass spectroscopy.
SOURCE: Adapted from Carr and Frei (1999).

creased chromosome breaks and Anderson et al. (1997) reported no effects on DNA damage but increased chromosome aberrations. Since the findings of these studies were inconsistent, ex vivo damage cannot be used to estimate a vitamin C requirement.

Cancer Biomarkers

Effects of vitamin C intakes on surrogate markers and biomarkers of colorectal, gastric, and bladder cancer are shown in Table 5-2 and Table 5-7. Of six studies of patients with precancerous colon polyps, vitamin C treatment for 1 month to 3 years demonstrated variable results with regard to effect on polyp growth and cell proliferation (Table 5-7).

Biomarkers of gastric cancer after vitamin C treatment of patients with the precancerous conditions, gastritis, or *Helicobacter pylori* infections were measured in four studies (Table 5-2). Three studies showed positive results of vitamin C supplementation in vivo: Man-

TABLE 5-6 Vitamin C Intake and Ex Vivo Measures of Oxidative DNA Damage in Humans

Reference	Subjects	Vitamin C Dose (mg/d)
Pohl and Reidy, 1989	8 subjects	0 100 1,000
Green et al., 1994	5 nonsmokers 1 smoker	2,400
Anderson et al., 1997	48 nonsmokers (24 females)	60 or 6,000
Panayiotidis and Collins, 1997	6 nonsmokers 6 smokers	1,000 or 3,000
Crott and Fenech, 1999	11 male nonsmokers	2,000

[a] DNA = deoxyribonucleic acid.
[b] H_2O_2 = hydrogen peroxide.
[c] CBMN = cytokinesis-block micronucleus.
SOURCE: Adapted from Carr and Frei (1999).

TABLE 5-7 Vitamin C Intake and Colorectal Polyps

Reference	Subjects	Vitamin C Dose (mg/d)
DeCosse et al., 1975	5 patients with familial polyps	3,000
Bussey et al., 1982	36 patients with colon polyps	3,000
McKeown-Eyssen et al., 1988	137 patients with colon polyps	400 + 400 mg/d vitamin E
Cahill et al., 1993	40 patients with colon polyps, 20 normal subjects	750
Greenberg et al., 1994	380 patients with diagnosed colon adenomas	1,000 + 400 mg vitamin E or 1,000 + 400 mg vitamin E + 25 mg β-carotene
Hofstad et al., 1998	116 patients with colon polyps	150 + 75 mg vitamin E + 15 mg β-carotene + 101 µg Se + 1.6 g Ca

Duration	Findings
2 wk	↓ Lymphocyte chromosome breaks after bleomycin treatment,
2 wk	average breaks per cell:
2 wk	0.289
	0.208
	0.184
Single dose	↓ Lymphocyte DNA[a] strand breaks in unirradiated and irradiated blood (comet assay)
2 wk	No effect on DNA damage (comet assay)
	↑ Chromosome aberrations after bleomycin treatment
Single dose	↓ Lymphocyte DNA strand breaks in both groups after ex vivo H_2O_2[b] oxidant stress (comet assay)
Single dose	No effect on DNA damage (CBMN[c] assay)

Duration	Findings
4–13 mo	Complete polyp regression in two patients, partial regression in two, and increased polyps in one
2 y	↓ Polyp area
2 y	Nonsignificant in ↓ polyp recurrence
1 mo	↓ Total colonic crypt cell proliferation
4 y	No change in incidence of adenomas, polyp frequency, or size
3 y	↓ Number of new adenomas. No effect on growth of existing polyps

nick et al. (1996) reported decreased gastric mucosal nitrotyrosine (a measure of RNS activity); Dyke et al. (1994a) reported decreased mucosal DNA damage in one group of gastric cancer patients and subsequently found increased mucosal O^6-alkyltransferase, a DNA repair enzyme in a second group of patients with gastric cancer (Dyke et al. 1994b). Leaf et al. (1987) found decreased nitrosation in men after vitamin C supplementation. Drake et al. (1996) used electron paramagnetic resonance to demonstrate the presence of the ascorbyl radical in 82 unsupplemented patients with dyspepsia and showed that ascorbyl radical concentrations correlated with ROS activity. Gastric muscosal concentrations of ascorbyl radical, ROS, and malondialdehyde (a measure of lipid peroxidation) were higher in patients with gastritis and *Helicobacter pylori* infections compared to patients with normal mucosal histology. Young et al. (1990) found decreased β-glucuronidase activity (linked to bladder cancer) after in vivo supplementation of apparently healthy men with 1,500 mg/day of vitamin C for 1 week.

Summary

For the three studies shown in Table 5-4 in which only vitamin C intake was varied, some markers of cellular DNA damage showed no change with increased vitamin C intake, two markers decreased, and one increased. Urinary measures of oxidized DNA products showed no change attributable to vitamin C intake (Table 5-5). Two of three studies of ex vivo DNA damage showed a benefit of vitamin C supplementation (Table 5-6); however, the relation of these results to the in vivo situation is uncertain. Studies of surrogate markers and biomarkers in precancerous colonic and gastric patients show beneficial or no effects of vitamin C supplementation. However, the interpretation of these endpoints and the relevance of the results to apparently healthy individuals are questionable. The study of dyspepsia patients indicates that vitamin C acts as an antioxidant in the gastric mucosa and prevents oxidative damage by scavenging ROS (Drake et al., 1996). This is consistent with previous findings that substantial amounts of ascorbic acid are secreted into the digestive tract (Dabrowski, 1990; Waring et al., 1996) and that vitamin C supplementation decreases gastric mucosal DNA adduct formation (Dyke et al., 1994a).

Overall, the results do not provide compelling evidence that vitamin C intakes of 60 to 6,000 mg/day reduce in vivo DNA oxidative damage in apparently healthy individuals. Hence, present data cannot be used to estimate a vitamin C requirement using the end-point of reduction of oxidative damage to DNA and chromosomes.

Immune Function

As summarized in Table 5-8, vitamin C has been shown to affect various components of the human immune response, including antimicrobial and natural killer cell activities, lymphocyte proliferation, chemotaxis, and delayed dermal sensitivity (DDS). Except for the metabolic unit study of Jacob et al. (1991) and the study of patients with furunculosis (Levy et al., 1996), the studies involved apparently healthy free-living populations supplemented with from 200 mg/day to 6 g/day of vitamin C in addition to dietary vitamin intake. Hence, the results relate largely to the pharmacological range of vitamin C intakes rather than the nutritional range of intakes usually provided from food alone.

As seen from analysis of Table 5-8, vitamin C supplementation resulted about equally in improved or little change in frequently used measures of immune function: lymphocyte proliferation, chemotaxis, and DDS response. The decrease in DDS during vitamin C depletion of men in a metabolic unit cannot be ascribed solely to changes in ascorbate status because the DDS did not increase again upon repletion for 4 weeks with 60 to 250 mg/day of the vitamin (Jacob et al., 1991). The only negative effect of intakes in the range of 600 to 10,000 mg/day was the decrease in ex vivo bactericidal activity found after apparently healthy men received 2,000 (but not 200) mg/day of the vitamin for 4 weeks (Shilotri and Bhat, 1977).

Few controlled studies of the effect of vitamin C intake on infectious episodes in humans have been reported, except for studies of the common cold (covered later under "Common Cold" in the section "Relationship of Vitamin C Intake to Chronic Disease"). Peters et al. (1993) reported a significantly decreased incidence of post-race upper respiratory infections in marathon runners receiving 600 mg/day of vitamin C compared to control runners taking a placebo.

Results from some studies show improvement in indices of immune function due to increased vitamin C intake, whereas other studies show no effect. The lack of effect may be due to the use of subject populations whose baseline vitamin C status is already adequate, because leukocytes saturate with vitamin C at a lower intake than is required to saturate plasma, about 100 mg/day (Levine et al., 1996a). Nevertheless, the existing data do not provide convincing evidence that supplemental vitamin C has a significant effect on

TABLE 5-8 Vitamin C Intake and Measures of Immune Function in Humans

Reference	Subjects	Vitamin C Dose (mg/d)
Shilotri and Bhat, 1977	5 healthy men, aged 23–28 y	200 2,000
Ludvigsson et al., 1979	24 healthy women	1,000–4,000
Anderson et al., 1980	5 healthy adults	1,000–3,000
Panush et al., 1982	28 healthy young adults	1,000–10,000
Kennes et al., 1983	Elderly adults, aged >70 y	500 IM[c]
Delafuente et al., 1986	15 elderly adults without acute illness	2,000
Vogel et al., 1986	9 healthy men and 2 healthy women, aged 22–28 y	1,500
Jacob et al., 1991	8 healthy men, aged 25–43 y	5–20 60–250
Johnston, 1991	14 healthy women and men	1,500
Johnston et al., 1992	10 adults	2,000
Peters et al., 1993	46 runners and 46 control subjects	600
Levy et al., 1996	23 patients with furunculosis (boils)	1,000

[a] PMN = polymorphonuclear leukocytes.
[b] DDS = delayed dermal sensitivity.
[c] IM = intramuscular.

immune functions in humans. Therefore, data from currently available immune function studies cannot be used to estimate the vitamin C requirement.

Other Indicators

Collagen Metabolism

Ascorbic acid is required along with iron as a cofactor for the post-translational hydroxylation of proline and lysine to effect cross-

Duration	Findings
2 wk	No change in bactericidal activity of leukocytes measured ex vivo
2 wk	↓ Ex vivo bactericidal activity of leukocytes
5 wk	No change in leukocyte ascorbate concentration or function
1–3 wk	↑ Mitogen-stimulated in vitro lymphocyte proliferation and PMN[a] chemotaxis. No change in other cellular or humoral immune functions
1 wk	↑ Mitogen-stimulated in vitro lymphocyte proliferation and DDS[b] response to skin antigens
1 mo	↑ Mitogen-stimulated in vitro lymphocyte proliferation and DDS response. No changes in serum immunoglobulins
3 wk	No change in mitogen-stimulated in vitro lymphocyte proliferation or DDS response
90 d	No change in PMN chemotaxis or response to experimental gingivitis
60 d	No changes in in vitro mitogen-stimulated lymphocyte proliferation
4 wk	↓ In DDS response with vitamin C intakes of 5–20 mg/d
4 wk	No change in plasma complement C1q
2 wk	No effect on PMN chemotaxis ↓ Blood histamine
21 d	↓ Incidence and severity of upper-respiratory-tract infections
4–6 wk	Improvement in PMN functions and clinical response in patients with low baseline PMN functions

linking of mature collagen (Englard and Seifter, 1986). Lack of this function due to ascorbate deficiency results in defective collagen formation and the physical symptoms of scurvy. However, serum or urinary levels of proline or lysine, their hydroxylated forms, or other measures of collagen metabolism have not been shown to be reliable markers of ascorbate status (Hevia et al., 1990). Therefore, despite the important role of the vitamin in collagen formation, no collagen-related measures are available to use as a functional indicator for the dietary vitamin C requirement.

Carnitine Biosynthesis

Ascorbate is required along with iron at two steps in the pathway of carnitine biosynthesis in reactions similar to the hydroxylation of proline during collagen formation. Muscle carnitine is significantly depleted in scorbutic guinea pigs, suggesting that loss of energy derived from carnitine-related β-oxidation of fatty acids may explain the fatigue and muscle weakness observed in human scurvy (Jacob and Pianalto, 1997; Rebouche, 1995). However, neither guinea pig nor human studies show a consistent relationship between vitamin C status and carnitine levels (Davies et al., 1987; Jacob and Pianalto, 1997; Johnston et al., 1996). Although vitamin C deficiency appears to alter carnitine metabolism, the specific interactions and their relevance to functional carnitine status in humans are unclear. Therefore, measures of carnitine status cannot be used as an indicator for estimating the vitamin C dietary requirement.

Periodontal Health

The gingival and dental pathology that accompanies scurvy has prompted numerous investigations of the relationship between ascorbic acid and periodontal health. Epidemiological studies have failed to demonstrate an association between vitamin C intake and periodontal disease (Alvares, 1997; Russell, 1967). Controlled experimental studies of patients with gingivitis and apparently healthy adults with vitamin C intakes of 5 to 1,500 mg/day have shown mixed results with regard to the influence of vitamin C status on periodontal integrity (Leggott et al., 1986, 1991; Vogel et al., 1986; Woolfe et al., 1984). Other studies, with animals and humans, have shown that vitamin C intake can affect the structural integrity of gingival tissue, including permeability of the gingival sulcular epithelium (Alvares, 1997).

Overall, while evidence suggests that vitamin C deficiency is linked to some aspects of periodontal disease, the relationship of vitamin C intake to periodontal health in the population at large is unclear. Beyond the amount needed to prevent scorbutic gingivitis (less than 10 mg/day) (Baker et al., 1971), the results from current studies are not sufficient to reliably estimate the vitamin C requirement for apparently healthy individuals based on oral health endpoints.

Relationship of Vitamin C Intake to Chronic Disease

Cardiovascular Disease

As suggested earlier, there is reason to expect that the antioxidant vitamins should decrease the risk of cardiovascular disease (Gey, 1995; Jha et al., 1995; Simon, 1992). Several studies have considered the association between vitamin C concentrations in blood and the risk of cardiovascular disease. Singh et al. (1995) found that the risk of coronary artery disease was approximately two times less among the top compared to the bottom quintile of plasma vitamin C concentrations in Indian subjects. A prospective study of 1,605 Finnish men showed that those with increased plasma vitamin C (greater than 11.4 µmol/L [0.2 mg/dL]) had a 60 percent decreased risk of coronary heart disease (Nyyssonen et al., 1997a). The Basel Prospective Study of 2,974 Swiss men reported that plasma vitamin C concentrations greater than 23 µmol/L (0.4 mg/dL) were associated with nonsignificant reductions in the risk of coronary artery disease (Eichholzer et al., 1992) and stroke (Gey et al., 1993). In a 20-year follow-up of 730 elderly adults in Britain, plasma vitamin C concentrations greater than 28 µmol/L (0.5 mg/dL) were associated with a 30 percent decreased risk of death from stroke compared with concentrations less than 12 µmol/L (0.2 mg/dL) (Gale et al., 1995). In a similar study, cross-sectional in design, in 6,624 men and women in the Second National Health and Nutrition Examination Survey, the relative risk of coronary heart disease and stroke was decreased about 26 percent with serum vitamin C concentrations of 63 to 153 µmol/L (1.1 to 2.7 mg/dL) compared with concentrations of 6 to 23 µmol/L (0.1 to 0.4 mg/dL) (Simon et al., 1998).

In addition, several prospective cohort studies have shown that vitamin C intakes between 45 and at least 113 mg/day are associated with reduced risk of cardiovascular disease (Gale et al., 1995; Knekt et al., 1994; Pandey et al., 1995). Gale et al. (1995) reported that in 730 elderly British men and women, vitamin C intakes greater than 45 mg/day were associated with a 50 percent lower risk of stroke than were intakes less than 28 mg/day. There was a nonsignificant 20 percent decrease in the risk of coronary artery disease in this study. Knekt et al. (1994) studied more than 5,000 Finnish men and women and found that women consuming more than 91 mg/day vitamin C had a lower risk of coronary artery disease than those consuming less than 61 mg/day. However, a similar association was not found in the men. In the Western Electric study in Chicago, a cohort of 1,556 middle-aged men consuming greater than 113 mg/day of vitamin C had a 25 percent lower risk of coronary artery disease than those consuming less than 82 mg/day (Pandey et al., 1995).

Other prospective studies have looked at higher levels of vitamin C intake and have reported similar findings. The First National Health and Nutrition Examination Survey Epidemiologic Follow-up Study cohort of more than 11,000 adults showed a reduction in cardiovascular disease of 45 percent in men and 25 percent in women whose vitamin C intakes were approximately 300 mg/day from food and supplements (Enstrom et al., 1992). Sahyoun et al. (1996) studied 725 elderly Massachusetts adults and reported a 62 percent lower risk of cardiovascular disease in those whose vitamin C intakes were more than 388 mg/day compared to those whose intakes were less than 90 mg/day. Kritchevsky et al. (1995) reported a negative association between vitamin C intake and carotid artery wall thickness in men and women more than 55 years of age in the Atherosclerosis Risk in Communities Study. Women consuming more than 728 mg/day and men consuming at least 982 mg/day of vitamin C had decreased intima thickness compared to women with intakes of less than 64 mg/day and men with intakes of less than 56 mg/day vitamin C.

In contrast to the above studies, several studies have reported no association between vitamin C intake and risk of cardiovascular disease. In a cohort composed of 3,119 residents of Alameda County, California, vitamin C intakes were not associated with a reduction in risk for cardiovascular disease (Enstrom et al., 1986). In the Established Populations for Epidemiologic Studies of the Elderly with more than 11,000 adults 65 years of age and older (Losonczy et al., 1996) and in the Iowa Women's Heath Study of 34,486 postmenopausal women (Kushi et al., 1996b), vitamin C intake was not associated with an alteration in risk of coronary heart disease mortality in these older age groups. Similarly, the U.S. Health Professionals Follow-up Study of nearly 40,000 male health professionals found that increased intakes of vitamin C (ranging from 92 to 1,162 mg/day) were not associated with a lower risk of coronary heart disease (Rimm et al., 1993).

Although many of the above studies suggest a protective effect of vitamin C against cardiovascular disease, the data are not consistent or specific enough to estimate a vitamin C requirement based on any of these specific biomarkers for cardiovascular disease.

Cancer

As a possible protectant against cancer, vitamin C has engendered a great deal of interest. Block (1991) has reported that the epidemiologic evidence is strongly suggestive of a protective effect, especially for the non-hormone-dependent cancers. However, Ames et al. (1995) have cautioned that the evidence to date of a protective effect for any of the antioxidants is far from complete. Available studies assessing the role of vitamin C in specific cancers by site are evaluated in the following section.

Breast Cancer. A combined meta-analysis, based upon data from 12 case-control studies, found vitamin C to be the micronutrient most strongly associated with breast cancer risk (Howe et al., 1990). According to Howe and colleagues's statistical analyses, each 300-mg increase in vitamin C intake was associated with a 37 percent decrease in the risk of postmenopausal, but not premenopausal, breast cancer. The Iowa Women's Health Study (Kushi et al., 1996a) found a 20 percent decrease in breast cancer risk with greater than 500 mg/day of vitamin C intake from supplements; in contrast, the Nurses Health Study, which used the same dietary assessment instrument, found no decreased risk of breast cancer at intakes greater than 359 mg/day (Hunter et al., 1993). Similarly, a Finnish cohort study (Jarvinen et al., 1997) of 4,697 women aged 15 years and older and the New York State Cohort Study (Graham et al., 1992) of more than 18,000 postmenopausal women with vitamin C intakes up to 498 mg/day found no association between vitamin C intake and breast cancer risk.

Cervical Cancer. In a case-control study, Wassertheil-Smoller et al. (1981) found high plasma vitamin C concentrations to be associated with decreased cervical cancer risk. Similarly Romney et al. (1985) reported a case-control study showing a negative association between increasing plasma vitamin C concentrations and cervical dysplasia.

Colorectal Cancer. In a large case-control study, Freudenheim et al. (1990) reported that increased intakes of vitamin C from food and supplements were associated with decreased risk of rectal cancer. In contrast, the Iowa Women's Cohort Study found no association between vitamin C intake and colon cancer risk at intakes from food and supplements of approximately 300 mg/day vitamin C (Bostick et al., 1993). However, in the women consuming more than 60 mg/day vitamin C from supplements compared with no supplements, the risk was decreased by 30 percent.

Pancreatic Cancer. Two separate case-control studies in Poland (Zatonski et al., 1991) and in Canada (Ghadirian et al., 1991) found that an elevated intake of vitamin C was associated with a decreased risk of pancreatic cancer. A study in the Netherlands, using a similar design, found a protective effect of vitamin C on pancreatic cancer in women but not in men (Bueno de Mesquita et al., 1991). A collaborative pooling of these and other case-control studies in 1992 found evidence overall of an inverse relationship between vitamin C and pancreatic cancer (Howe et al., 1992).

Lung Cancer. Several studies have considered whether vitamin C might be protective against lung cancer. The results of two large case-control studies in Hawaii found no association between dietary vitamin C intake and lung cancer (Hinds et al., 1984; Le Marchand et al., 1989). In contrast, Fontham et al. (1988) reported that vitamin C intake of approximately 140 mg/day was associated with protection for lung cancer among men and women in Louisiana who were non- or light smokers. Similarly, data from the First National Health and Nutrition Examination Survey Epidemiologic Follow-up Study of more than 10,000 men and women indicated that dietary vitamin C intakes greater than 133 mg/day were inversely associated with lung cancer risk (Yong et al., 1997). There was no additional protective effect of vitamin C supplements. This association between vitamin C intake and risk of lung cancer was weaker but still in a protective direction in several studies: a Finnish cohort study of 4,538 men (Knekt et al., 1991); a Dutch cohort study of 561 men (Ocke et al., 1997); a United States prospective study of 3,102 men (Shekelle et al., 1981); and the New York State Cohort Study of 27,544 men (Bandera et al., 1997).

Gastric Cancer. Epidemiological and experimental evidence has suggested that vitamin C may protect against the development of gastric cancer by inhibiting formation of carcinogenic N-nitroso compounds or by scavenging ROS/RNS in the gastric mucosa (Fontham, 1994; Mirvish, 1994; O'Toole and Lombard, 1996). As noted earlier and summarized in Table 5-2, several experimental studies have linked increased vitamin C status to decreased ROS/RNS activity and oxidant damage products in the gastric mucosa of patients with gastritis and *Helicobacter pylori* infection (Drake et al., 1996; Dyke et al., 1994a; Mannick et al., 1996). Gastric juice ascorbate concentrations of patients with *H. pylori* infection and chronic gastritis, risk factors for gastric cancer, are low compared to those of apparently healthy individuals and are increased by eradication of the *H. pylori* infection or by vitamin C supplementation (Rokkas et al., 1995; Waring et al., 1996). However, *H. pylori* infection and accompanying inflammation do not alter vitamin C levels or antioxidant potential in the gastroduodenal mucosa (Phull et al., 1999). Despite the epidemiological associations and the evidence that gastric juice vitamin C is protective against nitrosation and oxidant damage, the two vitamin C supplementation studies conducted to date have not shown a subsequent decrease in gastric cancer incidence (Blot et al., 1993; O'Toole and Lombard, 1996).

Although many of the above studies suggest a protective effect of vitamin C against specific cancers by site, the data are not consistent or specific enough to estimate a vitamin C requirement based on cancer.

Cataract

Ocular tissue concentrates vitamin C, which might suggest, teleologically, that the tissue needs this vitamin (Rose et al., 1998). It is reasonable to expect, therefore, that oxidative damage to ocular tissue is an important source of degenerative eye disease and that supplementation by vitamin C would be an effective means of lessening the risk of diseases such as cataract.

In a case-control comparison of 77 subjects with cataract and 35 control subjects with clear lenses, vitamin C intakes of greater than 490 mg/day were associated with a 75 percent decreased risk of cataracts compared with intakes of less than 125 mg/day (Jacques and Chylack, 1991). Similarly, vitamin C intakes greater than 300 mg/day were associated with a 70 percent reduced risk of cataracts (Robertson et al., 1989). In a second case-control comparison with 1,380 cataract patients and 435 control subjects, similar results were found: although intake numbers were not reported, above-median vitamin C intake was associated with a 20 percent decrease in the risks of cataracts (Leske et al., 1991). In contrast, an analysis of data derived from the Baltimore Longitudinal Study on Aging found no increased association between 260 mg/day of vitamin C and risk of cataracts compared to 115 mg/day (Vitale et al., 1993).

In an 8-year prospective study, Hankinson et al. (1992) evaluated the experience of more than 50,000 nurses in the Nurses Health Study. Dietary vitamin C intakes were not associated with a decreased risk of cataract, but cataract risk was 45 percent lower among the nurses who consumed vitamin C supplements for 10 or more years. With a cohort of 247 nurses from the above study, vitamin C supplement use, in amounts ranging from less than 400 mg/day to greater than 700 mg/day for 10 years or more, was associated with a statistically significant protective effect on lens opacities (Jacques et al., 1997). Women who consumed vitamin C supplements for less than 10 years were not protected.

Although many of the above studies suggest a protective effect of vitamin C against cataracts, the data are not consistent or specific enough to estimate the vitamin C requirement based on cataracts.

Asthma and Obstructive Pulmonary Disease

It is suspected that vitamin C may decrease the risk of asthma and other related pulmonary conditions (Hatch, 1995). Two cross-sectional studies suggest that high plasma vitamin C concentrations or intakes protect or perhaps enhance respiratory function in men but not in women (Ness et al., 1996) and in both men and women (Britton et al., 1995). Similarly, dietary vitamin C intake was positively associated with enhanced pulmonary function in 2526 adult men and women participants in the First National Health and Nutrition Survey Epidemiological Follow-up Study (Schwartz and Weiss, 1994). In another study, 20 middle-aged men and women patients with mild asthma had decreased ascorbate and α-tocopherol concentrations in lung lining fluid, while blood levels were normal (Kelly et al., 1999). These findings and the presence of increased oxidized glutathione in the airways indicate an increased oxidative stress in asthma patients.

A series of small, clinical experiments reported that vitamin C supplementation of 2 g/day may be protective against airway responsiveness to viral infections, allergens, and irritants (Bucca et al., 1992). In contrast, a clinical experiment testing the blocking effect of 2 g/day vitamin C against exercise-induced asthma found little evidence of such an effect (Cohen et al., 1997).

Although many of the above studies suggest a protective effect of vitamin C against asthma and obstructive pulmonary disease, the data are not consistent or specific enough to estimate the vitamin C requirement based on asthma or pulmonary disease.

Common Cold

There has been a great deal of interest in the use of vitamin C to protect against the common cold, much of this research stimulated by the views put forth by the late Linus Pauling (Hemila and Herman, 1995). Reviews of numerous studies generally conclude that vitamin C megadoses have no significant effect on incidence of the common cold, but do provide a moderate benefit in terms of the duration and severity of episodes in some groups (Chalmers, 1975; Jariwalla and Harakeh, 1996; Ludvigsson et al., 1977). The often-reported improvement in severity of colds after vitamin C ingestion may be due to the antihistaminic action of the vitamin at pharmacological doses (Johnston et al., 1992). One early study comparing 44 school-aged twins in vulnerability to colds found no significant over-all treatment effect of vitamin C intakes at doses of 500 to 1,000 mg/day (Miller et al., 1977). Other trials came to similar conclusions (Coulehan et al., 1976; Ludvigsson et al., 1977). Some reviews have stated that any impact of vitamin C is slight or that it is protective only among some subgroups of people (Hemila, 1996, 1997). Others view the accumulated results as so incomplete and flawed as to offer no evidence of protective effects (Herbert, 1995). Thus, the data are not consistent or specific enough to estimate the vitamin C requirement based on the common cold.

Cognitive Function and Memory

Although vitamin C's role as an antioxidant and cofactor for catecholamine biosynthesis might suggest that it protects cognitive function, there is little valid evidence that it does. One study found no association between cognitive function and vitamin C intake (range 84 to 147 mg/day) in 5,182 Dutch residents aged 55 to 95 years (Jama et al., 1996). Another study of 442 men and women, aged 65 to 94 years, reported that higher plasma ascorbate levels were associated with better memory performance (Perrig et al., 1997).

Summary

Although several studies have reported an inverse correlation between vitamin C intake and cardiovascular disease, some types of cancer, and cataracts, others have failed to do so. Very little variation in risk is seen based on the intake of vitamin C for chronic obstructive pulmonary disease, cold or infectious disease, or cognitive function and memory. Also it is important that, for all their power, human-based observational or epidemiological studies imply but do not prove cause and effect. Such studies do not rule out the impact of unidentified factors. In a recent review of epidemiological studies, Gey (1998) suggested that plasma vitamin C concentrations as low as 50 µmol/L (1.0 mg/dL) provide the optimal benefits with regard to cardiovascular disease and cancer. This plasma vitamin C concentration is achieved at a dietary intake of approximately 90 mg/day vitamin C (Levine et al., 1996a). Thus, in the United States or Canada, it may be difficult to do a large-scale trial that demonstrates a health benefit for vitamin C unless the subjects are prescreened to have dietary intakes less than 90 mg/day and plasma levels less than than 50 μmol/L (1.0 mg/dL) of vitamin C.

FACTORS AFFECTING THE VITAMIN C REQUIREMENT

Bioavailability

Some 70 to 90 percent of usual dietary intakes of ascorbic acid (30 to 180 mg/day) are absorbed, although absorption decreases to about 50 percent and less with single doses above 1 g (Kallner et al., 1979; Levine et al., 1996b). The type of food consumed has not been shown to have a significant effect on absorption of either intrinsic or supplemental vitamin C. The bioavailability of the vitamin naturally found in foods or in the form of a supplement has not been shown to be significantly different from that of pure synthetic ascorbic acid (Johnston and Luo, 1994; Mangels et al., 1993).

Nutrient-Nutrient Interactions

Vitamin C participates in redox reactions with many other dietary and physiological compounds, including glutathione, tocopherol, flavonoids, and the trace metals iron and copper (Jacob, 1995).

Glutathione

Interactions of ascorbate with the endogenous antioxidant glutathione have been shown in both rodents and humans. In apparently healthy men fed a low-ascorbate diet of 5 to 20 mg/day, plasma total glutathione (reduced [GSH] and oxidized [GSSG] forms) and the ratio of GSH/GSSG, both indicators of oxidative stress, were significantly decreased (Henning et al., 1991). In apparently healthy adults supplemented with 500 mg/day of ascorbic acid, erythrocyte glutathione rose significantly (Johnston et al., 1993). The results indicate that ascorbate may contribute to antioxidant protection by maintaining reduced glutathione.

Tocopherol and Flavonoids

Evidence from in vitro and animal studies has shown that vitamin C can regenerate or spare α-tocopherol (Halpner et al., 1998), but studies in guinea pigs and humans have not confirmed that this interaction occurs to a significant extent in vivo (Jacob et al., 1996). Calculation of redox potentials indicates that ascorbate can recycle the flavonoid radical (Bors et al., 1995), and Skaper et al. (1997) showed that ascorbic acid acts synergistically with the flavonoid quercetin, to protect cutaneous tissue cells in culture against oxidative damage induced by glutathione deficiency.

Iron and Copper

A variety of interactions of ascorbate with the redox-active trace metals iron and copper have been reported (the potential pro-oxidant effects are discussed later in the section "Pro-oxidant Effects"). Ascorbic acid is involved in the regulation of iron metabolism at a number of points. Ascorbate-related reduction of iron to the ferrous state is involved in iron transfer and storage pathways. Ascorbic acid added to meals facilitates intestinal absorption of nonheme iron, possibly due to lowering of gastrointestinal iron to the more absorbable ferrous state or amelioration of the effect of dietary iron absorption inhibitors (Hallberg, 1985). However, studies in which the vitamin is added to meals over long periods have not shown significant improvement of body iron status, indicating that ascorbic acid has less effect on iron bioavailability than has been predicted from tests with single meals (Hunt et al., 1994).

Some evidence indicates that excess ascorbic acid intake may affect copper metabolism in a variety of ways, including inhibition of intestinal absorption and ceruloplasmin oxidase activity and labilization of ceruloplasmin-bound copper for cellular transport (Harris and Percival, 1991). High concentrations of plasma ascorbate in premature infants has been suggested to decrease ceruloplasmin ferroxidase activity and thereby compromise antioxidant protection (Powers et al., 1995). However, the significance of these effects in humans is questionable, because high ascorbate intakes among men on a metabolic unit did not inhibit copper absorption (Jacob et al., 1987b). In addition, the findings of decreased ceruloplasmin ferroxidase activity due to high physiologic ascorbate concentrations have been attributed to an artifact of nonphysiological assay pH (Løvstad, 1997).

Smoking

Nearly all studies show that smokers have decreased plasma and leukocyte ascorbate levels compared to nonsmokers. Part of this difference may be attributable to a lower intake of fruits and vegetables among smokers than among nonsmokers (Dallongeville et al., 1998; Marangon et al., 1998). However, studies that have adjusted for differences in vitamin C intake (Marangon et al., 1998) and those which have assessed populations with similar fruit and vegetable intakes (Lykkesfeldt et al., 2000) still find that smokers have lower plasma vitamin C concentrations than nonsmokers. This indicates that smoking per se predisposes to lower vitamin C status.

Vitamin C Turnover

The mechanism by which smoking compromises vitamin C status has not been well established. A radioisotope-labeled ascorbic acid dilution study showed that the metabolic turnover of the vitamin in smokers averaged about double that of nonsmokers: 70.0 versus 35.7 mg/day (Kallner et al., 1981). Increased ascorbate turnover in smokers is likely due to the increased oxidative stress from substances in smoke that are directly oxidizing or that stimulate oxidizing inflammatory responses (Elneihoum et al., 1997; Lehr et al., 1997; Pryor, 1997). This hypothesis is supported by the finding that the ratio of dehydroascorbic acid (DHA) to ascorbate in plasma of smokers is increased compared to that in nonsmokers (Lykkesfeldt et al., 1997).

Most studies have found that smokers suffer increased in vivo oxidation of susceptible biological molecules, including lipids (Morrow et al., 1995; Reilly et al., 1996), lipoproteins (Sasaki et al., 1997), and deoxyribonucleic acid (DNA) (Asami et al., 1997; Panayiotidis and Collins, 1997). In many but not all of these studies, intervention with administration of vitamin C or cessation of smoking decreased the oxidant damage measured. Supplementation of smokers with vitamin C (2 g/day) reduced elevated levels of urinary isoprostanes, a measure of in vivo lipid peroxidation (Reilly et al., 1996). This is consistent with earlier findings that either endogenous or in vitro added ascorbic acid uniquely protected plasma lipids against oxidative damage caused by cigarette smoke (Frei et al., 1991). Large doses of vitamin C (1 g/day or more) provided protection against lymphocyte DNA strand break damage induced ex vivo by radiation with H_2O_2 (hydrogen peroxide) (Green et al., 1994;

Panayiotidis and Collins, 1997). Endogenous DNA strand breaks (in the absence of added H_2O_2) were not different between smokers and nonsmokers; however, DNA damage due to ex vivo H_2O_2 addition was significantly greater in smokers than in nonsmokers. Vitamin C at 1 g/day decreased ex vivo DNA damage by about 20 percent in both groups (Panayiotidis and Collins, 1997).

A few studies have shown no effect of smoking or vitamin C supplementation on oxidizable biomolecules (Marangon et al., 1997, 1998). Supplementation of 21 male smokers with 500 mg/day of vitamin C for 2 months had no effect on urinary excretion of 8-hydroxy-7, 8-dihydro-2'-deoxyguanosine (8-oxodG), a product of oxidative DNA damage (Prieme et al., 1997).

Endothelial and Hemostatic Dysfunction

Smokers also suffer from endothelial and hemostatic dysfunctions that are reported to be ameliorated by vitamin C. Some evidence suggests that ascorbate in neurons modulates synthesis of the vasodilator nitric oxide (NO) (Millar, 1995). Since endothelium-dependent, but not endothelium-independent, vasodilation was improved by vitamin C administration in smokers, Heitzer et al. (1996) concluded that vitamin C acts to decrease oxidative stress within the vasculature of smokers by directly scavenging reactive oxygen species (ROS), thereby protecting the endogenous vasodilator NO, among other hypothesized effects. Vitamin C in physiological amounts has been shown to increase by threefold the synthesis of NO by human endothelial cells in culture (Heller et al., 1999). Motoyama et al. (1997) reported that vitamin C infusion improved impaired endothelium-dependent vasodilation in the brachial arteries of smokers, along with a decrease in plasma thiobarbitutic acid reactive substances (TBARS), a nonspecific measure of lipid peroxidation. Smokers with low levels of plasma vitamin C compared to nonsmokers also had increased monocyte adhesion to endothelial cells, which was normalized to that of nonsmokers after oral supplementation with 2 g/day of vitamin C (Weber et al., 1996). A mechanism for the effect of vitamin C on diminishing leukocyte or platelet adhesion and aggregation in smokers is suggested by findings in hamsters, in which the vitamin decreases formation of oxidized phospholipids that induce intravascular adhesion, aggregation, and inflammation (Lehr et al., 1997).

Pregnancy

Cigarette smoking also promotes oxidant damage and disturbs vitamin C nutriture in pregnant women. Although vitamin C intakes and serum concentrations were not different between third trimester smokers compared to nonsmokers; breath ethane, a measure of lipid peroxidation, was increased in the smokers and correlated inversely with serum vitamin C in the smokers but not the nonsmokers (Schwarz et al., 1995). There are more than 10^{15} organic free radicals per puff in gas-phase cigarette smoke (Pryor, 1992). Given the time elapsed between the last cigarette smoked and the breath collection as well as the absence of correlation between breath ethane values and hours since the last cigarette smoked, the breath ethane in pregnant smokers was thought to originate from peroxidation of the smoker's body lipids rather than the smoke itself. In Spanish women in their third trimester, serum vitamin C levels were not different between smokers and nonsmokers, but vitamin C levels were lower in the smokers' milk after parturition (Ortega et al., 1998).

Environmental Tobacco Smoke

Increased oxidative stress and ascorbate turnover have also been shown in nonsmoking individuals who are regularly exposed to tobacco smoke in their environment. Environmental or sidestream tobacco smoke provokes oxidant damage similar to mainstream cigarette smoke (Bermudez et al., 1994; Pryor et al., 1983). Plasma ascorbate concentrations of passive smokers were intermediate between those of active smokers and nonsmokers who were not exposed to environmental tobacco smoke, despite similar vitamin C intakes (Tribble et al., 1993). Hypovitaminosis C (plasma ascorbate concentrations less than 23 μmol/L [0.5 mg/dL]) was found in 24 percent of the active smokers and 12 percent of passive smokers and indicated that both passive and active smoke exposure lowered body ascorbate pools. Exposure of nonsmokers to secondhand smoke for 30 minutes in a smoke-filled room resulted in a significant decline in serum ascorbate, increased lipid peroxidation, and oxidatively modified low-density lipoprotein (LDL) (Valkonen and Kuusi, 1998). Although the above data are insufficient to estimate a special requirement for nonsmokers regularly exposed to tobacco smoke, these individuals are urged to ensure that they meet the Recommended Dietary Allowance (RDA) for vitamin C.

Gender

In both observational and intervention studies, human plasma or serum ascorbate levels are usually found to be higher in females than in males of the same population. Serum ascorbate concentrations of adult females aged 19 and older were greater than those of males in the same age category as reported in the Third National Health and Nutrition Examination Survey (NHANES III) (Appendix Table F-1). A minority of studies has reported no gender difference in plasma vitamin C levels (Johnston and Thompson, 1998). Although the reported gender differences in blood vitamin C concentrations may be attributed in part to differences in vitamin C intake, studies of elderly populations show that the difference exists over a wide range of vitamin C intakes and remains significant when males and females consuming similar amounts of the vitamin are compared (Garry et al., 1982; Itoh et al., 1989; Jacob et al., 1988; VanderJagt et al., 1987). In a population of elderly English adults (75 years and older), higher fruit consumption by women contributed to but did not entirely account for their higher plasma and leukocyte ascorbate levels compared to men (Burr et al., 1974). However, the latter finding of higher leukocyte ascorbate in women compared to men was not confirmed in a subsequent study, which found no gender differences in leukocyte ascorbate concentrations (Evans et al., 1982).

Part of the gender difference could be attributed to the larger body and fat-free mass of men compared to women (Baker et al., 1962; Blanchard, 1991a,b; Jacob et al., 1987a). However, since differences in fat-free mass accounted for only 10 to 31 percent of the variation in plasma vitamin C parameters, other unknown gender-related variables such as hormonal or metabolic effects are needed to explain fully the observed gender differences in vitamin C metabolism (Blanchard, 1991a). The differences are not explained by renal handling of ascorbic acid, since renal clearance parameters of ascorbic acid for both young and elderly adults showed no gender-related differences (Oreopoulos et al., 1993).

Overall, the data indicate that women maintain higher plasma ascorbate levels than men at a given vitamin C intake. Although studies were not found that directly compare the vitamin C requirements for men and women, a difference in average vitamin C requirements of men and women is assumed based on mean differences in body size, total body water, and lean body mass.

FINDINGS BY LIFE STAGE AND GENDER GROUP

Infants Ages 0 through 12 Months

Method Used to Set the Adequate Intake

No functional criteria of vitamin C status have been demonstrated that reflect response to dietary intake in infants. Thus, recommended intakes of vitamin C are based on an Adequate Intake (AI) that reflects the observed mean vitamin C intake of infants fed principally with human milk.

Human Milk. Human milk is recognized as the optimal milk source for infants throughout at least the first year of life; it is recommended as the sole nutritional milk source for infants during the first 4 to 6 months of life (IOM, 1991). Therefore determination of the AI for vitamin C for infants is based on data from infants fed human milk as the principal fluid during the periods 0 through 6 months and 7 through 12 months of age. The AI is set at the mean value for observed intakes as determined from studies in which the intake of human milk was measured by test weighing volume and the intake of food was determined by dietary records.

A number of reports of vitamin C content of human milk are available (Table 5-9). In mothers not taking vitamin C supplements, vitamin C in human milk in the first 6 months of lactation varied from 34 mg/L (Bates et al., 1982) to 83 mg/L (Byerley and Kirksey, 1985). In mothers taking vitamin C supplements ranging from 45 to greater than 1,000 mg/day, vitamin C content of human milk varied from 45 to 115 mg/L (Byerley and Kirksey, 1985; Udipi et al., 1985). Thus, the influence of maternal vitamin C intake and its effect on the vitamin C content of human milk are inconclusive (Byerley and Kirksey, 1985; Sneed et al., 1981; Thomas et al., 1979, 1980). The vitamin C content of human milk appears to decline during the first year of life so that by the twelfth month of lactation the vitamin C content is about 8 to 12 percent lower (Karra et al., 1986; Salmenpera, 1984).

In a study of infantile vitamin C intake during prolonged lactation, mean human milk vitamin C concentration decreased from 49.7 ± 10.6 mg/L (SD) at at 4 months of lactation to 44.6 ± 5.6 mg/L (SD) at 9 months of lactation (Salmenpera, 1984). Calculated from the milk concentrations and volumes, the average daily vitamin C intake by these infants was 36 mg/day at 4 and 6 months, and 42 mg/day at 9 months. The plasma concentrations of vitamin C of all infants studied were in the normal range, greater than 34 μmol/ L (0.6 mg/dL) indicating that exclusively human milk-fed infants are well protected against vitamin C deficiency.

Ages 0 through 6 Months. The AI for infants 0 through 6 months is based on the average volume of milk intake of 0.78 L/day (Allen et al., 1991; Butte et al., 1984; Heinig et al., 1993), and an average concentration of vitamin C in human milk of 50 mg/L. This is the average vitamin C content of mature milk as assessed by Salmenpera (1984), Sneed et al. (1981), and George and De Francesca (1989) and is in the range of vitamin C content measured in the other studies (Table 5-9). Multiplying this amount by the average intake of human milk at 0 through 6 months, the AI would be 50 mg/L × 0.78 L/day = 39 mg/day vitamin C. Therefore the AI for vitamin C for infants 0 through 6 months of age is 40 mg/day, after rounding.

This amount is lower than the median intake of 75 mg/day of vitamin C for infants 1 through 6 months as reported in the U.S. Department of Agriculture 1994–1996 Continuing Survey of Food Intake by Individuals (CSFII) where intake data ranged from 4 to 273 mg, (Appendix Table D-1). The latter figure is probably higher than that calculated for an infant fed human milk because the data in CSFII are based on consumption of infant formula plus solid food, and the vitamin C content of proprietary infant formulas is approximately 50 mg/L (FDA, 1985). However, the proposed AI is comparable to vitamin C intakes from human milk-fed German infants whose median intakes were 41 mg/day at 6 months of age (Alexy et al., 1999). These figures are much higher than the amount of vitamin C shown to protect infants from scurvy (7 mg/day) in early studies determining amounts necessary to prevent deficiencies (Goldsmith, 1961; Rajalakshmi et al., 1965; Van Eekelen, 1953).

Ages 7 through 12 Months. During the second 6 months of life, solid foods become a more important part of the infant diet and add a significant but poorly defined amount of vitamin C to the diet. Although limited data are available for typical vitamin C intakes from foods by infants fed human milk, mean vitamin C intakes from solid foods are 22 mg/day for formula-fed infants (Montalto et al., 1985). For purposes of developing an AI for this age group, it is assumed that infants who are fed human milk have intakes of solid food similar to formula-fed infants of the same age group (Specker et al., 1997). Based on data of Dewey et al. (1984), mean human milk intake during the second 6 months of life would be 0.6 L/day. Thus, vitamin C intake from human milk with a vita-

TABLE 5-9 Vitamin C Content in Human Milk

Reference	Stage of Lactation (mg/d)	Vitamin C Content in Milk (mg/L)	Maternal Vitamin C Intake (mg/d)
Thomas et al., 1979	1 and 6 wk pp[a]	68[b] 73[b]	190 (diet only) 148 (diet) + 90 (supplement)
Thomas et al., 1980[c]	6 mo pp	35.2 ± 12.0 (SD[d]) 38.4 ± 12.3 (SD)	131 (diet only) 153 (diet) + 90 (supplement)
Sneed et al., 1981	1 and 6 wk pp	57[b] 68[b]	118 (diet only)[b] 108 (diet) + 90 (supplement)
Bates et al., 1982	Not Reported	34 45	No diet intake data reported 35 as supplement
Salmenpera, 1984	3–4 d pp 2 mo 4 mo 6 mo 9 mo 12 mo	61.8 ± 0.99 (SD) 59.1 ± 1.18 (SD) 49.7 ± 1.06 (SD) 46.8 ± 1.02 (SD) 44.6 ± 0.56 (SD) 41.4 ± 1.13 (SD)	48–277 (mean 138) (no supplements were taken)
Byerley and Kirksey, 1985[c]	7–13 wk lactation	83.3 104.1 114.7	<100 100–999 1,000
Udipi et al., 1985	1–6 d lactation 7–10 d 13–15 d 20–22 d 28–31 d	90[b] 95[b] 105[b] 120[b] 115[b]	198, range 60–270 (extradietary intake only)
Karra et al., 1986	7–12 mo lactation	90[b]	Not reported

[a] pp = postpartum.

[b] Values were estimated from graphs.

[c] Lack of correlation between maternal intake and breast milk concentration of vitamin C in human milk.

[d] SD = standard deviation.

Methods

$n = 17$ healthy women, aged 18–35 y
Intake was analyzed based on three 4-d diet records.
There was no significant difference in milk content between the two groups.
Plasma vitamin C levels were significantly lower at 7 d pp in the unsupplemented group; at 6 weeks, there was no difference. Serum concentrations were lower in the supplemented group

$n = 12$ healthy women, aged 18–35 y
Intake based on 4-d diet records

$n = 16$ low-socioeconomic women; aged 18–32 y
Intake was analyzed based on two 4-d diet records.
There was no significant difference in milk content between the two groups.
Also measured plasma concentration of ascorbic acid—found no significant difference

$n = 168$ Gambian women

$n = 200$ healthy nonsmoking mothers and full-term infants
Infants were exclusively fed human milk for at least 3 mo (range 3–12 mo)
Intake based on 7-d food records kept by a subset of mothers
Milk volumes (mL/d) based on 3-d averages were
calculated:
790 (510–1,120) at 4 mo lactation
800 (500–1,025) at 6 mo lactation
890 (655–1,100) at 9 mo lactation

$n = 25$ healthy women aged 20–36 yrs, and their infants
Milk concentration was calculated from estimates of the volume of milk intake of infants and infant intake of vitamin C

$n = 12$ healthy women; aged 21–35 y
Found significantly lower milk concentration on days 1–6 than on days 13–15 and 28–31

$n = 55$ women; aged 21–38 y
Found 8% decrease in Vit C milk levels between 7 and 12 mo lactation

min C concentration of about 45 mg/L at 9 months (the midpoint of this age group) of lactation (Salmenpera, 1984) would be approximately 27 mg/day. Adding the intake from milk (27 mg/day) and food (22 mg/day), the total AI for vitamin C is rounded to 50 mg/day.

An alternative method to calculate vitamin C intake is to use the method described in Chapter 3 to extrapolate from the AI for infants ages 0 through 6 months who receive human milk. Utilizing this method, the AI for the older infants is rounded up to 50 mg/day of vitamin C. This is comparable to the value calculated above utilizing human milk and solid food.

The 1994 to 1996 CSFII data for infants 7 through 12 months of age ranged from 21 to 293 mg/day, with median 106 mg/day of vitamin C (Appendix Table D-1).

Vitamin C AI Summary, Ages 0 through 12 Months

AI for Infants
0–6 months	**40 mg (227 μmol)/day of vitamin C**	**≈6 mg/kg**
7–12 months	**50 mg (256 μmol)/day of vitamin C**	**≈6 mg/kg**

Children and Adolescents Ages 1 through 18 Years

Evidence Considered in Estimating the Average Requirement

No direct data were found on which to base an Estimated Average Requirement (EAR) for vitamin C for children ages 1 through 18 years. In the absence of additional information, and because vitamin C is a water-soluble vitamin and males have a larger lean body mass and total body water than women, EARs for children and adolescents have been estimated on the basis of relative body weight as described in Chapter 3 using reference weights from Chapter 1 (Table 1-1).

The Recommended Dietary Allowances (RDAs) estimated below for children 1 through 13 years of age are lower than the AIs calculated above for infants 0 through 12 months of age. The reason an AI may be higher than an RDA lies in the way they are determined (see "Differences Between the AI and the RDA" in Chapter 1). The AI is based on data on milk composition and volume of milk consumed to calculate an adequate intake of infants. The vitamin C RDA, in the case of 1- through 13-year-old children, is based on assumed differences in body weight from adults for whom there are some data. Thus, the data that are utilized to estimate the AI and RDA are different and cannot be compared.

Vitamin C EAR and RDA Summary, Ages 1 through 18 Years

EAR for Children

1–3 years	13 mg (74 µmol)/day of vitamin C
4–8 years	22 mg (125 µmol)/day of vitamin C

EAR for Boys

9–13 years	39 mg (222 µmol)/day of vitamin C
14–18 years	63 mg (358 µmol)/day of vitamin C

EAR for Girls

9–13 years	39 mg (222 µmol)/day of vitamin C
14–18 years	56 mg (318 µmol)/day of vitamin C

The RDA for vitamin C is set by assuming a coefficient of variation (CV) of 10 percent (see Chapter 1) because information is not available on the standard deviation of the requirement for vitamin C; the RDA is defined as equal to the EAR plus twice the CV to cover the needs of 97 to 98 percent of the individuals in the group (therefore, for vitamin C the RDA is 120 percent of the EAR). The calculated values for RDAs have been rounded to the nearest 5 mg.

RDA for Children

1–3 years	15 mg (85 µmol)/day of vitamin C
4–8 years	25 mg (142 µmol)/day of vitamin C

RDA for Boys

9–13 years	45 mg (256 µmol)/day of vitamin C
14–18 years	75 mg (426 µmol)/day of vitamin C

RDA for Girls

9–13 years	45 mg (256 µmol)/day of vitamin C
14–18 years	65 mg (370 µmol)/day of vitamin C

Adults Ages 19 through 50 Years

Evidence Considered in Estimating the Average Requirement

Although it is known that the classic disease of severe vitamin C deficiency, scurvy, is rare in the United States and Canada, other human experimental data that can be utilized to set a vitamin C requirement, based on a biomarker other than scurvy, are limited. Values recommended here are based on an amount of vitamin C that is thought to provide antioxidant protection as derived from the correlation of such protection with neutrophil ascorbate concentrations.

It is recognized that there are no human data to quantify directly the dose-response relationship between vitamin C intake and in vivo antioxidant protection. In addition, only one study (Levine et al., 1996a) with seven apparently healthy males reported plasma, neutrophil, and urinary ascorbate concentrations during vitamin C depletion and repletion to steady state. Thus, there are wide uncertainties in the data utilized to estimate the vitamin C requirements. However, in the absence of other data, maximal neutrophil concentration with minimal urinary loss appears to be the best biomarker at the present time. It must be emphasized that research is urgently needed to explore the use of other biomarkers to assess vitamin C requirements.

Antioxidant Protection

The evidence summarized in the preceding sections indicates that vitamin C functions in vivo to scavenge reactive oxidants in activated leukocytes, lung, and gastric mucosa, and to protect against lipid peroxidation. Therefore, the determination of an EAR for vitamin C is based on an amount estimated to provide antioxidant protection. Evidence summarized in the earlier section "Antioxidant Functions in Leukocytes" indicates that the vitamin's antioxidant function in leukocytes, which includes neutrophils, lymphocytes, and monocytes, is especially important. In addition, studies with guinea pigs and monkeys show that the concentration of ascorbate in the leukocytes more accurately reflects liver and body pool ascorbate than does the concentration in plasma or erythrocytes (Omaye et al., 1987). The vitamin is transported into leukocytes by an energy-dependent transport system that concentrates the vitamin some 25, 40, and 80 times higher than plasma levels in neutrophils, platelets, and lymphocytes, respectively (Evans et al., 1982; Jacob et al., 1992; Levine et al., 1996a).

The cells actively concentrate the vitamin, which serves as a cellular reservoir of reducing capacity and scavenges damaging phagocyte-derived oxidants such as superoxide and myeloperoxidase-derived hypochlorus acid (HOCl) and reactive nitrogen species (RNS). In both the cell-free and the activated neutrophil systems described earlier, the protection of α-1-antiprotease against inactivation by HOCl (Halliwell et al., 1987) and the inhibition of superoxide production (Anderson and Lukey, 1987) were directly proportional to ascorbate concentrations within the normal range of plasma ascorbate concentrations (22 to 85 μmol/L [0.4 to 1.5 mg/dL]). Data plotted in Figure 5-2 show that superoxide production by activated neutrophils was inhibited 29, 44, 52, and 55 percent by extracellular ascorbate concentrations of 28, 57, 114, and 284 μmol/

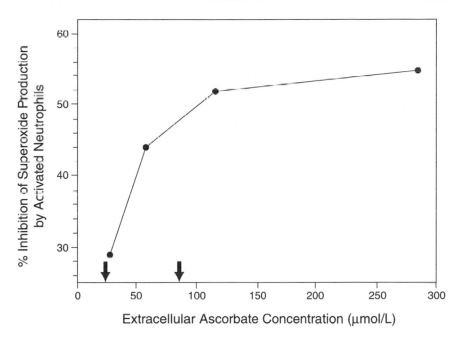

FIGURE 5-2 The effect of varying extracellular ascorbate concentrations on inhibition of superoxide produced by activated neutrophils. The range of normal human plasma ascorbate concentrations is shown within the arrows.
SOURCE: Adapted from Anderson and Lukey (1987).

L (0.5, 1.1, 2.2, and 5.0 mg/dL), respectively, without any effect on intracellular bacterial killing (Anderson and Lukey, 1987). This indicates that antioxidant protection is increasingly provided as ascorbate concentrations increase, with the greatest change in protection seen for ascorbate concentrations between 28 and 57 μmol/L (0.5 and 1.0 mg/dL).

Although similar dose-response data for leukocyte ascorbate levels are not available, the limited data from Levine et al. (1996a), seen in Figures 5-3 and 5-4, show that plasma and neutrophil ascorbate concentrations are both directly related to vitamin intake between about 50 and 90 mg/day. The concentrations were measured by a sensitive high-pressure liquid chromatography assay with electrochemical detection. Therefore, increasing neutrophil ascorbate concentrations within this range should provide for increased protection against phagocyte-derived oxidant damage.

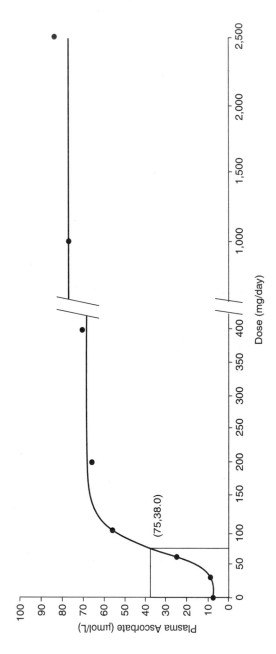

FIGURE 5-3 Steady-state plateau ascorbic acid concentrations (μmol/L) in plasma as a function of daily dose. Values are the means of plateau ascorbic acid concentrations from up to seven volunteers. SOURCE: Adapted from Levine et al. (1996a).

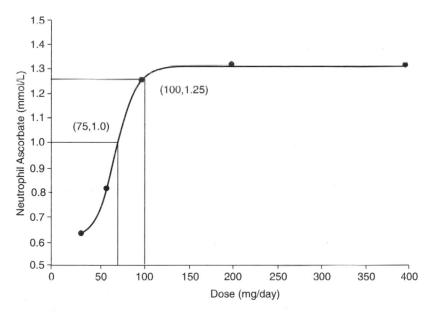

FIGURE 5-4 Neutrophil ascorbic acid concentrations (mmol/L) as a function of dose.
SOURCE: Adapted from Levine et al. (1996a).

There are no data to quantify directly the dose-response relation between vitamin C intake and in vivo antioxidant protection. Therefore, the criterion chosen for the EAR is the vitamin C intake that maintains near-maximal neutrophil vitamin C concentrations with minimal urinary loss. Since leukocyte ascorbate, which includes neutrophil ascorbate, correlates well with liver and body pool ascorbate (Omaye et al., 1987), this criterion should provide for adequate in vivo antioxidant protection to body tissues while minimizing excess urinary vitamin excretion. Vitamin C intakes greater than the urinary excretion threshold provide little or no increase in the ascorbate body pool (Baker et al., 1969; Kallner et al., 1979). A vitamin C intake that meets the above criteria is estimated from a controlled vitamin C dose-response study described below.

Depletion-Repletion Study

The requirement for vitamin C based on the above criteria can be estimated from the data reported by Levine et al. (1996a) in which plasma, neutrophil, and urinary ascorbate concentrations were determined during vitamin C depletion and repletion to steady-state. The rigorous criteria for achieving steady-state plasma concentrations (five daily samples that varied less than or equal to 10 percent) make the Levine et al. (1996a) data unique among depletion-repletion studies.

Seven apparently healthy male volunteers, aged 20 to 26 years, were studied as in-patients for 4 to 6 months. Subjects were depleted by being fed a diet containing less than 5 mg/day vitamin C. Depletion was defined as completed when plasma vitamin C concentrations ranged from 5 to 10 μmol/L (0.1 to 0.2 mg/dL) without signs or symptoms of scurvy. For repletion, seven consecutive doses of vitamin C (30, 60, 100, 200, 400, 1,000, and 2,500 mg/day) were given sequentially until steady-state plasma and leukocyte (neutrophils, monocytes, and lymphocytes) vitamin C concentrations were achieved at each dosage. The results for plasma and neutrophil concentrations can be seen in Figures 5-3 and 5-4, and Table 5-10.

As seen in Figure 5-4 and Table 5-10, the ascorbate saturation concentration in neutrophils was approximately 1.3 mmol/L. This was attained by four of the seven subjects at a vitamin C intake of 100 mg/day. Monocytes and lymphocytes also reached maximum concentrations at 100 mg/day (Levine et al., 1996a). However, at neutrophil saturation, about 25 percent of the doses were excreted in the urine, whereas at 60 percent of maximum ascorbate (dose of 60 mg/day), essentially no ascorbate was excreted.

No data from the Levine at al. (1996a) study are available for vitamin C intakes between 60 and 100 mg/day. However, because 60 percent of maximal ascorbate concentration in neutrophils would provide less antioxidant protection than 80 or 100 percent (Figure 5-2) (Anderson and Lukey, 1987), and since 25 percent of the dose is excreted at 100 percent of maximum neutrophil ascorbate concention, the midpoint 80 percent of maximum (1.0 mmol/L) was chosen. This is assuming that antioxidant protection in this range is linear. This point should better estimate an approximate neutrophil target concentration that fulfills the criteria of adequate in vivo antioxidant protection with little or no urinary loss. From the equation of Figure 5-4, 80 percent of maximal neutrophil concentration (1.0 mmol/L) is equivalent to a vitamin C intake of about 75 mg/day. This represents an EAR, because 80 percent (1.0 mmol/L) neutrophil concentration is an average value, estimated by regression analysis, for the men consuming 75 mg/day of vitamin C as shown in Table 5-10.

TABLE 5-10 Intracellular Ascorbic Acid Concentration in Neutrophils of Depleted Subjects Given Increasing Doses of Vitamin C (mmol/L)

Subject		Dose							
		30 mg	60 mg	75 mg[a]	100 mg	200 mg	400 mg	1,000 mg	2,500 mg
1	Mean	0.60	0.96	1.15	1.36	1.32	1.26	1.36	–
	SD[b]	0.01	0.01		0.02	0.03	0.50	0.03	–
2	Mean	0.42	0.50	0.67	1.13	1.24	1.12	1.63	–
	SD	0.01	0.02		0.06	0.05	0.08	0.15	–
3	Mean	1.18	0.83	1.19	1.33	1.43	–	–	–
	SD	0.30	0.50		0.10	0.90	–	–	–
4	Mean	0.58	0.75	1.03	1.35	1.11	1.56	1.23	1.28
	SD	0.03	0.04		0.10	0.05	0.06	0.08	1.12
5	Mean	0.57	1.10	1.21	1.30	–	1.40	1.48	1.44
	SD	0.02	0.05		0.03	–	0.05	0.11	0.13
6	Mean	0.61	0.93	1.01	1.24	–	0.96	0.95	–
	SD	0.01	0.03		0.05	–	0.14	0.16	–
7	Mean	0.42	0.54	0.77	1.02	1.46	–	1.23	–
	SD	0.01	0.02		0.05	0.12	–	0.06	–
	Average	0.63	0.81	1.00	1.25	1.31	1.26	1.31	1.36
	SD	0.26	0.20		0.12	0.13	0.23	0.21	0.80

[a] These values are neutrophil ascorbate concentrations corresponding to an intake of 75 mg/d calculated for each individual by regression analysis.
[b] SD = standard deviation.
SOURCE: Levine et al. (1996b).

Relevancy of Above EAR to Other Possible Vitamin C Biomarkers

Scurvy. As discussed earlier, scurvy occurs at plasma concentrations of less than 10 µmol/L. At an EAR of 75 mg/day, scurvy would be prevented for more than a month if vitamin C ingestion were to cease suddenly (Levine et al., 1996b).

Body Pool Saturation. Kallner et al. (1979) previously reported that the body pool of vitamin C was saturated at an intake of 100 mg/day in healthy non-smoking men; thus, an average intake at the EAR of 75 mg/day would not provide body pool saturation of vitamin C.

Antioxidant Role. At a vitamin C intake of 90 mg/day, the plasma ascorbate concentration reaches 50 µmol/L which has been shown to inhibit LDL oxidation in vitro in both cellular and cell free systems (Jialal et al., 1990). Although it is not known whether vitamin C prevents LDL oxidation in vivo, if it does this might be relevant in the prevention of heart disease (Jialal et al., 1990). Also, as discussed earlier, since neutrophils are at 80 percent saturation at an EAR of 75 mg/day, this should potentially protect intracellular proteins from oxidative injury when these cells are activated during infectious and inflammatory processes (Anderson and Lukey, 1987; Halliwell et al., 1987).

Plasma Vitamin C Concentrations. Based on data from the Third National Health and Nutrition Examination Survey (NHANES III), although more than 75 percent of adult men have dietary vitamin C intakes higher than the EAR of 75 mg/day (Appendix Table C-1), only 50 percent have plasma vitamin C concentrations greater than 38 µmol/L (0.67 mg/dL) (Appendix Table F-1). This plasma concentration is estimated from the data of Levine et al. (1996a) to correspond to an intake of 75 mg/day of vitamin C (Figure 5-3). This finding is not surprising since the NHANES III vitamin C plasma concentrations are for both smokers and nonsmokers, and it is known that plasma vitamin C concentrations are reduced by about 40 percent in male smokers (Pelletier, 1977; Weber et al., 1996). In addition, as discussed in the earlier section "Environmental Tobacco Smoke," exposure of nonsmokers to environmental tobacco smoke can result in a decline in plasma ascorbate concentrations (Tribble et al., 1993; Valkonen and Kuusi, 1998). Findings from the first three years (1988 to 1991) of NHANES III indicate that 38 percent of the participants were smokers and an additional 23 percent were nonsmokers exposed to environmental tobacco smoke at home or work (Pirkle et al., 1996).

Vitamin C EAR and RDA Summary, Ages 19 through 50 Years

Based on vitamin C intakes sufficient to maintain near-maximal neutrophil concentrations with minimal urinary loss, the data of Levine et al. (1996a) support an EAR of 75 mg/day of vitamin C for men. Since the data were based on men and no similar data are available for women at the present time, it is assumed that women will have a lower requirement due to their smaller lean body mass, total body water, and body size. This assumption is supported by the findings previously discussed that women maintain higher plasma ascorbate concentrations than men at a given vitamin C intake. Thus, the requirement for women is extrapolated based on body weight differences from those established for men (see Table 1-1).

EAR for Men
    19–30 years   **75 mg (426 μmol)/day of vitamin C**
    31–50 years   **75 mg (426 μmol)/day of vitamin C**
EAR for Women
    19–30 years   **60 mg (341 μmol)/day of vitamin C**
    31–50 years   **60 mg (341 μmol)/day of vitamin C**

The RDA for vitamin C is set by assuming a coefficient of variation (CV) of 10 percent (see Chapter 1) because information is not available on the standard deviation of the requirement for vitamin C; the RDA is defined as equal to the EAR plus twice the CV to cover the needs of 97 to 98 percent of the individuals in the group (therefore, for vitamin C the RDA is 120 percent of the EAR). Due to the many assumptions and approximations involved, the RDA for women is rounded up to 75 mg from its calculated value of 72 mg/day.

RDA for Men
    19–30 years   **90 mg (511 μmol)/day of vitamin C**
    31–50 years   **90 mg (511 μmol)/day of vitamin C**
RDA for Women
    19–30 years   **75 mg (426 μmol)/day of vitamin C**
    31–50 years   **75 mg (426 μmol)/day of vitamin C**

Adults Ages 51 Years and Older

Evidence Considered in Estimating the Average Requirement

Some cross-sectional studies have shown that vitamin C status, as measured by plasma and leukocyte ascorbate concentrations, is lower in the elderly, especially institutionalized elderly, than in young adults (Burr et al., 1974; Cheng et al., 1985). Low blood vitamin C concentrations in institutionalized and chronically ill elderly were normalized to those of active elderly and young adults by increasing their dietary vitamin C intake, suggesting that the low levels were primarily due to poor intake (Newton et al., 1985). However, Davies et al. (1984) found that intestinal absorption of a 500-mg oral dose of ascorbic acid, as measured by urinary ascorbate excretion, was significantly less in elderly (mean age 83 years) than in younger subjects (mean age 22 years). Although this dose (500 mg/day) was about 5 times higher than the vitamin C intake of many elderly individuals, it prompted the suggestion that impaired intestinal absorption may be an important causative factor in low blood concentrations of vitamin C in the elderly.

However, other studies, both cross-sectional and longitudinal, of apparently healthy, well-nourished elderly populations in the United States have not found evidence of a greater incidence of vitamin C deficiency among the elderly compared to young adults and no decrease in plasma ascorbate with advancing age (Garry et al., 1982, 1987; Jacob et al., 1988). Measurement of plasma, leukocyte, and urine ascorbate concentrations in a series of studies in elderly and young men and women showed no differences due to age (Blanchard, 1991a; Blanchard et al., 1989, 1990a,b). These studies included pharmacokinetic measures related to vitamin C absorption, depletion, repletion, and renal clearance. Consistent with these findings, a later study that measured maximal renal tubular reabsorption and excretion thresholds of ascorbic acid in apparently healthy elderly and young adults found no differences in renal handling of the vitamin between the two groups (Oreopoulos et al., 1993).

Older age groups, both men and women, have decreased lean body mass compared to younger individuals and thus, potentially a lower requirement for vitamin C. However, the vitamin C requirement of the elderly may be increased due to the oxidative stress of inflammatory and infectious conditions often found in this population (Cheng et al., 1985). As previously discussed, older adults have similar or lower plasma ascorbate concentrations than young adults. Therefore, the estimated requirement for vitamin C for individuals 51 years and older will remain the same as that of the younger adult.

Vitamin C EAR and RDA Summary, Ages 51 Years and Older

In summary, no consistent differences in the absorption or metabolism of ascorbic acid due to aging have been demonstrated at median vitamin C intakes. This suggests that the reports of low blood vitamin C concentrations in elderly populations may be due to poor dietary intakes, chronic disease or debilitation, or other factors, rather than an effect of aging per se. Therefore, for the older adults, no additional vitamin C allowance beyond that of younger adults is warranted.

EAR for Men
51–70 years	**75 mg (426 µmol)/day of vitamin C**
>70 years	**75 mg (426 µmol)/day of vitamin C**

EAR for Women
      51–70 years   60 mg (341 μmol)/day of vitamin C
      >70 years   60 mg (341 μmol)/day of vitamin C

The RDA for vitamin C is set by assuming a coefficient of variation (CV) of 10 percent (see Chapter 1) because information is not available on the standard deviation of the requirement for vitamin C; the RDA is defined as equal to the EAR plus twice the CV to cover the needs of 97 to 98 percent of the individuals in the group (therefore, for vitamin C the RDA is 120 percent of the EAR). As with the RDA for younger women, the calculated RDA of 72 mg has been rounded up to 75 mg/day.

RDA for Men
      51–70 years   90 mg (511 μmol)/day of vitamin C
      >70 years   90 mg (511 μmol)/day of vitamin C
RDA for Women
      51–70 years   75 mg (426 μmol)/day of vitamin C
      >70 years   75 mg (426 μmol)/day of vitamin C

Pregnancy

Evidence Considered in Estimating the Average Requirement

Plasma vitamin C concentration decreases with the progression of pregnancy, probably secondary to hemodilution (Morse et al., 1975) as well as active transfer to the fetus (Choi and Rose, 1989). This decrease in plasma concentration has not been shown to be associated with poor pregnancy outcomes. The placenta apparently clears oxidized ascorbic acid from the maternal circulation and delivers it in the reduced form to the fetus (Choi and Rose, 1989). Ascorbic acid deficiency during pregnancy is associated with increased risk of infections, premature rupture of the membranes (Casanueva et al., 1993; Pfeffer et al., 1996), premature birth (Casanueva et al., 1993; Tlaskal and Novakova, 1990), and eclampsia (Jendryczko and Tomala, 1995). In addition, both serum and amniotic fluid concentrations of ascorbic acid are decreased in pregnant smokers compared to nonsmokers (Barrett et al., 1991).

Vitamin C EAR and RDA Summary, Pregnancy

Although the amount of vitamin C required by the growing fetus is unknown, it is known that maternal plasma vitamin C concentration decreases with the progression of pregnancy due to hemodilution as well as active transfer to the fetus. Therefore, in order to transfer adequate vitamin C to the fetus, additional vitamin C is needed during pregnancy. In the absence of data on near maximal neutrophil saturation during pregnancy, the method of determining the EAR for pregnancy is based on adding the EAR for near-maximal neutrophil concentration of the nonpregnant woman to the amount of vitamin C necessary to transfer adequate vitamin C to the fetus. In the absence of precise data regarding transfer of maternal vitamin C to the fetus, and with the knowledge that intakes of 7 mg/day of vitamin C will prevent young infants from developing scurvy (Goldsmith, 1961; Rajalakshmi et al., 1965; van Eekelen, 1953), the EAR for pregnancy was estimated to increase 10 mg/day over the vitamin C requirement for the nonpregnant woman.

EAR for Pregnancy
    14–18 years   **66 mg (375 µmol)/day of vitamin C**
    19–30 years   **70 mg (398 µmol)/day of vitamin C**
    31–50 years   **70 mg (398 µmol)/day of vitamin C**

The RDA for vitamin C is set by assuming a coefficient of variation (CV) of 10 percent (see Chapter 1) because information is not available on the standard deviation of the requirement for vitamin C; the RDA is defined as equal to the EAR plus twice the CV to cover the needs of 97 to 98 percent of the individuals in the group (therefore, for vitamin C the RDA is 120 percent of the EAR). The calculated values for the pregnancy RDA have been rounded up to the nearest 5 mg.

RDA for Pregnancy
    14–18 years   **80 mg (454 µmol)/day of vitamin C**
    19–30 years   **85 mg (483 µmol)/day of vitamin C**
    31–50 years   **85 mg (483 µmol)/day of vitamin C**

Special Considerations

Certain subpopulations of pregnant women may have increased requirements for vitamin C. This group includes users of street drugs and cigarettes, heavy users of alcohol, and regular users of aspirin (Flodin, 1988). Women who smoke more than 20 cigarettes per day may require twice as much vitamin C as nonsmokers to maintain a replete body pool of vitamin C (Kallner et al., 1981). It has been reported that plasma vitamin C in pregnant smokers exhibited an indirect correlation with the breath content of ethane, a volatile marker of lipid peroxidation, even though the pregnant women were receiving supplements with 320 mg/day of vitamin C (Schwarz et al., 1995). Thus, pregnant women in these special sub-populations should consume additional vitamin C.

Lactation

Evidence Considered in Estimating the Average Requirement

As indicated earlier, infants fed human milk are estimated to consume on average 40 mg/day vitamin C during the first 6 months of life. Salmenpera (1984) reported that the vitamin C intake of 47 mothers during prolonged lactation ranged from 48 to 277 mg/day, mean 138 mg/day. Three mothers in this study who consumed less than 100 mg/day of vitamin C demonstrated plasma ascorbate values below the lower limit of normal [less than 10 µmol/L (0.2 mg/dL)]. Women who consumed 100 to 199 mg/day of vitamin C produced milk with 100 mg/L of vitamin C (Byerley and Kirksey, 1985). Maternal vitamin C intake in excess of 200 mg/day resulted in increased urinary excretion of vitamin C but did not increase the content of the vitamin in human milk (Byerley and Kirksey, 1985). It is thought that a regulatory mechanism in the mammary gland prevents the elevation of milk vitamin C concentrations beyond that level seen when urinary execretion increases representing blood saturation (Byerley and Kirksey, 1985).

Vitamin C EAR and RDA Summary, Lactation

To estimate the EAR for lactation, the average vitamin C produced in milk, 40 mg/day during the first 6 months of lactation, is added to the EAR for the nonlactating women. Although the vitamin C content of human milk declines with length of lactation and milk volume declines with the addition of solid foods, the EAR is not decreased for longer periods of lactation.

EAR for Lactation
14–18 years	96 mg (545 µmol)/day of vitamin C
19–30 years	100 mg (568 µmol)/day of vitamin C
31–50 years	100 mg (568 µmol)/day of vitamin C

The RDA for vitamin C is set by assuming a coefficient of variation (CV) of 10 percent (see Chapter 1) because information is not available on the standard deviation of the requirement for vitamin C; the RDA is defined as equal to the EAR plus twice the CV to cover the needs of 97 to 98 percent of the individuals in the group (therefore, for vitamin C the RDA is 120 percent of the EAR).

RDA for Lactation

14–18 years	**115 mg (653 µmol)/day of vitamin C**
19–30 years	**120 mg (682 µmol)/day of vitamin C**
31–50 years	**120 mg (682 µmol)/day of vitamin C**

Special Considerations

Smokers

Evidence that smokers have lower vitamin C status than nonsmokers, even with comparable vitamin C intakes, is summarized in the preceding section "Factors Affecting the Vitamin C Requirement." The data also show that the metabolic turnover of ascorbate in smokers is about 35 mg/day greater than in nonsmokers (Kallner et al., 1981), apparently due to increased oxidative stress and other metabolic differences. These findings indicate that smokers need additional vitamin C to provide comparable nutriture to nonsmokers.

From analysis of NHANES II data on vitamin C intakes and serum concentrations, Schectman et al. (1991) estimated that the average intake of smokers needed to be at least 200 mg/day of vitamin C in order to attain serum ascorbate concentrations equivalent to those of nonsmokers who meet the 1989 RDA of 60 mg/day (NRC, 1989). Use of population survey data to estimate an increased ascorbate requirement for smokers is questionable, because the cause and significance of the observed differences in serum ascorbate concentrations between smokers and nonsmokers are largely unknown.

From in vitro data on the loss of ascorbate in plasma exposed to cigarette smoke, it was estimated that one cigarette may consume about 0.8 mg of ascorbate, or about 32 mg/day for a two-pack-a-day smoker (Cross and Halliwell, 1993). More precise data were obtained from an experimental study of 17 apparently healthy male smokers who were administered radiolabeled tracer ascorbic acid at steady-state intakes of 30 to 180 mg/day to allow kinetic calculations of ascorbate metabolism and body pools. Results were compared with a similar protocol for nonsmokers (Kallner et al., 1979, 1981). Metabolic turnover of the vitamin was about 35 mg/day greater in smokers than in nonsmokers. Thus, to obtain a near maximal steady-state ascorbate body pool equivalent to that of nonsmokers, smokers would require an additional 35 mg/day of vitamin C over that needed by nonsmokers.

Passive Smokers

Environmental or sidestream tobacco smoke provokes oxidant damage similar to mainstream cigarette smoke (Bermudez et al., 1994; Pryor et al., 1983). Hypovitaminosis C (plasma ascorbate concentrations less than 23 µmol/L [0.5 mg/dL]) was found in 24 percent of the active smokers and 12 percent of passive smokers and indicated that both passive and active smoke exposure lowered body ascorbate pools (Tribble et al., 1993). Exposure of nonsmokers to secondhand smoke for 30 minutes in a smoke-filled room resulted in a significant decline in serum ascorbate, increased lipid peroxidation, and oxidatively modified low-density lipoprotein (LDL) (Valkonen and Kuusi, 1998). Although the above data are insufficient to estimate a special requirement for nonsmokers regularly exposed to tobacco smoke, these individuals are urged to ensure that they meet the Recommended Dietary Allowance (RDA) for vitamin C.

Exercise and Stress

The role of ascorbate as a cofactor for biosynthesis of carnitine, steroid hormones, and neurotransmitters provides a theoretical basis for increased requirements of the vitamin in persons under excessive physical and emotional stress. Studies of vitamin C status and physical activity in humans have shown mixed results, such that no definitive conclusion regarding vitamin C and exercise can be derived (Keith, 1994). For example, Fishbaine and Butterfield (1984) reported that blood vitamin C was higher in runners compared to sedentary control subjects, while a later study found that the vitamin C status of highly trained athletes was not significantly different from control subjects (Rokitzki et al., 1994). A cross-sectional study of physical activity, fitness, and serum ascorbate in 1,600 apparently healthy Irish adults provided no evidence that active people had different ascorbate status than inactive, and thus no justification for supplementation of exercisers (Sharpe et al., 1994). No substantial evidence that mental or emotional stress increases vitamin C turnover or requirement in apparently healthy persons has been reported. In sum, none of the above types of stress has been demonstrated to affect the human requirement for vitamin C.

INTAKE OF VITAMIN C

Food Sources

Almost 90 percent of vitamin C in the typical diet comes from fruits and vegetables, with citrus fruits, tomatoes and tomato juice, and potatoes being major contributors (Sinha et al., 1993). Other sources include brussel sprouts, cauliflower, broccoli, strawberries, cabbage, and spinach. Vitamin C is also added to some processed foods as an antioxidant. Values for the vitamin C content of foods can vary depending on the growing conditions, season of the year, stage of maturity, location, cooking practices, and storage time prior to consumption (Erdman and Klein, 1982).

Dietary Intake

Data from nationally representative U.S. and Canadian surveys are available to estimate vitamin C intakes (Appendix Tables C-1, D-1, and E-1). In the United States, the median dietary intake of vitamin C by adult men from 1988 to 1994 was about 105 mg (596 µmol)/day and median total intake (including supplements, see Appendix Table C-2) is about 120 mg (682 µmol)/day. For women, the median intake was estimated to be 90 mg (511 µmol)/day and median total intake (including supplements) is about 108 mg (613 µmol)/day. (See Chapter 9 for vitamin C intake of men and women who smoke.) In Canada, the median dietary intake of vitamin C for adult men and woman was lower than in the United States with intake estimated to be about 70 mg (397 µmol)/day (Appendix Table E-1). Although most Americans consume fewer than the minimum of five daily servings of fruits and vegetables recommended by the U.S. Department of Agriculture and the National Cancer Institute, estimated median daily vitamin C consumption is above the Estmated Average Requirement (EAR). Five servings of most fruits and vegetables provide more than 200 mg (1,136 µmol)/day of vitamin C per day.

The Boston Nutritional Status Survey of the Elderly estimated that among this relatively advantaged group of people over aged 60, those who were not taking supplements had a median vitamin C intake of 132 mg/day for males and 128 mg/day for females (Hartz et al., 1992).

Intake from Supplements

Information from the Boston Nutritional Status Survey of the Elderly estimated that 35 and 44 percent of the males and females, respectively, took some form of vitamin C supplements; while 19 percent of males and 15 percent of females surveyed who took supplements had intakes greater than 1,000 mg (5,680 μmol)/day. Approximately 31 percent of all adults in one 1986 survey reported taking a vitamin C supplement (Moss et al., 1989). Total vitamin C intakes from food plus supplements from the Third National Health and Nutrition Examination Survey (NHANES III) are found in Appendix Table C-2.

TOLERABLE UPPER INTAKE LEVELS

The Tolerable Upper Intake Level (UL) is the highest level of daily nutrient intake that is likely to pose no risk of adverse health effects in almost all individuals. Although members of the general population should be advised not to exceed the UL routinely, intake above the UL may be appropriate for investigation within well-controlled clinical trials. In light of evaluating possible benefits to health, clinical trials of doses above the UL should not be discouraged, as long as subjects participating in these trials have signed informed consent documents regarding possible toxicity and as long as these trials employ appropriate safety monitoring of trial subjects. Also, the UL is not meant to apply to individuals who are receiving vitamin C under medical supervision.

Hazard Identification

Adverse Effects

Many people believe vitamin C to be nontoxic and beneficial to health; therefore, the vitamin is often taken in large amounts. There is no evidence suggesting that vitamin C is carcinogenic or teratogenic or that it causes adverse reproductive effects. Reviews of high vitamin C intakes have indicated low toxicity (Johnston, 1999); adverse effects have been reported primarily after very large doses (greater than 3 g/day). Data show little increase in plasma steady-state concentrations at intakes above 200 mg/day (Figure 5-3), and saturable intestinal absorption and renal tubular reabsorption data suggest that overload of ascorbic acid is unlikely in humans (Blanchard et al., 1997; Levine et al., 1996a). Possible adverse effects associated with very high intakes have been reviewed and include:

diarrhea and other gastrointestinal disturbances, increased oxalate excretion and kidney stone formation, increased uric acid excretion, pro-oxidant effects, systemic conditioning ("rebound scurvy"), increased iron absorption leading to iron overload, reduced vitamin B_{12} and copper status, increased oxygen demand, and erosion of dental enamel (Hornig and Moser, 1981; Rivers, 1987). The data on these adverse effects are reviewed below. The UL for vitamin C applies to intake from both food and supplements.

Gastrointestinal Effects. Gastrointestinal disturbances such as nausea, abdominal cramps, and diarrhea are the most common adverse effects of high vitamin C intake (Hoffer, 1971). These effects are attributed to the osmotic effect of unabsorbed vitamin C passing through the intestine. Intestinal absorption of ascorbic acid occurs by a saturable process (Rumsey and Levine, 1998; Tsao, 1997). The remainder is not absorbed and is eliminated in the stool. The evidence of gastrointestinal disturbances following high vitamin C intakes is primarily from uncontrolled case reports (Hoffer, 1971; Hoyt, 1980). However, some studies have been conducted to evaluate gastrointestinal effects. Cameron and Campbell (1974) reported diarrhea, transient colic, and flatulent distension in normal healthy volunteers at doses of 3 to 4 g/day. Another study, which evaluated the adverse effects of 1-, 5-, and 10-g/day supplemental ascorbate for 5 days in apparently healthy adults, reported diarrhea in 2 of 15 subjects at 10 g/day (Wandzilak et al., 1994). Stein et al. (1976) reported mild diarrhea in one of three subjects following ingestion of 4 g of ascorbic acid.

Increased Oxalate Excretion and Kidney Stone Formation. Controversy exists as to whether increased intake of vitamin C can significantly increase urinary excretion of oxalate and, therefore, lead to an increase in the potential for renal calcium oxalate stone formation. The findings from studies evaluating the effect of vitamin C intake (0.03 to 10 g/day) on urinary oxalate excretion in apparently healthy individuals are conflicting (Hughes et al., 1981; Lamden and Chrystowski, 1954; Levine et al., 1996a; Mitch et al., 1981; Schmidt et al., 1981; Tiselius and Almgard, 1977; Tsao and Salimi, 1984; Wandzilak et al., 1994). An intervention study by Hughes et al. (1981) reported significant increases in mean urinary oxalate excretion in 39 apparently healthy adults consuming 1, 3, 6, and 9 g/day of ascorbic acid. However, Tsao and Salimi (1984) reported normal plasma oxalate concentrations in healthy subjects ingesting 3–10 g/day of ascorbic acid for at least two years, and no significant change in urinary oxalate excretion in five of six subjects who consumed 10 g/day of vitamin C over 1 day. Levine et al. (1996a) showed increased urinary oxalate excretion in apparently healthy male volunteers consuming 1 g/day of ascorbic acid; however, mean oxalate concentrations remained within the reference range. None of these studies showed oxalate excretion above normal.

Reports of kidney stone formation associated with excess ascorbic acid intake are limited to individuals with renal disease (see Sauberlich, 1994 for a review). Data from epidemiological studies do not support an association between excess ascorbic acid intake and kidney stone formation in apparently healthy individuals (Curhan et al., 1996, 1999; Fellstrom et al., 1989). A prospective cohort study by Curhan et al. (1996) of 45,000 men aged 40 to 70 years with no history of renal calculi showed that vitamin C intake was not significantly associated with the risk of stone formation. In fact, the age-adjusted relative risk for men consuming 1,500 mg/day or more compared to less than 250 mg/day was 0.78. In addition, vitamin C intake was not associated with kidney stone formation in women (Curhan et al., 1999). The lack of findings on oxalate excretion and kidney stone formation may be explained by the limited absorption of vitamin C at doses greater than 200 mg/day (Levine et al., 1996a). Because of the limited intestinal absorption, limited amounts of vitamin C are metabolized to oxalate in the urine. In addition, the large majority of excess absorbed vitamin C is excreted in the urine as ascorbic acid rather than its degradation products.

Increased Uric Acid Excretion. Similarly, the effect of high ascorbic acid intake on urate excretion has been studied (Berger et al., 1977; Fituri et al., 1983; Hatch et al., 1980; Herbert, 1978; Levine et al., 1996a; Mitch et al., 1981; Schmidt et al., 1981; Stein et al., 1976). Theoretically, increased uric acid excretion could be an important factor in the formation of uric acid stones especially in subjects who normally excrete large amounts of uric acid. The findings are conflicting. Levine et al. (1996a) reported significantly increased uric acid excretion above the normal range following ascorbic acid intakes of 1 g/day or more in 7 apparently healthy male subjects. Another study reported a 70 to 90 percent increase in the fractional clearance of uric acid following a single 4-g dose in nine subjects (Stein et al., 1976). Other studies have shown no significant effect of ascorbic acid intakes up to 12 g/day on uric acid excretion in apparently healthy subjects (Fituri et al., 1983; Hatch et al., 1980; Herbert, 1978; Mitch et al., 1981; Schmidt et al., 1981).

Excess Iron Absorption. Another possible adverse effect of high vitamin C intake is enhanced iron absorption leading to iron overload. Bendich and Cohen (1990) evaluated 24 studies to determine whether daily ascorbic acid intakes (ranging from 1 to 1,000 mg, with most in the 10- to 100-mg range) could increase iron stores above recommended levels in apparently healthy individuals. They found that vitamin C intakes did not increase the number of high iron absorbers, and limited data involving ascorbic acid intakes above 100 mg/day showed no change in iron absorption values. Another study by Cook et al. (1984) showed no increase in iron stores following vitamin C intakes up to 2 g/day (taken with meals for 20 months) in iron-replete subjects who consumed foods that contain iron. This suggests that vitamin C does not induce excess iron absorption in apparently healthy individuals. However, it is unknown if individuals with hereditary hemochromatosis, which affects between 1 in 200 and 1 in 400 persons of northern European descent (Bacon et al., 1999), could be adversely affected by long-term ingestion of large doses of vitamin C (McLaran et al., 1982).

Lowered Vitamin B_{12} Levels. An in vitro study showed that increasing destruction of vitamin B_{12} was associated with increasing vitamin C levels (Herbert and Jacob, 1974). However, when this study was performed using different analytical procedures, no loss of vitamin B_{12} was observed (Newmark et al., 1976). In a review of the stability of cobalamins under varying conditions, Hogenkamp (1980) found that only aquocobalamin was decreased and destroyed by ascorbic acid. Aquocobalamin is not a major cobalamin in biological tissues. Furthermore, results of in vivo studies in human subjects have shown that vitamin C intakes up to 4 g/day did not induce vitamin B_{12} deficiency (Afroz et al., 1975; Ekvall et al., 1981).

Systemic Conditioning. Evidence of systemic conditioning (the accelerated metabolism or excretion of ascorbic acid) exists from uncontrolled observations in humans following abrupt discontinuation of prolonged, high-dose vitamin C supplementation (Rhead and Schrauzer, 1971; Siegel et al., 1982). Omaye et al. (1986) showed increased turnover of plasma ascorbic acid in apparently healthy human adults who abruptly decreased their vitamin C intake from 605 to 5 mg/day. Two other studies showed that high intakes resulted in increased clearance but did not result in blood levels lower than normal (Schrauzer and Rhead, 1973; Tsao and Leung, 1988). Other studies have reported no rebound scurvy or excessive lowering of ascorbate blood levels after cessation of high intakes (Hoffer, 1973; Ludvigsson et al., 1979). Evidence that rebound scurvy may appear in infants whose mothers ingested large doses of vitamin C during pregnancy is limited to one anecdotal report of 2 infants (Cochrane, 1965). Overall, the evidence is inconsistent and does not suggest that systemic conditioning occurs to any significant extent in infants and adults.

Pro-oxidant Effects. Under certain conditions, ascorbate can act as a pro-oxidant by reducing iron and copper ions, which catalyze production of the hydroxyl radical via Fenton chemistry (Buettner and Jurkiewicz, 1996). The combination of ascorbic acid and redox-active (non-protein-bound) iron can promote lipid peroxidation in vitro (Laudicina and Marnett, 1990). In vivo however, iron is bound to proteins such as transferrin and ferritin and therefore is not normally available for such catalytic functions. Nevertheless, the strong pro-oxidant nature of the iron-ascorbate complex in vitro raises concern that consumption of vitamin C supplements by individuals with high iron stores may contribute to oxidative damage in vivo. In addition, dietary ascorbic acid can enhance the intestinal absorption of nonheme iron (Hallberg, 1985).

Concerns for a possible in vivo pro-oxidant effect of the iron-ascorbate couple were heightened by the report of a fatal cardiomyopathy in a patient with hemochromatosis who ingested excessive vitamin C (McLaran et al., 1982). Also, an association between myocardial infarctions and serum ferritin levels has been reported in a Finnish population (Salonen et al., 1992). Other studies have not supported the latter finding that high iron stores were associated with increased risk of heart disease (Baer et al., 1994) and have not indicated that excess vitamin C intakes have contributed significantly to iron overload or oxidant damage in normal healthy people. Controlled human studies in which supplemental vitamin C was added to the meals of apparently healthy adults for periods of up to 2 years showed little or no change in iron status measures including serum ferritin (Cook et al., 1984; Hunt et al., 1994). Data on iron-ascorbate combinations in the plasma of normal healthy adults and preterm infants with high plasma ascorbate levels showed that high plasma ascorbate concentrations in the presence of redox-active iron did not cause either lipid or protein oxidation. In addition, the endogenous ascorbate prevented rather than promoted lipid peroxidation in iron-overloaded plasma (Berger et al., 1997).

Similarly, concern for an in vivo pro-oxidant action of vitamin C in concert with copper has been suggested but not substantiated. Possible increased oxidant damage in premature infants had been attributed to the effect of high serum ascorbate levels inhibiting ceruloplasmin ferroxidase activity, thereby creating an excess of reactive ferrous ions (Powers et al., 1995). This result and other reports of ascorbate inhibition of ceruloplasmin ferroxidase activity (Gutteridge, 1991) have subsequently been attributed to an artifact of using a nonphysiological pH buffer in the ceruloplasmin ferroxidase assay (Løvstad, 1997).

Results of studies testing the effects of supplemental vitamin C intake on markers of oxidant damage to deoxyribonucleic acid (DNA) and chromosomes are discussed in an earlier section and are summarized in Tables 5-4, 5-5, and 5-6. The results are mixed, with studies showing a decrease, increase, or no change in oxidant damage measures. A study of 30 apparently healthy adults supplemented with 500 mg/day of vitamin C for 6 weeks reported an increase in 8-oxoadenine, but a decrease in the more mutagenic DNA lesion, 8-oxoguanine (Podmore et al., 1998). Supplementation of apparently healthy volunteers with vitamin C and iron resulted in increases in some DNA damage markers, decreases in others, and a rise in total DNA base damage at 6 weeks, which disappeared at 12 weeks (Rehman et al., 1998). Other evidence from in vitro and in vivo data as well as epidemiological studies have not shown increased oxidative DNA damage or increased cancer risk associated with high intakes of vitamin C (Block, 1991; Fontham, 1994; Fraga et al., 1991; Rifici and Khachadurian, 1993).

Other Adverse Effects. Other adverse effects observed following high vitamin C intakes include diminished high-altitude resistance (Schrauzer et al., 1975), delayed-type allergic response (Metz et al., 1980), and erosion of dental enamel (Giunta, 1983). Additional studies confirming these findings were not found.

Identification of Distinct and Highly Sensitive Subpopulations. Data show that individuals with hemochromatosis, glucose-6-phosphate dehydrogenase deficiency, and renal disorders may be susceptible to adverse effects from excess vitamin C intake. Vitamin C may enhance iron absorption and exacerbate iron-induced tissue damage in individuals with hemochromatosis (McLaran et al., 1982). Individuals with renal disorders may have increased risk of oxalate kidney stone formation from excess vitamin C intake (Auer et al., 1998; Ono, 1986; Urivetzky et al., 1992). Hemolysis has been associated with ascorbic acid administration in newborns with glucose-6-phosphate dehydrogenase deficiency and in normal premature infants (Ballin et al., 1988; Mentzer and Collier, 1975). There is also anecdotal evidence of hemolysis following ascorbic acid intake in adults with glucose-6-phosphate dehydrogenase deficiency (Campbell et al., 1975; Rees et al., 1993). However, a clinical study does not support the association (Beutler, 1991).

Summary

Based on considerations of causality, relevance, and the quality and completeness of the database, osmotic diarrhea and related gastrointestinal disturbances were selected as the critical endpoints on which to base a UL. The in vivo data do not clearly show a causal relationship between excess vitamin C intake by apparently healthy individuals and other adverse effects (i.e., kidney stone formation, excess iron absorption, reduced vitamin B_{12} and copper levels, increased oxygen demand, systemic conditioning, pro-oxidant effects, dental enamel erosion, or allergic response) in adults and children.

The data regarding possible vitamin C deficiency in two newborns resulting from abrupt withdrawal from mothers consuming high levels of vitamin C during pregnancy were considered too anecdotal and uncertain to warrant derivation of a separate UL for pregnant women.

Dose-Response Assessment

Adults

Data Selection. The data on osmotic diarrhea and gastrointestinal disturbances were selected as most relevant on which to base a UL for apparently healthy adults. The effects are generally not serious and are self-limiting; individuals experiencing them may easily eliminate them by reducing supplemental vitamin C intakes.

Identification of a No-Observed-Adverse-Effect Level (NOAEL) and Lowest-Observed-Adverse-Effect Level (LOAEL). A LOAEL of 3 g/day can be identified based on the data of Cameron and Campbell (1974). These investigators reported symptoms of flatulent distension, transient colic, and diarrhea at doses of 3 to 4 g/day in normal healthy volunteers (number of volunteers not stated). The volunteers increased oral ascorbic acid intake by increments of 1 g/day in successive weeks. Supporting evidence is provided by case reports (Hoffer, 1971; Hoyt, 1980), a graded dose study by Stein et al. (1976), and a multiple crossover study by Wandzilak et al. (1994). Stein et al. (1976) gave three patients 8 g/day in four divided doses of 2 g for 3 to 7 days. This study reported mild diarrhea in one of three subjects following ingestion of 4 g/day of ascorbic acid. Wandzilak et al. (1994) investigated the effect of high-dose ascorbic acid intake on 15 apparently healthy volunteers. Subjects ingested 1, 5, and 10 g/day supplemental ascorbate at mealtime for 5 days, separated by 5 days of no supplementation. This study reported diarrhea in 2 of the 15 subjects taking 10 g/day. These subjects were unable to continue at this dose

The above human data suggest that an intake of vitamin C greater than 3 g/day is likely to cause osmotic diarrhea in many individuals, although some reports involving a few individuals suggest this may occur at 3 g/day. Thus, the 3-g/day intake is considered a LOAEL.

Uncertainty Assessment. There is little uncertainty regarding the range of vitamin C intakes that are likely to induce osmotic diarrhea. An uncertainty factor (UF) of 1.5 was selected to extrapolate the LOAEL to a NOAEL. Thus, the 3 g/day intake is considered a LOAEL, and a NOAEL of 2 g/day is estimated for adult humans. Because the database has no other significant sources of uncertainty and because of the mild, reversible nature of osmotic diarrhea caused by high vitamin C intakes, no further uncertainty factors are necessary.

Derivation of a UL. The LOAEL of 3 g/day was divided by the UF of 1.5 to obtain a NOAEL and UL value of 2 g/day.

$$UL = \frac{LOAEL}{UF} = \frac{3\,g/day}{1.5} = 2\,g/day$$

Vitamin C UL Summary, Ages 19 Years and Older

UL for Adults
   19 years and older   2,000 mg (11,360 µmol)/day of vitamin C

Other Life Stage Groups

Infants. For infants, the UL was judged not determinable because of insufficient data on adverse effects in this age group and concern about the infant's ability to handle excess amounts. Potential concerns for high vitamin C concentrations in infants stem from isolated reports of anecdotal rebound scurvy, oxidative damage, and hemolysis (Ballin et al., 1988; Cochrane, 1965; Powers et al., 1995). To prevent high levels of intake, the only source of intake for infants should be that available from food and formula.

Children and Adolescents. Limited data exist on vitamin C toxicity in toddlers, children, and adolescents. Ludvigsson et al. (1977) conducted a double-blind, 7-week pilot study and a 3-month main study evaluating the prophylactic effect of 1,000 mg/day of vitamin C on colds in 172 and 642 children, respectively, ages 8 to 9 years. Reported side effects, including stomach pains, skin rash, headache, diarrhea, and nausea, were observed in about 3 percent of the children, which was no different from the control group and was not dose related. Therefore, this study could be used to support a NOA-EL of 1,000 mg/day.

Another study tested the effectiveness of a megavitamin regimen including 3 g/day of ascorbic acid for 3 months on attention deficit disorder (ADD) in 41 children ages approximately 7 to 11 years (Haslam et al., 1984). Forty-two percent of the children developed elevation of serum aminotransferases, and it was concluded that the regimen (which was ineffective) should not be used to treat ADD. It is unlikely that the increases in serum aminotransferases were due to the high acsorbic acid intake since no such effects of high vitamin C intakes have been reported by other investigators. Nevertheless, this study appears consistent with the adult data indicating a LOEAL at intakes of 3 g/day. However, this study cannot be utilized to establish a UL for children as the vitamin C was part of a megavitamin and the contribution of vitamin C to the results cannot be determined.

Because the results of these studies (particularly the study by Ludvigsson et al., 1977) are consistent with the data on adverse effects in adults on a body weight basis, the UL values for toddlers, children, and adolescents are extrapolated based on body weight differences from those established for adults as described in Chapter 4 using reference weights from Chapter 1 (Table 1-1). The calculated UL is rounded to the nearest 50 mg.

Pregnancy. No evidence of maternal toxicity of excess vitamin C intakes was found. However, because vitamin C is actively transported from maternal to fetal blood, there could be a potential for maternal intake of megadoses of vitamin C during pregnancy to lead to markedly elevated concentrations of vitamin C in the fetus. There is one anecdotal report (Cochrane, 1965) of possible fetal vitamin C dependence induced in utero in two infants, whose mothers consumed 400 mg/day of vitamin C during pregnancy. Although the infants developed scurvy during the first few weeks of life, the observation was complicated by the relatively high incidence of scurvy in the region of Canada in which the infants were born. Other concerns for high vitamin C concentrations in infants stem from reports of hemolysis (Ballin et al., 1988) and possible increased oxidative damage (Powers et al., 1995) in premature infants. However, these effects are not well documented, and do not warrant a separate UL for pregnant females.

Lactation. Byerley and Kirksey (1985) noted that the vitamin C composition of human milk was not affected by maternal vitamin C intake ranging from 156 to 1,123 mg/day and that urinary excretion increased as intake increased over 200 mg/day, suggesting that mammary tissue becomes saturated with vitamin C. One woman ingested 4,000 mg/day of vitamin C as a supplement; no toxic effects of the excess vitamin intake were noted in the mother. Her milk content of vitamin C was 100.5 mg/L, which was on the high end of values reported for human milk, but not reflective of the high intake (Anderson and Pittard, 1985). Based on these findings, the ULs for lactating adolescents and women are not different from those of nonlactating females.

Vitamin C UL Summary, Ages 1 through 18 Years, Pregnancy, Lactation

UL for Infants
    0–12 months   **Not possible to establish; source of intake should be formula and food only**

UL for Children
    1–3 years   **400 mg (2,272 µmol)/day of vitamin C**
    4–8 years   **650 mg (3,692 µmol)/day of vitamin C**
    9–13 years   **1,200 mg (6,816 µmol)/day of vitamin C**

UL for Adolescents
    14–18 years   **1,800 mg (10,224 µmol)/day of vitamin C**

UL for Pregnancy
    14–18 years   **1,800 mg (10,224 µmol)/day of vitamin C**
    19 years and older **2,000 mg (11,360 µmol)/day of vitamin C**

UL for Lactation
    14–18 years   **1,800 mg (10,224 µmol)/day of vitamin C**
    19 years and older **2,000 mg (11,360 µmol)/day of vitamin C**

Special Considerations

Individuals with hemochromatosis, glucose-6-phosphate dehydrogenase deficiency, and renal disorders may be especially susceptible to adverse effects of excess vitamin C intake and therefore should be cautious about ingesting more vitamin C than the Recommended Dietary Allowance (RDA). Vitamin C intakes of 250 mg/day or higher have been associated with false-negative results for detecting stool and gastric occult blood (Gogel et al., 1989; Jaffe et al., 1975). Therefore, high-dose vitamin C supplements should be discontinued at least 2 weeks before physical exams because they may interfere with blood and urine tests.

Intake Assessment

Based on data from the Third National Health and Nutrition Examination Survey (NHANES III), the highest mean intake of vitamin C from diet and supplements for any gender and lifestage group was estimated to be about 200 mg (1,136 µmol)/day (Appendix Table C-2). This was the intake of males aged 51 through 70 years and females aged 51 years and older. The highest reported intake at the ninety-ninth percentile was greater than 1,200 mg (6,816 µmol)/day in males aged 31 through 70 years and in females aged 51 through 70 years (Appendix Table C-2).

Risk Characterization

The risk of adverse effects resulting from excess intake of vitamin C from food and supplements appears to be very low at the highest intakes noted above. Although members of the general population should be advised not to exceed the UL routinely, intake greater than the UL may be appropriate for investigation within well-controlled clinical trials. Clinical trials of doses above the UL should not be discouraged, as long as subjects participating in these trials have signed informed consent documents regarding possible toxicity and as long as these trials employ appropriate safety monitoring of trial subjects. In addition, the UL is not meant to apply to individuals who are receiving vitamin C under medical supervision.

RESEARCH RECOMMENDATIONS FOR VITAMIN C

• Despite the many known biochemical roles of ascorbic acid, no reliable biochemical or physiologically based functional measures of vitamin C nutriture have been established. As a result, vitamin C intake requirements in adults have been based on estimates of body pool or tissue ascorbate deemed adequate to provide antioxidant protection. Knowledge of vitamin C intakes needed to fulfill specific functional roles of ascorbate will allow more accurate and precise determinations of the individual and average population requirements of the vitamin. Some current candidates that could be used as functional measures include pathways related to collagen and carnitine metabolism, oxidative damage, and oral health indices; however, research on new functions of the vitamin is also needed. Determination of vitamin C requirements based on antioxidant functions will require development of more reliable tests for in vivo oxidative damage and further understanding of the interactions of ascorbate with other physiological antioxidants. Additionally, a practical method for measuring the vitamin C body pool is needed as a standard of comparison against proposed functional measures and measures of health or disease endpoints.

• Since the requirements for children ages 1 through 18 years are extrapolated from the adult Estimated Average Requirements (EARs), it is critically important to conduct large-scale studies with children using state-of-the-art biomarkers to assess their vitamin C requirement.

• Many studies that provided vitamin C supplements to apparently healthy well-nourished populations were investigating pharmacological (at or above the point where body tissues are saturated) rather than nutritional effects of the vitamin. This may obscure possible relationships between vitamin C intake and disease risk in the range of dietary intakes. Therefore, population studies on the relationship of vitamin C nutriture and chronic disease should focus more on individuals or populations who eat few fruits and vegetables and are marginally deficient in vitamin C. Attention also has to be given to methods for sorting out the effects of vitamin C intake from those of other dietary and life-style factors that may also affect disease risk.

• While the evidence of adverse effects due to intakes of vitamin C supplements is at this time limited to osmotic diarrhea and gastrointestinal disturbances which are self-limiting, the frequency of high intakes of the vitamin in the North American population warrants further investigation. The well known pro-oxidant effects of the iron-ascorbate couple in vitro suggest that further research be done on possible related in vivo reactions—for example, during simultaneous supplement ingestion, iron overload, and inflammation or tissue trauma where non-protein-bound iron may be released.

• A small number of isolated reports raise concern that high vitamin C intakes during pregnancy may expose the fetus or neonate to risks of withdrawal symptoms, hemolysis, or oxidant damage. Further research is needed to confirm or refute these concerns.

REFERENCES

Afroz M, Bhothinard B, Etzkorn JR, Horenstein S, McGarry JD. 1975. Vitamins C and B$_{12}$. *J Am Med Assoc* 232:246.

Alexy U, Kersting M, Sichert-Hellert W, Manz F, Schöch G. 1999. Vitamin intake of 3- to 36-month-old German infants and children— Results of the DONALD study. *Int J Vitam Nutr Res* 69:285–291.

Allen JC, Keller RP, Archer P, Neville MC. 1991. Studies in human lactation: Milk composition and daily secretion rates of macronutrients in the first year of lactation. *Am J Clin Nutr* 54:69–80.

Alvares O. 1997. Ascorbic acid and periodontal disease. In: Packer L, Fuchs J, eds. *Vitamin C in Health and Disease.* New York: Marcel Dekker. Pp. 505–516.

Ames BN, Gold LS, Willett WC. 1995. The causes and prevention of cancer. *Proc Natl Acad Sci USA* 92:5258–5265.

Anderson D, Phillips BJ, Yu T, Edwards AJ, Ayesh R, Butterworth KR. 1997. The effects of vitamin C supplementation on biomarkers of oxygen radical generated damage in human volunteers with "low" or "high" cholesterol levels. *Environ Mol Mutagen* 30:161–174.

Anderson DM, Pittard WB. 1985. Vitamin E and C concentrations in human milk with maternal megadosing. A case report. *J Am Diet Assoc* 85:715–717.

Anderson R, Lukey, PT. 1987. A biological role for ascorbate in the selective neutralization of extracellular phagocyte-derived oxidants. *Ann NY Acad Sci* 498:229–247.

Anderson R, Oosthuizen R, Maritz R, Theron A, Van Rensburg AJ. 1980. The effects of increasing weekly doses of ascorbate on certain cellular and humoral immune function in normal volunteers. *Am J Clin Nutr* 33:71–76.

Asami S, Manabe H, Miyake J, Tsurudome Y, Hirano T, Yamaguchi R, Itoh H, Kasai H. 1997. Cigarette smoking induces an increase in oxidative DNA damage, 8-hydroxydeoxyguanosine, in a central site in the human lung. *Carcinogenesis* 18:1763–1766.

Auer BL, Auer D, Rodgers AL. 1998. Relative hyperoxaluria, crystalluria and haematuria after megadose ingestion of vitamin C. *Eur J Clin Invest* 28:695–700.

Bacon BR, Olynyk JK, Brunt EM, Britton RS, Wolff RK. 1999. *HFE* genotype in patients with hemochromatosis and other liver diseases. *Ann Int Med* 130:953–962.

Baer DM, Tekawa IS, Hurley LB. 1994. Iron stores are not associated with acute myocardial infarction. *Circulation* 89:2915–2918.

Baker EM, Sauberlich HE, Wolfskill SJ, Wallace WT, Dean EE. 1962. Tracer studies of vitamin C utilization in men: Metabolism of D-glucuronolactone-6-C^{14}, D-glucuronic-6-C^{14} acid and L-ascorbic-1-C^{14} acid. *Proc Soc Exp Biol Med* 109:737–741.

Baker EM, Hodges RE, Hood J, Sauberlich HE, March SC. 1969. Metabolism of ascorbic-1-C^{14} acid in experimental human scurvy. *Am J Clin Nutr* 22:549–558.

Baker EM, Hodges RE, Hood J, Sauberlich HE, March SC, Canham JE. 1971. Metabolism of ^{14}C- and ^{3}H-labeled L-ascorbic acid in human scurvy. *Am J Clin Nutr* 24:444–454.

Ballin A, Brown EJ, Koren G, Zipursky A. 1988. Vitamin C-induced erythrocyte damage in premature infants. *J Pediatr* 113:114–120.

Bandera EV, Freudenheim JL, Marshall JR, Zielezny M, Priore RL, Brasure J, Baptiste M, Graham S. 1997. Diet and alcohol consumption and lung cancer risk in the New York State Cohort. *Cancer Causes Control* 8:828–840.

Barrett B, Gunter E, Jenkins J, Wang M. 1991. Ascorbic acid concentration in amniotic fluid in late pregnancy. *Biol Neonate* 60:333–335.

Bates CJ, Prentice AM, Prentice A, Paul AA, Whitehead RG. 1982. Seasonal variations in ascorbic acid status and breast milk ascorbic acid levels in rural Gambian women in relation to dietary intake. *Trans Royal Soc Trop Med Hyg* 76:341–347.

Belcher JD, Balla J, Balla G, Jacobs DR Jr, Gross M, Jacob HS, Vercellotti GM. 1993. Vitamin E, LDL, and endothelium. Brief oral vitamin supplementation prevents oxidized LDL-mediated vascular injury in vitro. *Arterioscler Thromb* 13: 1779–1789.

Bendich A, Cohen M. 1990. Ascorbic acid safety: Analysis of factors affecting iron absorption. *Toxicol Lett* 51:189–201.

Berger L, Gerson CD, Yu TF. 1977. The effect of ascorbic acid on uric acid excretion with a commentary on the renal handling of ascorbic acid. *Am J Med* 62:71–76.

Berger TM, Polidori MC, Dabbagh A, Evans PJ, Halliwell B, Morrow JD, Roberts LJ II, Frei B. 1997. Antioxidant activity of vitamin C in iron-overloaded human plasma. *J Biol Chem* 272:15656–15660.

Berliner JA, Heinecke JW. 1996. The role of oxidized lipoproteins in atherogenesis. *Free Radic Biol Med* 20:707–727.

Bermudez E, Stone K, Carter KM, Pryor WA. 1994. Environmental tobacco smoke is just as damaging to DNA as mainstream smoke. *Environ Hlth Perspect* 102:870–874.

Beutler E. 1991. Glucose-6-phosphate dehydrogenase deficiency. *N Engl J Med* 324:169–174.

Blanchard J. 1991a. Depletion and repletion kinetics of vitamin C in humans. *J Nutr* 121:170–176.

Blanchard J. 1991b. Effects of gender on vitamin C pharmacokinetics in man. *J Am Coll Nutr* 10:453–459.

Blanchard J, Conrad KA, Watson RR, Garry PJ, Crawley JD. 1989. Comparison of plasma, mononuclear and polymorphonuclear leucocyte vitamin C levels in young and elderly women during depletion and supplementation. *Eur J Clin Nutr* 43:97–106.

Blanchard J, Conrad KA, Garry PJ. 1990a. Effects of age and intake on vitamin C disposition in females. *Eur J Clin Nutr* 44:447–460.

Blanchard J, Conrad KA, Mead RA, Garry PJ. 1990b. Vitamin C disposition in young and elderly men. *Am J Clin Nutr* 51:837–845.

Blanchard J, Tozer TN, Rowland M. 1997. Pharmacokinetic perspectives on megadoses of ascorbic acid. *Am J Clin Nutr* 66:1165–1171.

Block G. 1991. Vitamin C and cancer prevention: The epidemiologic evidence. *Am J Clin Nutr* 53:270S–282S.

Blot WJ, Li J-Y, Taylor PR, Guo W, Dawsey S, Wang G-Q, Yang CS, Zheng S-F, Gail M, Li G-Y, Yu Y, Liu B-Q, Tangrea J, Sun Y-H, Liu F, Fraumeni JF Jr, Zhang Y-H, Li B. 1993. Nutrition intervention trials in Linxian, China: Supplementation with specific vitamin/mineral combinations, cancer incidence, and disease-specific mortality in the general population. *J Natl Cancer Inst* 85: 1483–1492.

Bors W, Michel C, Schikora S. 1995. Interaction of flavonoids with ascorbate and determination of their univalent redox potentials: A pulse radiolysis study. *Free Radic Biol Med* 19:45–52.

Bostick RM, Potter JD, McKenzie DR, Sellers TA, Kushi LH, Steinmetz KA, Folsom AR. 1993. Reduced risk of colon cancer with high intake of vitamin E: The Iowa Women's Health Study. *Cancer Res* 53:4230–4237.

Britton JR, Pavord ID, Richards KA, Knox AJ, Wisniewski AF, Lewis SA, Tattersfield AE, Weiss ST. 1995. Dietary antioxidant vitamin intake and lung function in the general population. *Am J Respir Crit Care Med* 151:1383–1387.

Bucca C, Rolla G, Farina JC. 1992. Effect of vitamin C on transient increase of bronchial responsiveness in conditions affecting the airways. *Ann NY Acad Sci* 669:175–187.

Bueno de Mesquita HB, Maisonneuve P, Runia S, Moerman CJ. 1991. Intake of foods and nutrients and cancer of the exocrine pancreas: A population-based case-control study in The Netherlands. *Int J Cancer* 48:540–549.

Buettner GR. 1993. The pecking order of free radicals and antioxidants: Lipid peroxidation, alpha-tocopherol, and ascorbate. *Arch Biochem Biophys* 300:535–543.

Buettner GR, Jurkiewicz BA. 1996. Catalytic metals, ascorbate and free radicals: Combinations to avoid. *Radiat Res* 145:532–541.

Burr ML, Elwood PC, Hole DJ, Hurley RJ, Hughes RE. 1974. Plasma and leukocyte ascorbic acid levels in the elderly. *Am J Clin Nutr* 27:144–151

Bussey HJ, DeCosse JJ, Deschner EE, Eyers AA, Lesser ML, Morson BC, Ritchie SM, Thomson JP, Wadsworth J. 1982. A randomized trial of ascorbic acid in polyposis coli. *Cancer* 50:1434–1439.

Butte NF, Garza C, Smith EO, Nichols BL. 1984. Human milk intake and growth in exclusively breast-fed infants. *J Pediatr* 104:187–195.

Byerley LO, Kirksey A. 1985. Effects of different levels of vitamin C intake on the vitamin C concentration in human milk and the vitamin C intakes of breast-fed infants. *Am J Clin Nutr* 41:665–671.

Byun J, Mueller DM, Fabjan JS, Heinecke JW. 1999. Nitrogen dioxide radical generated by the myeloperoxidase-hydrogen peroxide-nitrite system promotes lipid peroxidation of low density lipoprotein. *FEBS Lett* 455:243–246.

Cadenas S, Rojas C, Méndez J, Herrero A, Barja G. 1996. Vitamin E decreases urine lipid peroxidation products in young healthy human volunteers under normal conditions. *Pharmacol Toxicol* 79:247–253.

Cahill RJ, O'Sullivan KR, Mathias PM, Beattie S, Hamilton H, O'Morain C. 1993. Effects of vitamin antioxidant supplementation on cell kinetics of patients with adenomatous polyps. *Gut* 34:963–967.

Cameron E, Campbell A. 1974. The orthomolecular treatment of cancer. II. Clinical trial of high-dose ascorbic acid supplements in advanced human cancer. *Chem Biol Interact* 9:285–315.

Campbell GD Jr, Steinberg MH, Bower JD. 1975. Ascorbic acid-induced hemolysis in G-6-PD deficiency. *Ann Intern Med* 82:810.

Carr AC, Frei B. 1999. Toward a new recommended dietary allowance for vitamin C based on antioxidant and health effects in humans. *Am J Clin Nutr* 69:1086–1087.

Casanueva E, Polo E, Tejero E, Meza C. 1993. Premature rupture of amniotic membranes as functional assessment of vitamin C status during pregnancy. *Ann NY Acad Sci* 678:369–370.

Chalmers TC. 1975. Effects of ascorbic acid on the common cold. An evaluation of the evidence. *Am J Med* 58:532–536.

Chazan JA, Mistilis SP. 1963. The pathophysiology of scurvy. *Am J Med* 34:350–358.

Cheng L, Cohen M, Bhagavan HN. 1985. Vitamin C and the elderly. In: Watson RR, ed. *CRC Handbook of Nutrition in the Aged*. Boca Raton, FL: CRC Press. Pp. 157–185.

Choi JL, Rose RC. 1989. Transport and metabolism of ascorbic acid in human placenta. *Am J Physiol* 257:C110–C113.

Cochrane WA. 1965. Overnutrition in prenatal and neonatal life: A problem? *Can Med Assoc J* 93:893–899.

Cohen HA, Neuman I, Nahum H. 1997. Blocking effect of vitamin C in exercise-induced asthma. *Arch Pediatr Adolesc Med* 151:367–370.

Cook JD, Watson SS, Simpson KM, Lipschitz DA, Skikne BS. 1984. The effect of high ascorbic acid supplementation on body iron stores. *Blood* 64:721–726.

Cooke MS, Evans MD, Podmore ID, Herbert KE, Mistry N, Mistry P, Hickenbotham PT, Hussieni A, Griffiths HR, Lunec J. 1998. Novel repair action of vitamin C upon in vivo oxidative DNA damage. *FEBS Lett* 439:363–367.

Coulehan JL, Eberhard S, Kapner L, Taylor F, Rogers K, Garry P. 1976. Vitamin C and acute illness in Navajo school children. *N Engl J Med* 295:973–977.

Cross CE, Halliwell B. 1993. Nutrition and human disease: How much extra vitamin C might smokers need? *Lancet* 341:1091.

Cross CE, Forte T, Stocker R, Louie S, Yamamoto Y, Ames BN, Frei B. 1990. Oxidative stress and abnormal cholesterol metabolism in patients with adult respiratory distress syndrome. *J Lab Clin Med* 115:396–404.

Crott JW, Fenech M. 1999. Effect of vitamin C supplementation on chromosome damage, apoptosis and necrosis ex vivo. *Carcinogenesis* 20:1035–1041.

Curhan GC, Willett WC, Rimm EB, Stampfer MJ. 1996. A prospective study of the intake of vitamins C and B_6, and the risk of kidney stones in men. *J Urol* 155:1847–1851.

Curhan GC, Willett WC, Speizer FE, Stampfer MJ. 1999. Intake of vitamins B_6 and C and the risk of kidney stones in women. *J Am Soc Nephrol* 10:840–845.

Dabrowski K. 1990. Gastro-intestinal circulation of ascorbic acid. *Comp Biochem Physiol* 95A:481–486.

Dallongeville J, Marécaux N, Fruchart J-C, Amouyel P. 1998. Cigarette smoking is associated with unhealthy patterns of nutrient intake: A meta-analysis. *J Nutr* 128:1450–1457.

Davies HE, Davies JE, Hughes RE, Jones E. 1984. Studies on the absorption of L-xyloascorbic acid (vitamin C) in young and elderly subjects. *Hum Nutr Clin Nutr* 38C:463–471.

Davies HE, Gruffudd S, Hughes RE, Jones E. 1987. Ascorbic acid and carnitine in man. *Nutr Report Int* 36:941–948.

DeCosse JJ, Adams MB, Kuzma JF, LoGerfo P, Condon RE. 1975. Effect of ascorbic acid on rectal polyps of patients with familial polyposis. *Surgery* 78:608–612.

Delafuente JC, Prendergast JM, Modigh A. 1986. Immunologic modulation by vitamin C in the elderly. *Int J Immunopharmacol* 8:205–211.

Delamere NA. 1996. Ascorbic acid and the eye. *Subcell Biochem* 25:313–329.

Devaraj S, Jialal I. 1996. Oxidized low-density lipoprotein and atherosclerosis. *Int J Clin Lab Res* 26:178–184.

Dewey KG, Finley DA, Lonnerdal B. 1984. Breast milk volume and composition during late lactation (7–20 months). *J Pediatr Gastroenterol Nutr* 3:713–720.

Drake IM, Davies MJ, Mapstone NP, Dixon MF, Schorah CJ, White KLM, Chalmers DM, Axon ATR. 1996. Ascorbic acid may protect against human gastric cancer by scavenging mucosal oxygen radicals. *Carcinogenesis* 17:559–562.

Duthie SJ, Ma A, Ross MA, Collins AR. 1996. Antioxidant supplementation decreases oxidative DNA damage in human lymphocytes. *Cancer Res* 56:1291–1295.

Dyke GW, Craven JL, Hall R, Garner RC. 1994a. Effect of vitamin C supplementation on gastric mucosal DNA damage. *Carcinogenesis* 15:291–295.

Dyke GW, Craven JL, Hall R, Garner RC. 1994b. Effect of vitamin C upon gastric mucosal O^6-alkyltransferase activity and on gastric vitamin C levels. *Cancer Lett* 86:159–165.

Eichholzer M, Stahelin HB, Gey KF. 1992. Inverse correlation between essential antioxidants in plasma and subsequent risk to develop cancer, ischemic heart disease and stroke respectively: 12-year follow-up of the Prospective Basel Study. *Exp Suppl* 62:398–410.

Ekvall S, Chen IW, Bozian R. 1981. The effect of supplemental ascorbic acid on serum vitamin B_{12} levels in myelomenigocele patients. *Am J Clin Nutr* 34:1356–1361.

Elneihoum AM, Falke P, Hedblad B, Lindgarde F, Ohlsson K. 1997. Leukocyte activation in atherosclerosis: Correlation with risk factors. *Atherosclerosis* 131:79–84.

Englard S, Seifter S. 1986. The biochemical functions of ascorbic acid. *Annu Rev Nutr* 6:365–406.

Enstrom JE, Kanim LE, Breslow L. 1986. The relationship between vitamin C intake, general health practices, and mortality in Alameda County, California. *Am J Pub Hlth* 76:1124–1130.

Enstrom JE, Kanim LE, Klein MA. 1992. Vitamin C intake and mortality among a sample of the United States population. *Epidemiology* 3:194–202.

Erdman JW Jr, Klein BP. 1982. The influence of harvesting, processing, and cooking on vitamin C in foods. In: Seib PA, Tolbert BM, eds. *Ascorbic Acid: Chemistry, Metabolism and Uses*. Washington, DC: American Chemical Society. Pp. 499–532.

Evans RM, Currie L, Campbell A. 1982. The distribution of ascorbic acid between various cellular components of blood in normal individuals, and its relation to the plasma concentration. *Br J Nutr* 47:473–482.

FDA (Food and Drug Adminstration). 1985. Nutrient requirements for infant formulas. *Fed Regis* 50:45106–45108.

Fellstrom B, Danielson BG, Karlstrom B, Lithell H, Ljunghall S, Vessby B. 1989. Dietary habits in renal stone patients compared with healthy subjects. *Br J Urol* 63:575–580.

Fishbaine B, Butterfield G. 1984. Ascorbic acid status of running and sedentary men. *Int J Vitam Nutr Res* 54:273.

Fituri N, Allawi N, Bentley M, Costello J. 1983. Urinary and plasma oxalate during ingestion of pure ascorbic acid: A re-evaluation. *Eur Urol* 9:312–315.

Flodin NW. 1988. *Pharmacology of Micronutrients*. New York: Alan R. Liss. Pp. 201–244.

Fontham ET. 1994. Vitamin C, vitamin C-rich foods, and cancer: Epidemiologic studies. In: Frei B, ed. *Natural Antioxidants in Human Health and Disease*. San Diego: Academic Press. Pp. 157–197.

Fontham ET, Pickle LW, Haenszel W, Correa P, Lin YP, Falk RT. 1988. Dietary vitamins A and C and lung cancer risk in Louisiana. *Cancer* 62:2267–2273.

Fraga CG, Motchnik PA, Shigenaga MK, Helbock HJ, Jacob RA, Ames BN. 1991. Ascorbic acid protects against endogenous oxidative DNA damage in human sperm. *Proc Natl Acad Sci USA* 88:11003–11006.

Frei B, Stocker R, Ames BN. 1988. Antioxidant defenses and lipid peroxidation in human blood plasma. *Proc Natl Acad Sci USA* 85:9748–9752.

Frei B, England L, Ames BN. 1989. Ascorbate is an outstanding antioxidant in human blood plasma. *Proc Natl Acad Sci USA* 86:6377–6381.

Frei B, Forte TM, Ames BN, Cross CE. 1991. Gas phase oxidants of cigarette smoke induce lipid peroxidation and changes in lipoprotein properties in human blood plasma. Protective effects of ascorbic acid. *Biochem J* 277:133–138.

Freudenheim JL, Graham S, Marshall JR, Haughey BP, Wilkinson G. 1990. A case-control study of diet and rectal cancer in western New York. *Am J Epidemiol* 131:612–624.

Fuller CJ, Grundy SM, Norkus EP, Jialal I. 1996. Effect of ascorbate supplementation on low density lipoprotein oxidation in smokers. *Atherosclerosis* 119:139–150.

Gale CR, Martyn CN, Winter PD, Cooper C. 1995. Vitamin C and risk of death from stroke and coronary heart disease in cohort of elderly people. *Br Med J* 310:1563–1566.

Garry PJ, Goodwin JS, Hunt WC, Gilbert BA. 1982. Nutritional status in a healthy elderly population: Vitamin C. *Am J Clin Nutr* 36:332–339.

Garry PJ, Vanderjagt DJ, Hunt WC. 1987. Ascorbic acid intakes and plasma levels in healthy elderly. *Ann NY Acad Sci* 498:90–99.

George DR, De Francesca BA. 1989. Human milk in comparison to cow milk. In: Lebenthal E, ed. *Textbook of Gastroenterology and Nutrition in Infancy and Childhood*, 2nd edition. New York: Raven Press. Pp. 242–243.

Gey KF. 1995. Ten-year retrospective on the antioxidant hypothesis of arteriosclerosis: Threshold plasma levels of antioxidant micronutrients related to minimum cardiovascular risk. *Nutr Biochem* 6:206–236.

Gey KF. 1998. Vitamins E plus C and interacting conutrients required for optimal health. A critical and constructive review of epidemiology and supplementation data regarding cardiovascular disease and cancer. *Biofactors* 7:113–174.

Gey KF, Stahelin HB, Eichholzer M. 1993. Poor plasma status of carotene and vitamin C is associated with higher mortality from ischemic heart disease and stroke: Basel Prospective Study. *Clin Invest* 71:3–6.

Ghadirian P, Boyle P, Simard A, Baillargeon J, Maisonneuve P, Perret C. 1991. Reported family aggregation of pancratic cancer within a population-based case-control study in the francophone community in Montreal, Canada. *Int J Pancreatol* 10:183–196.

Giunta JL. 1983. Dental erosion resulting from chewable vitamin C tablets. *J Am Dent Assoc* 107:253–256.

Gogel HK, Tandberg D, Strickland RG. 1989. Substances that interfere with guaiac card tests: Implications for gastric aspirate testing. *Am J Emerg Med* 7:474–480.

Goldsmith GA. 1961. Human requirements for vitamin C and its use in clinical medicine. *Ann NY Acad Sci* 92:230–245.

Gosiewska A, Mahmoodian F, Peterkofsky B. 1996. Gene expression of iron-related proteins during iron deficiency caused by scurvy in guinea pigs. *Arch Biochem Biophys* 325:295–303.

Graham S, Zielezny M, Marshall J, Priore R, Freudenheim J, Brasure J, Haughey B, Nasca P, Zdeb M. 1992. Diet in the epidemiology of postmenopausal breast cancer in the New York State Cohort. *Am J Epidemiol* 136:1327–1337.

Green MHL, Lowe JE, Waugh APW, Aldridge KE, Cole J, Arlett CF. 1994. Effect of diet and vitamin C on DNA strand breakage in freshly-isolated human white blood cells. *Mutat Res* 316:91–102.

Greenberg ER, Baron JA, Tosteson TD, Freeman DH, Beck GJ, Bond JH, Colacchio TA, Coller JA, Frankl HD, Haile RW, Mandel JS, Nierenberg DW, Rothstein R, Snover DC, Stevens MM, Summers RW, van Stolk RU. 1994. A clinical trial of antioxidant vitamins to prevent colorectal adenoma. *N Engl J Med* 331:141–147.

Gutteridge JMC. 1991. Plasma ascorbate levels and inhibition of the antioxidant activity of caeruloplasmin. *Clin Sci* 81:413–417.

Hallberg L. 1985. The role of vitamin C in improving the critical iron balance situation in women. *Int J Vitam Nutr Res* 27:177–187.

Halliwell B.1998. Can oxidative DNA damage be used as a biomarker of cancer risk in humans? *Free Radic Res* 29:469–486.

Halliwell B, Whiteman M. 1997. Antioxidant and prooxidant properties of vitamin C. In: Packer L, Fuchs J, eds. *Vitamin C in Health and Disease.* New York: Marcel Dekker. Pp. 59–73.

Halliwell B, Wasil M, Grootveld M. 1987. Biologically significant scavenging of the myeloperoxidase-derived oxidant hypochlorous acid by ascorbic acid. *FEBS Lett* 213:15–17.

Halpner AD, Handelman GJ, Belmont CA, Harris JM, Blumberg JB. 1998. Protection by vitamin C of oxidant-induced loss of vitamin E in rat hepatocytes. *J Nutr Biochem* 9:355–359.

Hankinson SE, Stampfer MJ, Seddon JM, Colditz GA, Rosner B, Speizer FE, Willett WC. 1992. Nutrient intake and cataract extraction in women: A prospective study. *Br Med J* 305:335–339.

Harats D, Ben-Naim M, Dabach Y, Hollander G, Havivi E, Stein O, Stein Y. 1990. Effect of vitamin C and E supplementation on susceptibility of plasma lipoproteins to peroxidation induced by acute smoking. *Atherosclerosis* 85:47–54.

Harats D, Chevion S, Nahir M, Norman Y, Sagee O, Berry EM. 1998. Citrus fruit supplementation reduces lipoprotein oxidation in young men ingesting a diet high in saturated fat: Presumptive evidence for an interaction between vitamins C and E in vivo. *Am J Clin Nutr* 67:240–245.

Harris ED, Percival SS. 1991. A role for ascorbic acid in copper transport. *Am J Clin Nutr* 54:1193S–1197S.

Hartz SC, Russell RM, Rosenberg IH. 1992. *Nutrition in the Elderly. The Boston Nutritional Status Survey.* London: Smith-Gordon. P. 38.

Haslam RH, Dalby JT, Rademaker AW. 1984. Effects of megavitamin therapy on children with attention deficit disorders. *Pediatrics* 74:103–111.

Hatch GE. 1995. Asthma, inhaled oxidants, and dietary antioxidants. *Am J Clin Nutr* 61:625S–630S.

Hatch M, Mulgrew S, Bourke E, Keogh B, Costello J. 1980. Effect of megadoses of ascorbic acid on serum and urinary oxalate. *Eur Urol* 6:166–169.

Hazell LJ, Arnold L, Flowers D, Waeg G, Malle E, Stocker R. 1996. Presence of hypochlorite-modified proteins in human atherosclerotic lesions. *J Clin Invest* 97:1535–1544.

Heinecke JW. 1997. Pathways for oxidation of low density lipoprotein by myeloperoxidase: Tyrosyl radical, reactive aldehydes, hypochlorous acid and molecular chlorine. *BioFactors* 6:145–155.

Heinig MJ, Nommsen LA, Peerson JM, Lonnerdal B, Dewey KG. 1993. Energy and protein intakes of breast-fed and formula-fed infants during the first year of life and their association with growth velocity: The DARLING Study. *Am J Clin Nutr* 58:152–161.

Heitzer T, Just H, Munzel T. 1996. Antioxidant vitamin C improves endothelial dysfunction in chronic smokers. *Circulation* 94:6–9.

Heller R, Munscher-Paulig F, Grabner R, Till U. 1999. L-Ascorbic acid potentiates nitric oxide synthesis in endothelial cells. *J Biol Chem* 274:8254–8260.

Hemila H. 1996. Vitamin C, the placebo effect, and the common cold: A case study of how preconceptions influence the analysis of results. *J Clin Epidemiol* 49: 1079–1084.

Hemila H. 1997. Vitamin C intake and susceptibility to the common cold. *Br J Nutr* 77:59–72.

Hemila H, Herman ZS. 1995. Vitamin C and the common cold: A retrospective analysis of Chalmers' review. *J Am Coll Nutr* 14:116–123.

Henning SM, Zhang JZ, McKee RW, Swendseid ME, Jacob RA. 1991. Glutathione blood levels and other oxidant defense indices in men fed diets low in vitamin C. *J Nutr* 121:1969–1975.

Herbert V. 1978. Risk of oxalate stones from large doses of vitamin C. *N Engl J Med* 298:856.

Herbert V. 1995. Vitamin C supplements and disease—Counterpoint. *J Am Coll Nutr* 14:112–113.

Herbert V, Jacob E. 1974. Destruction of vitamin B$_{12}$ by ascorbic acid. *J Am Med Assoc* 230:241–242.

Hevia P, Omaye ST, Jacob RA. 1990. Urinary hydroxyproline excretion and vitamin C status in healthy young men. *Am J Clin Nutr* 51:644–648.

Hinds MW, Kolonel LN, Hankin JH, Lee J. 1984. Dietary vitamin A, carotene, vitamin C and risk of lung cancer in Hawaii. *Am J Epidemiol* 119:227–237.

Hoffer A. 1971. Ascorbic acid and toxicity. *N Engl J Med* 285:635–636.

Hoffer A. 1973. Vitamin C and infertility. *Lancet* 2:1146.

Hofstad B, Almendingen K, Vatn M, Andersen S, Owen R, Larsen S, Osnes M. 1998. Growth and recurrence of colorectal polyps: A double-blind 3-year intervention with calcium and antioxidants. *Digestion* 59:148–156.

Hogenkamp HP. 1980. The interaction between vitamin B$_{12}$ and vitamin C. *Am J Clin Nutr* 33:1–3.

Hornig B, Arakawa N, Kohler C, Drexler H. 1998. Vitamin C improves endothelial function of conduit arteries in patients with chronic heart failure. *Circulation* 97:363–368.

Hornig D. 1975. Distribution of ascorbic acid, metabolites and analogues in man and animals. *Ann NY Acad Sci* 258:103–118.

Hornig DH, Moser U. 1981. The safety of high vitamin C intakes in man. In: Counsell JN, Hornig DH, eds. Vitamin C (Ascorbic Acid). London: Applied Science. Pp. 225–248.

Horrobin DF. 1996. Ascorbic acid and prostaglandin synthesis. *Subcell Biochem* 25:109–115.

Howe GR, Hirohata T, Hislop TG, Iscovich JM, Yuan JM, Katsouyanni K, Lubin F, Marubini E, Modan B, Rohan T. 1990. Dietary factors and risk of breast cancer: Combined analysis of 12 case-control studies. *J Natl Cancer Inst* 82:561–569.

Howe GR, Ghadirian P, Bueno de Mesquita HB, Zatonski WA, Baghurst PA, Miller AB, Simard A, Baillargeon J, de Waard F, Przewozniak K. 1992. A collaborative case-control study of nutrient intake and pancreatic cancer within the search programme. *Int J Cancer* 51:365–372.

Hoyt CJ. 1980. Diarrhea from vitamin C. *J Am Med Assoc* 244:1674.

Hughes C, Dutton S, Truswell AS. 1981. High intakes of ascorbic acid and urinary oxalate. *J Hum Nutr* 35:274–280.

Hunt JR, Gallagher SK, Johnson LK. 1994. Effect of ascorbic acid on apparent iron absorption by women with low iron stores. *Am J Clin Nutr* 59:1381–1385.

Hunter DJ, Manson JE, Colditz GA, Stampfer MJ, Rosner B, Hennekens CH, Speizer FE, Willett WC. 1993. A prospective study of the intake of vitamins C, E, and A and the risk of breast cancer. *N Engl J Med* 329:234–240.

IOM (Institute of Medicine). 1991. *Nutrition During Lactation*. Washington, DC: National Academy Press. P. 179.

Itoh R, Yamada K, Oka J, Echizen H, Murakami K. 1989. Sex as a factor in levels of serum ascorbic acid in a healthy elderly population. *Int J Vitam Nutr Res* 59:365–372.

Jacob RA. 1995. The integrated antioxidant system. *Nutr Res* 15:755–766.

Jacob RA. 1999. Vitamin C. In: Shils ME, Olson JA, Shike M, Ross AC, eds. *Modern Nutrition in Health and Disease*, 9th edition. Baltimore, MD: Williams & Wilkins. Pp. 467–483.

Jacob RA, Pianalto FS. 1997. Urinary carnitine excretion increases during experimental vitamin C depletion of healthy men. *J Nutr Biochem* 8:265–269.

Jacob RA, Skala JH, Omaye ST. 1987a. Biochemical indices of human vitamin C status. *Am J Clin Nutr* 46:818–826.

Jacob RA, Skala JH, Omaye ST, Turnlund JR. 1987b. Effect of varying ascorbic acid intakes on copper absorption and ceruloplasmin levels of young men. *J Nutr* 117:2109–2115.

Jacob RA, Otradovec CL, Russell RM, Munro HN, Hartz SC, McGandy RB, Morrow FD, Sadowski JA. 1988. Vitamin C status and nutrient interactions in a healthy elderly population. *Am J Clin Nutr* 48:1436–1442.

Jacob RA, Kelley DS, Pianalto FS, Swendseid ME, Henning SM, Zhang JZ, Ames BN, Fraga CG, Peters JH. 1991. Immunocompetence and oxidant defense during ascorbate depletion of healthy men. *Am J Clin Nutr* 54:1302S–1309S.

Jacob RA, Pianalto FS, Agee RE. 1992. Cellular ascorbate depletion in healthy men. *J Nutr* 122:1111–1118.

Jacob RA, Kutnink MA, Csallany AS, Daroszewska M, Burton GW. 1996. Vitamin C nutriture has little short-term effect on vitamin E concentrations in healthy women. *J Nutr* 126:2268–2277.

Jacques PF, Chylack LT Jr. 1991. Epidemiologic evidence of a role for the antioxidant vitamins and carotenoids in cataract prevention. *Am J Clin Nutr* 53:352S–355S.

Jacques PF, Taylor A, Hankinson SE, Willett WC, Mahnken B, Lee Y, Vaid K, Lahav M. 1997. Long-term vitamin C supplement use and prevalence of early age-related lens opacities. *Am J Clin Nutr* 66:911–916.

Jaffe RM, Kasten B, Young DS, MacLowry JD. 1975. False-negative stool occult blood tests caused by ingestion of ascorbic acid (vitamin C). *Ann Intern Med* 83:824–826.

Jama JW, Launer LJ, Witteman JC, den Breeijen JH, Breteler MM, Grobbee DE, Hofman A. 1996. Dietary antioxidants and cognitive function in a population-based sample of older persons. The Rotterdam Study. *Am J Epidemiol* 144:275–280.

Jariwalla RJ, Harakeh S. 1996. Antiviral and immunomodulatory activities of ascorbic acid. *Subcell Biochem* 25:213–231.

Jarvinen R, Knekt P, Seppanen R, Teppo L. 1997. Diet and breast cancer risk in a cohort of Finnish women. *Cancer Lett* 114:251–253.

Jendryczko A, Tomala J. 1995. The total free radical trapping ability of blood plasma in eclampsia. *Zentralbl Gynakol* 117:126–129.

Jha P, Flather M, Lonn E, Farkouh M, Yusuf S. 1995. The antioxidant vitamins and cardiovascular disease. A critical review of epidemiologic and clinical trial data. *Ann Intern Med* 123:860–872.

Jialal I, Devaraj S. 1996. The role of oxidized low density lipoprotein in atherogenesis. *J Nutr* 126:1053S–1057S.

Jialal I, Grundy SM. 1991. Preservation of the endogenous antioxidants in low density lipoprotein by ascorbate but not probucol during oxidative modification. *J Clin Invest* 87:597–601.

Jialal I, Vega GL, Grundy SM. 1990. Physiologic levels of ascorbate inhibit the oxidative modification of low density lipoprotein. *Atherosclerosis* 82:185–191.

Johnston CS. 1991. Complement component C1q unaltered by ascorbate supplementation in healthy men and women. *J Nutr Biochem* 2:499–501.

Johnston CS. 1999. Biomarkers for establishing a tolerable upper intake level for vitamin C. *Nutr Rev* 57:71–77.

Johnston CS, Luo B. 1994. Comparison of the absorption and excretion of three commercially available sources of vitamin C. *J Am Diet Assoc* 94:779–781.

Johnston CS, Thompson LL. 1998. Vitamin C status of an outpatient population. *J Am Coll Nutr* 17:366–370.

Johnston CS, Martin LJ, Cai X. 1992. Antihistamine effect of supplemental ascorbic acid and neutrophil chemotaxis. *J Am Coll Nutr* 11:172–176.

Johnston CS, Meyer CG, Srilakshmi JC. 1993. Vitamin C elevates red blood cell glutathione in healthy adults. *Am J Clin Nutr* 58:103–105.

Johnston CS, Solomon E, Corte C. 1996. Vitamin C depletion is associated with alterations in blood histamine and plasma free carnitine in adults. *J Am Coll Nutr* 15:586–591.

Kallner A, Hartmann D, Hornig D. 1979. Steady-state turnover and body pool of ascorbic acid in man. *Am J Clin Nutr* 32:530–539.

Kallner AB, Hartmann D, Hornig DH. 1981. On the requirements of ascorbic acid in man: Steady-state turnover and body pool in smokers. *Am J Clin Nutr* 34:1347–1355.

Karra MV, Udipi SA, Kirksey A, Roepke JL. 1986. Changes in specific nutrients in breast milk during extended lactation. *Am J Clin Nutr* 43:495–503.

Katsuki H. 1996. Vitamin C and nervous tissue: In vivo and in vitro aspects. *Subcell Biochem* 25:293–311.

Keith RE. 1994. Vitamins and physical activity. In: Wolinsky I, Hickson JF, eds. *Nutrition in Exercise and Sport,* 2nd edition. Boca Raton, FL: CRC Press. Pp. 159–183.

Kelly FJ, Mudway I, Blomberg A, Frew A, Sandstrom T. 1999. Altered lung antioxidant status in patients with mild asthma. *Lancet* 354:482–483.

Kennes B, Dumont I, Brohee D, Hubert C, Neve P. 1983. Effect of vitamin C supplements on cell-mediated immunity in old people. *Gerontology* 29:305–310.

Knekt P, Jarvinen R, Seppanen R, Rissanen A, Aromaa A, Heinonen OP, Albanes D, Heinonen M, Pukkala E, Teppo L. 1991. Dietary antioxidants and the risk of lung cancer. *Am J Epidemiol* 134:471–479.

Knekt P, Reunanen A, Jarvinen R, Seppanen R, Heliovaara M, Aromaa A. 1994. Antioxidant vitamin intake and coronary mortality in a longitudinal population study. *Am J Epidemiol* 139:1180–1189.

Kritchevsky SB, Shimakawa T, Tell G, Dennis B, Carpenter M, Eckfeldt JH, Peacher-Ryan H, Heiss G. 1995. Dietary antioxidants and carotid artery wall thickness. The ARIC Study. *Circulation* 92:2142–2150.

Kushi LH, Fee RM, Sellers TA, Zheng W, Folsom AR. 1996a. Intake of vitamins A, C, and E and postmenopausal breast cancer. The Iowa Women's Health Study. *Am J Epidemiol* 144:165–174.

Kushi LH, Folsom AR, Prineas RJ, Mink PJ, Wu Y, Bostick RM. 1996b. Dietary antioxidant vitamins and death from coronary heart disease in postmenopausal women. *N Engl J Med* 334:1156–1162.

Lamden MP, Chrystowski GA. 1954. Urinary oxalate excretion by man following ascorbic acid ingestion. *Proc Soc Exp Biol Med* 85:190–192.

Laudicina DC, Marnett LJ. 1990. Enhancement of hydroperoxide-dependent lipid peroxidation in rat liver microsomes by ascorbic acid. *Arch Biochem Biophys* 278:73–80.

Leaf CD, Vecchio AJ, Roe DA, Hotchkiss JH. 1987. Influence of ascorbic acid dose on *N*-nitrosoproline formation in humans. *Carcinogenesis* 8:791–795.

Leggott PJ, Robertson PB, Rothman DL, Murray PA, Jacob RA. 1986. The effect of controlled ascorbic acid depletion and supplementation on periodontal health. *J Periodontol* 57:480–485.

Leggott PJ, Robertson PB, Jacob RA, Zambon JJ, Walsh M, Armitage GC. 1991. Effects of ascorbic acid depletion and supplementation on periodontal health and subgingival microflora in humans. *J Dent Res* 70:1531–1536.

Lehr HA, Weyrich AS, Saetzler RK, Jurek A, Arfors KE, Zimmerman GA, Prescott SM, McIntyre TM. 1997. Vitamin C blocks inflammatory platelet-activating factor mimetics created by cigarette smoking. *J Clin Invest* 99:2358–2364.

Le Marchand L, Yoshizawa CN, Kolonel LN, Hankin JH, Goodman MT. 1989. Vegetable consumption and lung cancer risk: A population-based case-control study in Hawaii. *J Natl Cancer Inst* 81:1158–1164.

Lenton KJ, Therriault H, Fulop T, Payette H, Wagner JR. 1999. Glutathione and ascorbate are negatively correlated with oxidative DNA damage in human lymphocytes. *Carcinogenesis* 20:607–613.

Leske MC, Chylack LT Jr, Wu SY. 1991. The Lens Opacities Case-Control Study. Risk factors for cataract. *Arch Ophthalmol* 109:244–251.

Levine GN, Frei B, Koulouris SN, Gerhard MD, Keaney JF Jr, Vita JA. 1996. Ascorbic acid reverses endothelial vasomotor dysfunction in patients with coronary artery disease. *Circulation* 93:1107–1113.

Levine M, Dhariwal KR, Wang Y, Park JB, Welch RW. 1994. Ascorbic acid in neutrophils. In: Frei B, ed. *Natural Antioxidants in Health and Disease*. San Diego: Academic Press. Pp. 469–488.

Levine M, Conry-Cantilena C, Wang Y, Welch RW, Washko PW, Dhariwal KR, Park JB, Lazarev A, Graumlich JF, King J, Cantilena LR. 1996a. Vitamin C pharmacokinetics in healthy volunteers: Evidence for a recommended dietary allowance. *Proc Natl Acad Sci USA* 93:3704–3709.

Levine M, Rumsey S, Wang Y, Park J, Kwon O, Xu W, Amano N. 1996b. Vitamin C. In: Ziegler EE, Filer LJ Jr, eds. *Present Knowledge in Nutrition*, 7th edition. Washington, DC: ILSI Press. Pp. 146–159.

Levy R, Shriker O, Porath A, Riesenberg K, Schlaeffer F. 1996. Vitamin C for the treatment of recurrent furunculosis in patients with impaired neutrophil functions. *J Infect Dis* 173:1502–1505.

Loft S, Vistisen K, Ewertz M, Tjonneland A, Overvad K, Poulsen HE. 1992. Oxidative DNA damage estimated by 8-hydroxydeoxyguanosine excretion in humans: Influence of smoking, gender and body mass index. *Carcinogenesis* 13: 2241–2247.

Losonczy KG, Harris TB, Havlik RJ. 1996. Vitamin E and vitamin C supplement use and risk of all-cause and coronary heart disease mortality in older persons: The Established Populations for Epidemiologic Studies of the Elderly. *Am J Clin Nutr* 64:190–196.

Løvstad RA. 1997. A study on ascorbate inhibition of ceruloplasmin ferroxidase activity. *BioMetals* 10:123–126.

LSRO/FASEB (Life Sciences Research Office/ Federation of American Societies for Experimental Biology). 1989. *Nutrition Monitoring in the United States: An Update Report on Nutrition Monitoring.* Prepared for the U.S. Department of Agriculture and the U.S. Department of Health and Human Services. DHHS Publication No. (PHS) 89-1255. Washington, DC: U.S. Government Printing Office.

Ludvigsson J, Hansson LO, Tibbling G. 1977. Vitamin C as a preventive medicine against common colds in children. *Scand J Infect Dis* 9:91–98.

Ludvigsson J, Hansson LO, Stendahl O. 1979. The effect of large doses of vitamin C on leukocyte function and some laboratory parameters. *Int J Vitam Nutr Res* 49:160–165.

Lunec J, Blake DR. 1985. The determination of dehydroascorbic acid and ascorbic acid in the serum and synovial fluid of patients with rheumatoid arthritis. *Free Radic Res Commun* 1:31–39.

Lykkesfeldt J, Loft S, Nielsen JB, Poulsen HE. 1997. Ascorbic acid and dehydroascorbic acid as biomarkers of oxidative stress caused by smoking. *Am J Clin Nutr* 65:959–963.

Lykkesfeldt J, Christen S, Wallock LM, Change HH, Jacob RA, Ames BN. 2000. Ascorbate is depleted by smoking and repleted by moderate supplementation: A study in male smokers and nonsmokers with matched dietary antioxidant intakes. *Am J Clin Nutr* 71:530–536.

Mangels AR, Block G, Frey CM, Patterson BH, Taylor PR, Norkus EP, Levander OA. 1993. The bioavailability to humans of ascorbic acid from oranges, orange juice and cooked broccoli is similar to that of synthetic ascorbic acid. *J Nutr* 123:1054–1061.

Mannick EE, Bravo LE, Zarama G, Realpe JL, Zhang XJ, Ruiz B, Fontham ETH, Mera R, Miller MJS, Correa P. 1996. Inducible nitric oxide synthase, nitrotyrosine, and apoptosis in *Helicobacter pylori* gastritis: Effect of antibiotics and antioxidants. *Cancer Res* 56:3238–3243.

Marangon K, Herbeth B, Artur Y, Esterbauer H, Siest G. 1997. Low and very low density lipoprotein composition and resistance to copper-induced oxidation are not notably modified in smokers. *Clin Chim Acta* 265:1–12.

Marangon K, Herbeth B, Lecomte E, Paul-Dauphin A, Grolier P, Chancerelle Y, Artur Y. 1998. Diet, antioxidant status, and smoking habits in French men. *Am J Clin Nutr* 67: 231–239.

May JM, Cobb CE, Mendiratta S, Hill KE, Burk RF. 1998. Reduction of the ascorbyl free radical to ascorbate by thioredoxin reductase. *J Biol Chem* 273:23039–23045.

May JM, Mendiratta S, Qu ZC, Loggins E. 1999. Vitamin C recycling and function in human monocytic U-937 cells. *Free Radic Biol Med* 26:1513–1523.

McKeown-Eyssen G, Holloway C, Jazmaji V, Bright-See E, Dion P, Bruce WR. 1988. A randomized trial of vitamins C and E in the prevention of recurrence of colorectal polyps. *Cancer Res* 48:4701–4705.

McLaran CJ, Bett JHN, Nye JA, Halliday JW. 1982. Congestive cardiomyopathy and haemochromatosis—Rapid progression possibly accelerated by excessive ingestion of ascorbic acid. *Aust NZ J Med* 12:187–188.

Melethil S, Mason WD, Chang C-J. 1986. Dose-dependent absorption and excretion of vitamin C in humans. *Int J Pharmaceut* 31:83–89.

Mentzer WC, Collier E. 1975. Hydrops fetalis associated with erythrocyte G-6-PD deficiency and maternal ingestion of fava beans and ascorbic acid. *J Pediatr* 86:565–567.

Metz J, Hundertmark U, Pevny I. 1980. Vitamin C allergy of the delayed type. *Contact Dermatitis* 6:172–174.

Millar J. 1995. The nitric oxide/ascorbate cycle: How neurones may control their own oxygen supply. *Med Hypoth* 45:21–26.

Miller JZ, Nance WE, Norton JA, Wolen RL, Griffith RS, Rose RJ. 1977. Therapeutic effect of vitamin C. A co-twin control study. *J Am Med Assoc* 237:248–251.

Mirvish SS. 1994. Experimental evidence for inhibition of N-nitroso compound formation as a factor in the negative correlation between vitamin C consumption and the incidence of certain cancers. *Cancer Res* 54:1948S–1951S.

Mitch WE, Johnson MW, Kirshenbaum JM, Lopez RE. 1981. Effect of large oral doses of ascorbic acid on uric acid excretion by normal subjects. *Clin Pharmcol Ther* 29:318–321.

Montalto MB, Benson JD, Martinez GA. 1985. Nutrient intakes of formula-fed infants and infants fed cow's milk. *Pediatrics* 75:343–351.

Morrow JD, Frei B, Longmire AW, Gaziano JM, Lynch SM, Shyr Y, Strauss WE, Oates JA, Roberts LJ II. 1995. Increase in circulating products of lipid peroxidation (F_2-isoprostanes) in smokers. *N Engl J Med* 332:1198–1203.

Morse EH, Clark RP, Keyser DE, Merrow SB, Bee DE. 1975. Comparison of the nutritional status of pregnant adolescents with adult pregnant women. I. Biochemical findings. *Am J Clin Nutr* 28:1000–1013.

Moser U. 1987. Uptake of ascorbic acid by leukocytes. *Ann NY Acad Sci* 498:200–215.

Moss AJ, Levy AS, Kim I, Park YK. 1989. *Use of Vitamin and Mineral Supplements in the United States: Current Users, Types of Products, and Nutrients.* Advance Data, Vital and Health Statistics of the National Center for Health Statistics. Number 174. Hyattsville, MD: National Center for Health Statistics. Pp. 1–19.

Motoyama T, Kawano H, Kugiyama K, Hirashima O, Ohgushi M, Yoshimura M, Ogawa H, Yasue H. 1997. Endothelium-dependent vasodilation in the brachial artery is impaired in smokers: Effect of vitamin C. *Am J Physiol* 273:H1644–H1650.

Mudway IS, Krishna MT, Frew AJ, MacLeod D, Sandstrom T, Holgate ST, Kelly FJ. 1999. Compromised concentrations of ascorbate in fluid lining the respiratory tract in human subjects after exposure to ozone. *Occup Environ Med* 56:473–481.

Mulholland CW, Strain JJ, Trinick TR. 1996. Serum antioxidant potential, and lipoprotein oxidation in female smokers following vitamin C supplementation. *Int J Food Sci Nutr* 47:227–231.

Naidoo D, Lux O. 1998. The effect of vitamin C and E supplementation on lipid and urate oxidation products in plasma. *Nutr Res* 18:953–961.

Ness AR, Khaw KT, Bingham S, Day NE. 1996. Vitamin C status and respiratory function. *Eur J Clin Nutr* 50:573–579.

Newmark HL, Scheiner MS, Marcus M, Prabhudesai M. 1976. Stability of vitamin B_{12} in the presence of ascorbic acid. *Am J Clin Nutr* 29:645–649.

Newton HM, Schorah CJ, Habibzadeh N, Morgan DB, Hullin RP. 1985. The cause and correction of low blood vitamin C concentrations in the elderly. *Am J Clin Nutr* 42:656–659.

NRC (National Research Council). 1989. *Recommended Dietary Allowances,* 10th edition. Washington, DC: National Academy Press.

Nyyssonen K, Parviainen MT, Salonen R, Tuomilehto J, Salonen JT. 1997a. Vitamin C deficiency and risk of myocardial infarction: Prospective population study of men from eastern Finland. *Br Med J* 314:634–638.

Nyyssonen K, Poulsen HE, Hayn M, Agerbo P, Porkkala-Sarataho E, Kaikkonen J, Salonen R, Salonen JT. 1997b. Effect of supplementation of smoking men with plain or slow release ascorbic acid on lipoprotein oxidation. *Eur J Clin Nutr* 51:154–163.

Ocke MC, Bueno-de-Mesquita HB, Feskens EJ, van Staveren WA, Kromhout D. 1997. Repeated measurements of vegetables, fruits, beta-carotene, and vitamins C and E in relation to lung cancer. *Am J Epidemiol* 145:358–365.

Omaye ST, Skala JH, Jacob RA. 1986. Plasma ascorbic acid in adult males: Effects of depletion and supplementation. *Am J Clin Nutr* 44:257–264.

Omaye ST, Schaus EE, Kutnink MA, Hawkes WC. 1987. Measurement of vitamin C in blood components by high-performance liquid chromatography. Implication in assessing vitamin C status. *Ann NY Acad Sci* 498:389–401.

Ono K. 1986. Secondary hyperoxalemia caused by vitamin C supplementation in regular hemodialysis patients. *Clin Nephrol* 26:239–243.

Oreopoulos DG, Lindeman RD, VanderJagt DJ, Tzamaloukas AH, Bhagavan HN, Garry PJ. 1993. Renal excretion of ascorbic acid: Effect of age and sex. *J Am Coll Nutr* 12:537–542.

Ortega RM, Lopez-Sobaler AM, Quintas ME, Martinez RM, Andres P. 1998. The influence of smoking on vitamin C status during the third trimester of pregnancy and on vitamin C levels in maternal milk. *J Am Coll Nutr* 17:379–384.

O'Toole P, Lombard M. 1996. Vitamin C and gastric cancer: Supplements for some or fruit for all? *Gut* 39:345–347.

Panayiotidis M, Collins AR. 1997. Ex vivo assessment of lymphocyte antioxidant status using the comet assay. *Free Rad Res* 27:533–537.

Pandey DK, Shekelle R, Selwyn BJ, Tangney C, Stamler J. 1995. Dietary vitamin C and beta-carotene and risk of death in middle-aged men. The Western Electric Study. *Am J Epidemiol* 142:1269–1278.

Panush RS, Delafuente JC, Katz P, Johnson J. 1982. Modulation of certain immunologic responses by vitamin C. III. Potentiation of in vitro and in vivo lymphocyte responses. *Int J Vitam Nutr Res Suppl* 23:35–47.

Park JB, Levine M. 1996. Purification, cloning and expression of dehydroascorbic acid-reducing activity from human neutrophils: Identification as glutaredoxin. *Biochem J* 315:931–938.

Parkkinen J, Vaaranen O, Vahtera E. 1996. Plasma ascorbate protects coagulation factors against photooxidation. *Thromb Haemost* 75:292–297.

Pelletier O. 1977. Vitamin C and tobacco. *Int J Vitam Nutr Res Suppl* 16:147–170.

Perrig WJ, Perrig P, Stahelin HB. 1997. The relation between antioxidants and memory performance in the old and very old. *J Am Geriatr Soc* 45:718–724.

Peters EM, Goetzsche JM, Grobbelaar B, Noakes TD. 1993. Vitamin C supplementation reduces the incidence of postrace symptoms of upper-respiratory-tract infection in ultramarathon runners. *Am J Clin Nutr* 57:170–174.

Pfeffer F, Valdes-Ramos R, Avila-Rosas H, Meza C, Casanueva E. 1996. Iron, zinc and vitamin C nutritional status is not related to weight gain in pregnant women. *Nutr Res* 16:555–564.

Phull PS, Price AB, White KL, Schorah CJ, Jacyna MR. 1999. Gastroduodenal mucosal vitamin-C levels in *Helicobacter pylori* infection. *Scand J Gastroenterol* 34:361–366.

Pirkle JL, Flegal KM, Bernert JT, Brody DJ, Etzel RA, Maurer KR. 1996. Exposure of the US population to environmental tobacco smoke: The Third National Health and Nutrition Examination Survey, 1988 to 1991. *J Am Med Assoc* 275: 1233–1240.

Podmore ID, Griffiths HR, Herbert KE, Mistry N, Mistry P, Lunec J. 1998. Vitamin C exhibits pro-oxidant properties. *Nature* 392:559.

Pohl H, Reidy JA. 1989. Vitamin C intake influences the bleomycin-induced chromosome damage assay: Implications for detection of cancer susceptibility and chromosome breakage syndromes. *Mutat Res* 224:247–252.

Powers HJ, Loban A, Silvers K, Gibson AT. 1995. Vitamin C at concentrations observed in premature babies inhibits the ferroxidase activity of caeruloplasmin. *Free Radic Res* 22:57–65.

Prieme H, Loft S, Nyyssonen K, Salonen JT, Poulsen HE. 1997. No effect of supplementation with vitamin E, ascorbic acid, or coenzyme Q_{10} on oxidative DNA damage estimated by 8-hydroxy-7,8-dihydro-2'-deoxyguanosine excretion in smokers. *Am J Clin Nutr* 65:503–507.

Pryor WA. 1992. Biological effects of cigarette smoke, wood smoke, and the smoke from plastics: The use of electron spin resonance. *Free Radic Biol Med* 13:659–676.

Pryor WA. 1997. Cigarette smoke radicals and the role of free radicals in chemical carcinogenicity. *Environ Hlth Perspect* 105:875–882.

Pryor WA, Prier DG, Church DF. 1983. Electron-spin resonance study of mainstream and sidestream cigarette smoke: Nature of the free radicals in gasphase smoke and in cigarette tar. *Environ Hlth Perspect* 47:345–355.

Rajalakshmi R, Deodhar AD, Ramarkrishnan CV. 1965. Vitamin C secretion during lactation. *Acta Paediatr Scand* 54:375–382.

Rebouche CJ. 1995. Renal handling of carnitine in experimental vitamin C deficiency. *Metabolism* 44:1639–1643.

Rees DC, Kelsey H, Richards JDM. 1993. Acute haemolysis induced by high dose ascorbic acid in glucose-6-phosphate dehydrogenase deficiency. *Br Med J* 306: 841–842.

Rehman A, Collis CS, Yang M, Kelly M, Diplock AT, Halliwell B, Rice-Evans C. 1998. The effects of iron and vitamin C co-supplementation on oxidative damage to DNA in healthy volunteers. *Biochem Biophys Res Commun* 246:293–298.

✳ Reilly M, Delanty N, Lawson JA, Fitzgerald GA. 1996. Modulation of oxidant stress in vivo in chronic cigarette smokers. *Circulation* 94:19–25.

Rhead WJ, Schrauzer GN. 1971. Risks of long-term ascorbic acid overdosage. *Nutr Rev* 29:262–263.

Rifici VA, Khachadurian AK. 1993. Dietary supplementation with vitamins C and E inhibits in vitro oxidation of lipoproteins. *J Am Coll Nutr* 12:631–637.

Rimm EB, Stampfer MJ, Ascherio A, Giovannucci E, Colditz GA, Willett WC. 1993. Vitamin E consumption and the risk of coronary heart disease in men. *N Engl J Med* 328:1450–1456.

Rivers, JM. 1987. Safety of high-level vitamin C ingestion. *Ann NY Acad Sci* 498:445–454.

Robertson JM, Donner AP, Trevithick JR. 1989. Vitamin E intake and risk of cataracts in humans. *Ann NY Acad Sci* 570:372–382.

Rokitzki L, Hinkel S, Klemp C, Cufi D, Keul J. 1994. Dietary, serum and urine ascorbic acid status in male athletes. *Int J Sports Med* 15:435–440.

Rokkas T, Papatheodorou G, Karameris A, Mavrogeorgis A, Kalogeropoulos N, Giannikos N. 1995. *Helicobacter pylori* infection and gastric juice vitamin C levels. Impact of eradication. *Dig Dis Sci* 40:615–621.

Romney SL, Duttagupta C, Basu J, Palan PR, Karp S, Slagle NS, Dwyer A, Wassertheil-Smoller S, Wylie-Rosett J. 1985. Plasma vitamin C and uterine cervical dysplasia. *Am J Obstet Gynecol* 151:976–980.

Ronchetti IP, Quaglino D Jr, Bergamini G. 1996. Ascorbic acid and connective tissue. *Subcell Biochem* 25:249–264.

Rose RC, Richer SP, Bode AM. 1998. Ocular oxidants and antioxidant protection. *Proc Soc Exp Biol Med* 217:397–407.

Rumsey SC, Levine M. 1998. Absorption, transport, and disposition of ascorbic acid in humans. *J Nutr Biochem* 9:116–130.

Russell AL. 1967. Epidemiology of periodontal disease. *Int Dent J* 17:282–296.

Sahyoun NR, Jacques PF, Russell RM. 1996. Carotenoids, vitamins C and E, and mortality in an elderly population. *Am J Epidemiol* 144:501–511.

Salmenpera L. 1984. Vitamin C nutrition during prolonged lactation: Optimal in infants while marginal in some mothers. *Am J Clin Nutr* 40:1050–1056.

Salonen JT, Salonen R, Nyyssonen K, Korpela H. 1992. Iron sufficiency is associated with hypertension and excess risk of myocardial infarction: The Kuopio Ischemic Heart Disease Risk Factor Study (KIHD). *Circulation* 85:864–876.

Samman S, Brown AJ, Beltran C, Singh S. 1997. The effect of ascorbic acid on plasma lipids and oxidisability of LDL in male smokers. *Eur J Clin Nutr* 51:472–477.

Sasaki A, Kondo K, Sakamoto Y, Kurata H, Itakura H, Ikeda Y. 1997. Smoking cessation increases the resistance of low-density lipoprotein to oxidation. *Atherosclerosis* 130:109–111.

Satarug S, Haswell-Elkins MR, Tsuda M, Mairiang P, Sithithaworn P, Mairiang E, Esumi H, Sukprasert S, Yongvanit P, Elkins DB. 1996. Thiocyanate-independent nitrosation in humans with carcinogenic parasite infection. *Carcinogenesis* 17:1075–1081.

Sauberlich HE. 1994. Pharmacology of vitamin C. *Annu Rev Nutr* 14:371–391.

Scaccini C, Jialal I. 1994. LDL Modification by activated polymorphonuclear leukocytes: A cellular model of mild oxidative stress. *Free Radic Biol Med* 16:49–55.

Schectman G, Byrd JC, Hoffmann R. 1991. Ascorbic acid requirements for smokers: Analysis of a population survey. *Am J Clin Nutr* 53:1466–1470.

Schmidt KH, Hagmaier V, Hornig DH, Vuilleumier JP, Rutishauser G. 1981. Urinary oxalate excretion after large intakes of ascorbic acid in man. *Am J Clin Nutr* 34:305–311.

Schrauzer GN, Rhead WJ. 1973. Ascorbic acid abuse: Effects on long-term ingestion of excessive amounts on blood levels and urinary excretion. *Int J Vitam Nutr Res* 43:201–211.

Schrauzer GN, Ishmael D, Kiefer GW. 1975. Some aspects of current vitamin C usage: Diminished high altitude resistance following overdosage. *Ann NY Acad Sci* 258:377–381.

Schwartz J, Weiss ST. 1994. Relationship between dietary vitamin C intake and pulmonary function in the First National Health and Nutrition Examination Survey (NHANES I). *Am J Clin Nutr* 59:110–114.

Schwarz KB, Cox J, Sharma S, Witter F, Clement L, Sehnert SS, Risby TH. 1995. Cigarette smoking is pro-oxidant in pregnant women regardless of antioxidant nutrient intake. *J Nutr Environ Med* 5:225–234.

Sharpe PC, MacAuley D, McCrum EE, Stott G, Evans AE, Mulholland C, Boreham CA, Duly E, Trinick TR. 1994. Ascorbate and exercise in the Northern Ireland population. *Int J Vitam Nutr Res* 64:277–282.

Shekelle RB, Lepper M, Liu S, Maliza C, Raynor WJ, Rossof AH. 1981. Dietary vitamin A and risk of cancer in the Western Electric Study. *Lancet* 2:1185–1190.

Shilotri PG, Bhat KS. 1977. Effect of mega doses of vitamin C on bactericidal activity of leukocytes. *Am J Clin Nutr* 30:1077–1081.

Siegel C, Barker B, Kunstadter M. 1982. Conditioned oral scurvy due to megavitamin C withdrawal. *J Periodontol* 53:453–455.

Sies H, Stahl W. 1995. Vitamins E and C, beta-carotene, and other carotenoids as antioxidants. *Am J Clin Nutr* 62:1315S–1321S.

Simon JA. 1992. Vitamin C and cardiovascular disease: A review. *J Am Coll Nutr* 11:107–125.

Simon JA, Hudes ES, Browner WS. 1998. Serum ascorbic acid and cardiovascular disease prevalence in US adults. *Epidemiology* 9:316–321.

Singh RB, Ghosh S, Niaz MA, Singh R, Beegum R, Chibo H, Shoumin Z, Postiglione A. 1995. Dietary intake, plasma levels of antioxidant vitamins, and oxidative stress in relation to coronary artery disease in elderly subjects. *Am J Cardiol* 76:1233–1238.

Sinha R, Block G, Taylor PR. 1993. Problems with estimating vitamin C intakes. *Am J Clin Nutr* 57:547–550.

Skaper SD, Fabris M, Ferrari V, Carbonare MD, Leon A. 1997. Quercetin protects cutaneous tissue-associated cell types including sensory neurons from oxidative stress induced by glutathione depletion: Cooperative effects of ascorbic acid. *Free Radic Biol Med* 22:669–678.

Sneed SM, Zane C, Thomas MR. 1981. The effects of ascorbic acid, vitamin B_6, vitamin B_{12}, and folic acid supplementation on the breast milk and maternal nutritional status of low socioeconomic lactating women. *Am J Clin Nutr* 34:1338–1346.

Solzbach U, Hornig B, Jeserich M, Just H. 1997. Vitamin C improves endothelial dysfunction of epicardial coronary arteries in hypertensive patients. *Circulation* 96:1513–1519.

Specker BL, Beck A, Kalkwarf H., Ho M. 1997. Randomized trial of varying mineral intake on total body bone mineral accretion during the first year of life. *Pediatrics* 99:e12.

Stein HB, Hasan A, Fox IH. 1976. Ascorbic acid-induced uricosuria. *Ann Intern Med* 84:385–388.

Taddei S, Virdis A, Ghiadoni L, Magagna A, Salvetti A. 1998. Vitamin C improves endothelium-dependent vasodilation by restoring nitric oxide activity in essential hypertension. *Circulation* 97:2222–2229.

Thomas MR, Kawamoto J, Sneed SM, Eakin R. 1979. The effects of vitamin C, vitamin B_6, and vitamin B_{12} supplementation on the breast milk and maternal status of well-nourished women. *Am J Clin Nutr* 32:1679–1685.

Thomas MR, Sneed SM, Wei C, Nail PA, Wilson M, Sprinkle EE. 1980. The effects of vitamin C, vitamin B_6, vitamin B_{12}, folic acid, riboflavin, and thiamin on the breast milk and maternal status of well-nourished women at 6 months postpartum. *Am J Clin Nutr* 33:2151–2156.

Timimi FK, Ting HH, Haley EA, Roddy MA, Ganz P, Creager MA. 1998. Vitamin C improves endothelium-dependent vasodilation in patients with insulin-dependent diabetes mellitus. *J Am Coll Cardiol* 31:552–557.

Ting HH, Timimi FK, Boles KS, Creager SJ, Ganz P, Creager MA. 1996. Vitamin C improves endothelium-dependent vasodilation in patients with non-insulin-dependent diabetes mellitus. *J Clin Invest* 97:22–28.

Ting HH, Timimi FK, Haley EA, Roddy MA, Ganz P, Creager MA. 1997. Vitamin C improves endothelium-dependent vasodilation in forearm resistance vessels of humans with hypercholesterolemia. *Circulation* 95:2617–2622.

Tiselius HG, Almgard LE. 1977. The diurnal urinary excretion of oxalate and the effect of pyridoxine and ascorbate on oxalate excretion. *Eur Urol* 3:41–46.

Tlaskal P, Novakova V. 1990. Vitamins C and E in neonates and their mothers. *Cesk Pediatr* 45:339–343.

Tribble DL, Giuliano LJ, Fortmann SP. 1993. Reduced plasma ascorbic acid concentrations in nonsmokers regularly exposed to environmental tobacco smoke. *Am J Clin Nutr* 58:886–890.

Tsao CS. 1997. An overview of ascorbic acid chemistry and biochemistry. In: Packer L, Fuchs J, eds. *Vitamin C in Health and Disease.* New York: Marcel Dekker. Pp. 25–58.

Tsao CS, Leung PY. 1988. Urinary ascorbic acid levels following the withdrawal of large doses of ascorbic acid in guinea pigs. *J Nutr* 118:895–900.

Tsao CS, Salimi SL. 1984. Effect of large intake of ascorbic acid on urinary and plasma oxalic acid levels. *Int J Vitam Nutr Res* 54:245–249.

Udipi SA, Kirksey A, West K, Giacoia G. 1985. Vitamin B_6, vitamin C and folacin levels in milk from mothers of term and preterm infants during the neonatal period. *Am J Clin Nutr* 42:522–530.

Urivetzky M, Kessaris D, Smith AD. 1992. Ascorbic acid overdosing: A risk factor for calcium oxalate nephrolithiasis. *J Urol* 147:1215–1218.

Valkonen M, Kuusi T. 1998. Passive smoking induces atherogenic changes in low-density lipoprotein. *Circulation* 97:2012–2016.

VanderJagt DJ, Garry PJ, Bhagavan HN. 1987. Ascorbic acid intake and plasma levels in healthy elderly people. *Am J Clin Nutr* 46:290–294.

Van Eekelen M. 1953. Occurrence of vitamin C in foods. *Proc Nutr Soc* 12:228–232.

Vitale S, West S, Hallfrisch J, Alston C, Wang F, Moorman C, Muller D, Singh V, Taylor HR. 1993. Plasma antioxidants and risk of cortical and nuclear cataract. *Epidemiology* 4:195–203.

Vogel RI, Lamster IB, Wechsler SA, Macedo B, Hartley LJ, Macedo JA. 1986. The effects of megadoses of ascorbic acid on PMN chemotaxis and experimental gingivitis. *J Periodontol* 57:472–479.

Wandzilak TR, D'Andre SD, Davis PA, Williams HE. 1994. Effect of high dose vitamin C on urinary oxalate levels. *J Urol* 151:834–837.

Wang Y, Russo TA, Kwon O, Chanock S, Rumsey SC, Levine M. 1997. Ascorbate recycling in human neutrophils: Induction by bacteria. *Proc Natl Acad Sci USA* 94:13816–13819.

Waring AJ, Drake IM, Schorah CJ, White KL, Lynch DA, Axon AT, Dixon MF. 1996. Ascorbic acid and total vitamin C concentrations in plasma, gastric juice, and gastrointestinal mucosa: Effects of gastritis and oral supplementation. *Gut* 38:171–176.

Wassertheil-Smoller S, Romney SL, Wylie-Rosett J, Slagle S, Miller G, Lucido D, Duttagupta C, Palan PR. 1981. Dietary vitamin C and uterine cervical dysplasia. *Am J Epidemiol* 114:714–724.

Weber C, Wolfgang E, Weber K, Weber PC. 1996. Increased adhesiveness of isolated monocytes to endothelium is prevented by vitamin C intake in smokers. *Circulation* 93:1488–1492.

Wen Y, Cooke T Feely, J. 1997. The effect of pharmacological supplementation with vitamin C on low-density lipoprotein oxidation. *Br J Clin Pharmacol* 44:94–97.

Witt EH, Reznick AZ, Viguie CA, Starke-Reed P, Packer L. 1992. Exercise, oxidative damage and effects of antioxidant manipulation. *J Nutr* 122:766–773.

Witztum JL, Steinberg D. 1991. Role of oxidized low density lipoprotein in atherogenesis. *J Clin Invest* 88:1785–1792.

Woolfe SN, Kenney EB, Hume WR, Carranza FA Jr. 1984. Relationship of ascorbic acid levels of blood and gingival tissue with response to periodontal therapy. *J Clin Periodontol* 11:159–165.

Yong LC, Brown CC, Schatzkin A, Dresser CM, Slesinski MJ, Cox CS, Taylor PR. 1997. Intake of vitamins E, C, and A and risk of lung cancer. The NHANES I Epidemiologic Followup Study. *Am J Epidemiol* 146:231–243.

Young JC, Kenyon EM, Calabrese EJ. 1990. Inhibition of beta-glucuronidase in human urine by ascorbic acid. *Hum Exp Toxicol* 9:165–170.

Zatonski W, Przewozniak K, Howe GR, Maisonneuve P, Walker AM, Boyle P. 1991. Nutritional factors and pancreatic cancer: A case-control study from southwest Poland. *Int J Cancer* 48:390–394.

6

Vitamin E

SUMMARY

Vitamin E is thought to function primarily as a chain-breaking antioxidant that prevents the propagation of lipid peroxidation. Overt deficiency is very rare, seen only in individuals unable to absorb the vitamin or with inherited abnormalities that prevent the maintenance of normal blood concentrations. Thus, current dietary patterns appear to provide sufficient vitamin E to prevent deficiency symptoms such as peripheral neuropathy. Estimates of vitamin E intake are underreported, due in part to underreporting of amounts of dietary fat consumed and lack of specificity of sources in the diet. Data on human experimental vitamin E deficiency are very limited but provide some guidance as to the appropriate Recommended Dietary Allowance (RDA). The values recommended here are based largely on induced vitamin E deficiency in humans and the correlation between hydrogen peroxide-induced erythrocyte lysis and plasma α-tocopherol concentrations. The RDA for both men and women is 15 mg (35 μmol)/day of α-tocopherol. Vitamin E activity of α-tocopherol as defined in this report is limited to that available from the naturally occuring form (*RRR-*) and the other three synthetic 2*R*-stereoisomer forms (*RSR-*, *RRS-*, and *RSS-*) of α-tocopherol for purposes of establishing the human requirement for vitamin E. Other naturally occurring forms of vitamin E (β-, γ-, and δ-tocopherols and the tocotrienols) do not contribute toward meeting the vitamin E requirement because (although absorbed) they are not converted to α-tocopherol by humans and are recognized poorly by the α-tocopherol transfer protein (α-TTP) in the liver. Therefore, the RDA is based only on the α-tocopherol form of vitamin E which represents a change from most recent recommendations. A large and growing body of experimental evidence suggests that high intakes of vitamin E may lower the risk of some chronic diseases, especially heart disease. However, the limited and discordant clinical trial evidence available precludes recommendations at this time of higher vitamin E intakes to reduce chronic disease risk. The Tolerable Upper Intake Level (UL) for adults is set at 1,000 mg (2,325 μmol)/day of any form of supplemental α-tocopherol based on the adverse effect of increased tendency to hemorrhage.

BACKGROUND INFORMATION

Definition of Vitamin E

Of the eight naturally occurring forms of vitamin E (see section on "Naturally Occurring Forms" and Figure 6-1) only the α-tocopherol form of the vitamin is maintained in human plasma (Traber, 1999). Furthermore, the only forms of α-tocopherol that are maintained in plasma are *RRR*-α-tocopherol [2,5,7,8-tetramethyl-2*R*-(4′*R*, 8′*R*, 12′ trimethyltridecyl)-6-chromanol], the form of α-tocopherol that occurs naturally in foods, and the 2*R*-stereoisomeric forms of α-tocopherol (*RRR-*, *RSR-*, *RRS-*, and *RSS*-α-tocopherol) present in synthetic all racemic- (*all rac-*) α-tocopherol [2,5,7,8-tetramethyl-2*RS*-(4′*RS*, 8′*RS*, 12′ trimethyltridecyl)-6-chromanol (Traber, 1999) (Figure 6-2). Since the 2*S*-stereoisomers of α-tocopherol (*SRR-*, *SSR-*, *SRS-*, and *SSS*-α-tocopherol), part of the synthetic *all rac*-α-tocopherol, are not maintained in human plasma (Acuff et al., 1994; Kiyose et al., 1997; Traber, 1999) or tissues (Burton et al., 1998), they are not included in the definition of active components of vitamin E for humans. Therefore, vitamin E is defined in this report as limited to the 2*R*-stereoisomeric forms of α-tocopherol to establish recommended intakes. All forms of supplemental α-tocopherol are used as the basis of establishing the Tolerable Upper Intake Level (UL) for vitamin E. These recommended intakes and ULs are at variance with past definitions and recommendations for vitamin E (NRC, 1989).

Structure

Naturally Occurring Forms

Naturally occurring structures (Figure 6-1) classified in the past as having vitamin E antioxidant activity include 4 tocopherols (α-tocopherol, trimethyl [3 methyl groups on the chromanol ring]; β-

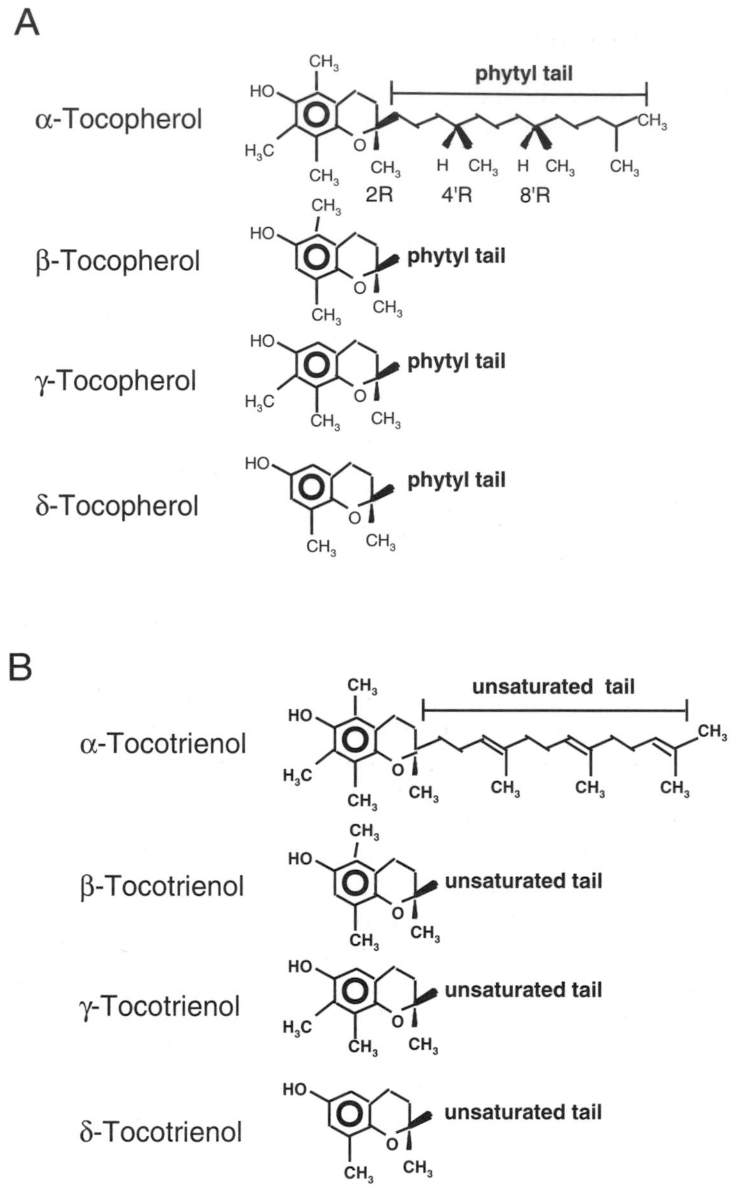

FIGURE 6-1 Structures of tocopherols and tocotrienols. The four tocopherols are shown in A and the four tocotrienols in B. All tocopherols are in the *RRR*-form. SOURCE: Adapted from Traber (1999).

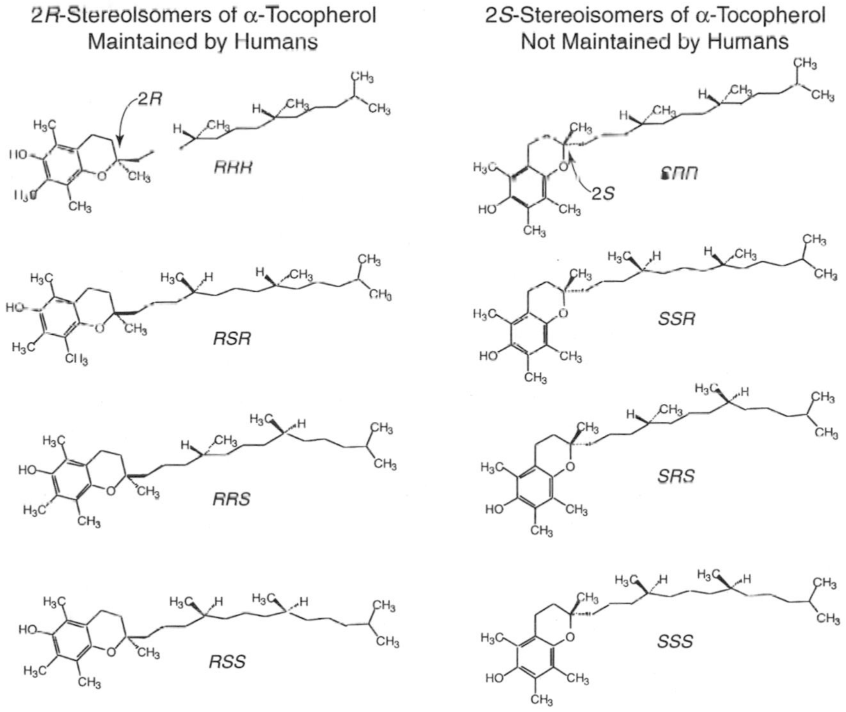

2*R*-Stereoisomers of α-Tocopherol
Maintained by Humans

2*S*-Stereoisomers of α-Tocopherol
Not Maintained by Humans

FIGURE 6-2 *all rac*-α-Tocopherol structures. Shown are the eight different stereo-isomers in synthetic vitamin E (*all rac* α-tocopherol): *RRR*, *RSR*, *RRS*, *RSS*, *SRR*, *SSR*, *SRS*, and *SSS*. All eight stereoisomers are formed in equal amounts. One stereoisomer, *RRR*-α-tocopherol, is also naturally present in food. The structure differences occur in the side chain and most importantly at the ring/tail junction.

or γ-tocopherols, dimethyl [2 methyl groups on the chromanol ring at different positions]; and δ-tocopherol, monomethyl [1 methyl group on the chromanol ring]) and 4 tocotrienols (α-tocotrienol, trimethyl; β- or γ-tocotrienols, dimethyl; and δ-tocotrienol, monomethyl) (IUPAC-IUB Joint Commission on Biochemical Nomenclature, 1974). The tocopherols are characterized by a substituted, hydroxylated ring system (chromanol ring) with a long, saturated (phytyl) side chain (Figure 6-1). Tocotrienols differ from tocopherols only in that they have an unsaturated side chain. All tocopherols that occur naturally in foods have the *RRR* stereochemistry in the side chain. However, the various forms of vitamin E are not interconvertible in the human and thus do not behave the same metabolically.

Synthetic Vitamin E

Synthetic forms of α-tocopherol are present in fortified foods and in vitamin supplements. Vitamin E supplements are sold as esters of either the natural *RRR-* or the synthetic mixture (*all rac-*) forms of α-tocopherol. Because α-tocopherol has three asymmetric carbon atoms, it has eight possible stereoisomers, seven of which are only found in synthetic preparations. Synthetic vitamin E, *all rac-α-*tocopherol (historically and incorrectly labeled *dl-α-*tocopherol) (Horwitt, 1976),[1] is produced by coupling trimethylhydroquinone with isophytol; it contains all eight stereoisomers in equal amounts (Figure 6-2). Four of the stereoisomers are in the 2*R*-stereoisomeric form (*RRR-, RSR-, RRS-,* and *RSS-α-*tocopherol) and four are in the 2*S*-stereoisomeric form (*SRR- SSR-, SRS-,* and *SSS-α-*tocopherol). Although *RRR-α-*tocopherol is the most biologically active of the eight stereoisomers in rats, the other 2*R*-stereoisomers generally have a higher activity than the 2*S* stereoisomers (Weiser and Vecchi, 1982; Weiser et al., 1986).

The naturally occurring stereoisomer is *RRR-α-*tocopherol (historically and incorrectly labeled *d-α-*tocopherol) (Horwitt, 1976). *RRR-α-*Tocopherol can be derived by methylating γ-tocopherol isolated from vegetable oil. This is labeled "natural source" vitamin E when marketed.

Esterification of the labile hydroxyl (OH) group on the chromanol ring of vitamin E prevents its oxidation and extends its shelf life. This is why esters of α-tocopherol are often used in vitamin E supplements and in fortified foods. In apparently healthy humans,

---

[1]The original international standard for vitamin E, *dl-α-*tocopheryl acetate (one asymmetric carbon atom in the 2 position on the chromal ring, ambo-α-tocopheryl acetate) is no longer commercially available. It was synthesized from natural phytol and was a mixture of two stereoisomers of α-tocopherols, *RRR-α-*tocopheryl acetate and *SRR-α-*tocopheryl acetate (Horwitt, 1976). For practical purposes at the time, the activity of 1 mg of *dl-α-*tocopheryl acetate was defined as equivalent to one IU of vitamin E. The *dl-α-*tocopheryl acetate of commerce currently available is synthesized from synthetic isophytol, has eight stereoisomers, and is labeled as *dl-α-*tocopheryl acetate. However, it is more accurately called *all rac-α-*tocopheryl acetate (AIN, 1990; IUPAC, 1974) because it contains three asymmetric carbon atoms in the 2, 4', and 8' positions (2*RS,* 4'*RS,* 8'*RS-α-*tocopherol). The *all rac* and ambo-α-tocopheryl acetates were shown to have the same biological activity in rats (Weiser et al., 1986).

the esters (e.g., α-tocopheryl acetate or α-tocopheryl succinate) are hydrolyzed and absorbed as efficiently as α-tocopherol (Cheeseman et al., 1995).

Interconversion of Vitamin E Units

Before 1980, for pharmacological uses, one international unit (IU) of vitamin E activity was defined as 1 mg of all rac-α-tocopheryl acetate by the United States Pharmacopeia (USP) (USP, 1979). Using the rat fetal resorption assay, 1 mg of RRR-α-tocopherol was calculated to be equivalent to 1.49 IU of vitamin E (Weiser and Vecchi, 1981).

After 1980, the IU was changed to the USP unit where one USP unit of vitamin E was still defined as having the activity of 1 mg of all rac-α-tocopheryl acetate, 0.67 mg RRR-α-tocopherol, or 0.74 mg RRR-α-tocopheryl acetate (USP, 1980). Although IUs are no longer recognized, many fortified foods and supplements still retain this terminology while USP units are now generally used by the pharmaceutical industry in labeling vitamin E supplements. Both systems are based on the same equivalency.

Since the USP unit was defined before studies were published indicating that the 2S-stereoisomers of all rac-α-tocopherol were not maintained in human plasma (Acuff et al., 1994; Kiyose et al., 1997: Traber, 1999) or in tissues (Burton et al., 1998), it is recommended that the present equivalency used in the USP system be redefined based on the definition presented in this report of what contributes to the active form of vitamin E in humans. Vitamin E is defined here as limited to the 2R-stereoisomeric forms of α-tocopherol (RRR-, RSR-, RRS-, and RSS-α-tocopherol) to establish recommended intakes. Based on this definition, all rac-α-tocopherol has one-half the activity of RRR-α-tocopherol found in foods or present with the other 2R stereoisomeric forms (RSR-, RRS- and RSS-) of α-tocopherol in fortified foods and supplements. Thus to achieve the RDA recommended in this report of 15 mg/day of α-tocopherol, a person can consume 15 mg/day of RRR-α-tocopherol or 15 mg/day of the 2R-stereoisomeric forms of α-tocopherol (e.g., 30 mg/day of all rac-α-tocopherol) or a combination of the two. The factors necessary to convert RRR- and all rac-α-tocopherol and their esters based on this new definition of vitamin E to USP units (IUs) are shown in Table 6-1.

TABLE 6-1 Factors for Converting International Units of Vitamin E[a] to α-Tocopherol[b] (mg) to Meet Recommended Intake

	USP Conversion Factors[c]		Molar Conversion Factors[d]	α-Tocopherol Conversion Factors[e]
	IU/mg	mg/IU	μmol/IU	mg/IU
Synthetic Vitamin E and Esters				
dl-α-Tocopheryl acetate	1.00	1.00	2.12	0.45
dl-α-Tocopheryl succinate	0.89	1.12	2.12	0.45
dl-α-Tocopherol[f]	1.10	0.91	2.12	0.45
Natural Vitamin E and Esters				
d-α-Tocopheryl acetate	1.36	0.74	1.56	0.67
d-α-Tocopheryl succinate	1.21	0.83	1.56	0.67
d-α-Tocopherol[g]	1.49	0.67	1.56	0.67

[a] Vitamin E supplements are historically and incorrectly labeled *d*- or *dl*-α-tocopherol. Vitamin E compounds include the *all racemic* (*all rac*)-α-tocopherol (*dl*-α-tocopherol [*RRR*-, *RRS*-, *RSR*-, *RSS*-, *SSS*-, *SRS*-, *SSR*-, and *SRR*-] or synthetic) form and its esters and the *RRR*-α-tocopherol (*d*-α-tocopherol or natural) form and its esters. All of these compounds of vitamin E may be present in fortified foods and multivitamins. Not all stereoisomers function to meet vitamin E requirements in humans.

[b] α-Tocopherol as defined in this report to meet recommended intakes includes *RRR*-α-tocopherol (historically and incorrectly labeled *d*-α-tocopherol) the only form of α-tocopherol that occurs naturally in foods, and the other 2*R*-stereoisomeric forms of α-tocopherol (*RSR*-, *RRS*-, and *RSS*-α-tocopherol) that are synthesized chemically and thus are found in fortified foods and supplements (Figure 6-2).

[c] Official United States Pharmacopeia (USP) conversions where one IU is defined as 1 mg of *all rac*-α-tocopheryl acetate (USP, 1979, 1999). All of the conversions are based on rat fetal resorption assays that were conducted in the 1940s. The amounts of the free and succinate forms have been adjusted for their different molecular weights relative to the *all rac*-α-tocopheryl acetate (incorrectly labeled *dl*-α-tocopheryl acetate).

[d] To convert mg to μmol divide the mg by the molecular weight of the vitamin E compound (α-tocopheryl acetate = 472; α-tocopheryl succinate = 530; α-tocopherol = 430) and multiply by 1,000. Because the amount of free and succinate compounds are adjusted for their different molecular weights relative to α-tocopheryl acetate, these forms have the same conversion factors as the corresponding tocopherol compounds.

[e] To convert the μmol of the vitamin E compound to mg of α-tocopherol, multiply the μmol by the molecular weight of α-tocopherol (430) and divide by 1,000. The activities of the three synthetic α-tocopherol compounds have been divided by 2 because the 2*S*-stereoisomers contained in synthetic-α-tocopherol are not maintained in the blood.

[f] *dl*-α-Tocopherol = *all rac*-(racemic) α-tocopherol = synthetic vitamin E; *all rac*-α-tocopherol = *RRR*-, *RRS*-, *RSR*-, *RSS*-, *SSS*-, *SRS*-, *SSR*-, and *SRR*-α-tocopherol isomers.

[g] *d*-α-Tocopherol = *RRR*-α-tocopherol = natural vitamin E.

Units of Vitamin E Activity

It is now known that vitamin E forms are not interconvertible in the human and that their plasma concentrations are dependent on the affinity of hepatic α-tocopherol transfer protein (α-TTP) for them (see section on "Hepatic α-Tocopherol Transfer Protein"). Kinetic studies have shown that while *RRR*-α-tocopherol concentrations are maintained in human plasma, the same is not true for either synthetic *SRR*-α-tocopherol or natural γ-tocopherol (Traber et al., 1990a, 1992). These compounds are efficiently absorbed and delivered to the liver in chylomicrons but are packaged poorly into newly secreted lipoproteins for delivery to peripheral tissues (see section on "Preferential Secretion of α-Tocopherol from the Liver"). In light of these new findings in humans, it becomes necessary to reevaluate the relative biological potencies of different forms of vitamin E. Therefore, it is best to measure and report the actual concentrations of each of the various vitamin E forms in food and biological samples.

Current information suggests that the number of methyl groups and the stereochemistry of the phytyl tail at the point where it meets the chromanol ring (2 position) determine the affinity of the α-TTP for the vitamin E form and that this protein in turn determines the effective vitamin E biological activity (Hosomi et al., 1997). Since the 2*S*-stereoisomers (Figure 6-2) are not maintained in human plasma or in tissues, the difference in relative activity of *all rac*-α-tocopherol compared to *RRR*-α-tocopherol is 50 percent as demonstrated in Figure 6-3.

Vitamin E activity in food is often reported as α-tocopherol equivalents (α-TE) (Bieri and Evarts, 1973, 1974; Eitenmiller and Landen, 1995) as have been dietary recommendations (NRC, 1989). Previously, factors for the conversion of the tocopherols and tocotrienols to α-TE units were based on the biological activity of the various forms as determined using the rat fetal resorption assay (Bieri and McKenna, 1981). α-TEs were defined as α-tocopherol, mg $\times$ 1.0; β-tocopherol, mg $\times$ 0.5; γ-tocopherol, mg $\times$ 0.1; δ-tocopherol, mg $\times$ 0.03; α-tocotrienol, mg $\times$ 0.3; and β-tocotrienol, mg $\times$ 0.05 (NRC, 1989). The biological activities of γ- and δ-tocotrienol were below detection.

Based on a review of the data, the 2*R*-stereoisomeric forms of α-tocopherol (*RRR*-, *RSR*-, *RRS*-, and *RSS*-α-tocopherol) are now used to estimate the vitamin E requirement. The 2*S*-stereoisomeric forms of α-tocopherol and the other tocopherols (β-, γ-,and δ-tocopherol) and the tocotrienols are not used to estimate the vitamin E require-

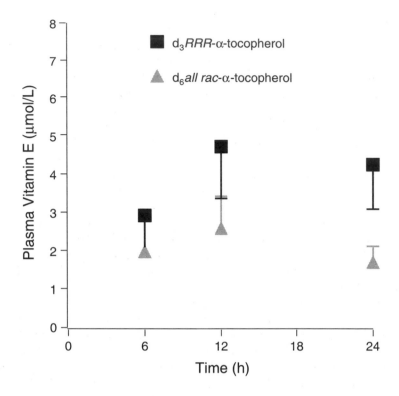

FIGURE 6-3 Plasma labeled (d_3 and d_6) α-tocopherols (means ± standard error, n = 6) following administration of a single dose containing 150 mg each d_3RRR-α- and d_6all rac-α-tocopherol acetates.
SOURCE: Adapted from Traber et al. (1998).

ment because of their failure to bind with the α-TTP. Thus, the Estimated Average Requirements (EARs), Recommended Dietary Allowances (RDAs), and Adequate Intakes (AIs) that follow apply only to intake of the 2R-stereoisomeric forms of α-tocopherol from food, fortified food, and multivitamins. The ULs apply to any forms of supplemental α-tocopherol.

Currently, most nutrient databases, as well as nutrition labels, do not distinguish between the different tocopherols in food. They often present the data as α-tocopherol equivalents and include the contribution of all eight naturally occurring forms of vitamin E (Figure 6-1), after adjustment for bioavailability of the various forms (see above). Because these other forms of vitamin E occur naturally in foods (e.g., γ-tocopherol is present in widely consumed oils such as soybean and corn oils), the intake of α-tocopherol equivalents is greater than the intake of α-tocopherol (2R-stereoisomeric forms) alone (see later section "Intake of Vitamin E" for suggested conversion factor).

Function

Unlike most nutrients, a specific role for vitamin E in a required metabolic function has not been found. Vitamin E's major function appears to be as a non-specific chain-breaking antioxidant.

Antioxidant Activity

Vitamin E is a chain-breaking antioxidant that prevents the propagation of free-radical reactions (Burton and Ingold, 1986; Burton et al., 1983; Ingold et al., 1987; Kamal-Eldin and Appelqvist, 1996; Packer, 1994; Tappel, 1962). The vitamin is a peroxyl radical scavenger and especially protects polyunsaturated fatty acids (PUFAs) within membrane phospholipids and in plasma lipoproteins (Burton et al., 1983). Peroxyl radicals (abbreviated ROO•) react with vitamin E (abbreviated Vit E-OH) 1,000 times more rapidly than they do with PUFA (abbreviated RH) (Packer, 1994). The phenolic hydroxyl group of tocopherol reacts with an organic peroxyl radical to form the corresponding organic hydroperoxide and the tocopheroxyl radical (Vit E-O•) (Burton et al., 1985):

In the presence of vitamin E: ROO• + Vit E-OH → ROOH + Vit E-O•

In the absence of vitamin E: ROO• + RH › ROOH + R•

R• + O$_2$ → ROO•

The tocopheroxyl radical can then undergo several possible fates. It can (1) be reduced by other antioxidants to tocopherol (see section on "Antioxidant Interactions"), (2) react with another tocopheroxyl radical to form non-reactive products such as tocopherol dimers, (3) undergo further oxidation to tocopheryl quinone (see section on "Metabolism"), and (4) act as a prooxidant and oxidize other lipids (see section on "Antioxidant Interactions").

Biochemical and Molecular Biologic Activities

In addition to its direct antioxidant function, α-tocopherol reportedly has specific molecular functions. α-Tocopherol inhibits protein kinase C activity, which is involved in cell proliferation and differentiation, in smooth muscle cells (Boscoboinik et al., 1991; Chatelain et al., 1993; Clement et al., 1997; Stauble et al., 1994; Tasinato et al., 1995), human platelets (Freedman et al., 1996), and monocytes (Cachia et al., 1998; Devaraj et al., 1996). Protein kinase C inhibition by α-tocopherol is in part attributable to its attenuating effect on the generation of membrane-derived diacylglycerol, a lipid that facilitates protein kinase C translocation, thus increasing its activity (Kunisaki et al., 1994; Tran et al., 1994).

Vitamin E enrichment of endothelial cells downregulates the expression of intercellular cell adhesion molecule (ICAM-1) and vascular cell adhesion molecule-1 (VCAM-1), thereby decreasing the adhesion of blood cell components to the endothelium (Cominacini et al., 1997). Vitamin E also upregulates the expression of cytosolic phospholipase A_2 (Chan et al., 1998a; Tran et al., 1996) and cyclooxygenase-1 (Chan et al., 1998b). The enhanced expression of these two rate-limiting enzymes in the arachidonic acid cascade explains the observation that vitamin E, in a dose-dependent fashion, enhanced the release of prostacyclin, a potent vasodilator and inhibitor of platelet aggregation in humans (Szczeklik et al., 1985; Tran and Chan, 1990).

Physiology of Absorption, Metabolism, and Excretion

Absorption and Transport

Intestinal Absorption. While the efficiency of vitamin E absorption is low in humans, the precise rate of absorption is not known with certainty. In the early 1970s, vitamin E absorption was estimated to be 51 to 86 percent, measured as fecal radioactivity following ingestion of α-tocopherol (Kelleher and Losowsky, 1970; MacMahon and Neale, 1970). However, when Blomstrand and Forsgren (1968) measured vitamin E absorption in two individuals with gastric carcinoma and lymphatic leukemia, respectively, they found fractional absorption in the lymphatics to be only 21 and 29 percent of label from meals containing α-tocopherol and α-tocopheryl acetate, respectively.

Vitamin E absorption from the intestinal lumen is dependent upon biliary and pancreatic secretions, micelle formation, uptake into enterocytes, and chylomicron secretion. Defects at any step lead to impaired absorption (Gallo-Torres, 1970; Harries and Muller, 1971; Sokol, 1993; Sokol et al., 1983, 1989). Chylomicron secretion is required for vitamin E absorption and was suggested by Muller et al. (1974) to be the most important factor for efficient vitamin E absorption. All of the various vitamin E forms studied, including α- and γ-tocopherols (Meydani et al., 1989; Traber and Kayden, 1989; Traber et al., 1992), *RRR*- and *SRR*-α-tocopherols (Kiyose et al., 1997; Traber et al., 1990a, 1992), or *RRR*- and *all rac*-α-tocopherols (Traber et al., 1994a), showed similar apparent efficiencies of intestinal absorption and subsequent secretion in chylomicrons. During chylomicron catabolism, some vitamin E is distributed to all of the circulating lipoproteins (Figure 6-4).

Preferential Secretion of α-Tocopherol from the Liver. Chylomicron remnants, containing newly absorbed vitamin E, are taken up by the liver. Vitamin E is secreted from the liver in very low density lipoproteins (VLDLs), as demonstrated in rats (Cohn et al., 1988), isolated rat hepatocytes (Bjørneboe et al., 1987; Cohn et al., 1988), and perfused monkey livers (Traber et al., 1990b). Plasma vitamin E concentrations depend upon the secretion of vitamin E from the liver, and only one form of vitamin E, α-tocopherol, is preferentially resecreted by the liver (Figure 6-5) (Traber, 1999). Thus, the liver, not the intestine, discriminates between tocopherols and is responsible for the preferential plasma enrichment with α-tocopherol. α-TTP is a likely candidate for this discriminatory function (see below).

Hepatic α-Tocopherol Transfer Protein (α-TTP). α-TTP was first identified (Catignani and Bieri, 1977), purified, and characterized from rat liver cytosol (Sato et al., 1991; Yoshida et al., 1992). It has also been isolated from human liver cytosol (Kuhlenkamp et al., 1993), and the human complementary deoxyribonucleic acid (cDNA) sequence has been reported (Arita et al., 1995). The human cDNA sequence (encoding 238 amino acids) has 94 percent homology to the rat sequence, and the some similarity to sequences for the retinaldehyde binding protein in the retina and to sec14, a phospholipid transfer protein (Arita et al., 1995).

In vitro, α-TTP transfers α-tocopherol between liposomes and microsomes (Hosomi et al., 1997; Sato et al., 1991). The relative affinities of α-TTP toward the various forms of vitamin E (calculated from the degree of competition with *RRR*-α-tocopherol) are *RRR*-α-tocopherol = 100 percent; *RRR*-β-tocopherol = 38 percent; *RRR*-γ-tocopherol = 9 percent; *RRR*-δ-tocopherol = 2 percent; α-tocopheryl acetate = 2 percent; α-tocopheryl quinone = 2 percent; *SRR*-α-tocopherol = 11 percent; α-tocotrienol = 12 percent; and Trolox = 9

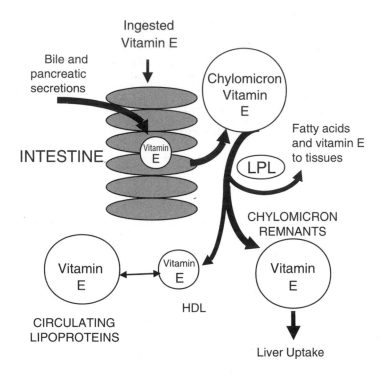

FIGURE 6-4 Vitamin E secretion in chylomicrons and distribution to circulating lipoproteins.
NOTE: HDL = high-density lipoprotein; LPL = lipoprotein lipase.
SOURCE: Adapted from Traber (1999).

percent (Hosomi et al., 1997). Data on the affinity of α-TTP for the other 2*R*-stereoisomers (*RSR-*, *RRS-*, and *RSS-*) of α-tocopherol has not been reported.

Plasma Vitamin E Kinetics. A kinetic model of vitamin E transport in human plasma has been developed using data from studies with deuterium-labeled stereoisomers of α-tocopherol (*RRR* and *SRR*) (Traber et al., 1994b). The apparent half-life of *RRR*-α-tocopherol in normal subjects was approximately 48 hours, consistent with the "slow" disappearance of *RRR*-α-tocopherol from the plasma, whereas the half-life for *SRR*-α-tocopherol was approximately 13 hours. The half-life of γ-tocopherol in normal subjects has been estimated to be approximately 15 hours (Acuff et al., 1997).

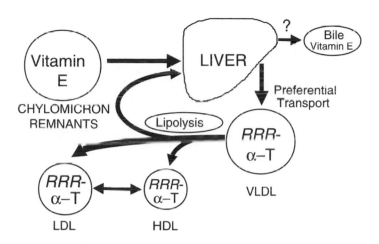

FIGURE 6-5 *RRR*-α-Tocopherol is preferentially resecreted by the liver and distributed to circulating lipoproteins. NOTE: HDL = high-density lipoprotein; LDL = low-density lipoprotein; VLDL = very low-density lipoprotein.
SOURCE: Adapted from Traber (1999).

In three people with ataxia and vitamin E deficiency (AVED) secondary to a defect in the α-TTP gene (Cavalier et al., 1998), the half-lives for both *RRR*- and *SRR*-α-tocopherols were approximately 13 hours (Traber et al., 1994b). These studies demonstrate that *RRR*- and *SRR*-α-tocopherols in the AVED patients disappear at the same rate as *SRR*-α-tocopherol in the control subjects. This suggests that α-TTP, which is defective in the AVED patients, is responsible for the longer half-life of *RRR*-α-tocopherol in the control subjects. It was estimated that resecretion of *RRR*-α-tocopherol by the liver in the control subjects resulted in the daily replacement of nearly all of the circulating *RRR*-α-tocopherol. Thus, the liver maintains plasma *RRR*-α-tocopherol concentrations by a continuous resecretion process. In contrast, other forms of vitamin E (e.g., *SRR*-α- and γ-tocopherols) are not resecreted into the plasma.

Metabolism

Oxidation Products. α-Tocopherol can be oxidized to the tocopheroxyl radical—one-electron oxidation product—which can be reduced back to the unoxidized form by reducing agents such as vitamin C. Further oxidation of the tocopheroxyl radical forms tocopheryl quinone, the two-election oxidation product. The tocopheryl quinone is not converted in any physiologically significant amounts back to tocopherol (Moore and Ingold, 1997). Other oxidation products, including dimers and trimers as well as adducts (Kamal-Eldin and Appelqvist, 1996), are formed during in vitro oxidation; their importance in vivo is unknown.

Other Metabolites. Vitamin E metabolites in human urine include both 2,5,7,8-tetramethyl-2-(2′-carboxyethyl)-6-hydroxychroman (α-CEHC) derived from α-tocopherol (Schultz et al., 1995, 1997) and 2,7,8-trimethyl-2-(2′-carboxyethyl)-6-hydroxychroman (γ-CEHC) derived from γ-tocopherol (Murray et al., 1997; Wechter et al., 1996). These metabolites result from degradation of the phytyl tail; the chromanol ring is unchanged and thus they are not oxidation products of vitamin E. It is unknown where these metabolites are formed.

Excretion

Urinary Excretion. Increasing doses of supplemental vitamin E in humans result in increasing urinary excretion of the α-CEHC metabolite (Schultz et al., 1995). Interestingly, three times as much *all rac*-α-tocopherol as compared with *RRR*-α-tocopherol is excreted as α-CEHC, while twice as much *RRR*-α-tocopherol is found in the plasma (Traber et al., 1998), suggesting that these urinary metabolites may be indicators of nonpreferentially utilized vitamin E forms. Indeed, Swanson et al. (1998, 1999) showed that about half of the ingested γ-tocopherol is metabolized and excreted as γ-CEHC. This metabolite has been reported to inhibit the potassium channel and increase urinary sodium excretion (Kantoci et al., 1997; Murray et al., 1997; Wechter et al., 1996). Thus, urinary excretion of CEHC may indicate excess vitamin E intake. However, this has yet to be definitively demonstrated, and no physiological role for the in vivo effects of γ-CEHC have been established.

Fecal Excretion. The major route of excretion of ingested vitamin E is fecal elimination because of its relatively low intestinal absorption. Excess α-tocopherol, as well as forms of vitamin E not preferentially used, are probably excreted unchanged in bile (Traber and Kayden, 1989). Leo et al. (1995) report α-tocopherol concentrations in human bile of 8.4 ± 0.9 (SD) μmol/L (361 ± 38.7 μg/dL) compared with 23.2 ± 1.7 (SD) μmol/L (998 ± 73 μg/dL) in plasma.

Storage

Tissues are dependent upon uptake of vitamin E from plasma (Traber, 1999). No specific plasma transport proteins have been described; therefore, it is likely that the mechanisms of lipoprotein metabolism determine the delivery of vitamin E to tissues. Tissues probably acquire vitamin E by several major routes: (1) during lipoprotein lipase mediated triglyceride-rich lipoprotein catabolism; (2) during low-density lipoprotein (LDL) uptake via the LDL receptor; (3) via high-density lipoprotein (HDL)-mediated delivery systems; and (4) by nonspecific transfers between lipoproteins and tissues. Vitamin E rapidly transfers between various lipoproteins and also between lipoproteins and membranes, which may enrich membranes with vitamin E. The human plasma phospholipid transfer protein accelerates this process (Kostner et al., 1995).

Human tissue vitamin E contents have been reported mostly from relatively easy-to-sample tissues (e.g., adipose tissue and buccal mucosal cells) (Handelman et al., 1994; Kayden et al., 1983; Parker, 1988; Peng et al., 1994; Traber and Kayden, 1987; Traber et al., 1987). To obtain a variety of human tissues, Burton et al. (1998) enlisted two terminally ill subjects who agreed to daily supplementation with deuterated (d_3-RRR- and d_6-all rac) α-tocopherols. At death, an autopsy was performed to obtain various tissues. One subject took 15 mg (32 μmol) d_3-RRR- and 15 mg (32 μmol) d_6-all rac-α-tocopheryl acetate for 361 days, while the other took 150 mg (320 μmol) d_3-RRR- plus 150 mg (320 μmol) d_6-all rac-α-tocopheryl acetates for 615 days. Tissue unlabeled α-tocopherol concentrations were generally similar in both patients. In the patient who consumed 30 mg (64 μmol)/day labeled vitamin E for 1 year, about 5.9 ± 2.2 (SD) percent of the tissue vitamin E was labeled, while about 65 ± 10 (SD) percent was labeled in the patient who consumed a total of 300 mg (640 μmol) daily for 2 years. The RRR/all rac ratios in plasma and tissues at autopsy were similar in both patients (2.06 and 1.71 ± 0.24 (SD), respectively, on the lower dose and 2.11 and 2.01 ± 0.17 (SD), respectively, on the higher dose).

The results indicate that the RRR-stereoisomer has roughly twice the availability of the all rac forms. The effect of 300 mg vitamin E supplementation was to increase plasma α-tocopherol concentrations threefold and to at least double most tissue concentrations, while supplementation with 30 mg had little effect on either plasma or tissue α-tocopherol concentrations. These data suggest that tissue α-tocopherol concentrations largely reflect changes in plasma concentrations of α-tocopherol and that larger doses increase tissue α-tocopherol concentrations, including those in the nervous tissues (Burton et al., 1998). Importantly, the lower dose, even though given for more than a year and a half, did not increase tissue α-tocopherol concentrations.

Clinical Effects of Inadequate Intake

Prevalence of Vitamin E Deficiency

Vitamin E deficiency occurs only rarely in humans, and overt deficiency symptoms in normal individuals consuming diets low in vitamin E have never been described. Vitamin E deficiency occurs only as a result of genetic abnormalities in α-TTP, as a result of various fat malabsorption syndromes (Rader and Brewer, 1993; Sokol, 1993), or as a result of protein-energy malnutrition (Kalra et al., 1998; Laditan and Ette, 1982).

Only a handful of families with clinically evident vitamin E deficiency due to a mutation of the α-TTP have been described (Cavalier et al., 1998). The prevalence of less drastic abnormalities in α-TTP, or the occurrence of heterozygotes for α-TTP gene defects, is not known. It is important to note that symptoms associated with α-TTP defects and malabsorption syndromes can be reversed by vitamin E supplementation if it is provided before irreversible neurological injury occurs (Kohlschütter et al., 1988; Muller et al., 1985; Schuelke et al., 1999; Sokol et al., 1985, 1988).

Clinical Signs of Deficiency

The primary human vitamin E deficiency symptom is a peripheral neuropathy characterized by the degeneration of the large-caliber axons in the sensory neurons (Sokol, 1988). Other vitamin E deficiency symptoms observed in humans include spinocerebellar ataxia, skeletal myopathy, and pigmented retinopathy (Sokol, 1993). Typical symptoms of vitamin E deficiency are given in Table 6-2.

A distinct pattern in the progression of neurologic symptoms resulting from vitamin E deficiency in humans has been described (Sokol, 1993). By the end of the first decade of life untreated patients with chronic cholestatic hepatobiliary disease have a combination of spinocerebellar ataxia, neuropathy, and ophthalmoplegia. However, the progression of neurological symptoms is slower in children with cystic fibrosis and abetalipoproteinemia. The symptomatology of vitamin E deficiency in AVED is similar to that found in these latter patients (Amiel et al., 1995; Sokol et al., 1988). These observations suggest that in patients with cholestatic liver disease, there is increased oxidative stress, perhaps as a result of copper accumulation in the liver (Bayliss et al., 1995).

Hemolysis, using hydrogen peroxide or other oxidants added in vitro, has been used as a test for vitamin E adequacy in subjects thought to be at risk for vitamin E deficiency (Boda et al., 1998; Farrell et al., 1977). These tests suggest that plasma α-tocopherol concentrations of 14 µmol/L (600 µg/dL) are sufficient to prevent hemolysis (Farrell et al., 1977).

SELECTION OF INDICATORS FOR ESTIMATING THE REQUIREMENT FOR α-TOCOPHEROL

Lipid Peroxidation Markers

Several biomarkers measured in plasma, urine, or breath have been used to reflect the degree of lipid peroxidation in vivo. These include thiobarbituric acid reactive substances (TBARS), malondialdehyde, conjugated dienes, pentane, ethane, and the F_2-isoprostanes.

Quantification of F_2-isoprostanes, isomers of prostaglandin F_2, has been suggested by a number of investigators as the most reliable index of in vivo free-radical generation and oxidative lipid damage (Morrow et al., 1999). The F_2-isoprostanes are formed in membranes from arachidonyl-containing lipids largely as a result of free radical-catalyzed lipid peroxidation (Klein et al., 1997; Moore and Roberts, 1998). The F_2-isoprostanes are increased in vitamin E-deficient rats (Awad et al., 1994). Importantly, their excretion was depressed in humans by consuming antioxidant vitamin supplements (Delanty et al., 1996; Reilly et al., 1996). Furthermore, in an animal atherosclerosis model, the apoE-deficient mouse, vitamin E supplementation not only suppressed F_2-isoprostane production but also decreased atherosclerotic lesion formation (Pratico et al., 1998).

In general, lipid peroxidation markers are elevated during vitamin E depletion and their levels can be normalized upon vitamin E repletion. However, these markers are not necessarily specific to vitamin E, since changes in intake of other antioxidants can also change the levels of these markers. At present, there is no evidence that lowering lipid peroxidation marker levels is associated with health benefits. Therefore, estimates of lipid peroxidation products have not been used for establishing α-tocopherol requirements.

TABLE 6-2 Vitamin E Deficiency Symptoms in Subjects with Ataxia with Vitamin E Deficiency

Reference	Country	Subjects	Clinical Features
Burck et al., 1981	Germany	n = 1 male; aged 12	Ataxia Sensory neuropathy Muscle hypertrophy
Laplante et al., 1984	Canada	n = 1 male; aged 10	Areflexia Gait and limb ataxia Muscle weakness Decreased vibration sense Decreased proprioception Limb dysmetria Babinski sign
Harding et al., 1985	United Kingdom	n = 1 female; aged 23 (aged 13 at onset)	Head titubation Reduced muscle tone Ataxia Areflexia Romberg sign Defective or absent vibration sense Impaired proprioception
Krendel et al., 1987	United States	n = 1 male; aged 19	Severe dysarthria Unintelligible speech Bradykinesia Absent tendon reflexes
Stumpf et al., 1987	Italy	n = 1 female; aged 30 (aged 4 at onset)	Dysarthria Dystonic smile Absent position sensation in leg and hands Absent tendon reflexes Mildly dysmetric Extensor plantar responses Moderately ataxic heel to shin movements Romberg sign

Genetic Abnormalities in α-TPP[a] Gene	Histological/Biochemical Features
530AG→6/530AG→6 mutation	Low serum vitamin E concentration: <2.3 μmol/L (1.0 μg/mL) (normal: 20.2 μmol/L [8.7 μg/mL])
R134X mutation	Low blood vitamin E concentration: <2.3 μmol/L (1.0 μg/mL) (normal: 12–28 μmol/L [5–12 μg/mL])
ND[b]	No detectable vitamin E in serum (normal: 12–35 μmol/L [5–15 μg/mL]) All other histologic and biochemical measurements were normal
ND	Low serum vitamin E concentration: 1.6 μmol/L (0.7 μg/mL) (normal: >12 μmol/L [5 μg/mL])
ND	Reduced sensory nerve amplitudes Low serum vitamin E concentration: <2.3 μmol/L (1.0 μg/mL) (normal: 12–46 μmol/L [5–20 μg/mL]) Low serum vitamin E to total serum lipids ratio: <0.15 mg/g (normal: >0.8 mg/g) Skeletal muscle changes characteristic of vitamin E deficiency (fiber size variation, coarse intra-myofibrillar network, fiber-type grouping, and lysosomal inclusions) Normal fat excretion, mitochondria function, cytochrome c oxidase activity, and ADP[c]:O[d] ratios

continued

TABLE 6-2 Continued

Reference	Country	Subjects	Clinical Features
Gotoda et al., 1995	Japan	*n* = 1 male; aged 62 (aged 52 at onset)	Unsteadiness in the dark Slurred and scanning speech Moderate ataxia in all extremities Flexor plantar responses Reduced reaction to touch and pinprick No joint position sense in toes Broad-based and ataxic gait Romberg sign No knee or ankle reflexes Numbness in fingers and toes
Kohlschütter et al., 1988	Germany	*n* = 1 male; aged 19	Ataxia Sensory neuropathy Lipopigment deposition
Sokol et al., 1988	United States	*n* = 1 male and 3 females; aged 21–30	Head titubation Intention tremor in hand Difficulty walking Progressive ataxia Dysarthria Vibratory and sensory loss Incontinence Pes cavus Position sense loss
Trabert et al., 1989	Germany	*n* = 1 male; aged 26	Cerebellar ataxia No tendon reflexes in lower limbs Vibration sense disturbances Babinsky sign Head titubation
Ben Hamida et al., 1993	Tunisia	*n* = 7 Friedreich's ataxia patients; aged 21–34	Severe cerebellar ataxia Severe dysarthria Slight deep sensory loss Slight Babinski signs Slight Pes cavus Slight kyphoscoliosis Absent to moderate cardiomyopathy[f]

Genetic Abnormalities in α-TPP[a] Gene	Histological/Biochemical Features
Homozygous for His101Gln point mutation	Low serum vitamin E concentration: 2.6 µmol/L (1.1 µg/mL) (normal: 12–46 µmol/L [5–20 µg/mL]) Low muscle vitamin E: 1.6 µg/g (normal: 10.5–25.7 µg/g) Low serum vitamin E to total lipid ratio: 0.19 mg/g (normal: >0.80 mg/g) Low vitamin E in erythrocytes: 0.5 µmol/L (0.2 µg/mL) (normal: 3.9–12.5 µmol/L [1.7–5.4 µg/mL]) Normal serum cholesterol and serum triglycerides
530AG→6/530AG→6 mutation	Subnormal serum vitamin E concentration: <2.3 µmol/L (1.0 µg/mL) (normal: 7–32 µmol/L [3–14 µg/mL]) Elevated TBARS[e]
R192H/513insTT mutation	Low serum vitamin E: 2.3–4.2 µmol/L (1.0–1.8 µg/mL) (normal: 10.9–47.1 µmol/L [4.7–20.3 µg/mL]) Low serum E to total lipids ratio: 0.13–0.38 mg/g (normal: >0.80 mg/g) Abnormal hydrogen peroxide hemolysis: 38–50% (normal: <10%) Low to reduced adipose tissue vitamin E content: 28–143 ng/mg (normal: 150–400 ng/mg) Low sural nerve vitamin E content: 0.8–2.9 ng/µg (normal: 2.1–62.5 ng/µg)
744delA mutation	Low vitamin E concentration: <2.3 µmol/L (1.0 µg/mL) (normal: 20.2 µmol/L [8.7 µg/mL])
744delA mutation	Very low serum vitamin E concentration: 0.72–2.02 µmol/L (0.31–0.87 µg/mL) (normal: 20.2 µmol/L [8.7 µg/mL])

continued

TABLE 6-2 Continued

Reference	Country	Subjects	Clinical Features
Shorer et al., 1996	Israel	$n = 4$ females (sisters); aged 11–24	Dysarthria Absent tendon reflexes Intention tremor Gait ataxia Pes cavus Hyperlordosis Retinopathy
Hammans and Kennedy, 1998	United Kingdom	$n = 1$; female; aged 16 (age 6 at onset)	Mild thoracic scoliosis Head titubation Gait and limb ataxia Areflexia Upgoing plantar responses Dysarthria
Martinello et al., 1998	Italy	$n = 1$ male; aged 26 (age 5 at onset)	Ataxia No deep tendon reflexes Decreased muscle strength Diminished trophism Bilateral Babinski's sign Scoliosis Reduced vibratory sensation Severe dysmetria and dysarthria Bilateral pes cavus Fasciculations of the tongue

NOTES: Lipid absorption was normal in all cases. There were no reports of anemia, lipid peroxidation products, or lipofuscin.

a α-TTP gene = α-tocopherol transfer protein gene.

b ND = not determined.

Oxidation Products of DNA or Proteins

Vitamin E has not been shown to directly protect deoxyribonucleic acid (DNA) or proteins against oxidative damage (Halliwell, 1999). Therefore, DNA adducts or protein carbonyls were not used to assess α-tocopherol requirements.

Vitamin E Metabolite Excretion

Excretion of vitamin E metabolites have been shown in one study to increase with increasing vitamin E intake in humans (Schultz et al., 1995). Increasing amounts of 2,5,7,8-tetramethyl-2-(2'-carboxy-

Genetic Abnormalities in α-TPP[a] Gene	Histological/Biochemical Features
Found no mutations or polymorphisms in the α-TTP gene	Low serum vitamin E concentration: 0.05–1.18 µmol/L (0.02–0.51 µg/mL) (normal: 12–46 µmol/L [5–20 µg/mL])
Found no mutations in the frataxin gene	Low serum vitamin E concentration: 2.8 and 5.3 µmol/L (1.2 and 2.3 µg/mL) (normal: 12–37 µmol/L [5–16 µg/mL]) Slightly low sensory action potentials
Homozygous for 513insTT mutation	Low serum vitamin E concentration: <5 µmol/L (2 µg/mL) (normal: 10–42 µmol/L [4–18 µg/mL])

[c] ADP = adenosine diphosphate.
[d] O = oxygen.
[e] TBARS = thiobarbituric acid reactive substances.
[f] This was the only report of any cardiomyopathy.

ethyl)-6-hydroxychroman (α-CEHC) were excreted in the urine when a plasma threshold of 30 µmol/L (1,290 µg/dL) of α-tocopherol was exceeded. However, the α-CEHC metabolite represents only a small fraction of the α-tocopherol consumed daily, and there are few data concerning its formation. Therefore, α-CEHC excretion has not been used as a basis for assessing the α-tocopherol requirement.

Vitamin E Biokinetics

Vitamin E kinetics, metabolism, and pool size determinations in humans have been limited. Therefore, insufficient data exist for assessing human requirements for the amounts needed to maintain body pools. Almost no data exist on pool sizes or tissue concentrations of vitamin E, especially the various forms of vitamin E. Studies using isotope-labeled vitamin E may provide kinetic data that can be used to determine daily α-tocopherol requirements in the future.

Vitamin E Deficiency Symptoms

Overt vitamin E deficiency is so rare in humans that signs of deficiency (e.g., neurological abnormalities) and comparisons of deficiency signs with dietary intakes are simply not available to serve as a basis for estimating requirements.

Plasma α-Tocopherol Concentration

Several studies have reported the determinants of plasma α-tocopherol, as measured by high-performance liquid chromatography methods, and provided mathematical models that attempted to correlate usual vitamin E intakes with normal plasma concentrations (Ascherio et al., 1992; Gascón-Vila et al., 1997; Kardinaal et al., 1995; Stryker et al., 1988). Kardinaal et al. (1995) reported that plasma α-tocopherol concentrations were not associated with dietary intake, whereas others (Ascherio et al., 1992; Stryker et al., 1988) report that associations seen were largely due to vitamin E supplement intake. Recently, Ford and Sowell (1999) reported that plasma α-tocopherol concentrations in the Third National Health and Nutrition Examination Survey (NHANES III) did not correlate with the 24-hour dietary recall data. In any case, the correlation between intake and normal vitamin E plasma concentrations (greater than 16 μmol/L [688 μg/dL]) is not strong and could not be used as the basis for estimating the α-tocopherol requirement. However, in vitamin E-depleted subjects a linear increase in plasma α-tocopherol concentration was found with increasing vitamin E intake up to 17 mg (39.5 μmol)/day (Horwitt, 1960).

Hydrogen Peroxide-Induced Hemolysis

Studies in children with cystic fibrosis and in vitamin E-depleted adults provide evidence for the relationship between vitamin E status, plasma α-tocopherol concentrations, and erythrocyte susceptibility to hydrogen peroxide-induced lysis (Farrell et al., 1977; Horwitt, 1960). The children become vitamin E deficient because the impaired secretion of pancreatic digestive enzymes causes steatorrhea and vitamin E malabsorption, even when pancreatic enzyme supplements are administered orally. More severe vitamin E deficiency symptoms, including neurological abnormalities, occur if bile secretion is also impaired in the children (Cynamon et al., 1988; Elias et al., 1981; Farrell et al., 1977; Sokol et al., 1989; Stead et al., 1986; Winklhofer-Roob et al., 1996a,b). Breath ethane, a lipid peroxidation marker, and erythrocyte susceptibility to in vitro hydrogen peroxide lysis have been inversely correlated with plasma α-tocopherol concentrations in children and adults with vitamin E deficiency as defined by low plasma vitamin E concentrations (Refat et al., 1991). Moreover, both the markers (breath ethane concentrations and erythrocyte lysis) and the symptoms of neurological abnormality can be corrected with supplemental vitamin E.

Relationship of Vitamin E Intake to Chronic Diseases

Cardiovascular Disease

The hypothesis that oxidized low-density lipoprotein (oxLDL) is a causative agent in the development of cardiovascular disease (Steinberg et al., 1989) continues to dominate experimental protocols aimed at understanding the cause, and potentially the prevention, of cardiovascular disease.

Vitamin E does inhibit LDL oxidation whether induced by cells in culture (Steinbrecher et al., 1984) or by copper ion in vitro (Dieber-Rotheneder et al., 1991; Jialal et al., 1995; Reaven et al., 1993). In addition, vitamin E could affect atherogenesis at a number of steps, based on the following in vitro observations:

- Vitamin E inhibits smooth muscle cell proliferation through the inhibition of protein kinase C (Azzi et al., 1995; Boscoboinik et al., 1991; Chatelain et al., 1993).
- Vitamin E inhibits platelet adhesion, aggregation, and platelet release reactions (Freedman et al., 1996; Higashi and Kikuchi, 1974; Ishizuka et al., 1998; Steiner and Anastasi, 1976).
- Vitamin E inhibits plasma generation of thrombin, a potent endogenous hormone that binds to platelet receptors and induces aggregation (Rota et al., 1998).
- Vitamin E decreases monocyte adhesion to the endothelium by downregulating expression of adhesion molecules (Devaraj et al., 1996; Faruqi et al., 1994; Islam et al., 1998; Martin et al., 1997; Molenaar et al., 1989) and decreasing monocyte superoxide production (Cachia et al., 1998; Islam et al., 1998).

- In human endothelial cells, vitamin E potentiates synthesis of prostacyclin, a potent vasodilator and inhibitor of platelet aggregation (Chan and Leith, 1981; Szczeklik et al., 1985; Thorin et al., 1994; Tran and Chan, 1990).
- Vitamin E mediates upregulation of the expression of cytosolic phospholipase A_2 and cyclo-oxygenase (Chan et al., 1998a,b; Tran et al., 1996).
- Vitamin E enrichment of endothelial cells in culture inhibits the expression of intracellular cell adhesion molecule (ICAM-1) and vascular cell adhesion molecule (VCAM-1) induced by exposure to oxLDL (Cominacini et al., 1997).

Inhibition of Atherogenesis in Animal Models. Studies of antioxidants and atherosclerosis have been conducted using LDL receptor-deficient rabbits, cholesterol-fed rabbits, cholesterol-fed monkeys, cholesterol-fed hamsters, apoE-deficient mice, and LDL receptor-deficient mice (see Steinberg, 1997, for list). It can be concluded that the antioxidant hypothesis of atherosclerosis is strongly supported by a large body of evidence in animal models (Parker et al., 1995; Pratico et al., 1999; Sparrow et al., 1992).

Observational Epidemiological Studies. As shown in Table 6-3, three large prospective cohort studies involving both men and women found an inverse association between estimated dietary intake of vitamin E and coronary heart disease (CHD) risk (Kushi et al., 1996; Rimm et al., 1993; Stampfer et al., 1993). One study (Rimm et al., 1993) included 39,910 male health professionals and found a nonsignificant reduction in CHD risk for both total vitamin E intake and intake of vitamin E from supplements. A second study (Stampfer et al., 1993) included 87,245 female nurses and found the reduction in CHD risk primarily for intake of vitamin E from supplements. In contrast, the third study, which was carried out among 34,486 postmenopausal women (Kushi et al., 1996), found the decrease in risk only for vitamin E intake from foods (*not* from supplements). Few women in the latter study took high doses of supplemental vitamin E, which may account for the difference in findings from the other two studies. Risk reductions of 30 to 60 percent were found for the highest, relative to the lowest, quintile of intake in these studies.

In a smaller cohort study in Finland (2,748 men, 2,385 women), a statistically significant inverse association between dietary intake of vitamin E and coronary mortality was found in both sexes (Knekt et al., 1994). Although the use of vitamin supplements was very low in this population, there was a suggested inverse association with supplemental vitamin E, as well.

Losonczy et al. (1996) examined vitamin E and vitamin C supplement use in 11,178 subjects (aged 67 to 105 years) who participated in the Established Populations for Epidemiological Studies of the Elderly. Vitamin E supplement use reduced the risk of all-cause mortality (relative risk [RR] = 0.66; 95 percent confidence interval [CI] 0.53 to 0.83) and risk of coronary disease mortality (RR = 0.53; 95 percent CI 0.34 to 0.84).

Additional data on the correlation between vitamin E and atherosclerosis were reported in the subjects who participated in the Cholesterol Lowering Atherosclerosis Study (CLAS), which was a randomized, placebo-controlled trial in men who had undergone coronary bypass surgery (Azen et al., 1996a,b; Hodis et al., 1995). Subjects were intensively treated with colestipol-niacin and advised to follow a cholesterol-lowering diet, or were given dietary counseling alone. Vitamin E intakes, obtained by dietary questionnaires, were inversely correlated with progression of atherosclerosis in coronary and carotid arteries. All subjects combined, those with supplementary vitamin E (100 IU/day or more) demonstrated significantly less coronary artery lesion progression than did subjects with lower vitamin E intakes from supplements (Hodis et al., 1995). Within the colestipol-niacin treated group, there was less coronary artery lesion progression among those taking vitamin E supplements (100 IU/day or more), but subjects in the placebo group showed no benefit of supplementary vitamin E (Hodis et al., 1995). A similar analysis was done on the progression of carotid artery atherosclerosis using ultrasound. Here there was no effect of vitamin E supplements in the drug-treated group, but there was an effect in the placebo group (i.e., opposite findings with respect to drug treatment and vitamin E interactions in the carotid artery from those in the coronary artery; Azen et al., 1996b).

Intervention Trials. Four large-scale, double-blind, randomized intervention trials using vitamin E have been reported. The first, the Alpha-Tocopherol Beta-Carotene (ATBC) Cancer Prevention Study (ATBC Cancer Prevention Study Group, 1994), was designed to determine whether α-tocopherol (50 mg/day of *all rac*-α-tocopherol acetate) and β-carotene (20 mg/day), alone or in combination, would reduce the incidence of lung cancer in a high-risk group of male smokers in Finland. Although vitamin E had no effect on the primary endpoint (lung cancer), the men taking α-tocopherol had a lower incidence of prostate cancer (see later sec-

TABLE 6-3 Vitamin E Intake and Risk of Coronary Heart Disease in Men and Women

Reference	Variable
Rimm et al., 1993	Intake from food (IU[a]/d)
	Relative risk of CHD[b]
	95% CI[c]
	Intake from supplements (IU/d)
	Relative risk of CHD
	95% CI
Stampfer et al., 1993	Intake from food (IU/d)
	Relative risk of CHD
	95% CI
	Intake from food and supplements (IU/d)
	Relative risk of CHD
	95% CI
Knekt et al., 1994	Intake from food (mg/d)
	Relative risk of CHD
	95% CI
Kushi et al., 1996	Intake from food (IU/d)
	Relative risk of CHD
	95% CI

[a] IU = international unit.
[b] CHD = coronary heart disease.

tion "Cancer"). The men who received α-tocopherol also had 50 percent higher mortality from hemorrhagic stroke (but 5 percent lower mortality from ischemic heart disease and 16 percent lower mortality from ischemic stroke) than the men who did not receive this supplement. In a subsequent analysis of individuals with previous myocardial infarction, vitamin E supplementation appeared to decrease the risk of nonfatal myocardial infarction by a nonstatistically significant 38 percent (Rapola et al., 1997).

In a trial in Great Britain, the Cambridge Heart Antioxidant Study (CHAOS), patients with angiographically proven coronary artery disease were randomized to receive either 400 or 800 international units (IU) (268 or 567 mg)/day of *RRR*-α-tocopherol or placebo (Stephens et al., 1996). The study was terminated early because there were statistically significant decreases in the occurrence of nonfatal myocardial infarctions (77 percent) and in total

Quintile/Tertile					
1	2	3	4	5	p Value for Trend
1.6–6.9	7.0–8.1	8.2–9.3	9.4–11.0	11.1	
1.0	1.10	1.17	0.97	0.79	
–	0.80–1.51	0.84–1.62	0.69–1.37	0.54–1.15	NS[d]
0	<25	25–99	100–249	≥250	
1.0	0.85	0.78	0.54	0.70	
–	0.69–1.05	0.59–1.08	0.33–0.88	0.55–0.89	NS
0.3–3.1	3.2–3.9	4.0–4.8	4.9–6.2	6.3–100	
1	1.04	0.77	1.14	0.95	
–	0.8–1.35	0.66–1.14	0.89–1.47	0.72–1.23	NS
1.2–3.5	3.6–4.9	5.0–8.0	8.1–21.5	21.6–1,000	
1	1	1.15	0.74	0.66	
–	0.78–1.28	0.9–1.48	0.57–0.98	0.5–0.87	<0.001
≤5.3	5.4–7.1	>7.1			
1	0.73	0.35			
–	0.38–1.39	0.14–0.88			<0.01
≤4.91	4.92–6.24	6.25–7.62	7.63–9.63	≥9.64	
1	0.70	0.76	0.32	0.38	
–	0.41–1.18	0.44–1.29	0.17–0.63	0.18–0.80	<0.004

[c] CI = confidence interval.

[d] NS = not significant.

(fatal plus nonfatal) myocardial infarctions (47 percent). However, there was a nonstatistically significant increase in fatal myocardial infarctions and no decrease in overall mortality. There were no differences reported between the two doses in the effects noted.

The third trial (GISSI-Prevenzione Investigators, 1999) was designed to determine whether 300 mg/day of *all rac-α*-tocopherol and 1 g/day of ω-3 polyunsaturated fatty acids (PUFA), alone or in combination, would reduce the risk of death, nonfatal myocardial infarction, and stroke in Italian patients surviving a recent myocardial infarction. After 3.5 years of supplementation, vitamin E had no benefit. Although ω-3 PUFA significantly decreased the rate of death, myocardial infarction, and stroke in these patients, the benefit was the same when the ω-3 PUFA was fed alone or in combination with vitamin E.

A study conducted in 19 countries, the Heart Outcomes Prevention Evaluation (HOPE) Study, evaluated more than 9,000 patients older than 55 years of age with a history of previous ischemic heart disease, stroke, or peripheral artery disease (HOPE Study Investigators, 2000). Similar to the GISSI-Prevenzione Trial, after 4.5 years of supplementation with either 400 IU (268 mg)/day of RRR-α-tocopherol or a placebo, vitamin E had a neutral effect on total mortality, cardiovascular death, myocardial infarction, or stroke. This study is continuing to determine whether any benefit of vitamin E in preventing cardiovascular disease outcomes or cancer will emerge after a longer duration of follow-up.

The discordant results of these four trials may be related to the different doses of vitamin E that were used, as it has been demonstrated that the effectiveness of vitamin E in protecting circulating LDL against ex vivo oxidation depends on both dose and experimental design. Some protection has been observed at doses as low as 25 IU/day (Princen et al., 1995), but a maximum degree of protection requires dosages greater than 200 IU/day (Jialal et al., 1995). At the ATBC Study dose of 50 mg/day, there is some protection, but it is minimal. However, at the GISSI Prevenzione trial dose of 300 mg/day and the HOPE Study dose of 400 IU (268 mg)/day, protection was neutral. Another possible difference between the four trials is that the coronary artery lesions in the Finnish smokers, Italians, and HOPE participants may have been much further advanced than those in the British population studied.

A smaller trial examined the effects of all rac-α-tocopherol supplementation (1,200 IU/day) for 4 months on re-stenosis after angioplasty (DeMaio et al., 1992) and found a small nonstatistically significant reduction in the treated group.

Summary. The hypothesis that reactive oxygen species (ROS) and reactive nitrogen species (RNS) play a role in atherosclerosis rests on a solid basic science foundation and is strongly supported by studies in animal models. At the clinical level, a variety of correlational studies and studies of biochemical markers are consistent with the hypothesis. However, only four published, large-scale, randomized, double-blind clinical intervention studies have tested the ability of vitamin E to prevent myocardial infarction. One of these, a secondary prevention trial supplementing with 400 or 800 IU (268 or 567 mg)/day of RRR-α-tocopherol, was strongly positive (Stephens et al., 1996). The other three, one carried out in a group of high-risk cigarette smokers using 50 mg/day of all rac-α-tocopherol (ATBC Cancer Prevention Study Group, 1994) and two carried out in high-risk cardiovascular patients supplemented with 300 mg/day of *all rac*-α-tocopherol (GISSI-Prevenzione Investigators, 1999) and 400 IU (268 mg)/day of *RRR*-α-tocopherol (HOPE Study Investigators, 2000), were neutral. As of this date there are insufficient data on which to base a recommendation of supplemental vitamin E as a heart disease preventative for the general population.

Diabetes Mellitus

Since cardiovascular complications account for the major causes of death in diabetes mellitus, it has been suggested that similar oxidative processes associated with cardiovascular disease may play a role in this chronic disease.

Oxidative Stress. It has been proposed that the development of the complications of diabetes mellitus may be linked to oxidative stress and therefore might be amenable to treatment with anti-oxidants (Baynes, 1991; Mullarkey et al., 1990; Semenkovich and Heinecke, 1997). Supplementation of either diabetic or nondiabetic subjects with α-tocopherol decreases the susceptibility of their LDL to ex vivo oxidation (Fuller et al., 1996; Reaven et al., 1995), but this treatment does not change blood glucose levels. Ceriello et al. (1991), using 600 and 1,200 mg/day of α-tocopherol, also observed decreases in labile hemoglobin A1 (HbA1) and plasma glycosylated proteins. While Jain et al. (1996a) found a decrease in glycosylated hemoglobin with α-tocopherol supplementation at a relatively low dose (100 IU/day), Reaven et al. (1995) using a much larger dose (1,600 IU/day of α-tocopherol) found no effects on glycosylated hemoglobin or other glycosylated plasma proteins. Paolisso et al. (1993), using 900 mg/day of α-tocopherol, reported minimal, but statistically significant, improvements in control of blood glucose. The reason for the above discordance in results is not apparent.

Vitamin E treatment has been reported to decrease TBARS reactivity in plasma of patients with diabetes, but this reaction is not highly specific to vitamin E (Jain et al., 1996b). Davi et al. (1999) did a comprehensive study using the urinary excretion of F_2-iso-prostanes (8-iso-prostaglandin F_2) as an indicator of oxidative stress. They found a highly significant increase in F_2-isoprostane excretion in diabetic subjects, and the level of excretion correlated inversely with the degree of control of blood glucose. When the subjects were supplemented with α-tocopherol acetate (600 mg/day for 14 days), they reported a statistically significant reduction (37 percent) in F_2-isoprostane excretion and also in the urinary excretion of 11-dehydrothromboxane B_2, the latter being an indicator of platelet activation.

Platelet Hyperactivity. Several studies have confirmed an increased tendency for aggregation of platelets from diabetic subjects, linking the tendency to increased thromboxane production and showing that prior treatment with α-tocopherol can ameliorate the increased tendency for platelet aggregation (Colette et al., 1988; Gisinger et al., 1988; Jain et al., 1998; Kunisaki et al., 1990). However, no clinical intervention trials have tested directly whether antioxidants can decrease the incidence of thrombosis in vivo.

Diabetic Neuropathy. Tutuncu et al. (1998) studied 21 subjects with type II diabetes and neuropathy, who were randomly assigned to receive either 900 mg/day of α-tocopherol or a placebo for 6 months. Although fasting and postprandial glucose were unchanged, nerve conduction velocity in the median motor nerve fibers and tibial motor nerve distal latency improved significantly with vitamin E treatment. The authors concluded that further studies with a larger number of patients for longer periods of time are needed.

Summary. The available data strongly suggest that individuals with diabetes are subject to increased oxidative stress. However, no clinical intervention trials have tested directly whether vitamin E can ameliorate the complications of diabetes mellitus. A gap remains between the effects of vitamin E treatment on biochemical markers of oxidative stress, clinical efficacy, and validation of a relationship between biomarkers and clinical outcomes. Studies in humans show that lipid and lipoprotein oxidation proceed more rapidly in patients with diabetes than in nondiabetic people and that treatment with vitamin E can partially reverse this process (Reaven, 1995; Yoshida et al., 1997). In theory then, intervention with vitamin E therapy to inhibit atherogenesis might be more effective in individual diabetics than in nondiabetics. However, as of this date there are insufficient data on which to base a recommendation of supplemental vitamin E in diabetics.

Cancer

Cancer is believed to develop as the result of an accumulation of mutations that are unrepaired. DNA is constantly undergoing damage due to interaction with free radicals, and therefore one mechanism by which vitamin E might inhibit cancer formation is by quenching these free radicals. An additional vitamin E chemoprevention mechanism that has been proposed is an effect on the immune system. Many compounds, including vitamin E, have been proposed as anticarcinogens (Ames et al., 1995).

Observational Epidemiological Studies. Epidemiological evidence for an association between vitamin E and cancer risk is limited. An analysis of vitamin E intake and lung cancer in the NHANES I Epidemiological Follow-up Study (Yong et al., 1997) showed a significant inverse association among current smokers in the lowest tertile of pack-years of smoking. A follow-up prospective cohort study found a weak inverse association between prediagnostic serum vitamin E levels and the incidence of lung cancer (Comstock et al., 1997).

A prospective cohort study in the Netherlands found no association between vitamin E intake and the incidence of breast cancer (Verhoeven et al., 1997). Similarly, a recent analysis from the Breast Cancer Serum Bank cohort study found no association of serum vitamin E with breast cancer risk (Dorgan et al., 1998). A multi-centered European case-control study of postmenopausal breast cancer found no relation between subcutaneous adipose tissue α-tocopherol levels and breast cancer risk (van 't Veer et al., 1996).

No association between dietary vitamin E and prostate cancer was found in a large case-control study in Sweden (Andersson et al., 1996). An inverse association between serum vitamin E levels in smokers and prostate cancer was found in a prospective cohort study in Switzerland (Eichholzer et al., 1996); however, earlier cohort studies reported no association of vitamin E with this cancer (Comstock et al., 1992; Knekt et al., 1988).

Intervention Trials. In an intervention trial in Finland among men who were heavy smokers, α-tocopherol supplements (50 mg/day) had no effect on risk for lung cancer, the primary endpoint of the study. However, a significant 34 percent lower incidence of prostate cancer was seen in the men who received this supplement (ATBC Cancer Prevention Study Group, 1994; Heinonen et al., 1998). Two small, short-term intervention trials found no effect of α-tocopherol supplementation on mammary dysplasia (London et al., 1985) or benign breast disease (Ernster et al., 1985). Several trials with vitamin E to prevent the recurrence of colorectal adenomatous polyps have been reported, but none found a beneficial effect (Chen et al.,

1988; DeCosse et al., 1989; Greenberg et al., 1994; Hofstad et al., 1998; McKeown-Eyssen et al., 1988).

Summary. Overall, the epidemiological evidence for an effect of vitamin E on cancer risk is weaker than that for vitamin E and cardiovascular disease. Observational epidemiological studies provide only limited evidence for a protective association and only for some cancer sites. At present, the data from intervention trials are most suggestive for the ability of vitamin E to prevent prostate cancer, but only a single trial has yet been reported, and prostate cancer was not the primary endpoint of that study.

Immune Function

It has been established that several aspects of immune function decline with increasing age (Bendich, 1994). Moreover, supplementation with vitamin E is able to reverse these deficits in some individuals. Meydani et al. (1997) studied a total of 88 free-living, apparently healthy subjects at least 65 years of age, who were randomly assigned to a placebo group or to groups consuming 60, 200, or 800 mg/day of vitamin E for 235 days. Subjects in the upper tertile of serum α-tocopherol concentrations (greater than 48.4 μmol/L [2.08 mg/dL] or approximately twice normal values) after supplementation with 200 or 800 mg/day of vitamin E had higher antibody responses to hepatitis B vaccine and delayed-type hypersensitivity (DTH) skin response. The 200-mg/day group also had a significant increase in antibody titer to tetanus vaccine. Recently, Pallast et al. (1999) reported that supplementation with 100 mg/day of vitamin E for 6 months may improve cellular immune function in apparently healthy elderly, but that the effect may be more pronounced in certain subgroups such as those who were physically less active or those with low baseline DTH reactivity.

Five subjects with tropical sprue for 8 to 10 years were found to have an abnormal delayed hypersensitivity response as well (Ghalaut et al., 1995). Moreover, their plasma vitamin E concentrations were approximately one-tenth of normal, and the subjects had a sensory neuropathy characteristic of vitamin E deficiency. Parenteral vitamin E therapy increased serum vitamin E concentrations to normal and improved neurological responses and response to the immune function skin test, suggesting that vitamin E may be important in immune function.

Whether or not increases in vitamin E intake have any effect on immune function in younger populations remains uncertain. However, the evidence is strong enough to warrant continued investigation.

Cataracts

There is a sound biochemical basis for the notion that the accumulation of damaged proteins in the lens leads to cataract formation and that free-radical damage contributes to this protein damage (Taylor, 1993). Studies in experimental animals show that antioxidant vitamins, including vitamin E, can protect against lens damage (Jacques et al., 1994).

At the epidemiological level, there have been nine studies relating vitamin E status to risk of at least one type of cataract. Five reported a protective association (Jacques and Chylack, 1991; Knekt et al., 1992; Leske et al., 1991; Robertson et al., 1989; Vitale et al., 1993), while four reported no association (Hankinson et al., 1992; Mares-Perlman et al, 1994a,b; Mohan et al., 1989).

Only one intervention study has been carried out to test the effects of α-tocopherol alone on the prevalence of cataracts (Teikari et al., 1998). A subgroup of men participating in the Finnish ATBC study were examined at the end of that study for cataracts. There were no differences in the prevalence of nuclear, cortical, or posterior subcapsular cataracts between control subjects and those taking 50 mg/day of α-tocopherol.

Central Nervous System Disorders

The most characteristic manifestation of vitamin E deficiency in humans is neuropathy affecting both the central and the peripheral nervous systems, particularly sensory axons (Sokol, 1988). The neuropathology associated with frank vitamin E deficiency has been discussed above. The discussion that follows focuses on neurological diseases in which free-radical damage has been proposed to play a role and in which vitamin E might therefore play a protective role.

Parkinson's Disease. Parkinson's disease is characterized by dopaminergic cell death in the substantia nigra. Reported local changes in the substantia nigra compatible with a role for oxidative stress in Parkinson's disease include signs of increases in lipid peroxidation, increases in iron concentration, and decreases in some of the antioxidant defense mechanisms (Muller, 1994). However, a placebo-controlled, double-blind study of 800 patients given 2,000 IU/day of *all rac*-α-tocopherol failed to show any beneficial effect (Parkinson Study Group, 1993). Follow-up publications reported again that α-tocopherol had no benefit (Shoulson, 1998) and had no effect on mortality (Parkinson Study Group, 1998). This did not appear to be a result of poor compliance because increases in vitamin E in cerebrospinal fluid in response to the supplement were reported (Vatassery et al., 1998).

Alzheimer's Disease and Down's Syndrome. Alzheimer's disease is a neurodegenerative disorder that appears to have an oxidative stress component; it is not clear if this is a cause or a consequence of the disease. The disease may be potentiated by an accumulation of redox-active metals (Cornett et al., 1998), especially iron (Smith et al., 1997). Additionally, amyloid β-peptide is a key factor in the neurotoxicity of Alzheimer's disease because it can initiate protein oxidation and lipid peroxidation (Keller et al., 1997), eventually leading to neuronal cell death. The free-radical dependence of β-amyloid-associated toxicity was confirmed by the ability of vitamin E to prevent the toxic effects of amyloid β-peptide in vitro (Subramaniam et al., 1998). These data are compatible with an etiology that includes oxidative damage, but other hypotheses are possible.

In a 2-year, double-blind, placebo-controlled, randomized, multi-center trial in 341 patients with moderately severe impairment from Alzheimer's disease, treatment with *all rac*-α-tocopherol (2,000 IU/day) significantly slowed the progression of disease (Sano et al., 1997).

A case can be made for a link between oxidative stress and neuropathology in Alzheimer's disease and Down's syndrome (Muller, 1994). In individuals dying from either disease, abnormalities in brain histology are remarkably similar. Down's syndrome is due to trisomy of chromosome 21, which carries the gene for superoxide dismutase (SOD). Interestingly, overexpression of human SOD in transgenic mice is associated with increased lipid peroxidation in the brain (Ceballos-Picot et al., 1991), perhaps secondary to SOD-induced conversion of the superoxide anion to hydrogen peroxide and water. Although these results are promising, it is still too early to draw any conclusions about the usefulness of vitamin E in Alzheimer's disease and Down's syndrome.

Tardive Dyskinesia (TD). TD is a neurologic disorder that develops in about 20 percent of patients treated long term with neuroleptic drugs. These drugs increase the turnover of brain catecholamines, particularly the neurotransmitter dopamine, and these are compounds that can give rise to ROS. TD is characterized by a variety of involuntary movements, especially of the face. It has been reported that the cerebrospinal fluid of patients with TD contains higher-than-normal concentrations of lipid peroxidation products (Lohr et al., 1990), and more recently, plasma also was found to have lipid peroxidation products (Brown et al., 1998). However, a causal relationship between these indicators of oxidative stress and the incidence or severity of tardive dyskinesia has not been established.

Some have reported short-term supplementation of TD patients with vitamin E (Egan et al., 1992; Elkashef et al., 1990; Lohr et al., 1987). The beneficial effects were minor, mostly limited to patients with recent onset of the disease, and the number of subjects was very small. Recently, in 40 patients who were supplemented with 1,600 IU/day of α-tocopherol or placebo for up to 36 weeks, there was a significant difference in mean Abnormal Involuntary Movements Scale scores, in those receiving vitamin E after 10 weeks of treatment (Adler et al., 1998).

Summary

A large number of studies have been carried out in the past decade that directly or indirectly concern the relationship between vitamin E intake and chronic disease. Among the effects of vitamin E intakes from supplements are inhibition of LDL oxidation both in vitro and in vivo; inhibition of smooth muscle cell proliferation through inhibition of protein kinase C; inhibition of platelet adhesion, aggregation, and platelet release reactions; and inhibition of plasma generation of thrombin. In addition, supplemental intakes of vitamin E decrease monocyte adhesion to endothelium, decrease monocyte superoxide production, potentiate the synthesis of prostacyclin, upregulate the expression of phospholipase A_2 and cyclooxygenase, and inhibit the expression of ICAM-1 and VCAM-1 induced by exposure to oxLDL. Many of these effects have been shown only in tissue culture and have not been studied in vivo. All of these actions could have an influence on health and the development of chronic disease. Some of these effects appear to be independent of the antioxidant properties of vitamin E. Thus, it must be recognized that consumption of large quantities of vitamin E will lead to multiple metabolic and cellular changes in humans. An important question is whether the net result of these changes will be beneficial when large amounts of vitamin E are consumed on a long-term basis.

Clinical trials are currently under way to determine whether high intakes of vitamin E will reduce the risk for certain diseases. Still, even a positive outcome of these trials may not necessarily lead to a change in recommended individual intakes for the whole population. These trials generally are targeting groups at high risk for particular diseases. If the results of these studies are positive, it is likely that initial recommendations for higher intakes will be limited in their application to high-risk populations. Because of the myriad of actions of high doses of vitamin E, recommendations of higher intakes for the general population undoubtedly will require extensive investigation of the long-term consequences of the multiple metabolic and cellular modifications.

FACTORS AFFECTING THE VITAMIN E REQUIREMENT

Bioavailability

Most dietary vitamin E is found in food that contains fat. It is clear that vitamin E absorption requires micelle formation and chylomicron secretion by the intestine (Muller et al, 1974), although the optimal amount of fat to enhance vitamin E absorption has not been reported. This is probably a more important issue for vitamin E supplement users than for nonsupplement users where all of the vitamin E is in a dietary fat-rich environment.

Nutrient-Nutrient Interactions

Antioxidant Interactions

When vitamin E intercepts a radical, a tocopheroxyl radical is formed (Burton and Ingold, 1981). This radical can be reduced by ascorbic acid or other reducing agents (Doba et al., 1985; Niki et al., 1982), thereby oxidizing the latter and returning vitamin E to its reduced state.

The ability of one antioxidant to regenerate another oxidized species is dependent on the redox potential of the antioxidant (Buettner, 1993). Biologically relevant electron donors that have been shown to regenerate α-tocopherol effectively from the α-tocopheroxyl radical include vitamin C (McCay, 1985), glutathione (Niki, 1987), and ubiquinols (Stoyanovsky et al., 1995). (For further information see "Nutrient-Nutrient Interactions" in Chapter 5.) Cellular redox cycling is coupled with the energy status of the organism. Thus, it can be expected that during prolonged energy deficit or inadequate production of nicotinamide adenine dinucleotide

(NADH), nicotinamide adenine dinucleotide phosphate (NADPH) or glutathione [GSSG] reductase due to dietary deficiencies of niacin (component of NADP or NADPH) or riboflavin (cofactor for GSSG reductase), the ability of the organism to produce sufficient reducing equivalents for recycling oxidized products will be compromised. Conversely, intakes of plant phenolic compounds and flavonoids may add to the total antioxidant pool (de Vries et al., 1998; Manach et al., 1998). The extent, involvement, and contribution of these newer compounds which may be acting as antioxidants to the redox cycling reactions in vitro and in vivo remain to be determined.

The regeneration of α-tocopherol from the α-tocopheroxyl radical may be faster than the further oxidation of the α-tocopheroxyl radical. The extent to which vitamin E is recycled in humans and which antioxidant species are preferentially used for recycling are not known. In human platelet homogenates, distinct chemical and enzymatic pathways for the regeneration of oxidized tocopherol, afforded by vitamin C and glutathione, have been identified (Chan et al., 1991). A metabolic study in humans designed to demonstrate the occurrence of vitamin E recycling by vitamin C had limitations since the body pools of vitamin C and E cannot be totally depleted (Jacob et al., 1996). Although the data were inconclusive, the authors did comment that there is "a trend towards sparing of tissue tocopherol by vitamin C" and that more study was warranted. This is an important area of investigation because the tocopheroxyl radical has been shown in vitro to increase lipid peroxidation in the absence of water-soluble antioxidants, and it has been proposed that this mechanism may be an important factor in potentiating in vivo atherogenesis (Stocker, 1999; Upston et al., 1999). However, there are still no data to determine whether this mechanism is operative in vivo.

Dietary Polyunsaturated Fat

Vitamin E requirements have been reported to increase when intakes of polyunsaturated fatty acids (PUFAs) are increased (Dam, 1962; Horwitt, 1962). Based on these data it was suggested that a ratio of at least 0.4 mg (1 µmol) α-tocopherol per gram of PUFA should be consumed by adults (Bieri and Evarts, 1973; Horwitt, 1974; Witting and Lee, 1975). However, the method of determining the vitamin E requirement generated by PUFA intakes is not universally accepted because the amount of vitamin E required to stabilize PUFAs in tissues is influenced to a greater extent by their degree of unsaturation than by their mass (Draper, 1993). Moreover, PUFAs are not deposited in the tissues in the same proportions that they occur in the diet. Finally, dietary PUFAs are modified by elongation and desaturation and are catabolized to various degrees depending on energy status (Jones and Kubow, 1999).

There are also data to suggest that low-density lipoprotein (LDL) oxidation susceptibility in vitro is dependent upon its PUFA content. A 10 percent PUFA diet with 34 percent of calories from fat increased LDL oxidation susceptibility compared to a 19 percent monosaturated fatty acid (MUFA) diet with 40 percent of the calories from fat, without changing the α-tocopherol content of the LDL (Schwab et al., 1998a). In a double-blind crossover trial in 48 postmenopausal women, supplementation with fish oil increased LDL oxidation susceptibility, while supplementation with both fish oil and α-tocopheryl acetate significantly decreased it (Wander et al., 1996).

The effect of the fatty acid composition of reduced-fat diets on the in vitro oxidation of LDL was also examined in 14 moderately hypercholesterolemic (LDL greater than 3.36 mmol/L) female and male subjects (aged 44 to 78 years). Each subject consumed each of five reduced-fat diets (30 percent of energy from total fat, 17 percent from protein, and 53 percent from carbohydrate) which included 20 percent of energy from beef tallow, canola oil, corn oil, olive oil, or rice bran oil for a period of 32 days. When the data from all dietary phases were pooled, LDL α-tocopherol levels and plasma 18:1/18:2 ratios were positively related to LDL oxidation resistance (Schwab et al., 1998b).

Although it is clear that the relationship between dietary PUFA and vitamin E needs is not simple, high PUFA intakes should certainly be accompanied by increased vitamin E intakes.

FINDINGS BY LIFE STAGE AND GENDER GROUP

Infants Ages 0 through 12 Months

Method Used to Set the Adequate Intake

No functional criteria of vitamin E status have been demonstrated which reflect response to dietary intake in infants. Thus recommended intakes of vitamin E are based on an Adequate Intake (AI) that reflects a calculated mean vitamin E intake of infants fed principally with human milk.

Human Milk. Human milk is recognized as the optimal milk source for infants throughout at least the first year of life and is recommended as the sole nutritional milk source for infants during the first 4 to 6 months of life (IOM, 1991). Therefore, determination of the AI for vitamin E for infants is based on data from infants fed human milk as the principal fluid during the periods 0 through 6 and 7 through 12 months of age. The AI is set for ages 0 through 6 months at the mean value calculated from studies in which the intake of human milk was measured by test weighing volume, and the average concentration of the nutrient in human milk was determined using average values from several reported studies.

In general, the total vitamin E content of colostrum is high (average content ranges from 6.8–23 mg/L) (Ali et al., 1986; Boersma et al., 1991; Chappell et al., 1985; Jansson et al., 1981; Kobayashi et al., 1975; Thomas et al., 1981); the concentration decreases in transitional milk, sampled at 6–10 days, and further decreases in mature milk, as shown in Table 6-4. The range of vitamin E concentrations in mature human milk after approximately 30 days of lactation varies from 1.8 mg/L (Kobayashi et al., 1975) to approximately 9 mg/L (Thomas et al., 1981).

Vitamin E concentrations are most accurately analyzed by high-performance liquid chromatography (HPLC). Therefore, reports of vitamin E concentrations in human milk utilizing non-HPLC methods (Ali et al., 1986; Kobayashi et al., 1975; and Thomas et al., 1981) are not used in this assessment. HPLC measurements of the average α-tocopherol content of mature human milk have yielded values of 2.3 (Lammi-Keefe et al., 1990), 3.5 (Chappell et al., 1985), 3.7 ± 0.6 (SD) (Lammi-Keefe et al., 1985), 7.2 ± 3.9 (SD) (Jansson et al., 1981), and 8 ± 5 mg/L (SD) (Boersma et al., 1991). The latter authors reported that the α-tocopherol amounts in human milk were nearly identical to the α-tocopherol equivalent amounts.

Data suggest that there is no difference in milk vitamin E content between mothers with preterm and term births (Lammi-Keefe et al., 1985; Thomas et al., 1981). In addition, there is no significant diurnal variation in the vitamin E content of human milk (Chappell et al., 1985).

Ages 0 through 6 Months. This recommendation is based on the mean volume of human milk intake of 0.78 L/day (Allen et al., 1991; Butte et al., 1984; Heinig et al., 1993), consumed by infants ages 0 through 6 months. The average concentration of α-tocopherol in human milk is approximately 4.9 mg/L as assessed by HPLC in the five studies cited above. If this amount is multiplied by the aver-

TABLE 6-4 Vitamin E Content in Human Milk

Reference	Vitamin E Content in Milk (mg/L ± SD[a])	Stage of Lactation
Kobayashi et al., 1975	7.8 (total tocopherol) 2.0 (total tocopherol) 1.8 (total tocopherol)	Days 2–7 Days 10–15 Days 30–39
Jansson et al., 1981	23.0 ± 12.6 (α-tocopherol) 10.4 ± 4.2 (α-tocopherol) 7.2 ± 3.9 (α-tocopherol)	Day 4 Days 6–10 Day 12–5th mo
Thomas et al., 1981[c]	20.4 ± 7.9 13.4 ± 3.9 10.2 ± 3.4 8.8 ± 2.2 9.5 ± 3.6 8.5 ± 3.6	Day 3 Day 9 Day 15 Day 21 Day 27 Day 33
Chappell et al., 1985[c]	15 7 5 3.5 3	Days 1-6 Day 7 2 wk 4 wk 5 wk
Lammi-Keefe et al., 1985	6.7 ± 0.5 (α-tocopherol) 4.0 ± 0.6 (α-tocopherol) 3.7 ± 0.5 (α-tocopherol) 3.7 ± 0.6 (α-tocopherol)	2 wk 6 wk 12 wk 16 wk
Ali et al., 1986	6.8 6.5 1.0–5.8	Day 1 Day 12 Days 1–12
Lammi-Keefe et al., 1990	2.3 (α-tocopherol) 0.85 (γ-tocopherol)	8 wk
Boersma et al., 1991	22 ± 14 (α-TE[d]) 14 ± 8 (α-TE) 8 ± 5 (α-TE)	Colostrum (0–4 d) Transitional (5–9 d) Mature (10 and 30 d)

[a] SD = standard deviation.
[b] HPLC = high-performance liquid chromatography.

Maternal Vitamin E Intake (mg/d)	Methods
Not reported	$n = 18$ samples Different individuals were sampled at each stage of lactation Thin-layer chromatography methods
Not reported	$n = 34$ donors Different individuals were sampled at each stage of lactation Milk was collected and stored at donor's home HPLC[b] methods
17.5 19.2 16.7	$n = 10$ mothers with term births Same individuals were sampled at each stage of lactation Non-HPLC methods Used diet records Found no difference in milk vitamin E content between mothers with preterm and term births Found that supplement use had no effect on milk content
15	$n = 12$ women with term births Same individuals were sampled at each stage of lactation HPLC methods Values are approximated from graph
Not reported	No description of the study population Same individuals were sampled at each stage of lactation HPLC methods
Not reported	$n - 1,034$ Malaysian women Non-HPLC methods Found that the ratio of milk vitamin E to total lipids dropped steadily over the 12-d period

Not reported	HPLC methods
	$n = 6$ breast-feeding mothers
	5 samples from each woman were taken in a single day at
	   different times.
	Found no significant variation in vitamin E content during
	   the day. There was considerable yet nonsignificant
	   variation in the total lipid content attributed to
	   individuality and within-day variation

Not reported	$n = 13$ well-nourished, healthy, breast-feeding mothers in
	   St. Lucia, West Indies and their term infants
	Same individuals were sampled at each stage of lactation
	HPLC methods
	Also measured α-, β-, and γ-tocopherol; α-tocopherol levels
	   were nearly identical to α-TE levels

[c] Lack of correlation between maternal intake and human milk concentration.
[d] TE = tocopherol equivalent.

age intake of human milk at 0 through 6 months, the AI would be 4.9 mg/L × 0.78 L/day = 3.8 mg/day of α-tocopherol. The AI is rounded up to 4 mg (9.3 μmol)/day of α-tocopherol.

This value is in the lower range of the Third National Health and Nutrition Examination Survey (NHANES III) data for intakes in this age group as shown in Appendix Table C-3. The mean of the reported intakes of infants 0 through 6 months of age was 12.3 mg (28.6 μmol)/day of α-tocopherol equivalents. The range of the 5th to the 95th percentile was 8.8–16.1 mg (20.5–37.4 μmol)/day. The mean reported intake is probably higher than that calculated for infants receiving solely human milk, because the NHANES III data include milk from infants fed formula which has a vitamin E content of approximately 7 mg/L of α-tocopherol (Thomas et al., 1981). However, this AI is comparable to vitamin E intakes from human milk-fed German infants whose median intakes of vitamin E were 2 mg/day at 3 months of age and 3 mg/day at 6 months of age (Alexy et al., 1999). Based on data from Boersma et al. (1991), it can be assumed that almost all of the α-tocopherol equivalents in human milk are from α-tocopherol.

Ages 7 through 12 Months. When the method described in Chapter 3 is used to extrapolate from the AI for infants ages 0 through 6 months receiving human milk and rounding, the AI for the older infants is rounded up to 5 mg (11.6 μmol)/day α-tocopherol.

The NHANES III data for infants 7 through 12 months of age range from 4.1 to 14.8 mg (11.2 to 34.4 μmol)/day, mean 8.5 mg (19.8 μmol)/day α-tocopherol equivalents (Appendix Table C-3).

Vitamin E AI Summary, Ages 0 through 12 Months

AI for Infants
  0–6 months   4 mg (9.3 μmol)/day of α-tocopherol   ≈0.6 mg/kg
  7–12 months 5 mg (11.6 μmol)/day of α-tocopherol   ≈0.6 mg/kg

Children and Adolescents Ages 1 through 18 Years

Evidence Considered in Estimating the Average Requirement

No data were found on which to base an Estimated Average Requirement (EAR) for vitamin E for apparently healthy children or adolescents. In the absence of additional information, EARs and Recommended Dietary Allowances (RDAs) for children and adolescents have been estimated using the metabolic formulas described in Chapter 3, which are extrapolated from adult values based on lean body mass and need for growth.

Vitamin E EAR and RDA Summary, Ages 1 through 18 Years

EAR for Children
1–3 years	5 mg (11.6 µmol)/day of α-tocopherol
4–8 years	6 mg (14.0 µmol)/day of α-tocopherol

EAR for Boys
9–13 years	9 mg (20.9 µmol)/day of α-tocopherol
14–18 years	12 mg (27.9 µmol)/day of α-tocopherol

EAR for Girls
9–13 years	9 mg (20.9 µmol)/day of α-tocopherol
14–18 years	12 mg (27.9 µmol)/day of α-tocopherol

The RDA for vitamin E is set by assuming a coefficient of variation (CV) of 10 percent (see Chapter 1) because information is not available on the standard deviation of the requirement for vitamin E; the RDA is defined as equal to the EAR plus twice the assumed CV to cover the needs of 97 to 98 percent of the individuals in the group (therefore, for vitamin E the RDA is 120 percent of the EAR). The calculated RDA in milligrams is rounded.

RDA for Children
1–3 years	6 mg (13.9 µmol)/day of α-tocopherol
4–8 years	7 mg (16.3 µmol)/day of α-tocopherol

RDA for Boys
9–13 years	11 mg (25.6 µmol)/day of α-tocopherol
14–18 years	15 mg (34.9 µmol)/day of α-tocopherol

RDA for Girls
9–13 years	11 mg (25.6 µmol)/day of α-tocopherol
14–18 years	15 mg (34.9 µmol)/day of α-tocopherol

Adults Ages 19 through 50 Years

Evidence Considered in Estimating the Average Requirement

As stated earlier, although it is known that humans require vitamin E (Cavalier et al., 1998; Hassan et al., 1966; Oski and Barness, 1967; Sokol et al., 1984), overt vitamin E deficiency (characterized by sensory neuropathy, increased erythrocyte fragility, and increased ethane and pentane production) is rare in the United States and

Canada. Thus, current dietary patterns appear to provide sufficient vitamin E to prevent deficiency symptoms such as peripheral neuropathy. However, since vitamin E intakes are underestimated, particularly with respect to estimates of intake associated with fats (see later section "Underreporting in Dietary Surveys"), an AI could not be reliably determined from the available data on intakes.

Data on human experimental vitamin E deficiency are very limited but do provide some guidance in estimating a requirement. The values recommended here are based largely on studies of induced vitamin E deficiency in humans and the correlation with hydrogen peroxide-induced erythrocyte lysis and plasma α-tocopherol concentrations.

Only one study has been carried out in apparently healthy human adults who were depleted of vitamin E over 6 years and then repleted (Horwitt, 1960, 1962; Horwitt et al., 1956). In response to vitamin E deficiency, increased erythrocyte fragility (as assessed by an in vitro test of hydrogen peroxide-induced hemolysis) was observed, which was reversed by vitamin E supplementation.

The hydrogen peroxide-induced hemolysis test has drawbacks in that it is critically dependent upon the concentration of hydrogen peroxide used, the erythrocyte content of catalase and antioxidants, and the precise incubation conditions. Nonetheless, it is one of the few tests in which the marker (erythrocyte lysis) has been correlated with a health deficit (decreased erythrocyte survival) that has been shown to be corrected by supplemental vitamin E. Therefore, the data from this study were used to estimate intakes for α-tocopherol requirements.

It is recognized that there are great uncertainties in the data utilized to set the α-tocopherol requirements. However, in the absence of other scientifically sound data, hydrogen peroxide-induced hemolysis is the best marker at the present time. It should be emphasized that research is urgently needed to explore the use of other biomarkers to assess vitamin E requirements.

Plasma α-Tocopherol Concentrations and Hydrogen Peroxide-Induced Hemolysis

The requirements for vitamin E intakes are therefore based primarily on studies in which plasma α-tocopherol concentrations and corresponding hydrogen peroxide-induced erythrocyte lysis were determined (Horwitt, 1960, 1962, 1974; Horwitt et al., 1956, 1963, 1972). Vitamin E depletion in 19 normal, adult men was studied by feeding them a 2,200-kcal diet containing 3 mg (7 μmol)/day (range

2 to 4 mg [4.7 to 9.3 µmol]) of α-tocopherol and 55 g/day of fat (30 g from vitamin E-free lard) for 2.5 years. After the first 2.5 years, serum α-tocopherol levels decreased further when thermally oxidized corn oil with the α-tocopherol removed was substituted for lard. By replacing lard with corn oil, the total intake of polyunsaturated fatty acids (PUFAs) was increased, thereby increasing the oxidant burden on the available vitamin E stores. Subjects were followed on the vitamin E-depleted diet for more than 6 years.

To establish a criterion for estimating the EAR, the biomarker selected was the plasma α-tocopherol concentration that limited hydrogen peroxide-induced hemolysis to 12 percent or less. Differences up to this amount are not significant unless special precautions are taken to age and standardize the hydrogen peroxide solutions (Horwitt et al., 1963). The data in Figure 6-6 comparing long-term vitamin E-depletion in four subjects (depleted for more than 72 months) with six control subjects (Horwitt et al., 1963) show that at some concentration of plasma α-tocopherol between 6 µmol/L (258 µg/dL) and 12 µmol/L (516 µg/dL), an increase in hydrogen peroxide-induced hemolysis above 12 percent was observed in vitro. Averaging the α-tocopherol concentrations in the six subjects with hemolysis values of 12 percent or less in Figure 6-6 results in an average α-tocopherol concentration of 16.2 µmol/L (697 µg/dL). This is higher than the results of Farrell et al. (1977), who suggested that plasma α-tocopherol concentrations of 14 µmol/L (600 µg/dL) are sufficient to prevent hydrogen peroxide-induced hemolysis. Although the exact plasma α-tocopherol concentration that allows hemolysis to take place is unknown, it appeared to be prudent to estimate the lowest known plasma α-tocopherol concentration as that cutoff point where hemolysis would take place in 50 percent of the population. Thus, a plasma concentration of 12 µmol/L (516 µg/dL) was chosen as the concentration of plasma α-tocopherol associated with normal in vitro hydrogen peroxide-induced hemolysis. Based on NHANES III data (Appendix Table F-2), more than 95 percent of the population surveyed would have plasma concentrations greater than 12 µmol/L (516 µg/dL), thus indicating that the American public is not vitamin E deficient by this criterion.

Plasma α-Tocopherol Repletion

The effect of vitamin E repletion of depleted subjects has been studied. Horwitt (1960) conducted a study in which each subject received a different amount of vitamin E supplement, ranging from

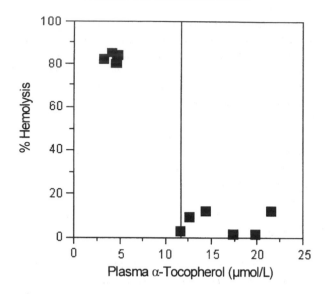

FIGURE 6-6 Relationship of plasma α-tocopherol concentrations and hemolysis in extensively vitamin E-depleted (>72 months) and control subjects.
SOURCE: Adapted from Horwitt et al. (1963).

0 to 320 mg (0 to 744 μmol)/day, for up to 138 days. For the purpose of keeping the various supplemental forms of vitamin E administered in the study equivalent, the amounts of *all rac*-α-tocopheryl acetate and *RRR*-α-tocopheryl acetate administered were converted to amounts of 2*R*-α-tocopherol forms for this analysis (see Table 6-1 for conversions). The criterion for vitamin E adequacy was defined as an intake sufficient to increase plasma α-tocopherol concentration to or above 12 μmol/L (516 μg/dL).

As shown in Figure 6-7 using the data for intakes generated above (Table 6-5), plasma α-tocopherol concentrations were linearly ($r^2 =$ 0.947) related to α-tocopherol intakes at intakes below 17 mg (40 μmol)/day. Using the limit of 12 μmol/L (516 μg/dL) plasma α-tocopherol as the criterion for the estimated vitamin E requirement generates a intake of 12 mg (28.2 μmol)/day α-tocopherol as the EAR.

Circulating Lipid Levels

Based on studies in normal and vitamin E-deficient children and adults, Horwitt et al. (1956), Farrell et al. (1982), and Sokol et al.

(1984) concluded that plasma tocopherol concentrations alone may be misleading in assessing human vitamin E status because their data have indicated a dependence of plasma tocopherol concentrations on the amount of circulating lipids. Moreover, Winklhofer-Roob et al. (1997) found that age was a significant predictor of plasma α-tocopherol concentrations in 208 Swiss subjects aged 0.4 to 38.7 years. This apparent relationship was attributed to an age-related increase in serum cholesterol concentrations. Sokol et al. (1993) reported that, because of the extremely high serum lipids in children with cholestasis, a ratio of serum α-tocopherol to serum total lipids of less than 0.6 mg/g indicated vitamin E deficiency, regardless of serum α-tocopherol concentrations.

When evaluating the vitamin E status of an individual, plasma lipid levels should be taken into account because all of the plasma vitamin E is transported in plasma lipoproteins (Traber et al., 1993). In subjects with normal serum lipid concentrations (328 to 573 mg/dL) (Sokol et al., 1984), corrections are not necessary to assess whether α-tocopherol concentrations are within the normal range.

PUFA Intake

As described earlier, high intakes of PUFAs are typically accompanied by increased vitamin E intakes. Using data from NHANES II, Murphy et al. (1990) reported that the mean PUFA intake in the United States was 16.3 g/day for men and 10.8 g/day for women. Based on a ratio of at least 1 μmol (0.4 mg) α-tocopherol per gram of PUFA when the primary dietary PUFA is linoleic acid, as in most U.S. diets (Bieri and Evarts, 1973; Horwitt, 1974; Witting and Lee, 1975), and a mean intake of 16.3 g PUFA, the lower boundary of required α-tocopherol intake is estimated to be 7 mg (16 μmol)/day. Thus, the amount of α-tocopherol required daily based on PUFA intakes would be met by the EAR of 12 mg (28.2 μmol)/day of α-tocopherol.

Vitamin E EAR and RDA Summary, Ages 19 through 50 Years

Based on the criterion of vitamin E intakes sufficient to prevent hydrogen peroxide-induced hemolysis, the data of Horwitt (1960) support an EAR of 12 mg (27.9 μmol) of α-tocopherol. The data were derived from studies in men only, and no similar data are available for women. However, there is no scientific basis for assuming different requirements for men and women, and although body

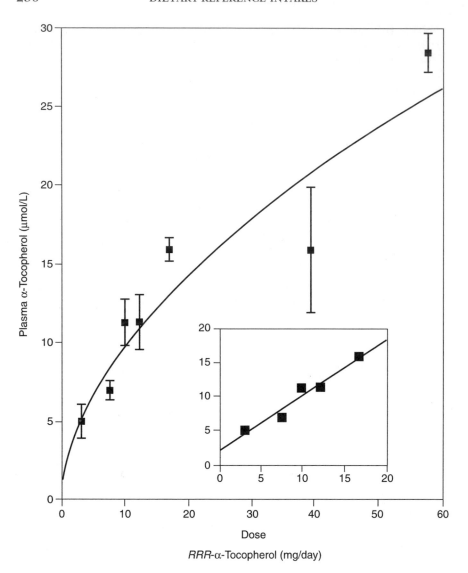

FIGURE 6-7 Relationship between serum α-tocopherol concentrations and dietary α-tocopherol intake in repleted subjects.
SOURCE: Adapted from Horwitt (1960).

TABLE 6-5 Effect of Vitamin E Supplements on Subjects Who Had Been on Basal Diet for 54 Months

Subject	α-Tocopherol Intake (mg/d)	Plasma Tocopherol + Standard Deviation[b] (μmol/L)
1	3.0	5.1 ± 1.1
2	7.6[a]	7.0 ± 0.6
3	9.8[a]	11.4 ± 1.5
4	12.1[a]	11.4 ± 1.7
5	16.7[a]	16.0 ± 0.7
6	39.4[a]	15.9 ± 4.0
7	57.7[a]	28.6 ± 1.2

[a] Intake was estimated from food and vitamin E supplements using conversion factors from Table 6-1.

[b] Plasma α-tocopherol concentrations were estimated for each individual by averaging the values on days 13, 21, 30, and 138.

SOURCE: Adapted from Horwitt (1960).

weights may be greater in men, women have larger fat masses as a percent of body weight, and thus may have similar requirements.

EAR for Men
    19–30 years   **12 mg (27.9 μmol)/day of α-tocopherol**
    31–50 years   **12 mg (27.9 μmol)/day of α-tocopherol**
EAR for Women
    19–30 years   **12 mg (27.9 μmol)/day of α-tocopherol**
    31–50 years   **12 mg (27.9 μmol)/day of α-tocopherol**

The RDA for vitamin E is set by assuming a coefficient of variation (CV) of 10 percent (see Chapter 1) because information is not available on the standard deviation of the requirement for vitamin E; the RDA is defined as equal to the EAR plus twice the CV to cover the needs of 97 to 98 percent of the individuals in the group (therefore, for vitamin E the RDA is 120 percent of the EAR). The calculated RDA in milligrams is rounded up.

RDA for Men
    19–30 years   **15 mg (34.9 μmol)/day of α-tocopherol**
    31–50 years   **15 mg (34.9 μmol)/day of α-tocopherol**
RDA for Women
    19–30 years   **15 mg (34.9 μmol)/day of α-tocopherol**
    31–50 years   **15 mg (34.9 μmol)/day of α-tocopherol**

Adults Ages 51 Years and Older

Evidence Considered in Estimating the Average Requirement

As discussed earlier, although vitamin E has been hypothesized to prevent myocardial infarction at the clinical level, only one of the four published large-scale, randomized, double-blind clinical secondary intervention studies that tested the ability of vitamin E to do this has been supportive of that hypothesis. This secondary prevention trial using 400 or 800 international units (IU) (268 or 567 mg)/day of *RRR*-α-tocopherol, was strongly positive (Stephens et al., 1996). The other three, one carried out in a group of high-risk cigarette smokers and using 50 mg/day of *all-rac*-α-tocopherol (ATBC Cancer Prevention Study Group, 1994) and two carried with groups of high-risk cardiovascular disease patients and using 300 mg/day of *all rac*-α-tocopherol (GISSI-Prevenzione Investigators, 1999) or 400 IU (268 mg)/day of *RRR*-α-tocopherol (HOPE Study Investigators, 2000), were neutral, with respect to coronary heart disease.

The limited clinical trial evidence precludes recommendations for higher vitamin E intakes at this time. Thus, adults ages 51 years and older appear to have the same vitamin E requirement as younger adults.

Vitamin E EAR and RDA Summary, Ages 51 Years and Older

There is no evidence that the aging process impairs vitamin E absorption or utilization. Therefore, for the age group 51 years and older an EAR of 12 mg (27.9 μmol)/day of α-tocopherol, the same as younger adults, is warranted.

EAR for Men
    51–70 years   12 mg (27.9 μmol)/day of α-tocopherol
    >70 years   12 mg (27.9 μmol)/day of α-tocopherol
EAR for Women
    51–70 years   12 mg (27.9 μmol)/day of α-tocopherol
    >70 years   12 mg (27.9 μmol)/day of α-tocopherol

The RDA for vitamin E is set by assuming a coefficient of variation (CV) of 10 percent (see Chapter 1) because information is not available on the standard deviation of the requirement for vitamin E. The RDA is defined as equal to the EAR plus twice the assumed CV to cover the needs of 97 to 98 percent of the individuals in the group (therefore, for vitamin E the RDA is 120 percent of the EAR). The calculated RDA in milligrams is rounded up.

RDA for Men
   51–70 years 15 mg (34.9 µmol)/day of α-tocopherol
   >70 years   15 mg (34.9 µmol)/day of α-tocopherol
RDA for Women
   51–70 years 15 mg (34.9 µmol)/day of α-tocopherol
   >70 years   15 mg (34.9 µmol)/day of α-tocopherol

Pregnancy

Evidence Considered in Estimating the Average Requirement

In contrast to the case for most nutrients, the blood concentration of α-tocopherol increases during pregnancy, in parallel with an increase in total lipids (Horwitt et al., 1972). Placental transfer of vitamin E from mother to fetus appears to be relatively constant as pregnancy progresses (Abbasi et al., 1990). Although vitamin E deficiency can occur in premature newborns, precipitating a hemolytic anemia (Oski and Barness, 1967; Ritchie et al., 1968), there are no reports of vitamin E deficiency during pregnancy and no evidence that maternal supplementation with vitamin E would prevent deficiency symptoms in premature offspring. Given the absence of data, it would appear that vitamin E supplementation of pregnant females is unwarranted.

Vitamin E EAR and RDA Summary, Pregnancy

Since there is no evidence at this time that the EAR for women during pregnancy should be increased above the level recommended for women in the nonpregnant state, the EAR for pregnancy is assumed to be the same and thus is 12 mg (27.9 µmol)/day of α-tocopherol.

EAR for Pregnancy
   14–18 years 12 mg (27.9 µmol)/day of α-tocopherol
   19–30 years 12 mg (27.9 µmol)/day of α-tocopherol
   31–50 years 12 mg (27.9 µmol)/day of α-tocopherol

The RDA for vitamin E is set by assuming a coefficient of variation (CV) of 10 percent (see Chapter 1) because information is not available on the standard deviation of the requirement for vitamin E; the RDA is defined as equal to the EAR plus twice the assumed CV to cover the needs of 97 to 98 percent of the individuals in the group (therefore, for vitamin E the RDA is 120 percent of the EAR). The calculated RDA in milligrams is rounded up.

RDA for Pregnancy
      14–18 years   **15 mg (34.9 µmol)/day of α-tocopherol**
      19–30 years   **15 mg (34.9 µmol)/day of α-tocopherol**
      31–50 years   **15 mg (34.9 µmol)/day of α-tocopherol**

Lactation

Evidence Considered in Estimating the Average Requirement

As indicated earlier in the section on infants, the estimated average amount of α-tocopherol secreted daily in human milk in the first 6 months of life is 4 mg (9.3 µmol). Thus, addition of this figure to the EAR for α-tocopherol for women, 12 mg (28.2 µmol)/day, would provide an EAR of 16 mg (37.5 µmol)/day of α-tocopherol in a lactating female.

The EAR is in excess of the median intake of 8.4 mg (19.5 µmol)/day for lactating women reported in the U.S. Department of Agriculture Continuing Survey of Food Intake by Individuals (CSFII) (Appendix Table D-2). Because estimates of vitamin E intake are underreported and vitamin E deficiency in infants receiving human milk is extremely rare, it is logical to postulate that lactating women are consuming more vitamin E than reported and that ingestion of supplements is unnecessary during lactation.

Vitamin E EAR and RDA Summary, Lactation

To estimate the EAR for lactation, the average vitamin E secreted in human milk, 4 mg (9.3 µmol) of α-tocopherol, is added to the EAR for the nonlactating woman, giving an EAR of 16 mg (37.2 µmol)/day of α-tocopherol.

EAR for Lactation
      14–18 years   **16 mg (37.2 µmol)/day of α-tocopherol**
      19–30 years   **16 mg (37.2 µmol)/day of α-tocopherol**
      31–50 years   **16 mg (37.2 µmol)/day of α-tocopherol**

The RDA for vitamin E is set by assuming a coefficient of variation (CV) of 10 percent (see Chapter 1) because information is not available on the standard deviation of the requirement for vitamin E; the RDA is defined as equal to the EAR plus twice the assumed CV to cover the needs of 97 to 98 percent of the individuals in the group (therefore, for vitamin E the RDA is 120 percent of the EAR). The calculated RDA in milligrams is rounded down.

RDA for Lactation

14–18 years	19 mg (44.2 µmol)/day of α-tocopherol
19–30 years	19 mg (44.2 µmol)/day of α-tocopherol
31–50 years	19 mg (44.2 µmol)/day of α-tocopherol

Special Considerations

Chronic Diseases

Data related to the effects of vitamin E on morbidity and mortality from chronic disease in the United States and Canada are limited. The evidence is strongest for prevention of coronary heart disease (CHD). However, even for this outcome, four double-blind, placebo-controlled trials have been reported, and only one of four, the Cambridge Heart Antioxidant Study (CHAOS) (Stephens et al., 1996), with prevention of heart disease as its primary aim, had a positive outcome. Two of the other trials, the GISSI-Prevenzione Trial and the Heart Outcomes Prevention Evaluation (HOPE) Study (GISSI-Prevenzione Investigators, 1999; HOPE Study Investigators, 2000), with prevention of heart disease as their primary aim, had neutral results. Similarly, the fourth trial, the Alpha-Tocopherol Beta-Carotene (ATBC) Cancer Prevention Study (ATBC Cancer Prevention Study Group, 1994), which had lung cancer as its primary outcome, reported no beneficial effect of vitamin E on myocardial infarction rates. Thus, a recommendation of high vitamin E intakes for the general population to decrease CHD risk is considered premature.

Some physicians caring for patients with coronary artery disease are already prescribing vitamin E at doses used in the CHAOS study, 400 or 800 IU (268 or 567 mg)/day of RRR-α-tocopherol. Precisely how vitamin E works at these high doses is not known but could include both antioxidant and nonantioxidant mechanisms. This is an active research area at both the molecular and the clinical levels, and further research is needed.

Currently, a number of other double-blind, placebo-controlled intervention trials of the efficacy of vitamin E to prevent or ameliorate CHD are in progress. If these studies result in positive outcomes, it may become necessary to review the recommendations for vitamin E intakes in some subgroups of the adult populations, especially those in the groups over 50 years of age because increasing age is an important risk factor for heart disease. Although there is a large and growing body of experimental evidence suggesting that vitamin E supplementation may reduce the risk of some chronic diseases, especially heart disease, the results of the GISSI Prevenzione Trial (GISSI-Prevenzione Investigators, 1999), the Heart Outcomes Prevention Evaluation (HOPE) study (HOPE Study Investigators, 2000), and the Alpha-Tocopherol Beta-Carotene (ATBC) Cancer Prevention Study (ATBC Cancer Prevention Study Group, 1994) preclude recommendations for higher vitamin E intakes at this time.

Exercise

High levels of physical activity and sports might increase oxidative damage and thus increase needs for antioxidants. It is unknown whether or the extent to which increased oxidative damage occurs in physical exercise. However, the Boston Nutritional Status Survey reported that plasma vitamin E concentrations increased slightly with regular exercise in adults 60 years of age and older (Hartz et al., 1992). It is, therefore, not known if any adjustment in vitamin E requirements is needed in response to strenuous or regular exercise.

Extreme Body Size and Composition

Given the minimal data available to develop the EAR, adjusting any recommendations for vitamin E requirements to meet expected needs for individuals with extreme variation for reference body size or composition must await additional data.

Cigarette Smokers

Potentially injurious free radicals are present in cigarette tar and smoke (Church and Pryor, 1985; Pryor and Stone, 1993). In addition, cigarette smokers have increased phagocyte activities (Eiserich et al., 1997). Smokers are therefore under a high and sustained free-radical load, both from cigarette smoke itself and from oxidants produced by activated phagocytes (Cross et al., 1997; Duthie et al., 1991; Eiserich et al., 1995).

Exposure to cigarette smoke damages antioxidant defenses. Low blood levels of vitamin C are a characteristic feature of heavy smokers (Duthie et al., 1995, 1996; Mezzetti et al., 1995; Ross et al., 1995). Cigarette smoke also damages low molecular weight thiols and especially thiol-containing proteins in human plasma (O'Neill et al.,

1994) and white blood cells (Tsuchiya et al., 1992). Plasma vitamin E is not routinely depleted in cigarette smokers relative to non-smokers. However, vitamin E supplementation of smokers has been shown to reduce indicators of lipid peroxidation (Mezzetti et al., 1995; Morrow et al., 1995; Pratico et al., 1998; Reilly et al., 1996), suggesting that plasma vitamin E may not be indicative of tissue stores.

It is unknown if any adjustment in vitamin E requirements is needed in those who smoke or are routinely exposed to smoke.

INTAKE OF VITAMIN E

As stated earlier, the Dietary Reference Intakes (DRIs) for vitamin E are based on α-tocopherol only and do not include amounts obtained from the other seven naturally occurring forms historically called vitamin E (β-, γ-, δ-tocopherol and the four tocotrienols). Because the different forms of vitamin E cannot be interconverted in the human, the Estimated Average Requirements (EARs), Recommended Dietary Allowances (RDAs), and Adequate Intakes (AIs) apply only to the intake of *RRR*-α-tocopherol from food and the 2*R*-stereoisomeric forms of α-tocopherol (*RRR*-, *RSR*-, *RRS*-, and *RSS*-α-tocopherol) that occur in fortified foods and supplements. Although both α- and γ-tocopherols are absorbed, only α-tocopherol is preferentially secreted by the liver into the plasma (because α-tocopherol transfer protein [α-TTP] recognizes only α-tocopherol) for transport to tissues while γ-tocopherol is preferentially metabolized and excreted. This implies that the body requires α-tocopherol for some special (as yet undefined) need and other forms of vitamin E do not qualify.

Currently, most nutrient databases, as well as nutrition labels, do not distinguish among the different tocopherols in food. Thus, the data below on intakes from surveys and nutrient content of foods are presented as α-tocopherol equivalents (α-TE) and thus include the contribution of all eight naturally occurring forms of vitamin E, after adjustment for bioavailability using previously determined equivalency (e.g., γ-tocopherol was assumed to have only 10 percent of the availability of α-tocopherol) based on fetal resorption assays (see earlier section on "Units of Vitamin E Activity"). Because other forms of vitamin E occur in foods (e.g., γ-tocopherol is present in widely consumed oils such as soybean and corn oils), the intake of α-TE is greater than the intake of α-tocopherol alone.

Vitamin E Conversion Factors

Food Sources of Vitamin E

The reported median vitamin E intake in the United States of all individuals surveyed in 1988 to 1994 in the Third National Health and Nutrition Examination Survey (NHANES III) was 9 mg (21 μmol)/day of α-TE (see Appendix Table C-3). Additional data from the NHANES III database indicate that α-tocopherol from food as defined in this report (the *RRR*-form) contributed approximately 7 mg/day of the 9 mg/day median intake of total α-TE (see Appendix Table C-4). Thus, based on NHANES III, approximately 80 percent of the α-TE from foods in the survey are reported to be contributed by foods containing α-tocopherol. Thus, to estimate the α-tocopherol intake from food surveys in the United States in which food intake data are presented as α-TE, the α-TE should be multiplied by 0.8:

$$\text{mg of α-tocopherol in a meal} =$$
$$\text{mg of α-tocopherol equivalents in a meal} \times 0.8.$$

If diets vary considerably from what might be considered typical in the United States and Canada, other factors may be more appropriate to use in place of 0.8.

Vitamin E Supplements

To determine the number of milligrams of α-tocopherol in a multiple-vitamin supplement labeled in international units (IUs), one of two conversion factors is used. If the form of the supplement is "natural" or RRR-α-tocopherol (historically and incorrectly labeled *d*-α-tocopherol) (Horwitt, 1976), the correct factor is 0.67 mg/IU (USP, 1999). Thus, 30 IUs of RRR-α-tocopherol (labeled as *d*-α-tocopherol) in a multivitamin supplement would equate to 20 mg of α-tocopherol (30 × 0.67). The same factor would be used for 30 IUs of either *RRR*-α-tocopherol acetate or *RRR*-α-tocopherol succinate, because the amount in grams of these forms in a capsule has been adjusted based on their molecular weight. If the form of the supplement is *all rac*-α-tocopherol (historically and incorrectly labeled *dl*-α-tocopherol) (Horwitt, 1976), the appropriate factor is 0.45 mg/IU, reflecting the inactivity of the 2*S*-stereoisomers. Thus, 30-IU of *all rac*-α-tocopherol (labeled as *dl*-α-tocopherol) in a multivitamin supplement would equate to 13.5 mg of α-tocopherol (30 ×

0.45). The same factor would be used for the *all rac*-α-tocopherol acetate and succinate forms as well. See Table 6-1 for more information on the derivation of these conversion factors to be used when estimating intake from these forms of α-tocopherol to meet requirements.

mg of α-tocopherol in food, fortified food, or multivitamin
= IU of the *RRR*-α-tocopherol compound × 0.67.

or

= IU of the *all rac*-α-tocopherol compound × 0.45.

Food Sources

The various vitamin E forms occur in different proportions in foods. The main dietary sources of vitamin E are edible vegetable oils (Dial and Eitenmiller, 1995; McLaughlin and Weihrauch, 1979; Sheppard et al., 1993) (Figure 6-8). At least half of the tocopherol content of wheat germ oil, sunflower oil, cottonseed oil, safflower oil, canola oil, and olive oil is in the form of α-tocopherol. Soybean and corn oils contain about 10 times as much γ-tocopherol as α-tocopherol. Palm and rice bran oils contain high proportions of α-tocopherol, as well as various tocotrienols (Dial and Eitenmiller, 1995). Other foods providing vitamin E include unprocessed cereal grains, nuts, fruits, vegetables, and meats, especially the fatty portion. As stated previously, all of the α-tocopherol present in these unfortified foods would be in the natural form, *RRR*-α-tocopherol and would contribute toward meeting the recommended dietary allowance. The other non-α-tocopherol forms of vitamin E present in food would not.

Dietary Intake

Dietary Surveys

According to the 1994 to 1996 Continuing Survey of Food Intakes by Individuals (CSFII) (Appendix Table D-2), the median reported dietary intakes of men and women aged 31 through 50 years are 9.3 mg (21.6 μmol)/day and 6.8 mg (15.8 μmol)/day, respectively, of α-TE. Using the factor (0.8) derived from NHANES III data to determine α-tocopherol intake from α-TE, the adjusted intakes would be 7.5 mg (17.4 μmol)/day for men (9.3 × 0.8) and 5.4 mg (12.6 μmol)/day for women (6.8 × 0.8).

Data from NHANES III (Appendix Tables C-3 and C-5) indicate a

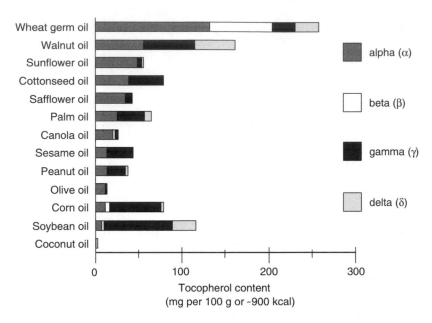

FIGURE 6-8 The various vitamin E forms in edible vegetable oils.
SOURCE: Data obtained from Dial and Eitenmiller (1995).

median total intake (including supplements) of 12.9 mg (30.0 µmol)/day of α-TE (10.3 mg [24.0 µmol]/day of α-tocopherol) and a median dietary intake from food alone of 11.7 mg (27.2 µmol)/day of α-TE (9.4 mg [21.9 µmol]/day of α-tocopherol) among men 31 through 50 years of age. Thus, these men are consuming 0.9 mg (10.3 minus 9.4 mg/day) of α-tocopherol from supplements. If the form of the supplement is *all rac*-α-tocopherol, the 0.9 mg (2.1 µmol)/day would be divided by 2 (see section on "Interconversion of Vitamin E Units"), which would result in an adjusted supplement intake of 0.4 mg (0.9 µmol)/day of α-tocopherol. Thus, the adjusted estimate for total intake from food (9.4 mg) and supplements (0.4 mg) is 9.8 mg (22.8 µmol)/day of α-tocopherol. If the form of the supplement is *RRR*-α-tocopherol, all of the 0.9 mg (2.1 µmol)/day of α-tocopherol in the multivitamin supplement contributes to meeting the requirement, and the total intake is 10.3 mg (24.0 µmol)/day of α-tocopherol. For women in this age range, the median total intake (including supplements) is 9.1 mg (21.2 µmol)/day of α-TE (7.3 mg [17.0 µmol] of α-tocopherol) and the median dietary intake is 8.0 mg (18.6 µmol)/day of α-TE (6.4 mg [14.9 µmol]/

day of α-tocopherol) from food alone. Thus, the adjusted median reported intake for these women would be 0.9 mg (7.3 minus 6.4 mg/day) of α-tocopherol from supplements. If the supplement is *all rac*-α-tocopherol, the 0.9 mg (2.1 μmol)/day would be divided by 2 (see section on "Interconversion of Vitamin E Units"), resulting in an adjusted median intake from supplements of 0.4 mg (0.9 μmol)/day of α-tocopherol. Thus, the total adjusted median intake reported from food (6.4 mg) and supplements (0.4 mg) is 6.8 mg (15.8 μmol)/day of α-tocopherol. Again, if the form of the supplement is *RRR*-α-tocopherol, all of the 0.9 mg (2.1 μmol)/day of α-tocopherol from the multivitamin supplement would contribute to meeting the requirement, and the total intake from diet and supplements remains 7.3 mg (17.0 μmol)/day of α-tocopherol.

Underreporting in Dietary Surveys

The above CSFII and NHANES III intake estimates may be low due to four sources of measurement error that are important with regard to vitamin E intake: (1) energy intake is underreported in the national surveys (Mertz et al., 1991), and fat intake (which serves as a major carrier for vitamin E) is likely to be more underreported than energy intake in the NHANES III survey (Briefel et al., 1997); (2) the amount of fats and oils added during food preparation (and absorbed into the cooked product) is difficult to assess using diet recall methodologies, yet contributes substantially to vitamin E intake; (3) uncertainties about the particular fats or oils consumed, particularly when food labels do not provide the specific fat or oil in the product (e.g., "this product may contain partially hydrogenated soybean and/or cottonseed oil or vegetable oil") necessitate a reliance on default selections (and thus assumptions about the relative content of α- and γ-tocopherols); and (4) because of the small number of samples, the vitamin E content of food sources in the CSFII and NHANES III databases are very variable (J. Holden, Agricultural Research Service, USDA, personal communication, April 13, 1999).

Recently, Haddad et al. (1999) reported vitamin E intakes of 25 vegans (defined as those who excluded all animal products from their diets) and 20 nonvegans between the ages of 20 and 60 years. The reported vitamin E intakes, based on 4-day food records, were 17 to 23 mg (40 to 53 μmol)/day of α-tocopherol equivalents. Using the factor (0.8) from NHANES III data to adjust for α-tocopherol equivalents, the above estimated intakes would equate to 13.6 to 18.4 mg (31.6 to 42.8 μmol)/day of α-tocopherol. Van het Hof et al. (1999) reported that conventional Dutch menus contained 20.9 mg

(48.7 µmol)/day of α-tocopherol when these diets were analyzed chemically. These two studies indicate that vitamin E intakes from the CSFII and NHANES III surveys are probably underestimated even with the adjustment factor (0.8) and suggest that mean intakes of apparently healthy adults in the United States and Canada are likely to be above the RDA of 15 mg (34.9 µmol)/day of α-tocopherol.

Most dietary vitamin E is present in fats and its oils (Sheppard et al., 1993); therefore, changes in dietary habits to decrease fat intake may have deleterious effects on vitamin E intake (Adam et al., 1995; Bae et al., 1993; Retzlaff et al., 1991; Sarkkinen et al., 1993; Velthuiste Wierik et al., 1996). Patients with coronary artery disease, who did not take vitamin supplements, had average dietary vitamin E intakes of 5.8 mg (13.4 µmol)/day of α-tocopherol equivalents (adjusted to 4.6 mg [10.8 µmol]/day of α-tocopherol) in a 25 percent fat diet containing 2,058 kcal (Mandel et al., 1997). This example demonstrates that low-fat diets can substantially decrease vitamin E intakes if food choices are not carefully made to enhance α-tocopherol intakes.

Dietary Vitamin E Sources

Murphy et al. (1990) evaluated vitamin E intakes from NHANES II. Fats and oils used as spreads, etc. contributed 20.2 percent of the total vitamin E; vegetables, 15.1 percent; meat, poultry, and fish, 12.6 percent; desserts, 9.9 percent; breakfast cereals, 9.3 percent; fruit, 5.3 percent; bread and grain products, 5.3 percent; dairy products, 4.5 percent; mixed main dishes, 4.0 percent; nuts and seeds, 3.8 percent; eggs, 3.2 percent; salty snacks, 3 percent; legumes, 2.1 percent; and soups, sauces, and gravies, 1.7 percent.

As indicated previously, estimation of dietary vitamin E intake is difficult because the source of oil is often not known with certainty. Lehmann et al. (1986) analyzed the foods used in a human diet study for vitamin E content. Each menu was designed to contain 2,400 kcal with 35 percent fat calories and included either 10 or 30 g/day of linoleic acid and 500 mg/day of cholesterol; the high linoleic acid diet contained 10 g of safflower oil. As shown in Figure 6-9, substituting various oils for the 10 g of safflower oil resulted in vitamin E intakes that varied from 6.9 to 13.8 mg (16 to 32 µmol)/day of α-TE depending on the source of the vegetable oil (vitamin E contents were estimated from Lehmann et al., 1986, and Dial and Eitenmiller, 1995).

Intake from Supplements

Vitamin E supplement use is high in the U.S. population (Hartz et al., 1988; Slesinski et al., 1996). Information from the Boston Nutritional Status Survey on use of supplemental vitamin E by a free-living population, 60 years of age and older, indicated that 38 percent of the men took a nutritional supplement and 68 percent of these users took a vitamin E supplement. Of the women, 49 percent used supplements with 73 percent of them taking a vitamin E supplement (Hartz et al., 1992). In the earlier 1986 National Health Interview Survey, 26 percent of all adults reported use of supplements containing vitamin E (Moss et al., 1989). Slesinski et al. (1996) examined supplement usage in over 11,000 adults who participated in the 1992 National Health Interview Survey Epidemiology Supplement and reported that diets of women utilizing supplements that contained vitamin E were higher in vitamin E compared with those of nonsupplement users. No differences in vitamin E intake were found in the men participating in the survey.

TOLERABLE UPPER INTAKE LEVELS

The Tolerable Upper Intake Level (UL) is the highest level of daily nutrient intake that is likely to pose no risk of adverse health effects in almost all individuals. Although members of the general population should be advised not to exceed the UL for vitamin E routinely, intake above the UL may be appropriate for investigation within well-controlled clinical trials. In light of evaluating possible benefits to health, clinical trials of doses above the UL should not be discouraged, as long as subjects participating in these trials have signed informed consent documents regarding possible toxicity, and as long as these trials employ appropriate safety monitoring of trial subjects. Also, the UL is not meant to apply to individuals who are receiving vitamin E under medical supervision.

Hazard Identification

Adverse Effects

There is no evidence of adverse effects from the consumption of vitamin E naturally occurring in foods. Therefore, this review is limited to evidence concerning intake of α-tocopherol as a supplement, food fortificant, or pharmacological agent. RRR-α-tocopheryl acetate (historically and incorrectly labeled d-α-tocopheryl acetate)

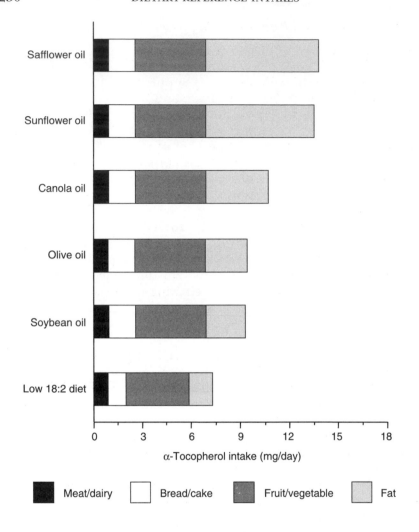

FIGURE 6-9 Variations in α-tocopherol content of diets containing different oils. A sample diet contained 2,400 kcal with 35 percent fat calories including either 10 or 30 g/day of linoleic acid (18:2) and 500 mg/day cholesterol; the high linoleic acid diet contained 10 g safflower oil. When various oils were substituted for the 10 g safflower oil, vitamin E intakes varied from 7 to 14 mg (16 to 33 μmol)/day of α-tocopherol depending on the source of the vegetable oil.
SOURCE: Lehmann et al. (1986) and Dial and Eitenmiller (1995).

(Horwitt, 1976) and *all rac*-α-tocopheryl acetate (historically and incorrectly labeled *dl*-α-tocopheryl acetate) (Horwitt, 1976) are the forms of synthetic vitamin E used almost exclusively in supplements, food fortification, and pharmacologic agents.

Animal studies show that α-tocopherol is not mutagenic, carcinogenic, or teratogenic (Abdo et al., 1986; Dysmsza and Park, 1975; Krasavage and Terhaar, 1977). Animals fed extremely high doses of α-tocopherol or α-tocopheryl acetate have been shown to experience a variety of adverse effects, but the relevance of some of this information to the human situation is questionable.

Little information exists on the adverse effects to humans that might result from ingestion of other forms of tocopherol, such as γ- or β-tocopherol, in amounts exceeding the levels normally found in foods. One study in humans given supplements of either *all rac*-α-tocopherol, *RRR*-α-tocopherol, or mixed tocopherols (α, β, and γ-tocopherol) demonstrated that all supplements yielded the same plasma α- and γ-tocopherol concentrations (Chopra and Bhagavan, 1999). Some data are available from animal studies, however. Clement and Bourre (1997) found that rats fed large amounts of γ tocopherol had increased concentrations of α-tocopherol in plasma and tissues. Although the fractional absorption of α-tocopherol was decreased when α-tocopherol supplements were given to thoracic duct-cannulated rats, no decrease was seen in γ-tocopherol absorption (Traber et al., 1986). Thus, it appears that absorption of the various forms of vitamin E is independent and unaffected by the presence of large amounts of the other forms.

Plasma α-tocopherol concentrations are not informative for assessing adverse effects because plasma concentrations reach a similar plateau (approximately 3 to 4 times unsupplemented concentrations) when humans consume supplements containing at least 200 mg (465 μmol)/day of either *RRR*- or *all rac*-α-tocopherol (Chopra and Bhagavan, 1999; Devaraj et al., 1997; Dimitrov et al., 1991, 1996; Jialal et al., 1995; Meydani et al., 1998; Princen et al., 1995). However, since all forms of vitamin E are absorbed, although are not maintained in the plasma (as discussed in the earlier section "Absorption and Transport" [Kiyose et al., 1997; Meydani et al., 1989; Traber and Kayden, 1989a; Traber et al., 1992, 1994a]), they all could contribute to vitamin E toxicity. These observations suggest that at doses at which adverse effects are observed, all the stereoisomers of α-tocopherol should be considered equivalent. A review of vitamin E toxicity studies concluded that humans show few side effects following supplemental doses below 2,100 mg (4,885 μmol)/day of *RRR*-α-tocopherol (Kappus and Diplock, 1992). However, most studies of the possible effects of supplemental α-tocopherol (all forms) on human health have been conducted over periods of a few weeks to a few months, so the possible chronic effects of lifetime exposures to high supplemental levels of α-tocopherol remain uncertain.

Hemorrhagic Toxicity—Humans. Three large-scale intervention trials, one supplementing with 400 or 800 IU (268 or 567 mg)/day of *RRR*-α-tocopherol for 1.4 years (Stephens et al., 1996), another supplementing with 300 mg/day of *all rac*-α-tocopherol for 3.5 years (GISSI-Prevenzione Investigators, 1999), and the third supplementing with 400 IU (268 mg)/day of *RRR*-α-tocopherol for 4.5 years (HOPE Study Investigators, 2000), reported no increased risk of stroke. However, another large-scale randomized trial, the Alpha-Tocopherol, Beta Carotene (ATBC) Cancer Prevention Study, in Finnish male smokers consuming 50 mg/day of *all rac*-α-tocopherol for 6 years, reported a significant 50 percent increase in mortality from hemorrhagic stroke (66 versus 44 strokes in the supplemented versus the control group) (ATBC Cancer Prevention Study Group, 1994). An increase in hemorrhagic strokes was not observed in another study that was designed to evaluate neurological function in 85 patients with Alzheimer's disease consuming 2,000 IU/day of supplemental *all rac*-α-tocopherol for 2 years (Sano et al., 1997). The number of subjects in this trial or the length of the trial may have been insufficient to detect an effect. The unexpected result in the ATBC study requires confirmation or additional refutation from several other ongoing, large-scale trials including the Women's Health Study, the Physicians' Health Study II, and the Women's Antioxidant Cardiovascular Study. If most of the evidence that develops from these ongoing randomized trials indicates an increased risk of hemorrhagic stroke from α-tocopherol, the recommended UL for α-tocopherol will have to be revised.

Hemorrhagic Toxicity—Animals. α-Tocopherol can cause hemorrhage, increase prothrombin time, and interrupt blood coagulation in experimental animals, but very high doses are required. The hemorrhagic toxicity of α-tocopherol has been observed in chicks (March et al., 1973) and rats (Abdo et al., 1986; Mellette and Leone, 1960; Takahashi et al., 1990; Wheldon et al., 1983; Yang and Desai, 1977). However, in both species, high doses of 500 mg/kg/day or more of *RRR*-α-tocopheryl acetate were necessary to induce the effects. Also, the hemorrhagic effects could be reversed by the administration of supplemental vitamin K (Abdo et al., 1986; March et al., 1973; Wheldon et al., 1983). Presumably, these hemorrhagic effects seen in experimental animals are relevant to humans, because similar abnormal blood coagulation has been observed in a patient receiving chronic warfarin therapy, which would interfere with vitamin K status (Corrigan and Marcus, 1974).

Platelet Effects. Evidence suggests that α-tocopherol inhibits platelet aggregation and adhesion in vitro (Calzada et al., 1997; Freedman et al., 1996; Higashi and Kikuchi, 1974; Steiner and Anastasi, 1976). However, it is not clear that these effects on platelet function are deleterious in normal healthy individuals at any dose. Oral administration of up to 600 mg/day of α-tocopherol up to three years did not result in any adverse blood coagulation effects in apparently healthy volunteers (Farrell and Bieri, 1975; Kitagawa and Mino, 1989). However, special consideration should be given to individuals who are deficient in vitamin K or who are on anticoagulant therapy. Administration of high doses of α-tocopherol may exacerbate the coagulation defects in these individuals (Corrigan and Marcus, 1974).

Other Adverse Effects in Humans. Uncontrolled studies have reported various other adverse effects associated with excess intake of α-tocopherol. These include fatigue, emotional disturbances, thrombophlebitis, breast soreness, creatinuria, altered serum lipid and lipoprotein levels, gastrointestinal disturbances, and thyroid effects (Anderson and Reid, 1974; Bendich and Machlin, 1988; Machlin, 1989; Tsai et al., 1978). However, none of these reported effects have been consistently observed or shown in controlled trials. Although side effects have been reported with extended intakes of 1,100 to 2,100 mg/day of *RRR*-α-tocopherol (Kappus and Diplock, 1992), these effects are not severe and subside rapidly upon reducing the dosage or discontinuing the administration of α-tocopherol. The lack of systematic observations of such effects in controlled clinical trails prevents any judgments regarding the risk of such effects in the normal healthy human population.

Adverse Effects in Premature Infants. In addition to the hemorrhagic effects described previously, an increased incidence of necrotizing enterocolitis (NEC) was observed in premature infants with birth weights of 1.5 kg or less who were given 200 mg/day of α-tocopheryl acetate (Finer et al., 1984). Johnson et al. (1985) also demonstrated an association between high serum vitamin E concentrations and increased incidence of sepsis and late-onset NEC in infants of less than 1.5-kg birth weight who were supplemented with α-tocopheryl acetate.

The incidence of intracranial hemorrhage in premature infants receiving supplemental intravenous or oral α-tocopheryl acetate has been reported as increased (Phelps et al., 1987), unchanged (Speer et al., 1984), or decreased (Speer et al., 1984) depending on the severity of the hemorrhage. It may well be that the small premature infant is particularly vulnerable to the toxic effects of vitamin E and that intravenous vitamin E is more toxic than the oral preparation.

Other Adverse Effects Seen in Animals. Many other adverse effects have been noted in various animal studies. For example, Abdo et al. (1986) observed lung lesions (chronic interstitial inflammation and adenomatous hyperplasia) in Fischer 344 rats in all treatment groups receiving α-tocopheryl acetate by gavage at doses as low as 125 mg/kg/day for 13 weeks. It is possible that the lung lesions may be the result of infusions into the lung from the gavage, rather than a vitamin E effect. However, this toxic effect was considered less relevant than the hemorrhagic effects seen because similar effects in the lung have not been noted in human trials or other animal studies.

Summary

Based on considerations of causality, relevance, and the quality and completeness of the database, hemorrhagic effects were selected as the critical endpoint on which to base the UL for vitamin E for adults. There is some evidence of an increased incidence of hemorrhagic effects in premature infants receiving supplemental α-tocopherol. However, the human data fail to demonstrate consistently a causal association between excess α-tocopherol intake in normal, apparently healthy individuals and any adverse health outcome. The unexpected finding of an increase in hemorrhagic stroke in the ATBC study was considered preliminary and provocative, but not convincing until it can be corroborated or refuted in further large-scale clinical trials. The human data demonstrating the safety of supplemental α-tocopherol have been accumulated primarily in small groups of individuals receiving supplemental doses of 3,200 mg/day of α-tocopherol or less (usually less than 2,000 mg/day) for relatively short periods of time (weeks to a few months). Thus, some caution must be exercised in judgments regarding the safety of supplemental doses of α-tocopherol over multiyear periods.

The hemorrhagic effects seen in experimental animals are encountered only with very high doses of α-tocopherol and can be corrected by administration of supplemental vitamin K. Similarly, it appears that in vitamin K-deficient humans these effects could occur if sufficiently high doses were obtained to overwhelm the protective effects of vitamin K. However, there is no direct evidence regarding the doses that might put normal apparently healthy humans at risk for such effects; these data show that individuals who are deficient in vitamin K are at increased risk of coagulation defects.

Adults

Data Selection. In the absence of human data pertaining to dose-response relationships, the data sets used to identify a no-observed-adverse-effect level (NOAEL) for α-tocopherol include studies showing hemorrhagic toxicity in rats (Abdo et al., 1986; Takahashi et al., 1990; Wheldon et al., 1983).

Dose-Response Assessment

Identification of NOAEL and Lowest-Observed-Adverse-Effect Level (LOAEL). A LOAEL of 500 mg/kg body weight/day can be identified based on a critical evaluation by Wheldon et al. (1983). They fed *all rac*-α-tocopheryl acetate to Charles River CD strain rats at levels of 500, 1,000, or 2,000 mg/kg body weight/day for 104 weeks. Hemorrhages from the gut, the urinary tract, the orbit and meninges, and the claws were observed in male rats only by week 15 in the highest-dose group, by week 16 in the intermediate-dose group, and by week 18 in the low-dose group. Prothrombin times were prolonged in males of all three treatment groups by week 4. However, additional vitamin K supplementation of the diets was initiated at week 24 and prothrombin times returned to normal by week 26. Although this was a chronic, 104-week study, the correction of vitamin K levels in the diet at week 24 means that the combined vitamin E–vitamin K effect was evaluated only on a subchronic basis.

Takahashi et al. (1990) supplemented the diets of male Sprague-Dawley rats with 600 or 1,000 mg/kg body weight/day *RRR*-α-tocopheryl acetate for 7 days. Despite the short duration of the feeding trial, a dose-dependent increase in prothrombin time and partial thromboplastin time was noted in rats receiving 600 and 1,000 mg/kg/day. The number of animals with hemorrhages was similar in both dose groups. No supplementation of vitamin K was attempted in this experiment. This study would yield a LOAEL of

600 mg/kg/day but is compromised by its short duration and by the fact that lower doses were not utilized.

Abdo et al. (1986) conducted a 13-week study administering *RRR*-α-tocopheryl acetate in corn oil by gavage to Fischer 344 rats at doses of 125, 500, and 2,000 mg/kg body weight/day. In males, high levels of *RRR*-α-tocopheryl acetate (2,000 mg/kg/day) caused prolongation of both prothrombin time and activated partial thromboplastin time (APTT), reticulocytosis, and a decrease in hematocrit values and hemoglobin concentrations. APTT was also lengthened in females at this dose level. Hemorrhagic diathesis was observed in both males and females at the highest dosage level (2,000 mg/kg/day). However, no adverse hemorrhagic effects, other than a minimal increase in activated partial thromboplastin time, were observed at a dose of 500 mg/kg/day.

While some differences were encountered among the results of these three key studies, they could be attributed to the dosage approach (gavage versus diet), the time period of dosing, the strain of rats, and possibly the level of vitamin K supplementation. The data of Wheldon et al. (1983) demonstrate that the hazard posed by excessive dietary intake of *all rac*-α-tocopheryl acetate can be overcome by administration of additional vitamin K. The Wheldon et al. (1983) study is considered the most definitive estimate because of the long exposure period of the dosage via diet. The LOAEL in this study was 500 mg/kg/day, the lowest dose tested. Thus, a precise NOAEL cannot be determined from the experiment. However, this LOAEL is consistent with the results of the shorter-term feeding study of Takahashi et al. (1990) with a LOAEL at 600 mg/kg/day, the lowest dose tested, and the gavage study of Abdo et al. (1986) with no adverse hemorrhagic effects at 125 mg/kg/day and only a minimal increase in activated partial thromboplastin time at 500 mg/kg/day of *RRR*-α-tocopherol acetate.

Uncertainty Assessment. When determining an uncertainty factor (UF) for α-tocopherol, several sources of uncertainty were considered and combined into the final UF (Table 6-6). A UF of 2 was used to extrapolate the LOAEL to a NOAEL. The severity of hemorrhagic effects justifies a UF greater than 1; however, the results of Abdo et al. (1986) showing no adverse effects at 125 mg/kg/day for hemorrhagic effects justify a UF of 2 to extrapolate from the LOAEL of 500 mg/kg body weight/day to the NOAEL of 250 mg/kg body weight/day. A UF of 2 was selected to extrapolate from subchronic to chronic intake, and a UF of 3 was selected to extrapolate from experimental animals to humans because of data showing

TABLE 6-6 Sources of Uncertainty Used to Determine UL for Vitamin E

	UF
LOAEL to NOAEL	2
Subchronic to chronic intake	2
Experimental animal to human	3
Interindividual variation in sensitivity	3
Final UF = 2 × 2 × 3 × 3 =	36

some similarities between the animal and human responses. Another UF of 3 was selected to account for interindividual variation in sensitivity. This value was deemed appropriate based on pharmacokinetic data showing plasma saturation of α-tocopherol concentrations with increasingly higher intakes in humans (Dimitrov et al., 1991, 1996; Jialal et al., 1995; Losowsky et al., 1972; Meydani et al., 1998; Princen et al., 1995). The various UFs are combined to yield an overall UF of 36 to extrapolate from the LOAEL in animals to derive a UL for humans.

Derivation of a UL. The LOAEL of 500 mg/kg/day was divided by the overall UF of 36 to obtain a UL value of 14 mg/kg/day for adult humans. The value of 14 mg/kg/day was multiplied by the average of the reference body weights for male and female adults, 68.5 kg, from Chapter 1 (Table 1-1). The resulting UL for adults is 959 mg/day (which was rounded to 1,000 mg/day):

$$UL = \frac{LOAEL}{UF} = \frac{500 \text{ mg / kg / day}}{36}$$

$$= 14 / \text{mg / kg / day} \times 68.5 \text{ kg} \approx 1,000 \text{ mg / day}.$$

Although adult males and females have different reference body weights, the uncertainties in the estimation of the UL were considerable, and distinction of separate ULs for male and female adults was therefore not attempted. This UL is consistent with the review by Kappus and Diplock (1992) that in humans, side effects occurred at doses of 1,100 to 2,100 mg (2,559 to 4,885 μmol)/day of *RRR*-α-tocopherol. At high doses all of the stereoisomers of α-tocopherol are considered equivalent given that all forms of vitamin E are absorbed (Kiyose et al., 1997; Meydani et al., 1989; Traber and Kayden, 1989a; Traber et al., 1992, 1994a). Thus, the UL applies to all eight stereoisomers of α-tocopherol.

Vitamin E UL Summary, Ages 19 Years and Older

UL for Adults
   19 years and older   **1,000 mg (2,326 μmol)/day of any**
                                   form of supplementary α-tocopherol

Other Life Stage Groups

Infants. For infants, the UL was judged not determinable be-cause of insufficient data on adverse effects in this age group and concern about the infant's ability to handle excess amounts. To prevent high levels of intake, the only source of intake for infants should be from food and formula.

Children and Adolescents. There are no reports of vitamin E toxic-ity in children and adolescents. Given the dearth of information, the UL values for children and adolescents are extrapolated from those established for adults. Thus, the adult UL of 1,000 mg (2,326 μmol)/day of α-tocopheryl was adjusted for children and adoles-cents on the basis of relative body weight as described in Chapter 4 using reference weights from Chapter 1 (Table 1-1). Values have been rounded.

Pregnancy and Lactation. There are no reports of vitamin E toxic-ity in pregnant or lactating women. One woman consumed 27 mg/day of α-tocopherol from the diet and 1,455 mg/day from supple-ments (Anderson and Pittard, 1985). Her milk α-tocopherol con-centrations were more than three times normal, which might in theory be dangerous for the infant, but the mother had no adverse effects. Given the dearth of information, it is recommended that the UL for pregnant and lactating females be the same as that for the nonpregnant and nonlactating female.

Vitamin E UL Summary, Ages 1 through 18 Years, Pregnancy, Lactation

UL for Infants
   0–12 months   **Not possible to establish; source of intake**
                            should be from food and formula only
UL for Children
   1–3 years   **200 mg (465 μmol)/day of any form of**
                            supplementary α-tocopherol
   4–8 years   **300 mg (698 μmol)/day of any form of**
                            supplementary α-tocopherol
   9–13 years   **600 mg (1,395 μmol)/day of any form of**
                            supplementary α-tocopherol

UL for Adolescents

14–18 years   800 mg (1,860 μmol)/day of any form of supplementary α-tocopherol

UL for Pregnancy

14–18 years   800 mg (1,860 μmol)/day of any form of supplementary α-tocopherol

19 years and older   1,000 mg (2,326 μmol)/day of any form of supplementary α-tocopherol

UL for Lactation

14–18 years   800 mg (1,860 μmol)/day of any form of supplementary α-tocopherol

19 years and older   1,000 mg (2,326 μmol)/day of any form of supplementary α-tocopherol

Special Considerations

Vitamin K Deficiency or Anticoagulant Therapy. The UL derived above pertains to individuals in the general population with adequate vitamin K intake. Individuals who are deficient in vitamin K or who are on anticoagulant therapy are at increased risk of coagulation defects. Patients on anticoagulant therapy should be monitored when taking vitamin E supplements as described by Kim and White (1996).

Premature Infants. As discussed above, the small premature infant is particularly vulnerable to the toxic effects of α-tocopherol. For premature infants, the UL of 14 mg/kg/day for adults would be equivalent to a UL of 21 mg/day for infants with birth weights of 1.5 kg. This UL seems prudent and appropriately conservative based on the observation by Phelps et al. (1987). Furthermore, the American Academy of Pediatrics states that "pharmacologic doses of vitamin E for the prevention or treatment of retinopathy of prematurity, bronchopulmonary dysplasia, and intraventricular hemorrhage are not recommended" (AAP, 1998). While it is recognized that hemolytic anemia due to vitamin E deficiency is frequently of concern in premature infants, its management via vitamin E supplementation must be carefully controlled.

Intake Assessment

Based on distribution data from the 1988 to 1994 Third National Health and Nutrition Examination Survey (NHANES III) (Appendix Table C-5), the highest mean reported intake of vitamin E from food and supplements for all life stage and gender groups was around 45 mg (104.7 μmol)/day of α-tocopherol equivalents. This was the mean intake reported by women 51 through 70 years of age. However, the intake distribution from food and supplements is extremely skewed because the median intake of these women was about 9 mg (20.9 μmol)/day in comparison with a mean intake of 45 mg (104.7 μmol)/day. This group also had the highest reported intake at the ninety-ninth percentile of 508 mg (1,181 μmol)/day of α-tocopherol equivalents, which is well below the UL of 1,000 mg/day of any form of α-tocopherol. Vitamin E supplement use is high in the U.S. population (Hartz et al., 1988; Slesinski et al., 1996). In the 1986 National Health Interview Survey, supplements containing vitamin E were used by 37 percent of young children, 23 percent of men, and 29 percent of all women in the United States (Moss et al., 1989).

Risk Characterization

The risk of adverse effects resulting from excess intake of α-tocopherol from food and supplements appears to be very low at the highest intakes noted above. Although members of the general population should be advised not to exceed the UL routinely, intakes above the UL for vitamin E may be appropriate for investigation within well-controlled clinical trials. In light of evaluating possible benefits to health, clinical trials of doses of α-tocopherol above the UL should not be discouraged, as long as subjects participating in these trials have signed informed consent documents regarding possible toxicity and as long as these trials employ appropriate safety monitoring of trial subjects. Also, the UL is not meant to apply to individuals who are receiving vitamin E under medical supervision.

RESEARCH RECOMMENDATIONS FOR VITAMIN E

• Biomarkers are needed for use in assessment of vitamin E intake and vitamin E status. What are the determinants of plasma concentrations of α-tocopherol, and are these concentrations regulated? Are plasma α-tocopherol concentrations the best parameter for assessing adequate plasma vitamin E status in apparently healthy individuals? Does an α-tocopherol/lipid (e.g., total lipid, triglyceride, or cholesterol) ratio better reflect optimal plasma vitamin E status?

• Since the Recommended Dietary Allowances (RDAs) for children ages 1 through 18 years are extrapolated from the adult RDAs, it is critically important to conduct large-scale studies with children using state-of-the-art biomarkers to assess their vitamin E requirements.

• Valid estimates are needed of vitamin E intakes. These estimates require identification of the specific fats and oils consumed, in addition to careful tabulation of all of the foods consumed, because the vitamin E content of various fats and oils differs widely and because vitamin E is widely distributed in many foods. Most individual foodstuffs consumed account for less than 1 percent of the daily intake of α-tocopherol. Calories are frequently underreported, as is dietary fat, and the form and quantity of fat consumed are unknown. Better methods for estimating vitamin E intakes are needed.

• Information on the relationship between oxidative stress and vitamin E status is needed. Some information is available about the dosage of vitamin E needed to achieve plasma levels that protect circulating low-density lipoprotein (LDL) from ex vivo oxidation. However, there are scant data on tissue levels of vitamin E at different levels of intake. Do the large doses that confer protection of circulating LDL also confer protection within tissues against lipid peroxidation or other manifestations of reactive oxygen species generation? Are there markers of oxidative stress that can be related to vitamin E status?

• Vitamin E kinetics and metabolism are promising areas of research. Can estimates of α-tocopherol requirements be made using stable isotopes? Are balance studies feasible that measure intake and output of stable isotope-labeled vitamin E? What is the turnover of α-tocopherol in various human tissues? In which tissues is it degraded and how rapidly? What are the major metabolic intermediates during degradation, and do they have biological function?

• Determination of the effects of vitamin E intake on the prevention of chronic disease is needed. There is a great deal of suggestive or indirect evidence that vitamin E intakes above those that can reasonably be obtained from foods may confer health benefits. Before clinical intervention trials can be interpreted properly, more knowledge about the relationship of vitamin E dosage to level of protection, or level of protection to plasma cholesterol or lipoprotein levels, is needed. Additional clinical trials to test directly whether or not supplementation with vitamin E can reduce the risk of coronary heart disease are needed. A number of trials already in progress are evaluating vitamin E effects in well over 100,000 individuals. However, whether the results are positive or negative, additional studies will be needed. For example, if the results are negative, the question will arise of whether treatment was instituted early enough and whether even longer trials starting at an earlier age are necessary to test the hypothesis properly. If the results are positive, the issue of dosage will arise. Most of these studies are supplementing with more than 200 mg/day of α-tocopherol, but this may be unnecessarily high. Again, if the results are positive, indicating that vitamin E does indeed offer protection, it will be important to determine if combinations of antioxidants in various dosages can further increase the beneficial effect. Possible interactions between cholesterol-lowering and antioxidant treatments should be studied to find the best algorithm for preventive management.

- More information is needed on the mechanisms of vitamin E function. It is unknown whether vitamin E functions solely as a relatively nonspecific antioxidant compound or whether it has some very specific modes of action, for which the precise structure of α-tocopherol is required. The mechanisms for regulation of tissue α-tocopherol are unknown. In fact, it is not known whether they are regulated at all. The relatively uniform concentrations in tissues from different individuals suggest that there may be regulation, but this may reflect differences in fat concentration. Additionally, the existence of α-tocopherol binding proteins in tissues other than the liver is being investigated. Do differences in depletion rates among various tissues reflect the functions of other tissue α-tocopherol binding proteins?

- More information is needed on the other forms of vitamin E. What is the biological potency of forms of vitamin E other than α-tocopherol in humans? Does γ-tocopherol have a role in humans? Does it function to act as a nitric oxide scavenger? What is the metabolic fate of γ-tocopherol in humans?

REFERENCES

AAP (American Academy of Pediatrics). 1998. *Pediatric Nutrition Handbook,* 4th edition. Elk Grove Village, IL: AAP. P. 67.

Abbasi S, Ludomirski A, Bhutani VK, Weiner S, Johnson L. 1990. Maternal and fetal plasma vitamin E to total lipid ratio and fetal RBC antioxidant function during gestational development. *J Am Coll Nutr* 9:314–319.

Abdo KM, Rao G, Montgomery CA, Dinowitz M, Kanagalingam K. 1986. Thirteen-week toxicity study of *d*-alpha-tocopheryl acetate (vitamin E) in Fischer 344 rats. *Food Chem Toxicol* 24:1043–1050.

Acuff RV, Thedford SS, Hidiroglou NN, Papas AM, Odom TA. 1994. Relative bioavailability of *RRR*- and *all-rac*-alpha-tocopheryl acetate in humans: Studies using deuterated compounds. *Am J Clin Nutr* 60:397–402.

Acuff RV, Webb LW, Brooks LJ, Papas AM, Lane JR. 1997. Pharmacokinetics of *RRR*-gamma-tocopherol in humans after a single dose administration of deuterium-labeled gamma-tocopherol in humans. *FASEB J* 11:A449.

Adam O, Lemmen C, Kless T, Adam P, Denzlinger C, Hailer S. 1995. Low fat diet decreases alpha-tocopherol levels, and stimulates LDL oxidation and cicosanoid biosynthesis in man. *Eur J Med Res* 1:65–71.

Adler LA, Edson R, Lavori P, Pesclow E, Duncan E, Rosenthal M, Rotrosen J. 1998. Long-term treatment effects of vitamin E for tardive dyskinesia. *Biol Psychiatry* 43:868–872.

AIN (American Institute of Nutrition). 1990. Nomenclature policy: Generic descriptors and trivial names for vitamins and related compounds. *J Nutr* 120:12–19.

Ali J, Kader HA, Hassan K, Arshat H. 1986. Changes in human milk vitamin E and total lipids during the first twelve days of lactation. *Am J Clin Nutr* 43:925–930.

Alexy U, Kersting M, Sichert-Hellert W, Manz F, Schöch G. 1999. Vitamin intake of 3- to 36-month-old German infants and children—Results of the DONALD-study. *Int J Vitam Nutr Res* 69:285–291.

Allen JC, Keller RP, Archer P, Neville MC. 1991. Studies in human lactation: Milk composition and daily secretion rates of macronutrients in the first year of lactation. *Am J Clin Nutr* 54:69–80.

Ames BN, Gold LS, Willett WC. 1995. The causes and prevention of cancer. *Proc Natl Acad Sci USA* 92:5258–5265.

Amiel J, Maziere J, Beucler I, Koenig M, Reutenauer L, Loux N, Bonnefont D, Feo C, Landrieu P. 1995. Familial isolated vitamin E deficiency. Extensive study of a large family with a 5-year therapeutic follow-up. *J Inherit Metab Dis* 18:333–340.

Anderson DM, Pittard WB. 1985. Vitamin E and C concentrations in human milk with maternal megadosing. A case report. *J Am Diet Assoc* 85:715–717.

Anderson TW, Reid DB. 1974. A double-blind trial of vitamin E in angina pectoris. *Am J Clin Nutr* 27:1174–1178.

Andersson SO, Wolk A, Bergstrom R, Giovannucci E, Lindgren C, Baron J, Adami HO. 1996. Energy, nutrient intake and prostate cancer risk: A population-based case-control study in Sweden. *Int J Cancer* 68:716–722.

Arita M, Sato Y, Miyata A, Tanabe T, Takahashi E, Kayden H, Arai H, Inoue K. 1995. Human alpha-tocopherol transfer protein: cDNA cloning, expression and chromosomal localization. *Biochem J* 306:437–443.

Ascherio A, Stampfer MJ, Colditz GA, Rimm EB, Litin L, Willett WC. 1992. Correlations of vitamin A and E intakes with the plasma concentrations of carotenoids and tocopherols among American men and women. *J Nutr* 122:1792–1801.

ATBC (Alpha-Tocopherol, Beta Carotene) Cancer Prevention Study Group. 1994. The effect of vitamin E and beta carotene on the incidence of lung cancer and other cancers in male smokers. *N Engl J Med* 330:1029–1035.

Awad JA, Morrow JD, Hill KE, Roberts LJ II, Burk RF. 1994. Detection and localization of lipid peroxidation in selenium- and vitamin E-deficient rats using F2-isoprostanes. *J Nutr* 124:810–816.

Azen SP, Mack WJ, Cashin-Hemphill L, LaBree L, Shircore AM, Selzer RH, Blankenhorn DH, Hodis HN. 1996a. Progression of coronary artery disease predicts clinical coronary events. Long-term follow-up from the Cholesterol Lowering Atherosclerosis Study. *Circulation* 93:34–41.

Azen SP, Qian D, Mack WJ, Sevanian A, Selzer RH, Liu CR, Liu CH, Hodis HN. 1996b. Effect of supplementary antioxidant vitamin intake on carotid arterial wall intima-media thickness in a controlled clinical trial of cholesterol lowering. *Circulation* 94:2369–2372.

Azzi A, Boscoboinik D, Marilley D, Ozer NK, Stauble B, Tasinato A. 1995. Vitamin E: A sensor and an information transducer of the cell oxidation state. *Am J Clin Nutr* 62:1337S–1346S.

Bae CY, Keenan JM, Fontaine P, Wenz J, Ripsin CM, McCaffrey DJ. 1993. Plasma lipid response and nutritional adequacy in hypercholesterolemic subjects on the American Heart Association Step-One Diet. *Arch Fam Med* 2:765–772.

Bayliss EA, Hambidge KM, Sokol RJ, Stewart B, Lilly JR. 1995. Hepatic concentrations of zinc, copper and manganese in infants with extrahepatic biliary atresia. *J Trace Elem Med Biol* 9:40–43.

Baynes JW. 1991. Role of oxidative stress in development of complications in diabetes. *Diabetes* 40:405–412.

Bendich A. 1994. Role of antioxidants in the maintenance of immune functions. In: Frei B, ed. *Natural Antioxidants in Human Health and Disease.* San Diego: Academic Press. Pp. 447–467.

Bendich A, Machlin LJ. 1988. Safety of oral intake of vitamin E. *Am J Clin Nutr* 48:612–619.

Ben Hamida M, Belal S, Sirugo G, Ben Hamida C, Panayides K, Ionannou P, Beckmann J, Mandel JL, Hentati F, Koenig M, Middleton L. 1993. Friedreich's ataxia phenotype not linked to chromosome 9 and associated with selective autosomal recessive vitamin E deficiency in two inbred Tunisian families. *Neurology* 43:2179–2183.

Bieri JG, Evarts RP. 1973. Tocopherols and fatty acids in American diets. The recommended allowance for vitamin E. *J Am Diet Assoc* 62:147–151.

Bieri JG, Evarts RP. 1974. Gamma-tocopherol: Metabolism, biological activity and significance in human vitamin E nutrition. *Am J Clin Nutr* 27:980–986.

Bieri JG, McKenna MC. 1981. Expressing dietary values for fat-soluble vitamins: Changes in concepts and terminology. *Am J Clin Nutr* 34:289–295.

Bjørneboe A, Bjørneboe GE, Hagen BF, Nossen JO, Drevon CA. 1987. Secretion of alpha-tocopherol from cultured rat hepatocytes. *Biochim Biophys Acta* 922:199–205.

Blomstrand R, Forsgren L. 1968. Labelled tocopherols in man. Intestinal absorption and thoracic-duct lymph transport of dl-alpha-tocopheryl-3,4-14C2 acetate dl-alpha-tocopheramine-3,4-14C2 dl-alpha-tocopherol-(5-methyl-3H) and N-(methyl-3H)-dl-gamma-tocopheramine. *Z Vitaminforsch* 38:328–344.

Boda V, Finckh B, Durken M, Commentz J, Hellwege HH, Kohlschutter A. 1998. Monitoring erythrocyte free radical resistance in neonatal blood microsamples using a peroxyl radical-mediated haemolysis test. *Scand J Clin Lab Invest* 58:317–322.

Boersma ER, Offringa PJ, Muskiet FA, Chase WM, Simmons IJ. 1991. Vitamin E, lipid fractions, and fatty acid composition of colostrum, transitional milk, and mature milk: An international comparative study. *Am J Clin Nutr* 53:1197–1204.

Boscoboinik D, Szewczyk A, Hensey C, Azzi A. 1991. Inhibition of cell proliferation by alpha-tocopherol. Role of protein kinase C. *J Biol Chem* 266:6188–6194.

Briefel RR, Sempos CT, McDowell MA, Chien S, Alaimo K. 1997. Dietary methods research in the Third National Health and Nutrition Examination Survey: Underreporting of energy intake. *Am J Clin Nutr* 65:1203S–1209S.

Brown K, Reid A, White T, Henderson T, Hukin S, Johnstone C, Glen A. 1998. Vitamin E, lipids, and lipid peroxidation products in tardive dyskinesia. *Biol Psychiatry* 43:863–867.

Buettner GR. 1993. The pecking order of free radicals and antioxidants: Lipid peroxidation, alpha-tocopherol, and ascorbate. *Arch Biochem Biophys* 300:535 543.

Burck U, Goebel HH, Kuhlendahl HD, Meier C, Goebel KM. 1981. Neuromyopathy and vitamin E deficiency in man. *Neuropediatrics* 12:267–278.

Burton GW, Ingold KU. 1981. Autoxidation of biological molecules. I. The antioxidant activity of vitamin E and related chain-breaking phenolic antioxidants in vitro. *J Am Chem Soc* 103:6472–6477.

Burton GW, Ingold KU. 1986. Vitamin E: Application of the principles of physical organic chemistry to the exploration of its structure and function. *Acc Chem Res* 19:194–201.

Burton GW, Joyce A, Ingold KU. 1983. Is vitamin E the only lipid-soluble, chain-breaking antioxidant in human blood plasma and erythrocyte membranes? *Arch Biochem Biophys* 221:281–290.

Burton GW, Doba T, Gabe EJ, Hughes L, Lee FL, Prasad L, Ingold KU. 1985. Autoxidation of biological molecules. 4. Maximizing the antioxidant activity of phenols. *J Am Chem Soc* 107:7053–7065.

Burton GW, Traber MG, Acuff RV, Walters DN, Kayden H, Hughes L, Ingold KU. 1998. Human plasma and tissue alpha-tocopherol concentrations in response to supplementation with deuterated natural and synthetic vitamin E. *Am J Clin Nutr* 67:669–684.

Butte NF, Garza C, Smith EO, Nichols BL. 1984. Human milk intake and growth in exclusively breast-fed infants. *J Pediatr* 104:187–195.

Cachia O, Benna JE, Pedruzzi E, Descomps B, Gougerot-Pocidalo MA, Leger CL. 1998. Alpha-tocopherol inhibits the respiratory burst in human monocytes. Attenuation of p47(phox) membrane translocation and phosphorylation. *J Biol Chem* 273:32801–32805.

Calzada C, Bruckdorfer R, Rice-Evans CA. 1997. The influence of antioxidant nutrients on platelet function in healthy volunteers. *Atherosclerosis* 128:97–105.

Catignani GL, Bieri JG. 1977. Rat liver alpha-tocopherol binding protein. *Biochim Biophys Acta* 497:349–357.

Cavalier L, Ouahchi K, Kayden HJ, DiDonato S, Reutenauer L, Mandel J-L, Koenig M. 1998. Ataxia with isolated vitamin E deficiency: Heterogeneity of mutations and phenotypic variability in a large number of families. *Am J Hum Genet* 62:301–310.

Ceballos-Picot I, Nicole A, Briand P, Grimber G, Delacourte A, Defossez A, Javoy-Agid F, Lafon M, Blouin JL, Sinet PM. 1991. Neuronal-specific expression of human copper-zinc superoxide dismutase gene in transgenic mice: Animal model of gene dosage effects in Down's syndrome. *Brain Res* 552:198–214.

Cerielло A, Giugliano D, Quatraro A, Donzella C, Dipalo G, Lefebvre PJ. 1991. Vitamin E reduction of protein glycosylation in diabetes. New prospect for prevention of diabetic complications? *Diabetes Care* 14:68–72.

Chan AC, Leith MK. 1981. Decreased prostacyclin synthesis in vitamin E-deficient rabbit aorta. *Am J Clin Nutr* 34:2341–2347.

Chan AC, Tran K, Raynor T, Ganz PR, Chow CK. 1991. Regeneration of vitamin E in human platelets. *J Biol Chem* 266:17290–17295.

Chan AC, Wagner M, Kennedy C, Chen E, Lanuville O, Mezl VA, Tran K, Choy PC. 1998a. Vitamin E up-regulates arachidonic acid release and phospholipase A^2 in megakaryocytes. *Mol Cell Biochem* 189:153–159.

Chan AC, Wagner M, Kennedy C, Mroske C, Proulx P, Laneuville O, Tran K, Choy PC. 1998b. Vitamin E up-regulates phospholipase A^2, arachidonic acid release and cyclooxygenasein endothelial cells. *Akt Ernahr-Med* 23:1–8.

Chappell JE, Francis T, Clandinin MT. 1985. Vitamin A and E content of human milk at early stages of lactation. *Early Hum Devel* 11:157–167.

Chatelain E, Boscoboinik DO, Bartoli GM, Kagan VE, Gey F, Packer L, Azzi A. 1993. Inhibition of smooth muscle cell proliferation and protein kinase C activity by tocopherols and tocotrienols. *Biochim Biophys Acta* 1176:83–89.

Cheeseman KH, Holley AE, Kelly FJ, Wasil M, Hughes L, Burton G. 1995. Biokinetics in humans of *RRR*-alpha-tocopherol: The free phenol, acetate ester, and succinate ester forms of vitamin E. *Free Radic Biol Med* 19:591–598.

Chen LH, Boissonneault GA, Glauert HP. 1988. Vitamin C, vitamin E and cancer. *Anticancer Res* 8:739-748.

Chopra RK, Bhagavan HN. 1999. Relative bioavailabilities of natural and synthetic vitamin E formulations containing mixed tocopherols in human subjects. *Int J Vitam Nutr Res* 69:92–95.

Church DF, Pryor WA. 1985. Free-radical chemistry of cigarette smoke and its toxicological implications. *Environ Hlth Perspect* 64:111–126.

Clement M, Bourre JM. 1997. Graded dietary levels of *RRR*-gamma-tocopherol induce a marked increase in the concentrations of alpha- and gamma-tocopherol in nervous tissues, heart, liver and muscle of vitamin-E-deficient rats. *Biochim Biophys Acta* 1334:173–1781.

Clement S, Tasinato A, Boscoboinik D, Azzi A. 1997. The effect of alpha-tocopherol on the synthesis, phosphorylation and activity of protein kinase C in smooth muscle cells after phorbol 12-myristate 13-acetate down-regulation. *Eur J Biochem* 246:745–749.

Cohn W, Loechleiter F, Weber F. 1988. Alpha-tocopherol is secreted from rat liver in very low density lipoproteins. *J Lipid Res* 29:1359–1366.

Colette C, Pares-Herbute N, Monnier LH, Cartry E. 1988. Platelet function in type I diabetes: Effects of supplementation with large doses of vitamin E. *Am J Clin Nutr* 47:256–261.

Cominacini L, Garbin U, Pasini AF, Davoli A, Campagnola M, Contessi GB, Pastorino AM, Lo Cascio V. 1997. Antioxidants inhibit the expression of intercellular cell adhesion molecule-1 and vascular cell adhesion molecule-1 induced by oxidized LDL on human umbilical vein endothelial cells. *Free Radic Biol Med* 22:117–127.

Comstock GW, Bush TL, Helzlsouer K. 1992. Serum retinol, beta-carotene, vitamin E, and selenium as related to subsequent cancer of specific sites. *Am J Epidemiol* 135:115–121.

Comstock GW, Alberg AJ, Huang HY, Wu K, Burke AE, Hoffman SC, Norkus EP, Gross M, Cutler RG, Morris JS, Spate VL, Helzlsouer KJ. 1997. The risk of developing lung cancer associated with antioxidants in the blood: Ascorbic acid, carotenoids, alpha-tocopherol, selenium, and total peroxyl radical absorbing capacity. *Cancer Epidemiol Biomarkers Prev* 6:907–916.

Cornett CR, Markesbery WR, Ehmann WD. 1998. Imbalances of trace elements related to oxidative damage in Alzheimer's disease brain. *Neurotoxicology* 19: 339–345.

Corrigan JJ Jr, Marcus FI. 1974. Coagulopathy associated with vitamin E ingestion. *J Am Med Assoc* 230:1300–1301.

Cross CE, Eiserich JP, Halliwell B. 1997. General biological consequences of inhaled environmental toxicants. In: Crystal RG, West JB, Barnes PJ, Weibel ER, eds. *The Lung: Scientific Foundations,* 2nd edition. Philadelphia: Lippincott-Raven. Pp. 2421–2437.

Cynamon HA, Milov DE, Valenstein E, Wagner M. 1988. Effect of vitamin E deficiency on neurologic function in patients with cystic fibrosis. *J Pediatr* 113:637–640.

Dam H. 1962. Interrelations between vitamin E and polyunsaturated fatty acids in animals. *Vitam Horm* 20:527–540.

Davi G, Ciabattoni G, Consoli A, Mezzetti A, Falco A, Santarone S, Pennese E, Vitacolonna E, Bucciarelli T, Costantini F, Capani F, Patrono C. 1999. In vivo formation of 8-iso-prostaglandin F2a and platelet activation in diabetes mellitus. Effects of improved metabolic control and vitamin E supplementation. *Circulation* 99:224–229.

DeCosse JJ, Miller HH, Lesser ML. 1989. Effect of wheat fiber and vitamins C and E on rectal polyps in patients with familial adenomatous polyposis. *J Natl Cancer Inst* 81:1290–1297.

Delanty N, Reilly M, Pratico D, FitzGerald DJ, Lawson JA, FitzGerald GA. 1996. 8-Epi PGF2 alpha: Specific analysis of an isoeicosanoid as an index of oxidant stress in vivo. *Br J Clin Pharmacol* 42:15–19.

DeMaio SJ, King SB 3rd, Lembo NJ, Roubin GS, Hearn JA, Bhagavan HN, Sgoutas DS. 1992. Vitamin E supplementation, plasma lipids and incidence of restenosis after percutaneous transluminal coronary angioplasty (PTCA). *J Am Coll Nutr* 11:68–73.

Devaraj S, Li D, Jialal I. 1996. The effects of alpha tocopherol supplementation on monocyte function. Decreased lipid oxidation, interleukin 1b secretion, and monocyte adhesion to endothelium. *J Clin Invest* 98:756–763.

Devaraj S, Adams-Huet B, Fuller CJ, Jialal I. 1997. Dose-response comparison of *RRR*-alpha-tocopherol and all-racemic alpha-tocopherol on LDL oxidation. *Arterioscler Thromb Vasc Biol* 17:2273–2279.

de Vries JH, Hollman PC, Meyboom S, Buysman MN, Zock PL, van Staveren WA, Katan MB. 1998. Plasma concentrations and urinary excretion of the antioxidant flavonols quercetin and kaempferol as biomarkers for dietary intake. *Am J Clin Nutr* 68:60–65.

Dial S, Eitenmiller RR. 1995. Tocopherols and tocotrienols in key foods in the U.S. diet. In: Ong ASH, Niki E, Packer L, eds. *Nutrition, Lipids, Health, and Disease.* Champaign, IL: AOCS Press. Pp. 327–342.

Dieber-Rotheneder M, Puhl H, Waeg G, Striegl G, Esterbauer H. 1991. Effect of oral supplementation with *d*-alpha-tocopherol on the vitamin E content of human low density lipoproteins and resistance to oxidation. *J Lipid Res* 32:1325–1332.

Dimitrov NV, Meyer C, Gilliland D, Ruppenthal M, Chenoweth W, Malone W. 1991. Plasma tocopherol concentrations in response to supplemental vitamin E. *Am J Clin Nutr* 53:723–729.

Dimitrov NV, Meyer-Leece C, McMillan J, Gilliland D, Perloff M, Malone W. 1996. Plasma alpha-tocopherol concentrations after supplementation with water- and fat-soluble vitamin E. *Am J Clin Nutr* 64:329–335.

Doba T, Burton GW, Ingold KU. 1985. Antioxidant and co-antioxidant activity of vitamin C. The effect of vitamin C, either alone or in the presence of vitamin E or a water-soluble vitamin E analogue, upon the peroxidation of aqueous multilamellar phospholipid liposomes. *Biochim Biophys Acta* 835:298–303.

Dorgan JF, Sowell A, Swanson CA, Potischman N, Miller R, Schussler N, Stephenson HE. 1998. Relationships of serum carotenoids, retinol, alpha-tocopherol, and selenium with breast cancer risk: Results from a prospective study in Columbia, Missouri (United States). *Cancer Causes Control* 9:89–97.

Draper HH. 1993. Interrelationships of vitamin E with other nutrients. In: Packer L, Fuchs J, eds. *Vitamin E in Health and Disease.* New York: Marcel Dekker. Pp. 53–61.

Duthie GG, Arthur JR, James WP. 1991. Effects of smoking and vitamin E on blood antioxidant status. *Am J Clin Nutr* 53:1061S–1063S.

Duthie SJ, Ross M, Collins AR. 1995. The influence of smoking and diet on the hypoxanthine phosphoribosyltransferase (hprt) mutant frequency in circulating T lymphocytes from a normal human population. *Mutat Res* 331:55–64.

Duthie SJ, Ma A, Ross MA, Collins AR. 1996. Antioxidant supplementation decreases oxidative DNA damage in human lymphocytes. *Cancer Res* 56:1291–1295.

Dysmsza HA, Park J. 1975. Excess dietary vitamin E in rats. *Fed Am Soc Exp Biol* 34:912.

Egan MF, Hyde TM, Albers GW, Elkashef A, Alexander RC, Reeve A, Blum A, Saenz RE, Wyatt RJ. 1992. Treatment of tardive dyskinesia with vitamin E. *Am J Psychiatry* 149:773–777.

Eichholzer M, Stahelin HB, Gey KF, Ludin E, Bernasconi F. 1996. Prediction of male cancer mortality by plasma levels of interacting vitamins: 17-year follow-up of the prospective Basel study. *Int J Cancer* 66:145–150.

Eiserich JP, van der Vliet A, Handelman GJ, Halliwell B, Cross CE. 1995. Dietary antioxidants and cigarette smoke-induced biomolecular damage: A complex interaction. *Am J Clin Nutr* 62:1490S–1500S.

Eiserich JP, Cross CE, Van der Vliet A. 1997. Nitrogen oxides are important contributors to cigarette smoke-induced ascorbate oxidation. In: Packer L, Fuchs J, eds. *Vitamin C in Health and Disease.* New York: Marcel Dekker. Pp. 399–412.

Eitenmiller RR, Landen WO Jr. 1995. Vitamins. In: Jeon IJ, Ikins WG, eds. *Analyzing Food for Nutrition Labeling and Hazardous Contaminants.* New York: Marcel Dekker. Pp. 195–281.

Elias E, Muller DP, Scott J. 1981. Association of spinocerebellar disorders with cystic fibrosis or chronic childhood cholestasis and very low serum vitamin E. *Lancet* 2:1319–1321.

Elkashef AM, Ruskin PE, Bacher N, Barrett D. 1990. Vitamin E in the treatment of tardive dyskinesia. *Am J Psychiatry* 147:505–506.

Ernster VL, Goodson WH, Hunt TK, Petrakis NL, Sickles EA, Miike R. 1985. Vitamin E and benign breast "disease": A double-blind, randomized clinical trial. *Surgery* 97:490–494.

Farrell PM, Bieri JG. 1975. Megavitamin E supplementation in man. *Am J Clin Nutr* 28:1381–1386.

Farrell PM, Bieri JG, Fratantoni JF, Wood RE, Di Sant'Agnese PA. 1977. The occurrence and effects of human vitamin E deficiency. A study in patients with cystic fibrosis. *J Clin Invest* 60:233–241.

Farrell PM, Mischler EH, Gutcher GR. 1982. Evaluation of vitamin E deficiency in children with lung disease. *Ann NY Acad Sci* 393:96–108.

Faruqi R, de la Motte C, DiCorleto PE. 1994. Alpha-tocopherol inhibits agonist-induced monocytic cell adhesion to cultured human endothelial cells. *J Clin Invest* 94:592–600.

Finer, NN, Peters, KL, Hayek, Z, Merkel, CL. 1984. Vitamin E and necrotizing enterocolitis. *Pediatrics* 73:387-93.

Ford ES, Sowell A. 1999. Serum alpha-tocopherol status in the United States population: Findings from the Third National Health and Nutrition Examination Survey. *Am J Epidemiol* 150:290-300.

Freedman JE, Farhat JH, Loscalzo J, Keaney JF Jr. 1996. Alpha-tocopherol inhibits aggregation of human platelets by a protein kinase C-dependent mechanism. *Circulation* 94:2434-2440.

Fuller CJ, Chandalia M, Garg A, Grundy SM, Jialal I. 1996. *RRR*-alpha-Tocopheryl acetate supplementation at pharmacologic doses decreases low-density-lipoprotein oxidative susceptibility but not protein glycation in patients with diabetes mellitus. *Am J Clin Nutr* 63:753-759.

Gallo-Torres HE. 1970. Obligatory role of bile for the intestinal absorption of vitamin E. *Lipids* 5:379-384.

Gascón-Vila P, Garcia-Closas R, Serra-Majem L, Pastor MC, Ribas L, Ramon JM, Marine-Font A, Salleras L. 1997. Determinants of the nutritional status of vitamin E in a non-smoking Mediterranean population. Analysis of the effect of vitamin E intake, alcohol consumption and body mass index on the serum alpha-tocopherol concentration. *Eur J Clin Nutr* 51:723-728.

Ghalaut VS, Ghalaut PS, Kharb S, Singh GP. 1995. Vitamin E in intestinal fat malabsorption. *Ann Nutr Metab* 39:296-301.

Gisinger C, Jeremy J, Speiser P, Mikhailidis D, Dandona P, Schernthaner G. 1988. Effect of vitamin E supplementation on platelet thromboxane A2 production in type I diabetic patients. Double-blind crossover trial. *Diabetes* 37:1260-1264.

GISSI-Prevenzione Investigators. 1999. Dietary supplementation with n-3 polyunsaturated fatty acids and vitamin E after myocardial infarction: Results of the GISSI-Prevenzione Trial. *Lancet* 354:447-455.

Gotoda T, Arita M, Arai H, Inoue K, Yokota T, Fukuo Y, Yazaki Y, Yamada N. 1995. Adult-onset spinocerebellar dysfunction caused by a mutation in the gene for the alpha-tocopherol-transfer protein. *N Engl J Med* 333:1313-1318.

Greenberg ER, Baron JA, Tosteson TD, Freeman DH, Beck GJ, Bond JH, Colacchio TA, Coller JA, Frankl HD, Haile RW, Mandel JS, Nierenberg DW, Rothstein R, Snover DC, Stevens MM, Summers RW, van Stolk RU. 1994. A clinical trial of antioxidant vitamins to prevent colorectal adenoma. *N Engl J Med* 331:141-147.

Haddad EH, Berk LS, Kettering JD, Hubbard RW, Peters WR. 1999. Dietary intake and biochemical, hematologic, and immune status of vegans compared with nonvegetarians. *Am J Clin Nutr* 70:586S-593S.

Halliwell B. 1999. Establishing the significance and optimal intake of dietary antioxidants: The biomarker concept. *Nutr Rev* 57:104-113.

Hammans SR, Kennedy CR. 1998. Ataxia with isolated vitamin E deficiency presenting as mutation negative Friedreich's ataxia. *J Neurol Neurosurg Psychiatry* 64:368-370.

Handelman GJ, Epstein WL, Peerson J, Spiegelman D, Machlin LJ, Dratz EA. 1994. Human adipose alpha-tocopherol and gamma-tocopherol kinetics during and after 1 y of alpha-tocopherol supplementation. *Am J Clin Nutr* 59:1025-1032.

Hankinson SE, Stampfer MJ, Seddon JM, Colditz GA, Rosner B, Speizer FE, Willett WC. 1992. Nutrient intake and cataract extraction in women: A prospective study. *Br Med J* 305:335-339.

Harding AE, Matthews S, Jones S, Ellis CJ, Booth IW, Muller DP. 1985. Spinocerebellar degeneration associated with a selective defect of vitamin E absorption. *N Engl J Med* 313:32–35.

Harries JT, Muller DP. 1971. Absorption of different doses of fat soluble and water miscible preparations of vitamin E in children with cystic fibrosis. *Arch Dis Child* 46:341–344.

Hartz SC, Otradovec CL, McGandy RB, Russell RM, Jacob RA, Sahyoun N, Peters H, Abrams D, Scura LA, Whinston-Perry RA. 1988. Nutrient supplement use by healthy elderly. *J Am Coll Nutr* 7:119–128.

Hartz SC, Russell RM, Rosenberg IH. 1992. *Nutrition in the Elderly. The Boston Nutritional Status Survey*. London: Smith-Gordon. P. 106–108.

Hassan H, Hashim SA, Van Itallie TB, Sebrell WH. 1966. Syndrome in premature infants associated with low plasma vitamin E levels and high polyunsaturated fatty acid diet. *Am J Clin Nutr* 19:147–157.

Heinig MJ, Nommsen LA, Peerson JM, Lonnerdal B, Dewey KG. 1993. Energy and protein intakes of breast-fed and formula-fed infants during the first year of life and their association with growth velocity: The DARLING Study. *Am J Clin Nutr* 58:152–161.

Heinonen OP, Albanes D, Virtamo J, Taylor PR, Huttunen JK, Hartman AM, Haapakoski J, Malila N, Rautalahti M, Ripatti S, Mäenpää H, Teerenhovi L, Koss L, Virolainen M, Edwards BK. 1998. Prostate cancer and supplementation with alpha-tocopherol and beta-carotene: Incidence and mortality in a controlled trial. *J Natl Cancer Inst* 90:440–446.

Higashi O, Kikuchi Y. 1974. Effects of vitamin E on the aggregation and the lipid peroxidation of platelets exposed to hydrogen peroxide. *Tohoku J Exp Med* 112:271–278.

Hodis HN, Mack WJ, LaBree L, Cashin-Hemphill L, Sevanian A, Johnson R, Azen SP. 1995. Serial coronary angiographic evidence that antioxidant vitamin intake reduces progression of coronary artery atherosclerosis. *J Am Med Assoc* 273:1849–1854.

Hofstad B, Almendingen K, Vatn M, Andersen S, Owen R, Larsen S, Osnes M. 1998. Growth and recurrence of colorectal polyps: A double-blind 3-year intervention with calcium and antioxidants. *Digestion* 59:148–156.

HOPE Study Investigators. 2000. Vitamin E supplementation and cardiovascular events in high-risk patients. *N Engl J Med* 342:154–160.

Horwitt MK. 1960. Vitamin E and lipid metabolism in man. *Am J Clin Nutr* 8:451–461.

Horwitt MK. 1962. Interrelations between vitamin E and polyunsaturated fatty acids in adult men. *Vitam Horm* 20:541–558.

Horwitt MK. 1974. Status of human requirements for vitamin E. *Am J Clin Nutr* 27:1182–1193.

Horwitt MK. 1976. Vitamin E: A reexamination. *Am J Clin Nutr* 29:569–578.

Horwitt MK, Harvey CC, Duncan GD, Wilson WC. 1956. Effects of limited tocopherol intake in man with relationships to erythrocyte hemolysis and lipid oxidations. *Am J Clin Nutr* 4:408–419.

Horwitt MK, Century B, Zeman AA. 1963. Erythrocyte survival time and reticulocyte levels after tocopherol depletion in man. *Am J Clin Nutr* 12:99–106.

Horwitt MK, Harvey CC, Dahm CH, Searcy MT. 1972. Relationship between tocopherol and serum lipid levels for determination of nutritional adequacy. *Ann NY Acad Sci* 203:223–236.

Hosomi A, Arita M, Sato Y, Kiyose C, Ueda T, Igarashi O, Arai H, Inoue K. 1997. Affinity for alpha-tocopherol transfer protein as a determinant of the biological activities of vitamin E analogs. *FEBS Lett* 409:105–108.

Ingold KU, Webb AC, Witter D, Burton GW, Metcalfe TA, Muller DPR. 1987. Vitamin E remains the major lipid-soluble, chain-breaking antioxidant in human plasma even in individuals suffering severe vitamin E deficiency. *Arch Biochem Biophys* 259:224–225.

IOM (Institute of Medicine). 1991. *Nutrition During Lactation*. Washington, DC: National Academy Press. P. 179.

Ishizuka T, Itaya S, Wada H, Ishizawa M, Kimura M, Kajita K, Kanoh Y, Miura A, Muto N, Yasuda K. 1998. Differential effect of the antidiabetic thiazolidinediones troglitazone and pioglitazone on human platelet aggregation mechanism. *Diabetes* 47:1494–1500.

Islam KN, Devaraj S, Jialal I. 1998. Alpha-tocopherol enrichment of monocytes decreases agonist-induced adhesion to human endothelial cells. *Circulation* 98:2255–2261.

IUPAC-IUB Commission on Biochemical Nomenclature. 1974. Nomenclature of tocopherols and related compounds. Recommendations 1973. *Eur J Biochem* 46:217–219.

Jacob RA, Kutnink MA, Csallany AS, Daroszewska M, Burton GW. 1996. Vitamin C nutriture has little short-term effect on vitamin E concentrations in healthy women. *J Nutr* 126:2268–2277.

Jacques PF, Chylack LT Jr. 1991. Epidemiologic evidence of a role for the antioxidant vitamins and carotenoids in cataract prevention. *Am J Clin Nutr* 53:352S–355S.

Jacques PF, Chylack LT Jr, Taylor A. 1994. Relationships between natural antioxidants and cataract formation. In: Frei B, ed. *Natural Antioxidants in Human Health and Disease*. San Diego: Academic Press. Pp. 515–529.

Jain SK, McVie R, Jaramillo JJ, Palmer M, Smith T. 1996a. Effect of modest vitamin E supplementation on blood glycated hemoglobin and triglyceride levels and red cell indices in type I diabetic patients. *J Am Coll Nutr* 15:458–461.

Jain SK, McVie R, Jaramillo JJ, Palmer M, Smith T, Meachum ZD, Little RL. 1996b. The effect of modest vitamin E supplementation on lipid peroxidation products and other cardiovascular risk factors in diabetic patients. *Lipids* 31:S87–S90.

Jain SK, Krueger KS, McVie R, Jaramillo JJ, Palmer M, Smith T. 1998. Relationship of blood thromboxane-B2 (TxB2) with lipid peroxides and effect of vitamin E and placebo supplementation on TxB2 and lipid peroxide levels in type 1 diabetic patients. *Diabetes Care* 21:1511–1516.

Jansson L, Akesson B, Holmberg L. 1981. Vitamin E and fatty acid composition of human milk. *Am J Clin Nutr* 34:8–13.

Jialal I, Fuller CJ, Huet BA. 1995. The effect of alpha-tocopherol supplementation on LDL oxidation. A dose-response study. *Arterioscler Thromb Vasc Biol* 15:190–198.

Johnson L, Bowen FW, Abbasi S, Herrmann N, Weston M, Sacks L, Porat R, Stahl G, Peckham G, Delivoria-Papadopoulos M, Quinn G, Schaffer D. 1985. Relationship of prolonged pharmacologic serum levels of vitamin E to incidence of sepsis and necrotizing enterocolitis in infants with birth weight 1,500 grams or less. *Pediatrics* 75:619–638.

Jones PJH, Kubow S. 1999. Lipids, sterols and their metabolism. In: Shils ME, Olson JA, Shike M, Ross AC, eds. *Modern Nutrition in Health and Disease, 9th edition.* Baltimore, MD: Williams & Wilkins. Pp. 347–362.

Kalra V, Grover J, Ahuja GK, Rathi S, Khurana DS. 1998. Vitamin E deficiency and associated neurological deficits in children with protein-energy malnutrition. *J Trop Pediatr* 44:291–295.

Kamal-Eldin A, Appelqvist LA. 1996. The chemistry and antioxidant properties of tocopherols and tocotrienols. *Lipids* 31:671–701.

Kantoci D, Wechter WJ, Murray ED Jr, Dewind SA, Borchardt D, Khan SI. 1997. Endogenous natriuretic factors 6: The stereochemistry of a natriuretic gamma-tocopherol metabolite LLU-alpha. *J Pharmacol Exp Ther* 282:648–656.

Kappus H, Diplock AT. 1992. Tolerance and safety of vitamin E: A toxicological position report. *Free Radic Biol Med* 13:55–74.

Kardinaal AF, van 't Veer P, Brants HA, van den Berg H, van Schoonhoven J, Hermus RJ. 1995. Relations between antioxidant vitamins in adipose tissue, plasma, and diet. *Am J Epidemiol* 141:440–450.

Kayden HJ, Hatam LJ, Traber MG. 1983. The measurement of nanograms of tocopherol from needle aspiration biopsies of adipose tissue: Normal and abetalipoproteinemic subjects. *J Lipid Res* 24:652–656.

Kelleher J, Losowsky MS. 1970. The absorption of alpha-tocopherol in man. *Br J Nutr* 24:1033–1047.

Keller JN, Pang Z, Geddes JW, Begley JG, Germeyer A, Waeg G, Mattson MP. 1997. Impairment of glucose and glutamate transport and induction of mitochondrial oxidative stress and dysfunction in synaptosomes by amyloid beta-peptide: Role of the lipid peroxidation product 4-hydroxynonenal. *J Neurochem* 69:273–284.

Kim JM, White RH. 1996. Effect of vitamin E on the anticoagulant response to warfarin. *Am J Cardiol* 77:545–546.

Kitagawa M, Mino M. 1989. Effects of elevated alpha (*RRR*)-tocopherol dosage in man. *J Nutr Sci Vitaminol* 35:133–142.

Kiyose C, Muramatsu R, Fujiyama-Fujiwara Y, Ueda T, Igarashi O. 1995. Biodiscrimination of alpha-tocopherol stereoisomers during intestinal absorption. *Lipids* 30:1015–1018.

Kiyose C, Muramatsu R, Kameyama Y, Ueda T, Igarashi O. 1997. Biodiscrimination of alpha-tocopherol stereoisomers in humans after oral administration. *Am J Clin Nutr* 65:785–789.

Klein T, Reutter F, Schweer H, Seyberth HW, Nusing RM. 1997. Generation of the isoprostane 8-epi-prostaglandin F2alpha in vitro and in vivo via the cyclooxygenases. *J Pharmacol Exp Ther* 282:1658–1665.

Knekt P, Aromaa A, Maatela J, Aaran RK, Nikkari T, Hakama M, Hakulinen T, Peto R, Saxen E, Teppo L. 1988. Serum vitamin E and risk of cancer among Finnish men during a 10-year follow-up. *Am J Epidemiol* 127:28–41.

Knekt P, Heliovaara M, Rissanen A, Aromaa A, Aaran RK. 1992. Serum antioxidant vitamins and risk of cataract. *Br Med J* 305:1392–1394.

Knekt P, Reunanen A, Jarvinen R, Seppanen R, Heliovaara M, Aromaa A. 1994. Antioxidant vitamin intake and coronary mortality in a longitudinal population study. *Am J Epidemiol* 139:1180–1189.

Kobayashi H, Kanno C, Yamauchi K, Tsugo T. 1975. Identification of alpha-, beta-, gamma-, and delta-tocopherols and their contents in human milk. *Biochim Biophys Acta* 380:282–290.

Kohlschütter A, Hubner C, Jansen W, Lindner SG. 1988. A treatable familial neuromyopathy with vitamin E deficiency, normal absorption, and evidence of increased consumption of vitamin E. *J Inher Metab Dis* 11:149 152.

Kostner GM, Oettl K, Jauhiainen M, Ehnholm C, Esterbauer H, Dieplinger H. 1995. Human plasma phospholipid transfer protein accelerates exchange/transfer of alpha-tocopherol between lipoproteins and cells. *Biochem J* 305:659–667.

Krasavage WJ, Terhaar CJ. 1977. d-alpha-Tocopheryl poly(ethylene glycol) 1000 succinate. Acute toxicity, subchronic feeding, reproduction, and teratologic studies in the rat. *J Agric Food Chem* 25:273–278.

Krendel DA, Gilchrist JM, Johnson AO, Bossen EII. 1987. Isolated deficiency of vitamin E with progressive neurologic deterioration. *Neurology* 37:538–540.

Kuhlenkamp J, Ronk M, Yusin M, Stolz A, Kaplowitz N. 1993. Identification and purification of a human liver cytosolic tocopherol binding protein. *Protein Expr Purif* 4:382–389.

Kunisaki M, Umeda F, Inoguchi T, Watanabe J, Nawata H. 1990. Effects of vitamin E administration on platelet function in diabetes mellitus. *Diabetes Res* 14:37–42.

Kunisaki M, Bursell SE, Umeda F, Nawata H, King GL. 1994. Normalization of diacylglycerol-protein kinase C activation by vitamin E in aorta of diabetic rats and cultured rat smooth muscle cells exposed to elevated glucose levels. *Diabetes* 43:1372–1377.

Kushi LH, Folsom AR, Prineas RJ, Mink PJ, Wu Y, Bostick RM. 1996. Dietary antioxidant vitamins and death from coronary heart disease in postmenopausal women. *N Engl J Med* 334:1156–1162.

Laditan AA, Ette SI. 1982. Plasma alpha-tocopherol (vitamin E) levels and tocopherol-lipid ratio among children with protein-energy malnutrition (PEM). *Ann Trop Paediatr* 2:85–88.

Lammi-Keefe CJ, Jensen RG, Clark RM, Ferris AM. 1985. Alpha tocopherol, total lipid and linoleic acid contents of human milk at 2, 6, 12, and 16 weeks. In: Schaub J, ed. *Composition and Physiological Properties of Human Milk*. New York: Elsevier Science. Pp. 241–245.

Lammi-Keefe CJ, Ferris AM, Jensen RG. 1990. Changes in human milk at 0600, 1000, 1400, 1800, and 2200 h. *J Pediatr Gastroenterol Nutr* 11:83–88.

Laplante P, Vanasse M, Michaud J, Geoffroy G, Brochu P. 1984. A progressive neurological syndrome associated with an isolated vitamin E deficiency. *Can J Neurol Sci* 11:561–564.

Lehmann J, Martin HL, Lashley EL, Marshall MW, Judd JT. 1986. Vitamin E in foods from high and low linoleic acid diets. *J Am Diet Assoc* 86:1208–1216.

Leo MA, Ahmed S, Aleynik SI, Siegel JH, Kasmin F, Lieber CS. 1995. Carotenoids and tocopherols in various hepatobiliary conditions. *J Hepatol* 23:550–556.

Leske MC, Chylack LT Jr, Wu SY. 1991. The Lens Opacities Case-Control Study. Risk factors for cataract. *Arch Ophthalmol* 109:244–251.

Lohr JB, Cadet JL, Lohr MA, Jeste DV, Wyatt RJ. 1987. Alpha-tocopherol in tardive dyskinesia. *Lancet* 1:913–914.

Lohr JB, Kuczenski R, Bracha HS, Moir M, Jeste DV. 1990. Increased indices of free radical activity in the cerebrospinal fluid of patients with tardive dyskinesia. *Biol Psychiatry* 28:535–539.

London RS, Sundaram GS, Murphy L, Manimekalai S, Reynolds M, Goldstein PJ. 1985. The effect of vitamin E on mammary dysplasia: A double-blind study. *Obstet Gynecol* 65:104–106.

Losonczy KG, Harris TB, Havlik RJ. 1996. Vitamin E and vitamin C supplement use and risk of all-cause and coronary heart disease mortality in older persons: The Established Populations for Epidemiologic Studies of the Elderly. *Am J Clin Nutr* 64:190–196.

Losowsky MS, Kelleher J, Walker BE, Davies T, Smith CL. 1972. Intake and absorption of tocopherol. *Ann NY Acad Sci* 203:212–222.

Machlin LJ. 1989. Use and safety of elevated dosages of vitamin E in adults. *Int J Vitam Nutr Res* 30:56-68.

MacMahon MT, Neale G. 1970. The absorption of alpha-tocopherol in control subjects and in patients with intestinal malabsorption. *Clin Sci* 38:197–210.

Manach C, Morand C, Crespy V, Demigne C, Texier O, Regerat F, Remesy C. 1998. Quercetin is recovered in human plasma as conjugated derivatives which retain antioxidant properties. *FEBS Lett* 426:331–336.

Mandel CH, Mosca L, Maimon E, Sievers J, Tsai A, Rock CL. 1997. Dietary intake and plasma concentrations of vitamin E, vitamin C, and beta carotene in patients with coronary artery disease. *J Am Diet Assoc* 97:655–657.

March BE, Wong E, Seier L, Sim J, Biely J. 1973. Hypervitaminosis E in the chick. *J Nutr* 103:371–377.

Mares-Perlman JA, Brady WE, Klein R, Klein BE, Palta M, Bowen P, Stacewicz-Sapuntzakis M. 1994a. Serum levels of carotenoids and tocopherols in people with age-related maculopathy. *Invest Ophthalmol Vis Sci* 35:2004.

Mares-Perlman JA, Klein BE, Klein R, Ritter LL. 1994b. Relation between lens opacities and vitamin and mineral supplement use. *Ophthalmology* 101:315–325.

Martin A, Foxall T, Blumberg JB, Meydani M. 1997. Vitamin E inhibits low-density lipoprotein-induced adhesion of monocytes to human aortic endothelial cells in vitro. *Arterioscler Thromb Vasc Biol* 17:429–436.

Martinello F, Fardin P, Ottina M, Ricchieri GL, Koenig M, Cavalier L, Trevisan CP. 1998. Supplemental therapy in isolated vitamin E deficiency improves the peripheral neuropathy and prevents the progression of ataxia. *J Neurol Sci* 156:177–179.

McCay PB. 1985. Vitamin E: Interactions with free radicals and ascorbate. *Annu Rev Nutr* 5:323–340.

McKeown-Eyssen G, Holloway C, Jazmaji V, Bright-See E, Dion P, Bruce WR. 1988. A randomized trial of vitamins C and E in the prevention of recurrence of colorectal polyps. *Cancer Res* 48:4701–4705.

McLaughlin PJ, Weihrauch JL. 1979. Vitamin E content of foods. *J Am Diet Assoc* 75:647–665.

Mellette SJ, Leone LA. 1960. Influence of age, sex, strain of rat and fat soluble vitamins on hemorrhagic syndromes in rats fed irradiated beef. *New Aspects Nutr* 19:1045–1049.

Mertz W, Tsui JC, Judd JT, Reiser S, Hallfrisch J, Morris ER, Steele PD, Lashley E. 1991. What are people really eating? The relation between energy intake derived from estimated diet records and intake determined to maintain body weight. *Am J Clin Nutr* 54:291–295.

Meydani M, Cohn JS, Macauley JB, McNamara JR, Blumberg JB, Schaefer EJ. 1989. Postprandial changes in the plasma concentration of alpha- and gamma-tocopherol in human subjects fed a fat-rich meal supplemented with fat-soluble vitamins. *J Nutr* 119:1252–1258.

Meydani SN, Meydani M, Blumberg JB, Leka LS, Siber G, Loszewski R, Thompson C, Pedrosa MC, Diamond RD, Stollar BD. 1997. Vitamin E supplementation and in vivo immune response in healthy elderly subjects. A randomized controlled trial. *J Am Med Assoc* 277:1380–1386.

Meydani SN, Meydani M, Blumberg JB, Leka LS, Pedrosa M, Diamond R, Schaefer EJ. 1998. Assessment of the safety of supplementation with different amounts of vitamin E in healthy older adults. *Am J Clin Nutr* 68:311–318.

Mezzetti A, Lapenna D, Pierdomenico SD, Calafiore AM, Costantini F, Riario-Sforza G, Imbastaro T, Neri M, Cuccurullo F. 1995. Vitamins E, C and lipid peroxidation in plasma and arterial tissue of smokers and non-smokers. *Atherosclerosis* 112:91–99.

Mohan M, Sperduto R, Angra S, Milton R, Mathur R, Underwood B, Jaffery N, Pandya C, Chhabra V, Vajpayee RB. 1989. India-US case-control study of age-related cataracts. India-US Case-Control Study Group. *Arch Ophthalmol* 107:670–676.

Molenaar R, Visser WJ, Verkerk A, Koster JF, Jongkind JF. 1989. Peroxidative stress and in vitro ageing of endothelial cells increases the monocyte-endothelial cell adherence in a human in vitro system. *Atherosclerosis* 76:193–202.

Moore AN, Ingold KU. 1997. Alpha-tocopheryl quinone is converted into vitamin E in man. *Free Radic Biol Med* 22:931–934.

Moore K, Roberts LJ II. 1998. Measurement of lipid peroxidation. *Free Radic Res* 28:659–671.

Morrow JD, Frei B, Longmire AW, Gaziano JM, Lynch SM, Shyr Y, Strauss WE, Oates JA, Roberts LJ II. 1995. Increase in circulating products of lipid peroxidation (F_2-isoprostanes) in smokers. *N Engl J Med* 332:1198–1203.

Morrow JD, Zackert WE, Yang JP, Kurhts EH, Callewaert D, Dworski R, Kanai K, Taber D, Moore K, Oates JA, Roberts LJ. 1999. Quantification of the major urinary metabolite of 15-F2t-isoprostane (8-iso-PGF2alpha) by a stable isotope dilution mass spectrometric assay. *Anal Biochem* 269:326–331.

Moss AJ, Levy AS, Kim I, Park YK. 1989. *Use of Vitamin and Mineral Supplements in the United States: Current Users, Types of Products, and Nutrients.* Advance Data, Vital and Health Statistics of the National Center for Health Statistics. Number 174. Hyattsville, MD: National Center for Health Statistics.

Mullarkey CJ, Edelstein D, Brownlee M. 1990. Free radical generation by early glycation products: A mechanism for accelerated atherogenesis in diabetes. *Biochem Biophys Res Commun* 173:932–939.

Muller DP. 1994. Vitamin E and other antioxidants in neurological function and disease. In: Frei B, ed. *Natural Antioxidants in Human Health and Disease.* San Diego: Academic Press. Pp. 535–565.

Muller DP, Harries JT, Lloyd JK. 1974. The relative importance of the factors involved in the absorption of vitamin E in children. *Gut* 15:966–971.

Muller DP, Lloyd JK, Wolff OH. 1985. The role of vitamin E in the treatment of the neurological features of abetalipoproteinaemia and other disorders of fat absorption. *J Inherit Metab Dis* 8:88–92.

Murphy SP, Subar AF, Block G. 1990. Vitamin E intakes and sources in the United States. *Am J Clin Nutr* 52:361–367.

Murray ED Jr, Wechter WJ, Kantoci D, Wang WH, Pham T, Quiggle DD, Gibson KM, Leipold D, Anner B. 1997. Endogenous natriuretic factors 7: Biospecificity of a natriuretic gamma-tocopherol metabolite LLU-alpha. *J Pharmacol Exp Ther* 282:657–662.

Niki E. 1987. Antioxidants in relation to lipid peroxidation. *Chem Phys Lipids* 44:227–253.

Niki E, Tsuchiya J, Tanimura R, Kamiya Y. 1982. Regeneration of vitamin E from alpha-chromanoxyl radical by glutathione and vitamin C. *Chem Lett* 6:789–792.

NRC (National Research Council). 1989. *Recommended Dietary Allowances*, 10th edition. Washington, DC: National Academy Press.

O'Neill CA, Halliwell B, van der Vliet A, Davis PA, Packer L, Tritschler H, Strohman WJ, Rieland T, Cross CE, Reznick AZ. 1994. Aldehyde-induced protein modifications in human plasma: Protection by glutathione and dihydrolipoic acid. *J Lab Clin Med* 124:359–370.

Oski FA, Barness LA. 1967. Vitamin E deficiency: A previously unrecognized cause of hemolytic anemia in the premature infant. *J Pediatr* 70:211–220.

Packer L. 1994. Vitamin E is nature's master antioxidant. *Sci Am Sci Med* 1:54–63.

Pallast EG, Schouten EG, de Waart FG, Fonk HC, Doekes G, von Blomberg BM, Kok FJ. 1999. Effect of 50- and 100-mg vitamin E supplements on cellular immune function in noninstitutionalized elderly persons. *Am J Clin Nutr* 69: 1273–1281.

Paolisso G, D'Amore A, Galzerano D, Balbi V, Giugliano D, Varricchio M, D'Onofrio F. 1993. Daily vitamin E supplements improve metabolic control but not insulin secretion in elderly type II diabetic patients. *Diabetes Care* 16:1433–1437.

Parker RA, Sabrah T, Cap M, Gill BT. 1995. Relation of vascular oxidative stress, alpha-tocopherol, and hypercholesterolemia to early atherosclerosis in hamsters. *Arterioscler Thromb Vasc Biol* 15:349–358.

Parker RS. 1988. Carotenoid and tocopherol composition of human adipose tissue. *Am J Clin Nutr* 47:33–36.

Parkinson Study Group. 1993. Effects of tocopherol and deprenyl on the progression of disability in early Parkinson's disease. *N Engl J Med* 328:176–183.

Parkinson Study Group. 1998. Mortality in DATATOP: A multicenter trial in early Parkinson's disease. *Ann Neurol* 43:318–325.

Peng Y-S, Peng Y-M, McGee D, Alberts D. 1994. Carotenoids, tocopherols, and retinoids in human buccal mucosal cells: Intra- and interindividual variability and storage stability. *Am J Clin Nutr* 59:636–643.

Phelps DL, Rosenbaum AL, Isenberg SJ, Leake RD, Dorey FJ. 1987. Tocopherol efficacy and safety for preventing retinopathy of prematurity: A randomized, controlled, double-masked trial. *Pediatrics* 79:489–500.

Pratico D, Tangirala RK, Rader DJ, Rokach J, FitzGerald GA. 1998. Vitamin E suppresses isoprostane generation in vivo and reduces atherosclerosis in ApoE-deficient mice. *Nat Med* 4:1189–1192.

Pratico D, Rokach J, Tangirala RK. 1999. Brains of aged apolipoprotein E-deficient mice have increased levels of F^2-isoprostanes, in vivo markers of lipid peroxidation. *J Neurochem* 73:736–741.

Princen HMG, van Duyvenvoorde W, Buytenhek R, van der Laarse A, van Poppel G, Gevers Leuven JA, van Hinsbergh VWM. 1995. Supplementation with low doses of vitamin E protects LDL from lipid peroxidation in men and women. *Arterioscler Thromb Vasc Biol* 15:325–333.

Pryor WA, Stone K. 1993. Oxidants in cigarette smoke. Radicals, hydrogen peroxide, peroxynitrate, and peroxynitrite. *Ann NY Acad Sci* 686:12–27.

Rader DJ, Brewer HB. 1993. Abetalipoproteinemia. New insights into lipoprotein assembly and vitamin E metabolism from a rare genetic disease. *J Am Med Assoc* 270:865–869.

Rapola JM, Virtamo J, Ripatti S, Huttunen JK, Albanes D, Taylor PR, Heinonen OP. 1997. Randomised trial of alpha-tocopherol and beta-carotene supplements on incidence of major coronary events in men with previous myocardial infarction. *Lancet* 349:1715–1720.

Reaven P. 1995. Dietary and pharmacologic regimens to reduce lipid peroxidation in non-insulin-dependent diabetes mellitus. *Am J Clin Nutr* 62:1483S–1489S.

Reaven PD, Khouw A, Beltz WF, Parthasarathy S, Witztum JL. 1993. Effect of dietary antioxidant combinations in humans. Protection of LDL by vitamin E but not by beta-carotene. *Arterioscler Thromb* 13:590–600.

Reaven PD, Herold DA, Barnett J, Edelman S. 1995. Effects of vitamin E on susceptibility of low-density lipoprotein and low-density lipoprotein subfractions to oxidation and on protein glycation in NIDDM. *Diabetes Care* 18:807–816.

Refat M, Moore TJ, Kazui M, Risby TH, Perman JA, Schwarz KB. 1991. Utility of breath ethane as a noninvasive biomarker of vitamin E status in children. *Pediatr Res* 30:396–403

Reilly M, Delanty N, Lawson JA, Fitzgerald GA. 1996. Modulation of oxidant stress in vivo in chronic cigarette smokers. *Circulation* 94:19–25.

Retzlaff BM, Dowdy AA, Walden CE, McCann BS, Gey G, Cooper M, Knopp RH. 1991. Changes in vitamin and mineral intakes and serum concentrations among free-living men on cholesterol-lowering diets: The Dietary Alternatives Study. *Am J Clin Nutr* 53:890–898.

Rimm EB, Stampfer MJ, Ascherio A, Giovannucci E, Colditz GA, Willett WC. 1993. Vitamin E consumption and the risk of coronary heart disease in men. *N Engl J Med* 328:1450–1456.

Ritchie JH, Fish MB, McMasters V, Grossman M. 1968. Edema and hemolytic anemia in premature infants. A vitamin E deficiency syndrome. *N Engl J Med* 279:1185–1190.

Robertson JM, Donner AP, Trevithick JR. 1989. Vitamin E intake and risk of cataracts in humans. *Ann NY Acad Sci* 570:372–382.

Ross MA, Crosley LK, Brown KM, Duthie SJ, Collins AC, Arthur JR, Duthie GG. 1995. Plasma concentrations of carotenoids and antioxidant vitamins in Scottish males: Influences of smoking. *Eur J Clin Nutr* 49:861–865.

Rota S, McWilliam NA, Baglin TP, Byrne CD. 1998. Atherogenic lipoproteins support assembly of the prothrombinase complex and thrombin generation: Modulation by oxidation and vitamin E. *Blood* 91:508–515.

Sano M, Ernesto C, Thomas RG, Klauber MR, Schafer K, Grundman M, Woodbury P, Growdon J, Cotman CW, Pfeiffer E, Schneider LS, Thal LJ. 1997. A controlled trial of selegiline, alpha-tocopherol, or both as treatment for Alzheimer's disease. The Alzheimer's Disease Cooperative Study. *N Engl J Med* 336:1216–1222.

Sarkkinen ES, Uusitupa MI, Nyyssonen K, Parviainen M, Penttila I, Salonen JT. 1993. Effects of two low-fat diets, high and low in polyunsaturated fatty acids, on plasma lipid peroxides and serum vitamin E levels in free-living hypercholesterolaemic men. *Eur J Clin Nutr* 47:623–630.

Sato Y, Hagiwara K, Arai H, Inoue K. 1991. Purification and characterization of the alpha-tocopherol transfer protein from rat liver. *FEBS Lett* 288:41–45.

Schuelke M, Mayatepek E, Inter M, Becker M, Pfeiffer E, Speer A, Hubner C, Finckh B. 1999. Treatment of ataxia in isolated vitamin E deficiency caused by alpha-tocopherol transfer protein deficiency. *J Pediatr* 134:240–244.

Schultz M, Leist M, Petrzika M, Gassmann B, Brigelius-Flohé R. 1995. Novel urinary metabolite of alpha-tocopherol, 2,5,7,8-tetramethyl-2(2′-carboxyethyl)-6-hydroxychroman, as an indicator of an adequate vitamin E supply? *Am J Clin Nutr* 62:1527S–1534S.

Schultz M, Leist M, Elsner A, Brigelius-Flohé R. 1997. Alpha-carboxyethyl-6-hydroxychroman as urinary metabolite of vitamin E. *Methods Enzymol* 282:297–310.

Schwab US, Sarkkinen ES, Lichtenstein AH, Li Z, Ordovas JM, Schaefer EJ, Uusitupa MI. 1998a. The effect of quality and amount of dietary fat on the susceptibility of low density lipoprotein to oxidation in subjects with impaired glucose tolerance. *Eur J Clin Nutr* 52:452–458.

Schwab US, Vogel S, Lammi-Keefe CJ, Ordovas JM, Schaefer EJ, Li Z, Ausman LM, Gualtieri L, Goldin BR, Furr HC, Lichtenstein AH. 1998b. Varying dietary fat type of reduced-fat diets has little effect on the susceptibility of LDL to oxidative modification in moderately hypercholesterolemic subjects. *J Nutr* 128: 1703–1709.

Semenkovich CF, Heinecke JW. 1997. The mystery of diabetes and atherosclerosis: Time for a new plot. *Diabetes* 46:327–334.

Sheppard AJ, Pennington JAT, Weihrauch JL. 1993. Analysis and distribution of vitamin E in vegetable oils and foods. In: Packer L, Fuchs J, eds. *Vitamin E in Health and Disease*. New York: Marcel Dekker. Pp. 9–31.

Shorer Z, Parvari R, Bril G, Sela BA, Moses S. 1996. Ataxia with isolated vitamin E deficiency in four siblings. *Pediatr Neurol* 15:340–343.

Shoulson I. 1998. DATATOP: A decade of neuroprotective inquiry. Parkinson Study Group. Deprenyl and Tocopherol Antioxidative Therapy of Parkinsonism. *Ann Neurol* 44:S160–S166.

Slesinski MJ, Subar AF, Kahle LL. 1996. Dietary intake of fat, fiber and other nutrients is related to the use of vitamin and mineral supplements in the United States: The 1992 National Health Interview Survey. *J Nutr* 126:3001–3008.

Smith MA, Harris PL, Sayre LM, Perry G. 1997. Iron accumulation in Alzheimer disease is a source of redox-generated free radicals. *Proc Natl Acad Sci USA* 94:9866–9868.

Sokol RJ. 1988. Vitamin E deficiency and neurologic disease. *Annu Rev Nutr* 8:351–373.

Sokol RJ. 1993. Vitamin E deficiency and neurological disorders. In: Packer L, Fuchs J, eds. *Vitamin E in Health and Disease*. New York: Marcel Dekker. Pp. 815–849.

Sokol RJ, Heubi JE, Iannaccone S, Bove KE, Balistreri WF. 1983. Mechanism causing vitamin E deficiency during chronic childhood cholestasis. *Gastroenterology* 85:1172–1182.

Sokol RJ, Heubi JE, Iannaccone ST, Bove KE, Balistreri WF. 1984. Vitamin E deficiency with normal serum vitamin E concentrations in children with chronic cholestasis. *N Engl J Med* 310:1209–1212.

Sokol RJ, Guggenheim M, Iannaccone ST, Barkhaus PE, Miller C, Silverman A, Balistreri WF, Heubi JE. 1985. Improved neurologic function after long-term correction of vitamin E deficiency in children with chronic cholestasis. *N Engl J Med* 313:1580–1586.

Sokol RJ, Kayden HJ, Bettis DB, Traber MG, Neville H, Ringel S, Wilson WB, Stumpf DA. 1988. Isolated vitamin E deficiency in the absence of fat malabsorption—Familial and sporadic cases: Characterization and investigation of causes. *J Lab Clin Med* 111:548–559.

Sokol RJ, Reardon MC, Accurso FJ, Stall C, Narkewicz M, Abman SH, Hammond KB. 1989. Fat-soluble-vitamin status during the first year of life in infants with cystic fibrosis identified by screening of newborns. *Am J Clin Nutr* 50:1064–1071.

Sokol RJ, Butler-Simon N, Conner C, Heubi JE, Sinatra FR, Suchy FJ, Heyman MB, Perrault J, Rothbaum RJ, Levy J, Iannaccone ST, Shneider BL, Koch TK, Narkewicz MR. 1993. Multicenter trial of *d*-alpha-tocopheryl polyethylene glycol 1000 succinate for treatment of vitamin E deficiency in children with chronic cholestasis. *Gastroenterology* 104:1727–1735.

Sparrow CP, Doebber TW, Olszewski J, Wu MS, Ventre J, Stevens KA, Chao YS. 1992. Low density lipoprotein is protected from oxidation and the progression of atherosclerosis is slowed in cholesterol-fed rabbits by the antioxidant *N,N'*-diphenyl-phenylenediamine. *J Clin Invest* 89:1885–1891.

Speer ME, Blifeld C, Rudolph AJ, Chadda P, Holbein ME, Hittner HM. 1984. Intraventricular hemorrhage and vitamin E in the very low-birth-weight infant: Evidence for efficacy of early intramuscular vitamin E administration. *Pediatrics* 74:1107–1112.

Stampfer MJ, Hennekens CH, Manson JE, Colditz GA, Rosner B, Willett WC. 1993. Vitamin E consumption and the risk of coronary disease in women. *N Engl J Med* 328:1444–1449.

Stauble B, Boscoboinik D, Tasinato A, Azzi A. 1994. Modulation of activator protein-1 (AP-1) transcription factor and protein kinase C by hydrogen peroxide and *d*-alpha-tocopherol in vascular smooth muscle cells. *Eur J Biochem* 226:393–402.

Stead RJ, Muller DP, Matthews S, Hodson ME, Batten JC. 1986. Effect of abnormal liver function on vitamin E status and supplementation in adults with cystic fibrosis. *Gut* 27:714–718.

Steinberg D. 1997. Oxidative modification of LDL and atherogenesis. *Circulation* 95:1062–1071.

Steinberg D, Parthasarathy S, Carew TE, Khoo JC, Witztum JL. 1989. Beyond cholesterol. Modifications of low-density lipoprotein that increase its atherogenicity. *N Engl J Med* 320:915–924.

Steinbrecher UP, Parthasarathy S, Leake DS, Witztum JL, Steinberg D. 1984. Modification of low density lipoprotein by endothelial cells involves lipid peroxidation and degradation of low density lipoprotein phospholipids. *Proc Natl Acad Sci USA* 81:3883–3887.

Steiner M, Anastasi J. 1976. Vitamin E. An inhibitor of the platelet release reaction. *J Clin Invest* 57:732–737.

Stephens NG, Parsons A, Schofield PM, Kelly F, Cheeseman K, Mitchinson MJ. 1996. Randomised controlled trial of vitamin E in patients with coronary disease: Cambridge Heart Antioxidant Study (CHAOS). *Lancet* 347:781–786.

Stocker R. 1999. The ambivalence of vitamin E in atherogenesis. *Trends Biochem Sci* 24:219–223.

Stoyanovsky DA, Osipov AN, Quinn PJ, Kagan VE. 1995. Ubiquinone-dependent recycling of vitamin E radicals by superoxide. *Arch Biochem Biophys* 323:343–351.

Stryker WS, Kaplan LA, Stein EA, Stampfer MJ, Sober A, Willett WC. 1988. The relation of diet, cigarette smoking, and alcohol consumption to plasma beta-carotene and alpha-tocopherol levels. *Am J Epidemiol* 127:283–296.

Stumpf DA, Sokol R, Bettis D, Neville H, Ringel S, Angelini C, Bell R. 1987. Friedreich's disease: V. Variant form with vitamin E deficiency and normal fat absorption. *Neurology* 37:68–74.

Subramaniam R, Koppal T, Green M, Yatin S, Jordan B, Drake J, Butterfield DA. 1998. The free radical antioxidant vitamin E protects cortical synaptosomal membranes from amyloid beta-peptide(25–35) toxicity but not from hydroxynonenal toxicity: Relevance to the free radical hypothesis of Alzheimer's disease. *Neurochem Res* 23:1403–1410.

Swanson JE, Ben R, Burton GW, Parker RS. 1998. Urinary excretion of 2,7,8-trimethyl-2-(beta-carboxyethyl)-6-hydroxychroman (gamma-CEHC) represents a major pathway of elimination of gamma-tocopherol in humans. *FASEB J* 12:A658.

Swanson JE, Ben RN, Burton GW, Parker RS. 1999. Urinary excretion of 2,7,8-trimethyl-2-(beta-carboxyethyl)-6-hydroxychroman is a major route of elimination of gamma-tocopherol in humans. *J Lipid Res* 40:665–671.

Szczeklik A, Gryglewski RJ, Domagala B, Dworski R, Basista M. 1985. Dietary supplementation with vitamin E in hyperlipoproteinemias: Effects on plasma lipid peroxides, antioxidant activity, prostacyclin generation and platelet aggregability. *Thromb Haemostasis* 54:425–430.

Takahashi O, Ichikawa H, Sasaki M. 1990. Hemorrhagic toxicity of *d*-alpha-tocopherol in the rat. *Toxicology* 63:157–165.

Tappel AL. 1962. Vitamin E as the biological lipid antioxidant. *Vitam Horm* 20:493–510.

Tasinato A, Boscoboinik D, Bartoli G, Maroni P, Azzi A. 1995. *d*-Alpha-tocopherol inhibition of vascular smooth muscle cell proliferation occurs at physiological concentrations, correlates with protein kinase C inhibition, and is independent of its antioxidant properties. *Proc Natl Acad Sci USA* 92:12190–12194.

Taylor A. 1993. Cataract: Relationship between nutrition and oxidation. *J Am Coll Nutr* 12:138–146.

Teikari JM, Rautalahti M, Haukka J, Jarvinen P, Hartman AM, Virtamo J, Albanes D, Heinonen O. 1998. Incidence of cataract operations in Finnish male smokers unaffected by alpha tocopherol or beta carotene supplements. *J Epidemiol Community Health* 52:468–472.

Thomas MR, Pearsons MH, Demkowicz M, Chan IM, Lewis CG. 1981. Vitamin A and vitamin E concentration of the milk from mothers of pre-term infants and milk of mothers of full term infants. *Acta Vitaminol Enzymol* 3:135–144.

Thorin E, Hamilton CA, Dominiczak MH, Reid JL. 1994. Chronic exposure of cultured bovine endothelial cells to oxidized LDL abolishes prostacyclin release. *Arterioscler Thromb* 14:453–459.

Traber MG. 1999. Vitamin E. In: Shils ME, Olson JA, Shike M, Ross AC, eds. *Modern Nutrition in Health and Disease*, 9th edition. Baltimore, MD: Williams & Wilkins. P. 347–362.

Traber MG, Kayden HJ. 1987. Tocopherol distribution and intracellular localization in human adipose tissue. *Am J Clin Nutr* 46:488–495.

Traber MG, Kayden HJ. 1989. Preferential incorporation of alpha-tocopherol vs gamma-tocopherol in human lipoproteins. *Am J Clin Nutr* 49:517–526.

Traber MG, Kayden HJ, Green JB, Green MH. 1986. Absorption of water-miscible forms of vitamin E in a patient with cholestasis and in thoracic duct-cannulated rats. *Am J Clin Nutr* 44:914–923.

Traber MG, Sokol RJ, Ringel SP, Neville HE, Thellman CA, Kayden HJ. 1987. Lack of tocopherol in peripheral nerves of vitamin E-deficient patients with peripheral neuropathy. *N Engl J Med* 317:262–265.

Traber MG, Burton GW, Ingold KU, Kayden HJ. 1990a. *RRR*- and *SRR*-alpha-tocopherols are secreted without discrimination in human chylomicrons, but *RRR*-alpha-tocopherol is preferentially secreted in very low density lipoproteins. *J Lipid Res* 31:675–685.

Traber MG, Rudel LL, Burton GW, Hughes L, Ingold KU, Kayden HJ. 1990b. Nascent VLDL from liver perfusions of cynomolgus monkeys are preferentially enriched in *RRR*- compared with *SRR*-alpha tocopherol: Studies using deuterated tocopherols. *J Lipid Res* 31:687–694.

Traber MG, Burton GW, Hughes L, Ingold KU, Hidaka H, Malloy M, Kane J, Hyams J, Kayden HJ. 1992. Discrimination between forms of vitamin E by humans with and without genetic abnormalities of lipoprotein metabolism. *J Lipid Res* 33:1171–1182.

Traber MG, Cohn W, Muller DP. 1993. Absorption, transport and delivery to tissues. In: Packer L, Fuchs J, eds. *Vitamin E in Health and Disease*. New York: Marcel Dekker. Pp. 35–51.

Traber MG, Rader D, Acuff R, Brewer HB, Kayden HJ. 1994a. Discrimination between *RRR*- and all racemic-alpha-tocopherols labeled with deuterium by patients with abetalipoproteinemia. *Atherosclerosis* 108:27–37.

Traber MG, Ramakrishnan R, Kayden HJ. 1994b. Human plasma vitamin E kinetics demonstrate rapid recycling of plasma *RRR*-alpha-tocopherol. *Proc Natl Acad Sci USA* 91:10005–10008.

Traber MG, Elsner A, Brigelius-Flohé R. 1998. Synthetic as compared with natural vitamin E is preferentially excreted as alpha-CEHC in human urine: Studies using deuterated alpha-tocopheryl acetates. *FEBS Lett* 437:145–148.

Trabert W, Stober T, Mielke U, Heck FS, Schimrigk K. 1989. Isolated vitamin E deficiency. *Fortschr Neurol Psychiatr* 57:495–501.

Tran K, Chan AC. 1990. *R,R,R*-alpha-tocopherol potentiates prostacyclin release in human endothelial cells. Evidence for structural specificity of the tocopherol molecule. *Biochim Biophys Acta* 1043:189–197.

Tran K, Proulx P, Chan AC. 1994. Vitamin E suppresses diacylglycerol (DAG) level in thrombin-stimulated endothelial cells through an increase of DAG kinase activity. *Biochim Biophys Acta* 1212:193–202.

Tran K, Wong JT, Lee E, Chan AC, Choy PC. 1996. Vitamin E potentiates arachidonate release and phospholipase A^2 activity in rat heart myoblastic cells. *Biochem J* 319:385–391.

Tsai AC, Kelley JJ, Peng B, Cook N. 1978. Study on the effect of megavitamin E supplementation in man. *Am J Clin Nutr* 31:831–837.

Tsuchiya M, Thompson DF, Suzuki YJ, Cross CE, Packer L. 1992. Superoxide formed from cigarette smoke impairs polymorphonuclear leukocyte active oxygen generation activity. *Arch Biochem Biophys* 299:30–37.

Tutuncu NB, Bayraktar M, Varli K. 1998. Reversal of defective nerve conduction with vitamin E supplementation in type 2 diabetes: A preliminary study. *Diabetes Care* 21:1915–1918.

USP (The United States Pharmacopeia). 1979. *The United States Pharmacopeia. National Formulary*. Rockville, MD: United States Pharmacopeial Convention.

USP (The United States Pharmacopeia). 1980. *The United States Pharmacopeia. National Formulary*. Rockville, MD: United States Pharmacopeial Convention.

USP (The United States Pharmacopeia). 1999. *The United States Pharmacopeia 24. National Formulary 19*. Rockville, MD: United States Pharmacopeial Convention.

Upston JM, Terentis AC, Stocker R. 1999. Tocopherol-mediated peroxidation of lipoproteins: Implications for vitamin E as a potential antiatherogenic supplement. *FASEB J* 13:977–994.

van het Hof KH, Brouwer IA, West CE, Haddeman E, Steegers-Theunissen RPM, van Dusseldorp M, Weststrate JA, Eskes TKAB, Hautvast JGAJ. 1999. Bioavailability of lutein from vegetables is 5 times higher than that of β-carotene. *Am J Clin Nutr* 70:261–268.

van 't Veer P, Strain JJ, Fernandez-Crehuet J, Martin BC, Thamm M, Kardinaal AF, Kohlmeier L, Huttunen JK, Martin-Moreno JM, Kok FJ. 1996. Tissue antioxidants and postmenopausal breast cancer: The European Community Multicentre Study on Antioxidants, Myocardial Infarction, and Cancer of the Breast (EURAMIC). *Cancer Epidemiol Biomarkers Prev* 5:441–447.

Vatassery GT, Fahn S, Kuskowski MA. 1998. Alpha tocopherol in CSF of subjects taking high-dose vitamin E in the DATATOP study. Parkinson Study Group. *Neurology* 50:1900–1902.

Velthuis-te Wierik EJ, van den Berg H, Weststrate JA, van het Hof KH, de Graaf C. 1996. Consumption of reduced-fat products: Effects on parameters of antioxidative capacity. *Eur J Clin Nutr* 50:214–219.

Verhoeven DT, Assen N, Goldbohm RA, Dorant E, van 't Veer P, Sturmans F, Hermus RJ, van den Brandt PA. 1997. Vitamins C and E, retinol, beta-carotene and dietary fibre in relation to breast cancer risk: A prospective cohort study. *Br J Cancer* 75:149–155.

Vitale S, West S, Hallfrisch J, Alston C, Wang F, Moorman C, Muller D, Singh V, Taylor HR. 1993. Plasma antioxidants and risk of cortical and nuclear cataract. *Epidemiology* 4:195–203.

Wander RC, Du SH, Ketchum SO, Rowe KE. 1996. Effects of interaction of *RRR*-alpha-tocopheryl acetate and fish oil on low-density-lipoprotein oxidation in postmenopausal women with and without hormone-replacement therapy. *Am J Clin Nutr* 63:184–193.

Wechter WJ, Kantoci D, Murray ED, D'Amico DC, Jung ME, Wang W-H. 1996. A new endogenous natriuretic factor: LLU-alpha. *Proc Natl Acad Sci USA* 93:6002–6007.

Weiser H, Vecchi M. 1981. Stereoisomers of alpha-tocopheryl acetate. Characterization of the samples by physico-chemical methods and determination of biological activities in the rat resorption-gestation test. *Int J Vitam Nutr Res* 51:100–113.

Weiser H, Vecchi M. 1982. Stereoisomers of alpha-tocopheryl acetate. II. Biopotencies of all eight stereoisomers, individually or in mixtures, as determined by rat resorption-gestation tests. *Int J Vitam Nutr Res* 52:351–370.

Weiser H, Vecchi M, Schlachter M. 1986. Stereoisomers of alpha-tocopheryl acetate. IV. USP units and alpha-tocopherol equivalents of all-rac-, 2-ambo- and RRR-alpha-tocopherol evaluated by simultaneous determination of resorption-gestation, myopathy and liver storage capacity in rats. *Int J Vitam Nutr Res* 56:45–56.

Wheldon GH, Bhatt A, Keller P, Hummler H. 1983. D,1-alpha-tocopheryl acetate (vitamin E): A long term toxicity and carcinogenicity study in rats. *Int J Vitam Nutr Res* 53:287–296.

Winklhofer-Roob BM, Tuchschmid PE, Molinari L, Shmerling DH. 1996a. Response to a single oral dose of *all-rac*-alpha-tocopheryl acetate in patients with cystic fibrosis and in healthy individuals. *Am J Clin Nutr* 63:717–721.

Winklhofer-Roob BM, van't Hof MA, Shmerling DH. 1996b. Long-term oral vitamin E supplementation in cystic fibrosis patients: *RRR*-alpha-tocopherol compared with *all-rac*-alpha-tocopheryl acetate preparations. *Am J Clin Nutr* 63:722–728.

Winklhofer-Roob BM, van't Hof MA, Shmerling DH. 1997. Reference values for plasma concentrations of vitamin E and A and carotenoids in a Swiss population from infancy to adulthood, adjusted for seasonal influences. *Clin Chem* 43:146–153.

Witting LA, Lee L. 1975. Dietary levels of vitamin E and polyunsaturated fatty acids and plasma vitamin E. *Am J Clin Nutr* 28:571–576.

Yang NY, Desai ID. 1977. Effect of high levels of dietary vitamin E on hematological indices and biochemical parameters in rats. *J Nutr* 107:1410–1417.

Yong LC, Brown CC, Schatzkin A, Dresser CM, Slesinski MJ, Cox CS, Taylor PR. 1997. Intake of vitamins E, C, and A and risk of lung cancer. The NHANES I Epidemiologic Followup Study. *Am J Epidemiol* 146:231–243.

Yoshida H, Yusin M, Ren I, Kuhlenkamp J, Hirano T, Stolz A, Kaplowitz N. 1992. Identification, purification and immunochemical characterization of a tocopherol-binding protein in rat liver cytosol. *J Lipid Res* 33:343–350.

Yoshida H, Ishikawa T, Nakamura H. 1997. Vitamin E/lipid peroxide ratio and susceptibility of LDL to oxidative modification in non-insulin-dependent diabetes mellitus. *Arterioscler Thromb Vasc Biol* 17:1438–1446.

7

Selenium

SUMMARY

Selenium functions through selenoproteins, several of which are oxidant defense enzymes. The Recommended Dietary Allowance (RDA) for selenium is based on the amount needed to maximize synthesis of the selenoprotein glutathione peroxidase, as assessed by the plateau in the activity of the plasma isoform of this enzyme. The RDA for both men and women is 55 µg (0.7 µmol)/day. The major forms of selenium in the diet are highly bioavailable. Selenium intake varies according to geographic location, but there is no indication of average intakes below the RDA in the United States or Canada. A study done in Maryland reported that adults consumed an average of 81 µg (1.0 µmol)/day of selenium (Welsh et al., 1981). A Canadian survey reported selenium intakes of 113 to 220 µg (1.4 to 2.8 µmol)/day (Thompson et al., 1975). The Tolerable Upper Intake Level (UL) for adults is set at 400 µg (5.1 µmol)/day based on selenosis as the adverse effect.

BACKGROUND INFORMATION

Most selenium in animal tissues is present as selenomethionine or selenocysteine. Selenomethionine, which cannot be synthesized by humans and is initially synthesized in plants, is incorporated randomly in place of methionine in a variety of proteins obtained from plant and animal sources. Selenium is present in varying amounts in these proteins, which are called selenium-containing proteins.

Selenomethionine is not known to have a physiological function separate from that of methionine.

Selenocysteine is present in animal selenoproteins that have been characterized (see below) and is the form of selenium that accounts for the biological activity of the element. In contrast to selenomethionine, there is no evidence that selenocysteine substitutes for cysteine in humans.

Function

Selenium functions largely through an association with proteins, known as selenoproteins (Stadtman, 1991), and disruption of their synthesis is lethal for embryos (Bösl et al., 1997). A selenoprotein is a protein that contains selenium in stoichiometric amounts. Fourteen selenoproteins have been characterized to date in animals. The four known selenium-dependent glutathione peroxidases designated as GSHPx 1 through 4 defend against oxidative stress (Flohe, 1988). Selenoproteins P and W are postulated to do so as well (Arteel et al., 1998; Burk et al., 1995; Saito et al., 1999; Sun et al., 1999). Three selenium-dependent iodothyronine deiodinases regulate thyroid hormone metabolism (Berry and Larsen, 1992). Three thioredoxin reductases have been identified (Sun et al., 1999). Their functions include reduction of intramolecular disulfide bonds and regeneration of ascorbic acid from its oxidized metabolites (May et al., 1998). The selenium-dependent isoform of selenophosphate synthetase participates in selenium metabolism (Guimaraes et al., 1996). Other selenoproteins have not yet been characterized to the same extent with respect to function (Behne et al., 1997). Thus, the known biological functions of selenium include defense against oxidative stress, regulation of thyroid hormone action, and regulation of the redox status of vitamin C and other molecules.

Physiology of Absorption, Metabolism, and Excretion

Absorption

Absorption of selenium is efficient and is not regulated. More than 90 percent of selenomethionine, the major dietary form of the element, is absorbed by the same mechanism as methionine itself (Swanson et al., 1991). Although little is known about selenocysteine absorption, it appears to be absorbed very well also.

An inorganic form of selenium, selenate (SeO_4^{2-}), is absorbed almost completely, but a significant fraction of it is lost in the urine before it can be incorporated into tissues. Another inorganic form of selenium, selenite (SeO_3^{2-}), has a more variable absorption, probably related to interactions with substances in the gut lumen, but it is better retained, once absorbed, than is selenate (Thomson and Robinson, 1986). Absorption of selenite is generally greater than 50 percent (Thomson and Robinson, 1986). Although selenate and selenite are not major dietary constituents, they are commonly used to fortify foods and as selenium supplements.

Body Stores

Two pools of reserve selenium are present in humans and animals. One of them, the selenium present as selenomethionine, depends on dietary intake of selenium as selenomethionine (Waschulewski and Sunde, 1988). The amount of selenium made available to the organism from this pool is a function of turnover of the methionine pool and not the organism's need for selenium.

The second reserve pool of selenium is the selenium present in liver glutathione peroxidase (GSHPx-1). In rats, 25 percent of total body selenium is present in this pool (Behne and Wolters, 1983). As dietary selenium becomes limiting for selenoprotein synthesis, this pool is downregulated by a reduction of GSHPx-1 messenger ribonucleic acid (RNA) concentration (Sunde, 1994). This makes selenium available for synthesis of other selenoproteins.

Metabolism

Selenomethionine, derived mainly from plants, enters the methionine pool in the body and shares the fate of methionine until catabolized by the transsulfuration pathway. The resulting free selenocysteine is further broken down with liberation of a reduced form of the element, which is designated selenide (Esaki et al., 1982). Ingested selenite, selenate, and selenocysteine are all apparently metabolized directly to selenide. This selenide may be associated with a protein that serves as a chaperone (Lacourciere and Stadtman, 1998). The selenide can be metabolized to selenophosphate, the precursor of selenocysteine in selenoproteins (Ehrenreich et al., 1992) and of selenium in transfer RNA (Veres et al., 1992), or it can be converted to excretory metabolites (Mozier et al., 1988), some of which have been characterized as methylated forms.

Excretion

The mechanism that regulates production of excretory metabolites has not been elucidated, but excretion has been shown to be responsible for maintaining selenium homeostasis in the animal

(Burk et al., 1972). The excretory metabolites appear in the urine primarily, but when large amounts of selenium are being excreted, the breath also contains volatile metabolites (e.g., dimethylselenide) (McConnell and Portman, 1952).

Clinical Effects of Inadequate Intake

In experimental animals, selenium deficiency decreases selenoenzyme activities, but if the animals are otherwise adequately nourished, it causes relatively mild clinical symptoms. However, certain types of nutritional, chemical, and infectious stresses lead to serious diseases in selenium-deficient animals. For example, induction of vitamin E deficiency in selenium-deficient animals causes lipid peroxidation and liver necrosis in rats and pigs and cardiac injury in pigs, sheep, and cattle (Van Vleet, 1980). Another example of this phenomenon is the conversion of a nonpathogenic strain of coxsackie B3 virus to a pathogenic one that causes myocarditis when it infects selenium-deficient mice (Beck and Levander, 1998).

Keshan disease, a cardiomyopathy that occurs only in selenium-deficient children, appears to be triggered by an additional stress, possibly an infection or a chemical exposure (Ge et al., 1983). Clinical thyroid disorders have not been reported in selenium-deficient individuals with adequate iodine intake, but based on observations in Africa, it has been postulated that infants born to mothers deficient in both selenium and iodine are at increased risk of cretinism (Vanderpas et al., 1992).

Kashin-Beck disease, an endemic disease of cartilage that occurs in preadolescence or adolescence, has been reported in some of the low-selenium areas of Asia (Yang et al., 1988). It is possible that this disease, like Keshan disease, occurs only in selenium-deficient people. However, there has been no demonstration that improvement of selenium nutritional status can prevent Kashin-Beck disease, so involvement of selenium deficiency in its pathogenesis remains uncertain.

These considerations indicate that selenium deficiency seldom causes overt illness when it occurs in isolation. However, it leads to biochemical changes that predispose to illness associated with other stresses.

SELECTION OF INDICATORS FOR ESTIMATING THE REQUIREMENT FOR SELENIUM

A search of the literature revealed several indicators that could be considered as the basis for deriving an Estimated Average Requirement (EAR) for selenium in adults. These included prevention of Keshan disease or various chronic diseases; concentration of selenium in blood, hair, and nails; concentration of selenoproteins in blood; and urinary excretion of the element.

Keshan Disease

Keshan disease, a cardiomyopathy that occurs almost exclusively in children, is the only human disease that is firmly linked to selenium deficiency (Keshan Disease Research Group, 1979). In addition to a low selenium intake, low blood and hair selenium concentrations are associated with Keshan disease. The disease occurs with varying frequency in areas of China where the population is severely selenium deficient (Ge et al., 1983). Based on these observations, the occurrence of Keshan disease in a population would indicate that the population is selenium deficient.

Selenium in Hair and Nails

Although the forms of selenium in hair and nails have not been characterized, some correlations between dietary intake of the element and hair and nail concentrations of selenium have been demonstrated. However, the use of hair and nail selenium as markers of selenium status has been limited because factors such as the form of selenium fed, the methionine content of the diet, and the color of the hair affect the deposition of selenium in these tissues (Salbe and Levander, 1990). In addition, some shampoos in the United States and Canada contain selenium. Therefore, only well-controlled studies can make use of hair and nail selenium concentrations, and these markers are of little value in determining selenium requirements across population groups.

Selenium in Blood

Several forms of selenium are present in blood and in metabolizing tissues; thus, they can be discussed together. Physiologically active forms include the selenoproteins and some as yet uncharacterized forms that are present in low abundance. These forms of selenium are under physiological regulation. Within a specific range of dietary selenium intakes, selenoprotein concentrations are a function of selenium intake. Above this range of intakes, selenoprotein concentrations become regulated only by genetic and environmental factors. This lack of selenium effect implies that the selenium requirement for selenoprotein synthesis has been met (Yang et al., 1987). At this plateau point, human plasma selenoproteins contain 0.8 to 1.1 µmol/L (7 to 9 µg/dL) of selenium (Hill et al., 1996). Thus, when tissue concentrations of selenium are below the level at which selenoproteins have plateaued, it can be stated with confidence that selenium supplies are limiting. Under these conditions, tissue (plasma) concentrations of the element are useful as indices of nutritional selenium status.

Above plateau concentration, however, the chemical form of selenium ingested and other factors become important in determining the tissue selenium concentration. Tissue (plasma) concentrations of selenium do not always correlate with selenium intake under these conditions (concentration greater than the plateau). As stated earlier, much of the dietary selenium supply is selenomethionine, which is synthesized by plants and appears to enter the methionine pool in animals where it is incorporated into protein randomly at methionine sites. Since selenomethionine is not subject to homeostatic regulation, blood levels of selenium will generally be higher when this form is consumed (Burk and Levander, 1999). The selenium released by the catabolism of selenomethionine will be present as selenocysteine in selenoproteins.

Based on these considerations, plasma selenium concentration has utility in assessing selenium intake of all forms of the element only when it is less than 0.8 µmol/L (7 µg/dL). Such values indicate that the synthesis of selenoproteins has not yet plateaued. Above these values, the plasma selenium concentration is highly dependent on the chemical form of the element ingested.

Glutathione Peroxidases and Selenoprotein P in Blood

Several selenoproteins are present in blood. Plasma contains the extracellular glutathione peroxidase (GSHPx-3) and selenoprotein P. Erythrocytes and platelets contain the most abundant form of selenium-containing glutathione peroxidase, intracellular glutathione peroxidase (GSHPx-1). Other selenoproteins have not been identified in blood. All three of these blood selenoproteins (GSHPx-3, selenoprotein P, and GSHPx-1) have been used to assess selenium status, but plasma GSHPx-3 has been preferred in recent years because its determination is more accurate than the determination of the erythrocyte enzyme GSHPx-1. Since hemoglobin interferes with the measurement of GSHPx-1 in the erythrocyte, use of this marker is problematic and consequently few data are available that can be used to set a selenium requirement. Also studies indicate that plasma GSHPx-3 activity reflects the activity of tissue selenoenzymes better than does GSHPx-1 activity in erythrocytes (Cohen et al., 1985).

The limited information available on selenoprotein P indicates that it is the major form of selenium in plasma and suggests that it will be as good an indicator of selenium status as plasma GSHPx-3 (Hill et al., 1996). However, since an assay for it is not widely available at present, the data for selenoprotein P are insufficient to use it to estimate a dietary requirement.

Cancer

In some animal models, high selenium intakes reduce the incidence of cancer (Ip, 1998). In these studies, selenium was fed in amounts greater than that needed to support maximum concentrations of selenoproteins. In humans, some but not all observational studies have shown that individuals who self-select diets that produce high plasma and nail selenium tend to have a lower incidence of cancer (Clark et al., 1991).

Randomized trial data are limited to three studies, one conducted with poorly nourished rural Chinese (Blot et al., 1995), another with U.S. patients with a history of treated nonmelanoma skin cancer (Clark et al., 1996), and a third with participants in the Health Professional Follow-up Study (Yoshizawa et al., 1999). In the China trial, among eight combinations tested, subjects assigned a daily combination of selenium (50 µg [0.6 µmol]), β-carotene (15 mg), and α-tocopherol (30 mg) achieved a significant (21 percent) decrease in gastric cancer mortality, resulting in a significant 9 percent decline in total all-cause mortality. However, these results cannot be attributed to selenium alone, because the individuals consumed selenium in combination with β-carotene and vitamin E.

In the second trial, 200 µg (2.5 µmol)/day of selenium administered in the form of yeast showed no effect on recurrence of nonmelanoma skin cancer compared to a similar placebo group (Clark et al., 1996). Although the numbers of subjects were small (1,312 patients randomly assigned to the supplement or a placebo, ≈ 75% male) and the outcomes not prespecified, significantly lower rates of prostate, colon, and total cancer were observed among those assigned to the selenium group.

Similar prostate cancer results were reported from a nested case-control design within the Health Professionals Follow-up Study; the risk of prostate cancer for men receiving 200 µg (2.5 µmol)/day of selenium was one-third that of men receiving the placebo (Yoshizawa et al., 1999). The inverse association seen between the selenium level in toenail clippings and the risk of advanced prostate cancer was not confounded by age, other dietary factors, smoking, body mass index, geographic region, family history of prostate cancer, or vasectomy.

Results of these three studies are compatible with the possibility that intakes of selenium above those needed to maximize seleno-proteins have an anticancer effect in humans. These findings support the need for large-scale trials. They can not, however, serve as the basis for determining dietary selenium requirements at this time.

Other Measurements

Urine

Attempts have been made to use urinary selenium excretion as an index of selenium status. While excretion of the element is proportional to selenium status, excretion is also sensitive to short-term changes in selenium intake (Burk et al., 1972). Thus, urinary excretion in selenium deficiency may reflect immediate selenium intake more than nutritional selenium status. This limits the utility of urinary selenium measurements.

Labeled Selenium

Uptake of selenium-75 (^{75}Se) by erythrocytes in vitro has been studied (Wright and Bell, 1963) as an indicator of selenium status. Although this method showed validity in sheep (Wright and Bell, 1963), its value in other species, including humans, has not been demonstrated (Burk et al., 1967).

FACTORS AFFECTING THE SELENIUM REQUIREMENT

Bioavailability

Most dietary selenium is highly bioavailable. Selenomethionine, which is estimated to account for at least half of the dietary selenium, is absorbed by the same mechanism as methionine, and its selenium is made available for selenoprotein synthesis when it is catabolized via the transsulfuration pathway (Esaki et al., 1982). The bioavailability of selenium in the form of selenomethionine is greater than 90 percent (Thomson and Robinson, 1986). The selenium in selenocysteine, another significant dietary form, is also highly bioavailable (Swanson et al., 1991). There appear to be some minor dietary forms of selenium (especially present in fish) that have relatively low bioavailability, but these forms have not been identified (Cantor and Tarino, 1982). Selenate and selenite, two inorganic forms of selenium, have roughly equivalent bioavailability which generally exceeds 50 percent (Thomson and Robinson, 1986). Although they are not major dietary constituents, these inorganic forms are commonly used as selenium supplements.

Gender

Earlier reports from China (Ge et al., 1983), from a time when selenium deficiency was more severe than in recent years, indicated that women of childbearing age were susceptible to developing Keshan disease, whereas men were resistant. However, cases of the disease reported in the past 20 years appear to be limited to children, with equal prevalence in boys and girls (Cheng and Qian, 1990). Thus, a gender effect in susceptibility to this disease may be present at extremely low selenium intakes, but no such effect has been demonstrated at current intakes. Given women's apparently increased susceptibility to Keshan disease, selenium requirements for the various age groups are based on male reference weights.

FINDINGS BY LIFE STAGE AND GENDER GROUP

Infants Ages 0 through 12 Months

Method Used to Set the Adequate Intake

No functional criteria of selenium status have been demonstrated that reflect response to dietary intake in infants. Thus, recommended intakes of selenium are based on an Adequate Intake (AI) that reflects the observed mean selenium intake of infants fed principally with human milk.

Human milk is recognized as the optimal milk source for infants throughout at least the first year of life and is recommended as the sole nutritional milk source for infants during the first 4 to 6 months of life (IOM, 1991). Therefore, determination of the AI for selenium for infants is based on data from infants fed human milk as the principal fluid during periods 0 through 6 and 7 through 12 months of age. The AI is the mean value of observed intakes as calculated from data on the selenium content of human milk and other studies which estimated the volume typically consumed as determined by test weighing of infants in the age category. In the age group 7 through 12 months, an amount is added for the contribution to intake of selenium obtained from weaning foods.

Average selenium concentrations of human milk consumed by infants at different ages are shown in Table 7-1. In general, the selenium content of human milk is highest in colostrum (33 to 80 µg [0.4 to 1.0 µmol]/L) (Ellis et al., 1990; Higashi et al., 1983; Hojo, 1986; Smith et al., 1982), whereas concentrations in transitional milk at 1 week (18 to 29 µg [0.2 to 0.4 µmol]/L) are less than half those of colostrum (Ellis et al., 1990; Higashi et al., 1983; Hojo, 1986). There is wide interindividual variation in the selenium content of human milk (Higashi et al., 1983), and the selenium content of hind milk (milk at the end of an infant feeding) is greater than that of the fore milk (milk at the beginning of the feeding) (Smith et al., 1982).

Selenium is also present in human milk in extracellular glutathione peroxidase (GSHPx-3) (Avissar et al., 1991), but the distribution of selenium among milk proteins needs further characterization. It is also likely that a large and variable fraction of milk selenium is present as selenomethionine substituting for methionine as has been described for plasma.

The average selenium content of mature human milk sampled between 2 and 6 months lactation appears to be relatively constant within a population group (Debski et al., 1989; Funk et al., 1990). However, human milk selenium varies with maternal selenium intake. Selenium concentrations in mature human milk in Finnish women consuming 30, 50, or 100 µg (0.4, 0.6, or 1.3 µmol)/day of selenium were 6, 11, or 14 µg (0.08, 0.14, or 0.18 µmol)/L of selenium, respectively (Kumpulainen et al., 1983, 1984, 1985). Other studies reported average selenium concentrations of mature human milk of 10 to 23 µg/L (with a range of 6 to 39 µg/L) (Cumming et al., 1992; Debski et al., 1989; Ellis et al., 1990; Funk et al., 1990; Higashi et al., 1983; Hojo, 1986; Levander et al., 1987; Mannan and Picciano, 1987; Smith et al., 1982).

The average selenium content of human milk from mothers in Canada and the United States was 15 to 20 µg (0.19 to 0.25 µmol)/L (Levander et al., 1987; Mannan and Picciano, 1987; Smith et al., 1982). An older study analyzed human milk samples from women living in 17 states in the United States. The authors reported mean milk selenium values to be 28 µg (0.35 µmol)/L in areas with high soil selenium content and 13 µg (0.16 µmol)/L in areas with low

TABLE 7-1 Selenium Content of Human Milk

Reference	Selenium Content of Milk (µg/L)	Stage of Lactation
Shearer and Hadjimarkos, 1975	18 (7–60)	17–869 d
Smith et al., 1982[a]	41.2 ± 17.3	1–4 d (colostrum), from a different sample of women
	18 ± 3.8	1 mo
	15.7 ± 4.6	2 mo
	15.1 ± 5.8	3 mo
Higashi et al., 1983[b]	80 (35–152)	Day 1 (colostrum)
	29 (15–79)	1 wk (transitional milk)
	18 (9–39)	1 mo
	17 (6–28)	3 mo
	18 (9–33)	5 mo
Kumpulainen et al., 1983	10.7 ± 1.6 (SD[c])	1 mo
	5.8 ± 1.2	3 mo
	5.6 ± 0.4	6 mo
Kumpulainen et al., 1984	11.8 ± 1.7	1 mo
	10.9 ± 1.9	2 mo
	10.0 ± 1.9	3 mo
Kumpulainen et al., 1985	13–14	2 mo
Hojo, 1986[e]	34.2 ± 12.8	4 d (colostrum)
	24.0 ± 4.2	7–8 d (transitional milk)
	22.5 ± 4.2	36–86 d
Levander et al., 1987	20 ± 1 (SEM[g])	1 mo
	15 ± 1	3 mo
	15 ± 1	6 mo

Maternal Selenium Intake (µg/d)	Methods
Not reported	$n = 241$ mothers from 17 states, ages 17–44
Not reported	$n = 8$ human milk-fed infants and their mothers who provided 72 milk samples Stage of lactation and time of day had no effect on milk Se
Not reported; thought to be comparable to American intakes	$n = 22$ Japanese healthy full-term infants and their mothers, aged 22–34 Women were from the same geographical area Wide interindividual variation in milk Se content Also measured serum level: mean serum level in mothers at 3 mo pp = 14.8 ± 4.7 µg/dL; level in control subjects = 13.5 ± 1.9 µg/dL
36 ± 13 (6–8 wk pp) 30 ± 12 (17–22 wk pp)	$n = 13$ Finnish human milk-fed infants and their mothers Dietary intake based on 7-d food records
50 (average Finnish dietary selenium intake)	$n = 46$ human milk samples from 31 Finnish mothers
100 (yeast-Se supplement)	$n = 200$ Finnish healthy full-term infants and their mothers Three groups: no supplement, 100 µg/d yeast-Se, and 100 µg/d selenite. Highest milk content values were found in the yeast-Se group. In the no-supplement group, the peak milk content (7.2) was reached at 6 mo pp[d]
Not reported	$n = 5$ Japanese healthy full-term infants and their mothers, aged 25–28 Also measured GSHPx[f] levels in milk. GSHPx levels were highest in colostrum and decreased with increasing time of lactation Urinary Se was not associated with milk Se or GSHPx
84 ± 4 84 ± 4 87 ± 4	$n = 23$ lactating mothers with healthy full-term deliveries, aged 18–36 Also examined 13 nonlactating women Dietary intake was based on duplicate food and drink composites and food records

continued

TABLE 7-1 Continued

Reference	Selenium Content of Milk (µg/L)	Stage of Lactation
Mannan and Picciano, 1987[a]	15.6 ± 0.4 (fore) 18.1 ± 0.6 (hind)	4, 8, 12, and 16 wk
Debski et al., 1989	22.2 ± 0.8 (SEM) (vegetarians) 16.8 ± 1.3 (nonvegetarians)	Any 9 consecutive mo during 1–26 mo lactation
Ellis et al., 1990	32.8 ± 3.2 26.4 ± 1.6 24.0 ± 1.6 21.6 ± 1.6	3 d 7 d 21 d 42 d
Funk et al., 1990	15.5 21.3 17.8 19.7	1–6 mo (rainy season) 1–6 mo (dry season) 13–19 mo (rainy season) 13–19 mo (dry season)
Cumming et al., 1992	11.9 ± 3.5 (SD)	6–12 wk
Jochum et al., 1995	9.9 ± 0.5	4 mo

[a] Hind milk selenium concentration greater than that in fore milk.
[b] Lack of correlation between human milk and serum selenium concentration.
[c] SD = standard deviation.
[d] pp = postpartum.

Maternal Selenium Intake (μg/d)	Methods
Not reported	n = 10 healthy mothers with normal term pregnancies, mean age = 30 Values from weeks 4, 8, 12, and 16 were pooled No Se supplements taken during pregnancy or lactation Measured GSHPx in milk—similar pattern as milk Se Also looked at plasma and erythrocyte levels of Se and GSHPx
101 ± 6 (vegetarians) 106 ± 5 (nonvegetarians)	n = 26 vegetarian and 12 nonvegetarian healthy lactating mothers, mean age = 29 Dietary intake based on 2-d intake records Milk Se content is based on undialyzed milk; values for dialyzed milk samples were similar for both vegetarians and nonvegetarians
Not reported	n = 10 term infants and their mothers Also examined preterm and very preterm infants Also measured GSHPx activity and protein content in milk
Food scarcity Food abundance Food scarcity Food abundance	n = 55 Gambian women; multiparous Milk Se was higher in the dry season Milk Se was lower in the rainy season, but only during early lactation (1–6 mo). The seasonal effect diminished during late lactation (13–19 mo) There was a negative correlation between parity and milk Se during late lactation regardless of season Protein, GSHPx, and Px were not affected by state of lactation or parity
Informal dietary assessment	n = 20 Australian human milk-fed infants and their mothers, aged 17–38 Hind milk Se was significantly greater than fore milk Se Blood and serum Se also measured
Not reported	n = 50 German healthy term infants exclusively fed human milk No change in plasma Se from birth to 4 mo Significant decrease in erythrocyte and plasma GSHPx activity from birth to 4 mo

[e] Positive correlation between human milk selenium and GSHPx.
[f] GSHPx = selenium-dependent glutathione peroxidases.
[g] SEM = standard error of the mean.

soil selenium content, with an overall average concentration of 18 µg (0.23 µmol)/L (Shearer and Hadjimarkos, 1975).

Ages 0 through 6 Months

There are no reports of full-term American or Canadian infants exclusively and freely fed human milk who manifest signs of selenium deficiency. The AI for infants ages 0 through 6 months is based on an average volume of milk intake for this age group of 0.78 L/ day (Allen et al., 1991; Butte et al., 1984; Heinig et al., 1993) and an average concentration of selenium in human milk of 18 µg (0.23 µmol)/L (Levander et al., 1987; Mannan and Picciano, 1987; Shearer and Hadjimarkos, 1975; Smith et al., 1982). Using the average selenium concentration of milk of well-nourished but unsupplemented mothers, 18 µg (0.23 µmol)/L, the AI for infants 0 through 6 months of age would be 18 µg/L × 0.78 L/day = 14 µg/day, rounded up to 15 µg (0.19 µmol)/day.

Ages 7 through 12 Months

One method of estimating the AI for infants in the second half of the first year of life is to utilize the method described in Chapter 3 to extrapolate from the AI for infants ages 0 through 6 months and rounding. By this method, the AI for infants ages 7 through 12 months is 20 µg (0.25 µmol)/day.

An alternative method is to calculate the estimated selenium intake from human milk and infant foods. The selenium content of mature human milk remains relatively constant during the first year of lactation (Debski et al., 1989; Funk et al., 1990). Therefore, if 18 µg (0.23 µmol)/L selenium is the average human milk content in the United States and Canada (Shearer and Hadjimarkos, 1975) and 0.6 L/day is the usual amount of human milk consumed by infants 7 through 12 months of age (Dewey et al., 1984), the selenium intake from human milk would be 11 µg (0.14 µmol)/day.

The selenium content of the usual intakes of complementary weaning foods can be calculated as follows. The average daily caloric intake in this age group is 845 kcal (Fomon and Anderson, 1974). Calories provided by human milk would be 450 kcal (0.6 L of human milk × 0.75 kcal/mL) (Fomon and Anderson, 1974). Thus, the caloric content of the usual intake of complementary weaning foods would be 845 − 450 = 395 kcal.

There is one report in which the selenium content of infant food was analyzed. The total selenium intake of 20 apparently healthy

German infants and children 5 to 20 months old was reported to be 34 µg (0.4 µmol)/day; the median selenium content of the food was 27 ng (0.34 nmol)/g wet weight (Lombeck et al., 1984). By using this same selenium content for U.S. infant food and assuming an average of 1 kcal/g in infant foods, the average daily selenium intake from infant food in the second half of the first year of life would be 11 µg (0.027 µg/kcal × 395 kcal). Thus, 11 µg (0.14 µmol) from food + 11 µg (0.14 µmol) from human milk = 22 µg (0.28 µmol)/day. This is comparable to the value calculated above by extrapolating from the AI for infants 0 through 6 months, and is in the same range as the amount calculated by Levander (1976) of 28 µg (0.35 µmol)/day for a 6 month old consuming whole milk and weaning foods.

Selenium AI Summary, Ages 0 through 12 Months

AI for Infants

0–6 months	**15 µg (0.19 µmol)/day of selenium**	**≈ 2.1 µg/kg**
7–12 months	**20 µg (0.25 µmol)/day of selenium**	**≈ 2.2 µg/kg**

Children and Adolescents Ages 1 through 18 Years

Evidence Considered in Estimating the Average Requirement

No data were found on which to base an Estimated Average Requirement (EAR) for selenium for children or adolescents. In the absence of additional information, EARs and Recommended Dietary Allowances (RDAs) for children and adolescents have been estimated using the method described in Chapter 3, which extrapolates from adult values. As noted above, most selenium in the diet is metabolized by a mechanism similar to that of methionine. Therefore, the formulas used for determining selenium requirements for children are the metabolic formulas rather than those based upon weights alone. Given the reported slightly increased susceptibility of females to developing Keshan disease, selenium requirements for the various age groups are based on the higher reference weights for males.

The EAR is thus determined based on the same criteria of adequacy as adults, that of selenium intakes that would be expected to maximize plasma glutathione peroxidase activity.

It is important to discuss these recommendations in the context of knowledge regarding the amount of dietary selenium necessary to prevent Keshan disease. This disease occurs in young selenium-deficient Chinese children, which suggests that these children have the greatest need for selenium of any individuals in the population. Studies in China indicate that Keshan disease does not occur in populations with a per capita adult selenium intake of 17 µg (0.22 µmol)/day or greater (Yang et al., 1987). Thus the calculated EARs listed below should be sufficient to prevent Keshan disease in all children.

Selenium EAR and RDA Summary, Ages 1 through 18 Years

EAR for Children
  1–3 years   17 µg (0.22 µmol)/day of selenium
  4–8 years   23 µg (0.29 µmol)/day of selenium
EAR for Boys
  9–13 years   35 µg (0.45 µmol)/day of selenium
  14–18 years   45 µg (0.57 µmol)/day of selenium
EAR for Girls
  9–13 years   35 µg (0.45 µmol)/day of selenium
  14–18 years   45 µg (0.57 µmol)/day of selenium

The RDA for selenium is set by assuming a coefficient of variation (CV) of 10 percent (see Chapter 1) because information is not available on the standard deviation of the requirement for selenium; the RDA is defined as equal to the EAR plus twice the CV to cover the needs of 97 to 98 percent of the individuals in the group (therefore, for selenium the RDA is 120 percent of the EAR). The calculated RDA is rounded to the nearest 5 µg.

RDA for Children
  1–3 years   20 µg (0.25 µmol)/day of selenium
  4–8 years   30 µg (0.38 µmol)/day of selenium
RDA for Boys
  9–13 years   40 µg (0.51 µmol)/day of selenium
  14–18 years   55 µg (0.70 µmol)/day of selenium
RDA for Girls
  9–13 years   40 µg (0.51 µmol)/day of selenium
  14–18 years   55 µg (0.70 µmol)/day of selenium

Adults Ages 19 through 50 Years

Evidence Considered in Estimating the Average Requirement

Twenty years ago, efforts to estimate human selenium requirements could produce only an estimated safe and adequate daily intake range that was based on extrapolations from experimentally determined selenium requirements of animals (NRC, 1980b). Since then, Keshan disease has been reported to be a disease of selenium deficiency in humans, and estimates of the selenium intake needed to prevent it have been made. Also, a number of selenoproteins, many of them enzymes with important functions, have been identified. These selenoproteins require selenium for their synthesis and for maintenance of their activities in tissues. As discussed earlier, two plasma selenoproteins (glutathione peroxidase and selenoprotein P) can serve as indices of selenium status and have been measured in individuals consuming varying amounts of selenium.

Surveys in China have compared per capita daily selenium intakes of adults in Keshan disease areas with intakes in adjacent areas that were free of the disease (Yang and Xia, 1995; Yang et al., 1987). Adult subjects living in the affected areas were found to have selenium intakes of 11 µg (0.14 µmol)/day or less, while those living in unaffected areas had intakes of 17 µg (0.22 µmol)/day or more. Thus, based on one Chinese study, no selenium-responsive disease is known to occur in populations with adult intakes as low as 17 µg (0.22 µmol)/day.

Additional results from China and elsewhere indicate that intakes of 20 µg (0.25 µmol)/day and greater protect adults against the development of Keshan disease (Yang et al., 1987). In New Zealand and Finland, intakes by adults as low as 25 µg (0.32 µmol)/day have been reported without the occurrence of Keshan disease (Griffiths, 1973; Varo et al., 1994).

Plasma glutathione peroxidase and selenoprotein P were measured in a population in which Keshan disease was endemic (Hill et al., 1996; Xia et al., 1989). Survey results estimated that per capita selenium intake of adults was 11 µg (0.14 µmol)/day in this population. Table 7-2 compares plasma selenium concentration, glutathione peroxidase activity, and selenoprotein P concentrations in boys aged 8 to 12 years and adult males residing in a Keshan disease area with corresponding values in a nearby area free of the disease. Males living in the disease-free area had been supplemented with inorganic selenium for 14 days (100 µg [1.3 µmol]/day for the boys and 200 µg [2.5 µmol]/day for the men). In the endemic area, selenoprotein P concentration in boys and men was 13 percent and 23 percent, respectively, of that in the unaffected selenium supplemented area. Glutathione peroxidase activities were 26 percent in the boys and 37 percent in the men, compared to these activities in the boys and men in the unaffected area. Plasma selenium concen-

TABLE 7-2 Plasma Selenium Indices in Boys and Men in Two Areas of China: (1) A Selenium-Deficient Area Where Keshan Disease Was Endemic and (2) an Area Supplemented with Inorganic Selenium

	Plasma Selenium (μg/dL)	Plasma Glutathione Peroxidase (U/L[a])	Plasma Selenoprotein P (U/L)
Boys (aged 8–12)			
Low-selenium area	1.3 ± 0.5	29 ± 15	0.10 ± 0.04
Supplemented area	6.3 ± 1.5	111 ± 21	0.76 ± 0.27
Low selenium/supplemented, %	21	26	13
Men (aged 17 and over)			
Low-selenium area	1.6 ± 0.4	51 ± 16	0.13 ± 0.04
Supplemented area	6.8 ± 1.0	137 ± 15	0.57 ± 0.13
Low selenium/supplemented, %	24	37	23

[a] Reference plasma contains 1 unit (U) selenoprotein P/L.
SOURCES: Hill et al. (1996); Xia et al. (1989).

trations were 21 percent of the supplemented values in the boys and 24 percent in the men.

These results show that biochemical functions of selenium are compromised in populations in which Keshan disease occurs. The results also show that development of the disease is possible in populations in which plasma glutathione peroxidase activities in adult males are as high as 37 percent of supplemented values. Finally, selenoprotein P concentrations appear to be more severely affected by selenium deficiency than is glutathione peroxidase activity.

Animal studies indicate that plasma selenoproteins reflect the activities of tissue selenoenzymes (Yang et al., 1989). It can therefore be argued that plateau concentrations of selenoenzymes in tissues would correlate with plateau concentrations of plasma selenoproteins. Xia et al. (1989) found that Keshan disease can occur in populations that have a plasma glutathione peroxidase activity in men that is 37 percent of maximum values. This would not leave a large margin of error if less than 100 percent of plasma glutathione peroxidase activity is deemed acceptable. For these two reasons, plateau concentration of plasma selenoproteins is chosen as the indicator for determining the selenium requirement.

Intervention Studies

Two intervention studies, one in China and one in New Zealand, have been done to assess the selenium intake required to achieve plateau concentrations of plasma selenoproteins.

China Study. In 1983, Yang et al. (1987) conducted an intervention study of selenium supplementation in China. Because the primary data from this study could not be obtained, interpretation of the results is based on a graph in the publication. The population consisted of men aged 18 to 42 years with dietary selenium intakes of 11 µg (0.14 µmol)/day and plasma glutathione peroxidase activities that were approximately 35 percent of the values reached after supplementation with the maximum amount of selenium. The men were studied in groups of eight to nine and were given selenium supplements of 0, 10, 30, 60, and 90 µg (0, 0.13, 0.38, 0.76, 1.14 µmol)/day as DL-selenomethionine for 8 months. Plasma glutathione peroxidase activities increased in all groups supplemented with selenium. The plasma enzyme activities in the groups given 30, 60, and 90 µg (0.38, 0.76, 1.14 µmol)/day increased and converged after the fourth month, whereas activities in the other two groups remained lower. This suggests that at a daily intake of 41 µg (0.52 µmol)/of selenium (11 µg [0.14 µmol] from diet plus 30 µg [0.38 µmol] from supplement), the activity of plasma glutathione peroxidase reaches a plateau in adult Chinese males with an estimated weight of 60 kg. With a weight adjustment for North American males (41 µg (0.52 µmol)/day × 76 kg/60 kg), this value would translate to 52 µg (0.66 µmol)/day.

New Zealand Study. A study in New Zealand examined 52 adults (17 men and 35 women) aged 19 to 59 years with a mean selenium intake of 28 ± 15 µg (standard deviation [SD]) (0.35 ± 0.19 µmol)/day and initial plasma glutathione peroxidase activities that were approximately 75 percent of the values after selenium supplementation. The subjects were given 0, 10, 20, 30, or 40 µg (0, 0.13, 0.25, 0.38, 0.51 µmol)/day of selenium as selenomethionine for 20 weeks (with about 10 subjects per group) (Duffield et al., 1999).

An independent analysis of the study data (Duffield et al., 1999), which were generously provided by the investigators, has been conducted for this report. Regression analysis indicates that plasma glutathione peroxidase activities of the supplemented groups were higher than those of the placebo group, although the magnitude of the differences was small relative to the variation of values between indi-

viduals in the same supplemented group. Selenium supplementation increased the plasma glutathione peroxidase activity because
the increase in the activity relative to presupplementation was apparent for nearly every supplemented individual. However, the increase
at the lowest level tested (10 µg [0.13 µmol]/day) could not be
statistically differentiated from the increase at the highest level tested (40 µg [0.51 µmol]/day). Thus, choosing to be conservative, an
EAR of 38 µg (0.48 µmol) (28 µg [0.35 µmol]/day from food + 10 µg
[0.13 µmol]/day from the lowest level supplemented) was selected.

Summary. Calculation of an EAR for selenium is based on the
results of two intervention studies that were done in different countries but had similar designs. The Chinese study suggests that a
plateau of plasma glutathione peroxidase activity was reached with
a selenium intake of 41 µg (0.52 µmol)/day. With a weight adjustment for North American males, the selenium intake was 52 µg
(0.66 µmol)/day. The New Zealand study can be interpreted to
suggest an EAR in the vicinity of 38 µg (0.48 µmol)/day. The average of those studies, 45 µg (0.57 µmol), has been chosen as the
EAR.

Selenium EAR and RDA Summary, Ages 19 through 50 Years

Based on the criterion of maximizing plasma glutathione peroxidase activity, the data described above support a selenium EAR of
45 µg/day for the age group 19 through 50 years based on the
weights of North American men. Given the reported greater susceptibility of women to develop Keshan disease and the fact that the
data used to set the EAR came largely from men, selenium requirements for both males and females are based on the higher reference weights for males.

EAR for Men
      19–30 years   **45 µg (0.57 µmol)/day of selenium**
      31–50 years   **45 µg (0.57 µmol)/day of selenium**
EAR for Women
      19–30 years   **45 µg (0.57 µmol)/day of selenium**
      31–50 years   **45 µg (0.57 µmol)/day of selenium**

The RDA for selenium is set by assuming a coefficient of variation
(CV) of 10 percent (see Chapter 1) because information is not available on the standard deviation of the requirement for selenium; the
RDA is defined as equal to the EAR plus twice the CV to cover the
needs of 97 to 98 percent of the individuals in the group (there-

fore, for selenium the RDA is 120 percent of the EAR). The calculated RDA is rounded to the nearest 5 µg.

RDA for Men
    19–30 years   55 µg (0.70 µmol)/day of selenium
    31–50 years   55 µg (0.70 µmol)/day of selenium
RDA for Women
    19–30 years   55 µg (0.70 µmol)/day of selenium
    31–50 years   55 µg (0.70 µmol)/day of selenium

Adults Ages 51 Years and Older

Evidence Considered in Estimating the Average Requirement

Adults ages 51 years and older appear to have the same selenium requirement as younger adults. No pathological conditions related to selenium insufficiency have been reported in older individuals, and markers of selenium status in blood do not differ by age or gender (Hill et al., 1996).

Selenium EAR and RDA Summary, Ages 51 Years and Older

Data from intervention studies support an EAR for the age group 51 years and older of 45 µg/day. The aging process does not appear to impair selenium absorption or utilization.

EAR for Men
    51–70 years   45 µg (0.57 µmol)/day of selenium
    >70 years   45 µg (0.57 µmol)/day of selenium
EAR for Women
    51–70 years   45 µg (0.57 µmol)/day of selenium
    >70 years   45 µg (0.57 µmol)/day of selenium

The RDA for selenium is set by assuming a coefficient of variation (CV) of 10 percent (see Chapter 1) because information is not available on the standard deviation of the requirement for selenium; the RDA is defined as equal to the EAR plus twice the CV to cover the needs of 97 to 98 percent of the individuals in the group (therefore, for selenium the RDA is 120 percent of the EAR). The calculated RDA is rounded to the nearest 5 µg.

RDA for Men
    51–70 years   55 µg (0.70 µmol)/day of selenium
    >70 years   55 µg (0.70 µmol)/day of selenium

RDA for Women
        51–70 years   55 µg (0.70 µmol)/day of selenium
        >70 years   55 µg (0.70 µmol)/day of selenium

Pregnancy

Evidence Considered in Estimating the Average Requirement

Few studies provide information about the selenium requirements of pregnant women. However, the pregnancy requirement should allow accumulation of enough selenium by the fetus to saturate its selenoproteins. Based on an estimated selenium content of 250 µg (3.2 µmol)/kg body weight (Schroeder et al., 1970), a 4-kg fetus would contain 1,000 µg (12.6 µmol) of selenium. This need could be met by an additional 4 µg (0.05 µmol)/day of selenium over the 270 days of the pregnancy. Based on this, an additional requirement of 4 µg (0.05 µmol)/day during pregnancy is estimated.

Reported selenium intakes of uncomplicated pregnancies have varied considerably. Levander et al. (1987) found that the average selenium intake of apparently healthy pregnant females in the United States was 73 µg (0.92 µmol)/day. Swanson et al. (1983) have shown that mean selenium retention in women fed a high-selenium diet (150 µg [1.9 µmol]/day) was 21 µg (0.27 µmol)/day in early pregnancy and 34 µg (0.43 µmol)/day in late pregnancy compared to 11 µg (0.14 µmol)/day for nonpregnant females. However, mean selenium intakes as low as 28 µg (0.35 µmol)/day have been reported for pregnant women in New Zealand without obvious ill effects for the newborn (Thomson and Robinson, 1980).

Selenium EAR and RDA, Pregnancy

Based on a fetal deposition of 4 µg (0.05 µmol)/day throughout pregnancy, the EAR is increased by 4 µg (0.05 µmol)/day during pregnancy. Since most selenium is highly bioavailable, no adjustment is made for absorption. No adjustment is made for the age of the mother.

EAR for Pregnancy
        14–18 years   49 µg (0.62 µmol)/day of selenium
        19–30 years   49 µg (0.62 µmol)/day of selenium
        31–50 years   49 µg (0.62 µmol)/day of selenium

The RDA for selenium is set by assuming a coefficient of variation (CV) of 10 percent (see Chapter 1) because information is not available on the standard deviation of the requirement for selenium; the RDA is defined as equal to the EAR plus twice the CV to cover the needs of 97 to 98 percent of the individuals in the group (therefore, for selenium the RDA is 120 percent of the EAR). The calculated RDA is rounded to the nearest 5 µg.

RDA for Pregnancy
14–18 years	60 µg (0.76 µmol)/day of selenium
19–30 years	60 µg (0.76 µmol)/day of selenium
31–50 years	60 µg (0.76 µmol)/day of selenium

Lactation

Evidence Considered in Estimating the Average Requirement

As previously noted, human milk selenium concentration appears to be about 18 µg (0.23 µmol)/L in Canada and the United States (Levander et al., 1987; Mannan and Picciano, 1987; Shearer and Hadjimarkos, 1975; Smith et al., 1982). The average daily milk consumption in months 2 to 6 of lactation by infants is 0.78 L, so the average amount of selenium secreted in milk would be 14 µg (0.18 µmol)/day. Since most selenium in human milk is present as selenomethionine, which has a bioavailability greater than 90 percent (Thomson and Robinson, 1980), no adjustment is made for absorption. Therefore an increment of 14 µg (0.18 µmol)/day of selenium over the adult EAR is set for lactation.

Although the amount of selenium in human milk varies with the mother's selenium intake, mean intakes as low as 4.7 µg (60 nmol)/day selenium in exclusively human milk-fed infants in Finland are not associated with selenium deficiency symptoms (Kumpulainen et al., 1983).

Selenium EAR and RDA Summary, Lactation

To estimate the EAR for lactation, 14 µg (0.18 µmol)/day of selenium is added to the EAR of 45 µg/day for the nonpregnant and nonlactating woman, giving an EAR of 59 µg (0.75 µmol)/day. No distinction is made for bioavailability or age of the mother.

EAR for Lactation
14–18 years	59 µg (0.75 µmol)/day of selenium
19–30 years	59 µg (0.75 µmol)/day of selenium
31–50 years	59 µg (0.75 µmol)/day of selenium

The RDA for selenium is set by assuming a coefficient of variation (CV) of 10 percent (see Chapter 1) because information is not available on the standard deviation of the requirement for selenium; the RDA is defined as equal to the EAR plus twice the CV to cover the needs of 97 to 98 percent of the individuals in the group (therefore, for selenium the RDA is 120 percent of the EAR). The calculated RDA is rounded to the nearest 5 µg.

RDA for Lactation

14–18 years	**70 µg (0.89 µmol)/day of selenium**
19–30 years	**70 µg (0.89 µmol)/day of selenium**
31–50 years	**70 µg (0.89 µmol)/day of selenium**

INTAKE OF SELENIUM

Food Sources

The selenium content of food varies depending on the selenium content of the soil where the animal was raised or the plant was grown: organ meats and seafood, 0.4 to 1.5 µg/g; muscle meats, 0.1 to 0.4 µg/g; cereals and grains, less than 0.1 to greater than 0.8 µg/g; dairy products, less than 0.1 to 0.3 µg/g; and fruits and vegetables, less than 0.1 µg/g (WHO, 1987). Thus the same foodstuffs may have more than a ten-fold difference in selenium content. Plants do not appear to require selenium and most selenium metabolism by plants occurs through sulfur pathways in which selenium substitutes for sulfur. Thus, plant content of selenium depends on the availability of the element in the soil where the plant was grown. This means that wheat grown in a low-selenium soil will have a low selenium content, whereas the same wheat variety grown in a high-selenium soil will have a high selenium content. For this reason, food tables that reflect average selenium contents are unreliable. Much plant selenium is in the form of selenomethionine, selenocysteine, or selenocysteine metabolites. Other organic forms of the element are known to exist, including some that have not yet been identified.

Unlike plants, animals require selenium. Meat and seafood are therefore reliable dietary sources of selenium. Meat and seafood contain selenium in its functional form as selenoproteins. Virtually all animal proteins contain selenomethionine obtained when the animal consumes selenium from plants. This means that meat varies in its selenium content depending largely on the selenomethionine intake of the animal.

Dietary Intake

Intake from Food

The dietary selenium intakes in the United States and Canada have been estimated in several studies. A detailed evaluation of diets consumed by 22 Maryland residents (using direct selenium analysis) indicated that selenium intake was 81 ± 41 (SD) µg (1.0 ± 0.5 µmol)/day (Welsh et al., 1981). The Food and Drug Administration analyzed food items purchased in different regions of the United States over the period 1982 to 1991 and calculated dietary selenium intake from those results (Pennington and Schoen, 1996). The median calculated intake was 87 µg (1.1 µmol)/day with a range of 79 to 104 µg (1.0 to 1.3 µmol)/day in different years. These results support those of the Maryland study generally, but do not provide an indication of the extremes of selenium intake in the United States.

The Third National Health and Nutrition Examination Survey (NHANES III) intake data (Appendix Tables C-6 and C-7) reported higher median selenium intakes of 106 µg (1.3 µmol)/day from food and 108 µg (1.4 µmol)/day from food and supplements for all individuals based on dietary recall and food tables, but this method has low accuracy as discussed earlier. Selenium intake in Canada has been reported to be somewhat higher than U.S. intake, 113 to 220 µg (1.4 to 2.8 µmol)/day (Thompson et al., 1975).

Dietary intake of selenium varies tremendously among different populations. Factors that affect the intake include the geographic origin of the food items and the meat content of the diet. The lowest selenium intakes are in populations that eat vegetarian diets consisting of plants grown in low-selenium areas. Selenium-deficient Chinese populations live in low-selenium areas and are generally too poor to eat meat or to purchase food grown in other regions. Dietary intake of selenium in the United States and Canada varies by region but is buffered by the food distribution system. Thus, extensive transport of food throughout Canada and the United States prevents low-selenium geographic areas from having low dietary selenium intakes.

Intake from Water

Drinking water has been analyzed in the United States and several countries and does not supply nutritionally significant amounts of selenium (Bratakos et al., 1988; NRC, 1980a; Robberecht et al.,

1983). Tap water is routinely used throughout the United States and Canada to raise selenium-deficient experimental animals. This is evidence that it contains very little selenium. In specific locales, however, water wells have been shown to supply much greater amounts of selenium. This is thought to result from irrigation practices, mining, or the presence of selenium-containing rocks (Valentine et al., 1978). Such high-selenium water supplies appear to be very limited and do not contribute to the selenium intake of large numbers of people (NRC, 1976).

Serum Concentrations

Information from NHANES III on serum selenium concentrations in a free-living population is given in Appendix Table F-3. Serum or plasma selenium concentrations greater than the 0.8 to 1.1 µmol/L (7 to 9 µg/dL) plateau concentration are associated with maximization of plasma selenoproteins (Hill et al., 1996). The NHANES III median serum selenium concentration was 1.4 µmol/L (12.4 µg/dL) for 17,630 subjects aged 9 to more than 70 years. The first percentile was 1.1 µmol/L (9.5 µg/dL) and the ninety-ninth percentile was 1.9 µmol/L (16.3 µg/dL). This shows that at least 99 percent of these subjects should have had maximal concentrations of plasma selenoproteins. Thus, the NHANES III serum data and dietary intake data (based on food tables) collected from 1988 to 1992 indicate that the selenium requirement of its participants was being met.

Intake from Supplements

In the United States or Canada, food is generally not fortified with selenium. An exception is proprietary infant formula that is designed to be the sole source of nutrients for the infant. Commercial formula manufacturers typically add selenium to ensure that infants consuming them will have an adequate selenium intake. Total selenium intakes from food plus supplements reported in NHANES III are found in Appendix Table C-7.

Selenium supplements of many strengths and types are available for purchase, and some popular multivitamin preparations contain selenium. However, according to NHANES III, selenium intake from both food (Appendix Table C-6) and food plus supplements (Appendix Table C-7) is above the EAR for most age groups in the United States. In the 1986 National Health Interview Survey, 9 percent of all adults reported use of supplements containing selenium (Moss et al., 1989).

TOLERABLE UPPER INTAKE LEVELS

Hazard Identification

The Tolerable Upper Intake Level (UL) is the highest level of daily nutrient intake that is likely to pose no risk of adverse health effects in almost all individuals. Although members of the general population should be advised not to exceed the UL for selenium routinely, intake above the UL may be appropriate for investigation within well-controlled clinical trials. In light of evaluating possible benefits to health, clinical trials of doses above the UL should not be discouraged, as long as subjects participating in these trials have signed informed consent documents regarding possible toxicity and as long as these trials employ appropriate safety monitoring of trial subjects. Also, the UL is not meant to apply to individuals who are receiving selenium under medical supervision.

Adverse Effects

The Tolerable Upper Intake Level (UL) for selenium pertains to selenium intake from food and supplements. As discussed earlier, drinking water does not contain nutritionally significant amounts of selenium. The data on chronic selenosis, acute toxicity, and biochemical indicators of toxicity are reviewed.

Chronic Selenosis. Chronic toxicity of selenium has been studied in animals and has been observed in humans. The limited data available in humans suggest that chronic toxicities from inorganic and organic forms have similar clinical features but differ in rapidity of onset and relationship to tissue selenium concentrations.

The most frequently reported features of selenosis (chronic toxicity) are hair and nail brittleness and loss (Yang et al., 1983). Other reported signs include gastrointestinal disturbances, skin rash, garlic breath odor (caused by selenium compounds), fatigue, irritability, and nervous system abnormalities (CDC, 1984; Helzlsouer et al., 1985; Jensen et al., 1984; Yang et al., 1983; G.-Q. Yang et al., 1989a).

The high prevalence of selenosis in Enshi, South China, provided an opportunity to study approximately 380 people with high selenium intakes (Yang and Zhou, 1994; G.-Q. Yang et al., 1989a, 1989b). Toxic effects occurred with increasing frequency in people with a blood selenium concentration greater than 12.7 µmol/L (100 µg/ dL), corresponding to a selenium intake above 850 µg/day.

Acute Toxicity Effects. There are a few reports in the literature of acute fatal or near-fatal selenium poisoning with either accidental or suicidal ingestion of selenium, usually in the form of gun blueing solution or sheep drench. Gun blue is a lubricant solution containing selenious acid, nitric acid, and copper nitrate (Ruta and Haider, 1989). Ingestion of this liquid, which would result in ingestion of gram quantities of selenium, is typically followed by severe gastrointestinal and neurological disturbances, acute respiratory distress syndrome, myocardial infarction, and renal failure (Carter, 1966; Lombeck et al., 1987; Matoba et al., 1986; Nantel et al., 1985; Pentel et al., 1985). Autopsy revealed necrosis of gut and kidney, cardiomyopathy, and severe pulmonary edema.

Biochemical Indicators of Selenium Toxicity. Biochemical assessment of high selenium intakes is more difficult than assessment of low intakes. The selenoproteins are maximized when nutritional requirements of the element have been met and do not rise further with additional increments in selenium intake. Thus, measurement of selenoproteins is not useful in assessing potential toxicity.

Measurement of total selenium concentrations in tissue (including plasma and blood) is helpful in assessing the risk of toxicity from dietary selenium. Chinese investigators have correlated blood selenium concentrations with dietary intakes from high-selenium foodstuffs (Yang and Zhou, 1994).

High intakes of selenium in the form of selenomethionine, the major form of selenium in food, lead to large increases in tissue selenium concentrations. These increases are caused by the random incorporation of selenomethionine into proteins in place of methionine as discussed earlier. In contrast, inorganic forms of selenium, usually present in supplements, typically do not cause such high tissue concentrations because these forms of selenium cannot enter the methionine pool. However, inorganic selenium can cause toxicity at tissue levels of selenium much lower than seen with similar intakes of dietary selenium as selenomethionine. Severe toxicity was reported from selenite ingestion that increased blood concentrations by only a small amount (CDC, 1984). Thus, it is necessary to know the chemical form of selenium being ingested in order to use the tissue level of the element to estimate selenium intake due to release of selenium as a result of normal protein metabolism.

Incorporation of dietary selenomethionine into protein delays selenium toxicity. This storage has created the impression that protein-bound dietary selenium is less toxic than inorganic selenium. Although inorganic selenium has greater immediate toxicity than does selenomethionine, both forms are likely to have similar toxicities under conditions of chronic intake.

Methylated selenium metabolites appear in the breath when large quantities of the element are ingested (McConnell and Portman, 1952). These metabolites are responsible for a garlic odor of the breath. Measurement of excretory metabolites of selenium, whether urinary or breath, is subject to significant error, because excretion by these routes is a function of recent intake as well as long-term selenium status. For example, selenium-deficient rats given a single large dose of selenium excrete part of that dose in the breath (Burk et al., 1972). In addition, quantitation of breath selenium excretion has never been linked to selenium toxicity. Based on these considerations, breath selenium cannot be used as an index of selenium toxicity at present, and urinary selenium excretion can be used as an index of toxicity only under carefully controlled conditions.

Summary

Based on considerations of causality, relevance, and the quality and completeness of the database, hair and nail brittleness and loss were selected as the critical endpoints on which to base a UL. Hair and nail brittleness and loss have been reported more frequently than other signs and symptoms of chronic selenosis. Biochemical markers have too much variation to be reliable except under controlled conditions.

Dose-Response Assessment

Adults

Data Selection. A useful data set for determining dose-response of selenium toxicity from food sources was reported by Chinese investigators (Yang and Zhou, 1994). That report consisted of a reexamination (in 1992) of five patients previously found (in 1986) to have overt signs of selenosis: hair loss and nail sloughing. Because the same patients were studied at different times while consuming the same food form of selenium, blood levels of selenium can be compared and dietary intakes can be inferred from blood selenium concentrations.

Identification of a No-Observed-Adverse-Effect Level (NOAEL) and a Lowest-Observed-Adverse-Effects Level (LOAEL). The lowest blood level of selenium measured in the five subjects at initial examination was 13.3 µmol/L (105 µg/dL), corresponding to a selenium intake of 913 µg (12 µmol)/day (range: 913 to 1,907 µg [12 to 24 µmol]/day). The average blood selenium level was 16.9 µmol/L (135 µg/dL). At the time of reexamination in 1992, all five patients were described as recovered from selenium poisoning, although their fingernails reportedly appeared brittle. The mean blood selenium level had decreased to 12.3 µmol/L (97 µg/dL), corresponding to a selenium intake of about 800 µg (10 µmol)/day (range 654 to 952 µg [8.3 to 12 µmol]/day). The lower limit of the 95 percent confidence interval was 600 µg (7.6 µmol)/day.

Yang and Zhou (1994) therefore suggested that 913 µg (12 µmol)/day of selenium intake represents an individual marginal toxic daily selenium intake or LOAEL. They further suggested that the mean selenium intake upon reexamination (800 µg [10 µmol]/day), represented a NOAEL, while 600 µg (7.6 µmol)/day of selenium intake was the lower 95 percent confidence limit for the NOAEL. These values appear reasonable, although the number of subjects was small. Nevertheless, the LOAEL for selenosis in this small data set appears to be representative of the larger data set, and the reexamination of the subjects provides valuable dose-response data. Uncertainty occurs because of the smallness of the data set and because the Chinese subjects may not be typical (e.g., they may be more or less sensitive to selenium than other populations).

Longnecker et al. (1991) studied 142 ranchers, both men and women, from eastern Wyoming and western South Dakota who were recruited to participate and were suspected of having high selenium intakes based on the occurrence of selenosis in livestock raised in that region. Average selenium intake was 239 µg (3 µmol)/day. Dietary intake and selenium in body tissues (whole blood, serum, urine, toenails) were highly correlated. Blood selenium concentrations in this western U.S. population were related to selenium intake in a similar manner to that found in the Chinese studies, presumably because the form of selenium ingested was selenomethionine. No evidence of selenosis was reported, nor were there any alterations in enzyme activities, prothrombin times, or hematology that could be attributed to selenium intake. The highest selenium intake in the study was 724 µg (9 µmol)/day.

It thus appears that a UL based on the Chinese studies is protective for the population in the United States and Canada. Therefore a NOAEL of 800 µg (10 µmol)/day is selected.

Uncertainty Assessment. An uncertainty factor (UF) of 2 was selected to protect sensitive individuals. The toxic effect is not severe, but may not be readily reversible, so a UF greater than 1 is needed.

Derivation of a UL. The NOAEL of 800 μg/day was divided by a UF of 2 to obtain a UL for adults as follows:

$$\frac{\text{NOAEL}}{\text{UF}} = \frac{800 \ \mu g \ / \ \text{day}}{2} = 400 \ \mu g \ / \ \text{day}.$$

Selenium UL Summary, Ages 19 Years and Older

UL for Adults
    19 years and older   **400 μg (5.1 μmol)/day of selenium**

Pregnancy and Lactation

Brätter et al. (1996) studied the effects of selenium intake on metabolism of thyroid hormones in lactating mothers in seleniferous regions in the foothills of the Venezuelan Andes. Selenium intakes ranged from 170 to 980 μg (2.2 to 12.4 μmol)/day. An inverse correlation between selenium intake and free triiodothyronine (FT_3) was observed, but all values were found to be within the normal range.

There are no reports of teratogenicity or selenosis in infants born to mothers with high but not toxic intakes of selenium. Therefore, ULs for pregnant and lactating women are the same as for nonpregnant and nonlactating women (400 μg [5.1 μmol]/day).

Selenium UL Summary, Pregnancy and Lactation

UL for Pregnancy
    14–18 years   **400 μg (5.1 μmol)/day of selenium**
    19 years and older   **400 μg (5.1 μmol)/day of selenium**
UL for Lactation
    14–18 years   **400 μg (5.1 μmol)/day of selenium**
    19 years and older   **400 μg (5.1 μmol)/day of selenium**

Infants and Children

Data Selection. There are several approaches for estimating a UL in human milk-fed infants (Levander, 1989). However, the most conservative approach is to use the data of Shearer and Hadjimarkos (1975).

Identification of a NOAEL. The data of Shearer and Hadjimarkos (1975) showed that a human milk selenium concentration of 60 µg (0.8 µmol)/L was not associated with known adverse effects. Thus, 60 µg (0.8 µmol)/L is the NOAEL selected. Multiplying the NOAEL for infants 0 through 6 months of age by the estimated average intake of human milk of 0.78 L/day results in a NOAEL of 47 µg (0.6 µmol) or approximately 7 µg (90 nmol)/kg/day. This is in agreement with another study by Brätter et al. (1991).

Brätter et al. (1991) studied effects of selenium intake on children in two seleniferous areas of the foothills of the Venezuelan Andes, using Caracas as a control. Mean human milk selenium content was 46 µg (0.6 µmol)/L in Caracas compared to 60 and 90 µg (0.8 and 1.1 µmol)/L in the two seleniferous areas. Mean selenium concentrations in infant blood in the area with the highest adult selenium intake were reported to be intermediate between those seen in the seleniferous and the nonseleniferous regions.

Uncertainty Assessment. There is no evidence that maternal intake associated with a human milk level of 60 µg (0.8 µmol)/L results in infant or maternal toxicity (Shearer and Hadjimarkos, 1975). Therefore, a UF of 1 is specified.

Derivation of a UL. The NOAEL of 47 µg (0.6 µmol)/day was divided by a UF of 1, resulting in a UL of 47 µg (0.6 µmol) or approximately 7 µg (90 nmol)/kg/day for 2 through 6-month-old infants. Thus, the infant UL and the adult UL are similar on a body weight basis. Also, there is no evidence indicating increased sensitivity to selenium toxicity for any age group. Thus, the UL of 7 µg/kg body weight/day was adjusted for older infants, children, and adolescents on the basis of relative body weight as described in Chapter 4 using reference weights from Chapter 1 (Table 1-1). Values have been rounded down to the nearest 5 µg.

Selenium UL Summary, Ages 0 Months through 18 Years

UL for Infants
      0–6 months   **45 µg (0.57 µmol)/day of selenium**
      7–12 months   **60 µg (0.76 µmol)/day of selenium**
UL for Children
      1–3 years   **90 µg (1.1 µmol)/day of selenium**
      4–8 years   **150 µg (1.9 µmol)/day of selenium**
      9–13 years   **280 µg (3.6 µmol)/day of selenium**
UL for Adolescents
      14–18 years   **400 µg (5.1 µmol)/day of selenium**

Intake Assessment

Selenium intake is primarily in the form of food. Reliance on foods grown in high-selenium areas causes selenosis in China (Yang et al., 1983). There are high-selenium areas in the United States, but the U.S. Department of Agriculture has identified them and proscribed their use for raising animals for food. The extensive food distribution system in Canada and the United States ensures that individuals do not eat diets that originate solely from one locality. This moderates the selenium content of diets, even in high-selenium areas.

The study of dietary selenium intake in a high-selenium area (western South Dakota and eastern Wyoming) indicated daily intakes of 68 to 724 µg (0.9 to 9.2 µmol) in 142 subjects (Longnecker et al., 1991). About half the subjects were consuming more than 200 µg (2.5 µmol)/day. No evidence of selenosis was found, even in the subjects consuming the most selenium.

Water selenium content is usually trivial compared to food selenium content. However, irrigation runoff water has been shown to contain significant amounts of selenium when the soil irrigated contains large amounts of the element (Valentine et al., 1978).

Selenium is available over the counter in many doses but usually under 100 µg (1.3 µmol)/dose. Some individuals may consume larger quantities than are recommended by the manufacturer. At least one manufacturing error has been reported to have led to selenium intoxication in 13 people who took a selenium supplement containing 27.3 mg, several hundred times the amount of selenium stated to be in the product (Helzlsouer et al., 1985).

Risk Characterization

The risk of selenium intake above the UL for the U.S. and Canadian populations appears to be small. There is no known seleniferous area in the United States and Canada where there have been recognized cases of selenosis.

Specifically as noted above, there have been no cases of selenosis in the high-selenium areas of Wyoming and South Dakota (Longnecker et al., 1991). There is some potential for selenium intake to exceed the UL in this area. These authors note that selenium intake exceeded 400 µg (5.1 µmol)/day in 12 subjects, with the highest intake being 724 µg (9.2 µmol)/day. Since 724 µg (9.2 µmol)/day is 3.4 standard deviations above the mean intake, intakes this high would be very rare. Even at this level, toxic effects would be unlikely, since the LOAEL is about 900 µg (11.4 µmol)/day, and many people would not be affected even at this level of intake.

Although intakes above the UL indicate an increased level of risk, these intakes—if below the LOAEL—would nevertheless be unlikely to result in observable clinical disease. This is especially true in a population that could self-select for high intake, so that people who might experience symptoms could alter their diets or move. In light of evaluating possible benefits to health, clinical trials at doses of selenium above the UL should not be discouraged, as long as subjects participating in these trials have signed informed consent documents regarding possible toxicity and as long as these trials employ appropriate safety monitoring of trial subjects. Also, the UL is not meant to apply to individuals who are receiving selenium under medical supervision.

RESEARCH RECOMMENDATIONS FOR SELENIUM

• Biomarkers for use in assessment of selenium status are needed to prevent selenium deficiency and selenium toxicity. The relationship of plasma selenoprotein concentrations to graded selenium intakes must be studied in a severely selenium-deficient population in order to establish a more precise dietary selenium requirement. Plasma selenium levels (and other measurements of the element) have to be carried out in subjects fed levels of selenium (both organic and inorganic forms) up to the Tolerable Upper Intake Level (UL). This could validate use of plasma selenium concentrations to assess high levels of selenium intake.

• Since the Recommended Dietary Allowances (RDAs) for children ages 1 through 18 years are extrapolated from the adult RDAs, it is critically important to conduct large-scale studies with children using state-of-the-art biomarkers to assess their selenium requirements.

• Selenium functions largely through selenoproteins. Although the functions of some selenoproteins are known, those of others are not. Moreover, there appear to be a number of selenoproteins that have not yet been characterized. Therefore, the functions of known and new selenoproteins need to be determined.

• At present the recommendation for selenium intake has been set at the amount needed to achieve a plateau of the plasma selenoprotein glutathione peroxidase. Most residents in Canada and the United States can reach this level of selenium intake with their usual diet, but residents of many regions of the world have lower selenium intakes. Research is needed to determine the health consequences of selenium intakes inadequate to allow full selenoprotein expression.

• Limited evidence has been presented that intakes of selenium greater than the amount needed to allow full expression of selenoproteins may have chemopreventive effects against cancer. Controlled intervention studies are needed to fully evaluate selenium as a cancer chemopreventive agent.

REFERENCES

Allen JC, Keller RP, Archer P, Neville MC. 1991. Studies in human lactation: Milk composition and daily secretion rates of macronutrients in the first year of lactation. *Am J Clin Nutr* 54:69–80.

Arteel GE, Mostert V, Oubrahim H, Briviba K, Abel J, Sies H. 1998. Protection by selenoprotein P in human plasma against peroxynitrite-mediated oxidation and nitration. *Biol Chem* 379:1201–1205.

Avissar N, Slemmon JR, Palmer IS, Cohen HJ. 1991. Partial sequence of human plasma glutathione peroxidase and immunologic identification of milk glutathione peroxidase as the plasma enzyme. *J Nutr* 121:1243–1249.

Beck MA, Levander OA. 1998. Dietary oxidative stress and the potentiation of viral infection. *Annu Rev Nutr* 18:93–116.

Behne D, Wolters W. 1983. Distribution of selenium and glutathione peroxidase in the rat. *J Nutr* 113:456–461.

Behne D, Kyriakopoulos A, Kalcklosch M, Weiss-Nowak C, Pfeifer H, Gessner H, Hammel C. 1997. Two new selenoproteins found in the prostatic glandular epithelium and in the spermatid nuclei. *Biomed Environ Sci* 10:340–345.

Berry MJ, Larsen PR. 1992. The role of selenium in thyroid hormone action. *Endocr Rev* 13:207–219.

Blot WJ, Li JY, Taylor PR, Guo W, Dawsey SM, Li B. 1995. The Linxian trials: Mortality rates by vitamin-mineral intervention group. *Am J Clin Nutr* 62:1424S–1426S.

Bösl MR, Takaku K, Oshima M, Nishimura S, Taketo MM. 1997. Early embryonic lethality caused by targeted disruption of the mouse selenocysteine tRNA gene (Trsp). *Proc Natl Acad Sci USA* 94:5531–5534.

Bratakos MS, Zafiropoulos TF, Siskos PA, Ioannou PV. 1988. Total selenium concentration in tap and bottled drinking water and coastal waters of Greece. *Sci Total Environ* 76:49–54.

Brätter P, Negretti de Brätter VE. 1996. Influence of high dietary selenium intake on the thyroid hormone level in human serum. *J Trace Elem Med Biol* 10:163–166.

Brätter P, Negretti de Brätter VE, Jaffe WG, Mendez Castellano H. 1991. Selenium status of children living in seleniferous areas of Venezuela. *J Trace Elem Electrolytes Hlth Dis* 5:269–270.

Burk RF, Brown DG, Seely RJ, Scaief CC III. 1972. Influence of dietary and injected selenium on whole-body retention, route of excretion, and tissue retention of $^{75}SeO_3^{2-}$ in the rat. *J Nutr* 102:1049–1055.

Burk RF, Hill KE, Awad JA, Morrow JD, Kato T, Cockell KA, Lyons PR. 1995. Pathogenesis of diquat-induced liver necrosis in selenium-deficient rats. Assessment of the roles of lipid peroxidation and selenoprotein P. *Hepatology* 21:561–569.

Burk RF, Levander OA. 1999. Selenium. In: Shils ME, Olson JA, Shike M, Ross AC, eds. *Modern Nutrition in Health and Disease,* 9th edition. Baltimore, MD: Williams & Wilkins. Pp. 265–276.

Burk RF, Pearson WN, Wood RP II, Viteri F. 1967. Blood selenium levels and in vitro red blood cell uptake of ^{75}Se in kwashiorkor. *Am J Clin Nutr* 20:723–733.

Butte NF, Garza C, Smith EO, Nichols BL. 1984. Human milk intake and growth in exclusively breast-fed infants. *J Pediatr* 104:187–195.

Cantor AH, Tarino JZ. 1982. Comparative effects of inorganic and organic dietary sources of selenium on selenium levels and selenium-dependent glutathione peroxidase activity in blood of young turkeys. *J Nutr* 112:2187–2196.

Carter RF. 1966. Acute selenium poisoning. *Med J Aust* 1:525–528.

CDC (Centers for Disease Control and Prevention). 1984. Selenium intoxication—New York. *Morbid Mortal Wkly Rep* 33:157–158.

Cheng Y-Y, Qian P-C. 1990. The effect of selenium-fortified table salt in the prevention of Keshan disease on a population of 1.05 million. *Biomed Environ Sci* 3:422–428.

Clark LC, Cantor KP, Allaway WH. 1991. Selenium in forage crops and cancer mortality in U.S. counties. *Arch Environ Health* 46:37–42.

Clark LC, Combs GF, Turnbull BW, Slate EH, Chalker DK, Chow J, Davis LS, Glover RA, Graham GF, Gross EG, Krongrad A, Lesher JL, Park HK, Sanders BB, Smith CL, Taylor JR. 1996. Effects of selenium supplementation for cancer prevention in patients with carcinoma of the skin. A randomized controlled trial. *J Am Med Assoc* 276:1957–1963.

Cohen HJ, Chovaniec ME, Mistretta D, Baker SS. 1985. Selenium repletion and glutathione peroxidase—Differential effects on plasma and red blood cell enzyme activity. *Am J Clin Nutr* 41:735–747.

Cumming FJ, Fardy JJ, Woodward DR. 1992. Selenium and human lactation in Australia: Milk and blood selenium levels in lactating women, and selenium intakes of their breast-fed infants. *Acta Paediatr* 81:292–295.

Debski B, Finley DA, Picciano MF, Lonnerdal B, Milner J. 1989. Selenium content and glutathione peroxidase activity of milk from vegetarian and nonvegetarian women. *J Nutr* 119:215–220.

Dewey KG, Finley DA, Lonnerdal B. 1984. Breast milk volume and composition during late lactation (7–20 months). *J Pediatr Gastroenterol Nutr* 3:713–720.

Duffield AJ, Thomson CD, Hill KE, Williams S. 1999. An estimation of selenium requirements for New Zealanders. *Am J Clin Nutr* 70:896–903.

Ehrenreich A, Forchhammer K, Tormay P, Veprek B, Böck A. 1992. Selenoprotein synthesis in *E. coli.* Purification and characterization of the enzyme catalysing selenium activation. *Eur J Biochem* 206:767–773.

Ellis L, Picciano MF, Smith AM, Hamosh M, Mehta NR. 1990. The impact of gestational length on human milk selenium concentration and glutathione peroxidase activity. *Pediatr Res* 27:32–35.

Esaki N, Nakamura T, Tanaka H, Soda K. 1982. Selenocysteine lyase, a novel enzyme that specifically acts on selenocysteine. Mammalian distribution and purification and properties of pig liver enzyme. *J Biol Chem* 257:4386–4391.

Flohe L. 1988. Glutathione peroxidase. *Basic Life Sci* 49:663–668.

Fomon SJ, Anderson TA. 1974. *Infant Nutrition,* 2nd edition. Philadelphia: WB Saunders. Pp. 104–111.

Funk MA, Hamlin L, Picciano MF, Prentice A, Milner JA. 1990. Milk selenium of rural African women: Influence of maternal nutrition, parity, and length of lactation. *Am J Clin Nutr* 51:220–224.

Ge K, Xue A, Bai J, Wang S. 1983. Keshan disease—An endemic cardiomyopathy in China. *Virchows Arch A Pathol Anat Histopathol* 401:1–15.

Griffiths NM. 1973. Dietary intake and urinary excretion of selenium in some New Zealand women. *Proc Univ Otago Med Sch* 51:8–9.

Guimaraes MJ, Peterson D, Vicari A, Cocks BG, Copeland NG, Gilbert DJ, Jenkins NA, Ferrick DA, Kastelein RA, Bazan JF, Zlotnik A. 1996. Identification of a novel selD homolog from eukaryotes, bacteria, and archaea: Is there an autoregulatory mechanism in selenocysteine metabolism? *Proc Natl Acad Sci USA* 93:15086–15091.

Heinig MJ, Nommsen LA, Peerson JM, Lonnerdal B, Dewey KG. 1993. Energy and protein intakes of breast-fed and formula-fed infants during the first year of life and their association with growth velocity: The DARLING Study. *Am J Clin Nutr* 58:152–161.

Helzlsouer K, Jacobs R, Morris S. 1985. Acute selenium intoxication in the United States. *Fed Proc* 44:1670.

Higashi A, Tamari H, Kuroki Y, Matsuda I. 1983. Longitudinal changes in selenium content of breast milk. *Acta Paediatr Scand* 72:433–436.

Hill KE, Xia Y, Åkesson B, Boeglin ME, Burk RF. 1996. Selenoprotein P concentration in plasma is an index of selenium status in selenium-deficient and selenium-supplemented Chinese subjects. *J Nutr* 126:138–145.

Hojo Y. 1986. Sequential study on glutathione peroxidase and selenium contents of human milk. *Sci Total Environ* 52:83–91.

IOM (Institute of Medicine). 1991. *Nutrition During Lactation*. Washington, DC: National Academy Press.

Ip C. 1998. Lessons from basic research in selenium and cancer prevention. *J Nutr* 128:1845–1854.

Jensen R, Closson W, Rothenberg R. 1984. Selenium intoxication—New York. *Morbid Mortal Wkly Rep* 33:157–158.

Jochum F, Fuchs A, Cser A, Menzel H, Lombeck I. 1995. Trace mineral status of full-term infants fed human milk, milk-based formula or partially hydrolysed whey protein formula. *Analyst* 120:905–909.

Keshan Disease Research Group. 1979. Observations on effect of sodium selenite in prevention of Keshan disease. *Chin Med J* 92:471–476.

Kumpulainen J, Vuori E, Kuitunen P, Makinen S, Kara R. 1983. Longitudinal study on the dietary selenium intake of exclusively breast-fed infants and their mothers in Finland. *Int J Vitam Nutr Res* 53:420–426.

Kumpulainen J, Vuori E, Siimes MA. 1984. Effect of maternal dietary selenium intake on selenium levels in breast milk. *Int J Vitam Nutr Res* 54:251–255.

Kumpulainen J, Salmenpera L, Siimes MA, Koivistoinen P, Perheentupa J. 1985. Selenium status of exclusively breast-fed infants as influenced by maternal organic or inorganic selenium supplementation. *Am J Clin Nutr* 42:829–835.

Lacourciere GM, Stadtman TC. 1998. The NIFS protein can function as a selenide delivery protein in the biosynthesis of selenophosphate. *J Biol Chem* 273:30921–30926.

Levander OA. 1976. Selenium in foods. In: *Proceedings of the Symposium on Selenium-Tellurium in the Environment*. South Bend, IN: University of Notre Dame.

Levander OA. 1989. Upper limit of selenium in infant formulas. *J Nutr* 119:1869–1873.

Levander OA, Moser PB, Morris VC. 1987. Dietary selenium intake and selenium concentrations of plasma, erythrocytes, and breast milk in pregnant and postpartum lactating and nonlactating women. *Am J Clin Nutr* 46:694–698.

Lombeck I, Ebert KH, Kasperek K, Feinendegen LE, Bremer HJ. 1984. Selenium intake of infants and young children, healthy children and dietetically treated patients with phenylketonuria. *Eur J Pediatr* 143:99–102.

Lombeck I, Menzel H, Frosch D. 1987. Acute selenium poisoning of a 2-year old child. *Eur J Pediatr* 146:308–312.

Longnecker MP, Taylor PR, Levander OA, Howe M, Veillon C, McAdam PA, Patterson KY, Holden JM, Stampfer MJ, Morris JS, Willett WC. 1991. Selenium in diet, blood, and toenails in relation to human health in a seleniferous area. *Am J Clin Nutr* 53:1288–1294.

Mannan S, Picciano MF. 1987. Influence of maternal selenium status on human milk selenium concentration and glutathione peroxidase activity. *Am J Clin Nutr* 46:95–100.

Matoba R, Kimura H, Uchima E, Abe T, Yamada T, Mitsukuni Y, Shikata I. 1986. An autopsy case of acute selenium (selenious acid) poisoning and selenium levels in human tissues. *Forensic Sci Int* 31:87–92.

May JM, Cobb CE, Mendiratta S, Hill KE, Burk RF. 1998. Reduction of the ascorbyl free radical to ascorbate by thioredoxin reductase. *J Biol Chem* 273:23039–23045.

McConnell KP, Portman OW. 1952. Excretion of dimethyl selenide by the rat. *J Biol Chem* 195:277–282.

Moss AJ, Levy AS, Kim I, Park YK. 1989. *Use of Vitamin and Mineral Supplements in the United States: Current Users, Types of Products, and Nutrients.* Advance Data, Vital and Health Statistics of the National Center for Health Statistics. Number 174. Hyattsville, MD: National Center for Health Statistics.

Mozier NM, McConnell KP, Hoffman JL. 1988. S-Adenosyl-L-methionine:thioether S-methyltransferase, a new enzyme in sulfur and selenium metabolism. *J Biol Chem* 263:4527–4531.

Nantel AJ, Brown M, Dery P, Lefebvre M. 1985. Acute poisoning by selenious acid. *Vet Hum Toxicol* 27:531–533.

NRC (National Research Council). 1976. *Selenium.* Washington, DC: National Academy of Sciences.

NRC (National Research Council). 1980a. *Drinking Water and Health*, Volume 3. Washington, DC: National Academy Press.

NRC (National Research Council). 1980b. *Recommended Dietary Allowances*, 9th edition. Washington, DC: National Academy Press.

Pennington JA, Schoen SA. 1996. Total diet study: Estimated dietary intakes of nutritional elements, 1982–1991. *Int J Vitam Nutr Res* 66:350–362.

Pentel P, Fletcher D, Jentzen J. 1985. Fatal acute selenium toxicity. *J Forensic Sci* 30:556–562.

Robberecht H, Van Grieken R, Van Sprundel M, Vanden Berghe D, Deelstra H. 1983. Selenium in environmental and drinking waters of Belgium. *Sci Total Environ* 26:163–172.

Ruta DA, Haider S. 1989. Attempted murder by selenium poisoning. *Br Med J* 299:316–317.

Saito Y, Hayashi T, Tanaka A, Watanabe Y, Suzuki M, Saito E, Takahashi K. 1999. Selenoprotein P in human plasma as an extracellular phospholipid hydroperoxide glutathione peroxidase. Isolation and enzymatic characterization of human selenoprotein P. *J Biol Chem* 274:2866–2871.

Salbe AD, Levander OA. 1990. Effect of various dietary factors on the deposition of selenium in the hair and nails of rats. *J Nutr* 120:200–206.

Schroeder HA, Frost DV, Balassa JJ. 1970. Essential trace metals in man: Selenium. *J Chronic Dis* 23:227–243.

Shearer RR, Hadjimarkos DM. 1975. Geographic distribution of selenium in human milk. *Arch Environ Hlth* 30:230–233.

Smith AM, Picciano MF, Milner JA. 1982. Selenium intakes and status of human milk and formula fed infants. *Am J Clin Nutr* 35:521–526.

Stadtman TC. 1991. Biosynthesis and function of selenocysteine-containing enzymes. *J Biol Chem* 266:16257–16260.

Sun QA, Wu Y, Zappacosta F, Jeang KT, Lee BJ, Hatfield DL, Gladyshev VN. 1999. Redox regulation of cell signaling by selenocysteine in mammalian thioredoxin reductases. *J Biol Chem* 274:24522–24530.

Sunde RA. 1994. Intracellular glutathione peroxidases—Structure, regulation, and function. In: Burk RF, ed. *Selenium in Biology and Human Health*. New York: Springer Verlag. Pp. 45–78.

Swanson CA, Reamer DC, Veillon C, King JC, Levander OA. 1983. Quantitative and qualitative aspects of selenium utilization in pregnant and nonpregnant women: An application of stable isotope methodology. *Am J Clin Nutr* 38:169–180.

Swanson CA, Patterson BH, Levander OA, Veillon C, Taylor PR, Helzlsouer K, McAdam PA, Zech LA. 1991. Human [74Se]selenomethionine metabolism: A kinetic model. *Am J Clin Nutr* 54:917–926.

Thompson JN, Erdody P, Smith DC. 1975. Selenium content of food consumed by Canadians. *J Nutr* 105:274–277.

Thomson CD, Robinson MF. 1980. Selenium in human health and disease with emphasis on those aspects peculiar to New Zealand. *Am J Clin Nutr* 33:303–323.

Thomson CD, Robinson MF. 1986. Urinary and fecal excretions and absorption of a large supplement of selenium: Superiority of selenate over selenite. *Am J Clin Nutr* 44:659–663.

Valentine JL, Kang HK, Spivey GH. 1978. Selenium levels in human blood, urine, and hair in response to exposure via drinking water. *Environ Res* 17:347–355.

Vanderpas JB, Dumont JE, Contempre B, Diplock AT. 1992. Iodine and selenium deficiency in northern Zaire. *Am J Clin Nutr* 56:957–958.

Van Vleet JF. 1980. Current knowledge of selenium-vitamin E deficiency in domestic animals. *J Am Vet Med Assoc* 176:321–325.

Varo P, Alfthan G, Huttunen JK, Aro A. 1994. Nationwide selenium supplementation in Finland—Effects on diet, blood and tissue levels, and health. In: Burk RF, ed. *Selenium in Biology and Human Health*. New York: Springer Verlag. Pp. 197–218.

Veres Z, Tsai L, Scholz TD, Politino M, Balaban RS, Stadtman TC. 1992. Synthesis of 5 methylaminomethyl-2-selenouridine in tRNAs: 31P NMR studies show the labile selenium donor synthesized by the selD gene product contains selenium bonded to phosphorus. *Proc Natl Acad Sci USA* 89:2975–2979.

Waschulewski IH, Sunde RA. 1988. Effect of dietary methionine on tissue selenium and glutathione peroxidase (EC 1.11.1.9) activity in rats given selenomethionine. *Br J Nutr* 60:57–68.

Welsh SO, Holden JM, Wolf WR, Levander OA. 1981. Selenium in self-selected diets of Maryland residents. *J Am Diet Assoc* 79:277–285.

WHO (World Health Organization). 1987. *Selenium. A Report of the International Programme on Chemical Safety.* Environmental Health Criteria 58. Geneva: WHO.

Wright PL, Bell MC. 1963. Selenium and vitamin E influence upon the in vitro uptake of Se[75] by ovine blood cells. *Proc Soc Exp Biol Med* 114:379–382 .

Xia YM, Hill KE, Burk RF. 1989. Biochemical studies of a selenium-deficient population in China: Measurement of selenium, glutathione peroxidase, and other oxidant defense indices in blood. *J Nutr* 119:1318–1326.

Yang G-Q, Xia YM. 1995. Studies on human dietary requirements and safe range of dietary intakes of selenium in China and their application in the prevention of related endemic diseases. *Biomed Environ Sci* 8:187–201.

Yang G-Q, Zhou R-H. 1994. Further observations on the human maximum safe dietary selenium intake in a seleniferous area of China. *J Trace Elem Electrolytes Hlth Dis* 8:159–165.

Yang G-Q, Wang S-Z, Zhou R-H, Sun S-Z. 1983. Endemic selenium intoxication of humans in China. *Am J Clin Nutr* 37:872–881.

Yang G-Q, Zhu L-Z, Liu S-J, Gu L-Z, Qian P-C, Huang J-H, Lu M-D. 1987. Human selenium requirements in China. In: Combs GF Jr, Levander OA, Spallholz JE, Oldfield JE, eds. *Selenium in Biology and Medicine.* New York: Avi. Pp. 589–607.

Yang G-Q, Ge K, Chen J, Chen X. 1988. Selenium-related endemic diseases and the daily selenium requirement of humans. *World Rev Nutr Diet* 55:98–152.

Yang G-Q, Yin S, Zhou R-H, Gu L, Yan B, Liu Y, Liu Y. 1989a. Studies of safe maximal daily dietary Se-intake in a seleniferous area in China. II. Relation between Se-intake and the manifestation of clinical signs and certain biochemical alterations in blood and urine. *J Trace Elem Electrolytes Hlth Dis* 3:123–130.

Yang G-Q, Zhou R, Yin S, Gu L, Yan B, Liu Y, Liu Y, Li X. 1989b. Studies of safe maximal daily dietary selenium intake in a seleniferous area in China. I. Selenium intake and tissue selenium levels of the inhabitants. *J Trace Elem Electrolytes Hlth Dis* 3:77–87.

Yang JG, Hill KE, Burk RF. 1989. Dietary selenium intake controls rat plasma selenoprotein P concentration. *J Nutr* 119:1010–1012.

Yoshizawa K, Willett WC, Morris SJ, Stampfer MJ, Spiegelman D, Rimm EB, Giovannucci E. 1999. Study of prediagnostic selenium level in toenails and the risk of advanced prostate cancer. *J Natl Cancer Inst* 90:1219–1224.

8

β-Carotene and Other Carotenoids

SUMMARY

Blood concentrations of carotenoids are the best biological markers for consumption of fruits and vegetables. A large body of observational epidemiological evidence suggests that higher blood concentrations of β-carotene and other carotenoids obtained from foods are associated with lower risk of several chronic diseases. This evidence, although consistent, cannot be used to establish a requirement for β-carotene or carotenoid intake because the observed effects may be due to other substances found in carotenoid-rich food, or to other behavioral correlates of increased fruit and vegetable consumption. While there is evidence that β-carotene is an antioxidant in vitro, its importance to health is not known. The one clear function of certain carotenoids that is firmly linked to a health outcome is the provitamin A activity of some dietary carotenoids (α-carotene, β-carotene, and β-cryptoxanthin) and their role in the prevention of vitamin A deficiency. Establishment of a requirement for carotenoids based upon vitamin A activity must be done in concert with the evaluation of Dietary Reference Intakes (DRIs) for vitamin A, which was not included in this report, but will be addressed in a subsequent DRI report. Although no DRIs are proposed for β-carotene or other carotenoids at the present time, existing recommendations for increased consumption of carotenoid-rich fruits and vegetables are supported. Based on evidence that β-carotene *supplements* have not been shown to confer any benefit for the prevention of the major chronic diseases and may cause harm in certain subgroups, it is concluded that β-carotene supplements are not advisable, other than as a provitamin

A source and for the prevention and control of vitamin A deficiency in at-risk populations.

BACKGROUND INFORMATION

The most prevalent carotenoids in North American diets include the following: α-carotene, β-carotene, lycopene, lutein, zeaxanthin, and β-cryptoxanthin. The structures of these carotenoids are shown in Figure 8-1. Three of these carotenoids, namely α-carotene, β-carotene, and β-cryptoxanthin, can be converted into retinol and are thus referred to as provitamin A carotenoids. Lycopene, lutein, and zeaxanthin have no vitamin A activity and are thus referred to as nonprovitamin A carotenoids. Most naturally occurring carotenoids are in the *all-trans*-configuration; but under conditions of heating, for example, *cis*-isomers such as 13-*cis*-β-carotene (Figure 8-1) are formed.

Functions and Actions

The various biological effects of carotenoids can be classified into functions, actions, and associations. Carotenoids function in plants and in photosynthetic bacteria as accessory pigments in photosynthesis and protect against photosensitization in animals, plants, and bacteria. In humans, the only known function of carotenoids is vitamin A activity (provitamin A carotenoids only).

Carotenoids also are thought to have a variety of different actions, including possible antioxidant activity, immunoenhancement, inhibition of mutagenesis and transformation, inhibition of premalignant lesions, quenching of nonphotochemical fluorescence, and activity as a pigment in primate macula (Olson, 1999). Carotenoids have also been associated with various health effects: decreased risk of macular degeneration and cataracts, decreased risk of some cancers, and decreased risk of some cardiovascular events (Olson, 1999).

However, as described above, the only known function of carotenoids in humans is to act as a source of vitamin A in the diet. This function, as well as carotenoid actions and associations, is reviewed elsewhere (Krinsky, 1993; Olson, 1989) and discussed in subsequent sections.

Physiology of Absorption, Metabolism, and Excretion

Absorption

The intestinal absorption of dietary carotenoids is facilitated by

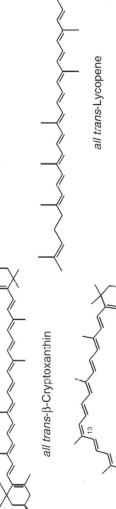

FIGURE 8-1 Structure of provitamin A and nonprovitamin A carotenoids.

Non provitamin A Carotenoids

all trans-Lutein

all trans-Zeaxanthin

all trans-Lycopene

Provitamin A Carotenoids

all trans-β-Carotene

all trans-α-Carotene

all trans-β-Cryptoxanthin

13-*cis*-β-Carotene

the formation of bile acid micelles. The hydrocarbon backbone of the carotenoids makes them insoluble in water, and like other non-polar lipids, they must be solubilized within micelles in the gastrointestinal tract to allow for absorption. Micellar solubilization facilitates the diffusion of lipids across the unstirred water layer. The presence of fat in the small intestine stimulates the secretion of bile acids from the gall bladder and improves the absorption of carotenoids by increasing the size and stability of micelles, thus allowing more carotenoids to be solubilized. The uptake of β-carotene by the mucosal cell is believed to occur by passive diffusion (Hollander and Ruble, 1978). Uptake by these cells, however, is not sufficient for absorption to be completed. Once inside the mucosal cell, carotenoids or their metabolic products (e.g., vitamin A) must also be incorporated into chylomicrons and released into the lymphatics. When mucosal cells are sloughed off due to cell turnover, spilling their contents into the lumen of the gastrointestinal tract, carotenoids that have been taken up by the cells but not yet incorporated into chylomicrons are lost into the lumen (Boileau et al., 1999).

Metabolism, Transport, and Excretion

Carotenoids may be either absorbed intact, or in the case of those possessing vitamin A activity, cleaved to form vitamin A prior to secretion into lymph. Portal transport of carotenoids is minimal due to the lipophilic nature of their structures. Some portal transport of more polar metabolites, such as retinoic acid, can occur (Olson, 1999).

Carotenoid cleavage is accomplished either by the intestinal mucosal enzyme β-carotene 15,15'-dioxygenase (EC 1.13.11.21) or by noncentral cleavage mechanisms (Boileau et al., 1999; Olson, 1999; Parker, 1996; Wang, 1994). The extent of conversion of a highly bioavailable source of dietary β-carotene to vitamin A in humans has been shown to be between 60 and 75 percent, with an additional 15 percent of the β-carotene absorbed intact (Goodman et al., 1966). However, absorption of most carotenoids from foods is considerably lower and can be as low as 2 percent (Rodriguez and Irwin, 1972). The effects of dietary and nondietary factors on the efficiency of carotenoid absorption are reviewed later.

Noncentral (or excentric) cleavage of carotenoids yields a wide variety of metabolic products, some of which are further metabolized. These cleavage products include aldehyde, acid, alcohol, and epoxide derivatives (Parker, 1996; Wang, 1994). Isomerization of carotenoids or their metabolic products may occur in vivo because isomers have been found upon extraction of carotenoids from human tissues (Clinton et al., 1996). Although little attention has been given to the study of carotenoid excretion pathways, epoxides and carotenoid metabolic products with less than 15 carbon chain lengths would presumably have no vitamin A activity. It is assumed that bile and urine would be excretion routes for metabolites (Olson, 1999).

The carotenoids are transported in blood exclusively by lipoproteins. The carotenoid content of individual lipoprotein classes is not homogeneous. In the fasted state, the hydrocarbon carotenoids such as α-carotene, β-carotene, and lycopene are carried predominantly by low-density lipoprotein. The remaining carotenoids, including the more polar xanthophylls such as lutein and zeaxanthin, are carried by high-density lipoprotein (HDL) and, to a lesser extent, by very low-density lipoprotein (Johnson and Russell, 1992; Parker, 1996; Traber et al., 1994). It is thought that β-carotene and other hydrocarbon carotenoids reside in the hydrophobic core of the particles, whereas the more polar xanthophylls reside closer to the surface (Parker, 1996).

β-Carotene is the most studied carotenoid in terms of metabolism and its potential effects on health. Lycopene, lutein, zeaxanthin, and α-carotene have received increasing attention in recent years. Much remains to be learned, however, about the relative metabolic effects of these carotenoids.

Body Stores

Recently, 34 carotenoids were identified in human serum and milk (Khachik et al., 1997b). Of these, 13 were geometrical isomers of their *all-trans* parent structures and 8 were metabolites. This finding is in contrast to the up to 50 carotenoids that have been identified in the U.S. diet and the more than 600 found in nature. The most prevalent carotenoids in human serum (Khachik et al., 1997b) are the same as those most commonly found in the diet: β-carotene, lycopene, and lutein (Nebeling et al., 1997). *Cis*-isomers of lycopene are commonly found in the serum and in fact have been shown to constitute more than 50 percent of the total serum lycopene (Stahl et al., 1992). In contrast, *cis*-isomers of β-carotene are considerably less common in serum with the *trans*-isomers being more common. In addition to these forms of α-carotene, β-carotene, lycopene, and zeaxanthin are also major serum carotenoids. The concentrations of various carotenoids in human serum and tissues are highly variable and likely depend on a number of factors such as food sources, efficiency of absorption, amount of fat in the diet, and so forth (Table 8-1).

The serum concentration of carotenoids after a single dose peaks at 24 to 48 hours post dose (Johnson and Russell, 1992). The earliest postprandial serum appearance of carotenoids is in the chylomicron fraction. It has been proposed that the increase in carotenoids in the triglyceride-rich lipoprotein fraction (primarily chylomicrons) be used for quantitating carotenoid absorption (van Vliet et al., 1995). This would provide a more direct measure of absorption because total serum carotenoid content is not an exclusive measure of newly absorbed carotenoids.

Data from the Third National Health and Nutrition Examination Survey (NHANES III) demonstrate the variability of normal serum carotenoid concentrations (Appendix Tables F-4 through F-8). This variability is attributed to a variety of life-style and physiological factors. In a recent population-based study, Brady et al. (1996) reported that lower serum concentrations of α-carotene, β-carotene, β-cryptoxanthin, lutein, and zeaxanthin, but not lycopene, were generally associated with male gender, smoking, younger age, lower non-HDL cholesterol, greater ethanol consumption, and higher body mass index.

The delivery of carotenoids to extrahepatic tissue is accomplished through the interaction of lipoprotein particles with receptors and the degradation of lipoproteins by extrahepatic enzymes such as lipoprotein lipase. Carotenoids are present in a number of human tissues including adipose, liver, kidney, and adrenal, but adipose tissue and liver appear to be the main storage sites (Parker, 1996). However, based on a wet tissue weight, the liver, adrenal gland, and testes contain the highest per-gram concentrations (Stahl et al., 1992). Similar to what is reported in serum, β-carotene, lutein, and lycopene are the main tissue carotenoids, although α-carotene, β-cryptoxanthin, and zeaxanthin are also present (Boileau et al., 1999). In contrast to serum profiles, 9-cis-β-carotene is consistently present in storage tissues. In both serum and tissue storage, lycopene cis-isomers constitute greater than 50 percent of the total lycopene present (Clinton et al., 1996; Stahl et al., 1992).

Clinical Effects of Inadequate Intake

If adequate retinol is provided in the diet, there are no known clinical effects of consuming diets low in carotenes over the short term. One study of premenopausal women consuming low-carotene diets in a metabolic ward reported skin lesions (Burri et al., 1993). However, this effect was not observed after 60 days of depletion in a subsequent β-carotene depletion study by the same group of investigators (Lin et al., 1998). These studies of carotene-deficient diets were reported to increase various measures of oxidative susceptibility (Dixon et al., 1994, 1998; Lin et al., 1998), but as discussed below, this is of uncertain relevance with regard to clinical outcomes.

SELECTION OF POSSIBLE INDICATORS FOR ESTIMATING THE REQUIREMENT FOR β-CAROTENE AND OTHER CAROTENOIDS

Vitamin A Equivalency

Vitamin A equivalency is a possible indicator for establishing requirements for provitamin A carotenoids. However, any such establishment of requirements for carotenoids based on vitamin A activity must be considered in concert with the evaluation of requirements for vitamin A. This information will be presented in a later Dietary Reference Intakes report.

Markers of Antioxidant Activity

The effect of increasing β-carotene intake on several markers of antioxidant activity has been investigated in a series of studies involving humans. These studies have examined antioxidant marker activity in apparently healthy men and women as well as in subjects who were physiologically challenged (i.e., smokers and patients with coronary disease or cystic fibrosis).

Studies of the effect of β-carotene intake on measures of antioxidant activity are summarized in Table 8-2. The dietary source of β-carotene ranged from modification of diets with normally consumed foods to giving supplements that provided as much as 120 mg/day of a highly bioavailable preparation. In general, subjects in most studies consumed β-carotene in amounts that would be difficult to achieve from foods alone and, as a result, relate to the pharmacological range of intakes.

The findings reported in Table 8-2 indicate that β-carotene supplementation did not alter, or inconsistently alter, markers of antioxidant activity, which were somewhat dependent on β-carotene intake. In studies in which subjects were fed less than 25 mg/day of β-carotene, either from foods or as a supplement, changes in the markers for antioxidant activity were minimal. Exceptions noted

TABLE 8-1 Concentrations of Selected Carotenoids in Human Serum and Tissues

Carotenoid	Serum (μmol/L)	Liver (μmol/g)
α-Carotene	0.02–0.47 (1.0–25.3 μg/dL)	0.075–10.8 (0.04–5.8 μg/g)
β-Carotene	0.04–2.26 (2.2–122.7 μg/dL)	0.39–19.4 (0.21–6.3 μg/g)
β-Cryptoxanthin	0.03–0.70 (1.4–38.2 μg/dL)	0.037–20.0 (0.05–11.0 μg/g)
Lutein	0.10–1.23 (5.8–69.8 μg/dL)	0.10–3.0 (0.06–6.9 μg/g)
Lycopene	0.05–1.05 (2.7–54.6 μg/dL)	0.20–17.2 (0.11–11.1 μg/g)

SOURCE: Data from Schmitz et al. (1991) and Kaplan et al. (1990) for tissues and Iowa State University Department of Statistics (1999) for serum.

were decreased deoxyribonucleic acid strand breaks observed when 22 mg/day of β-carotene was administered as carrot juice (Pool-Zobel et al., 1997) and lowered copper-induced oxidation of low-density lipoprotein when 12 or 24 mg/day of β-carotene was given along with vitamins C and E (Mosca et al., 1997). As shown in Table 8-2, feeding β-carotene in amounts greater than 25 mg/day generally resulted in inconsistent responses of the biological markers monitored. Administration of β-carotene to subjects with increased oxidative stress (e.g., smoking, cystic fibrosis) was associated with more consistent evidence of decreased lipid peroxidation compared to studies in which subjects without known additional oxidative stress were given β-carotene. In studies that involved depletion followed by repletion of body stores of β-carotene, as indicated by plasma concentrations, the biological markers that were negatively altered as a result of depleted body stores of β-carotene were restored to baseline values as a consequence of repletion (Table 8-2).

In summary, results from some studies show improvement of measures of antioxidant activity due to intake of relatively high levels of β-carotene, while studies that investigated low to modest levels of β-carotene show no or inconsistent changes in the same activities.

Kidney (μmol/g)	Lung (μmol/g)
0.037–1.5 (0.02–0.80 μg/g)	0.1–1.0 (0.05–0.54 μg/g)
0.093–2.8 (0.05–1.5 μg/g)	0.1–1.6 (0.05–0.86 μg/g)
0.019–3.9 (0.05–2.2 μg/g)	0.1–2.5 (0.05–1.4 μg/g)
0.037–2.1 (0.05–5.9 μg/g)	0.1–2.3 (0.05–1.3 μg/g)
0.093–2.4 (0.05–1.3 μg/g)	0.1–1.0 (0.05–2.3 μg/g)

Some benefit of feeding increased amounts of β-carotene was observed for several markers of antioxidant activity when body stores were relatively low or when an oxidant-type stress was present. These observations suggest that the lack of effect in some studies may be due to study populations whose baseline β-carotene status was already adequate. Nevertheless, current data do not provide convincing evidence that substantially increasing β-carotene intake above current dietary intakes has a significant effect on measures of antioxidant status. Also, none of these markers has been validated to be predictive of any known health outcomes. Therefore, these data are inadequate for the estimation of a requirement for β-carotene.

Gap Junctional Communication

Appropriate communication among cells is essential for the coordination of biochemical functions in complex, multicellular organisms. One theory suggests that failure of signaling is one cause of cell overgrowth and eventually cancer. Two research groups have demonstrated that carotenoids stimulate gap junction communication between cells in vitro (Sies and Stahl, 1997; Zhang et al., 1991).

TABLE 8-2 β-Carotene Intake and Measures of Antioxidant Activity in Selected Studies

Reference, Country	Subjects	β-Carotene Dose
Richards et al., 1990 South Africa	40 smokers, average age 33 y; received placebo and 20 received treatment	40 mg/d, Roche prep
Mobarhan et al., 1990; Gottlieb et al., 1993 United States	15 healthy men, aged 19–30 y; randomly assigned repletion levels	Carotene-free diet (depletion); Repletion: 15 mg/d or 120 mg/d, Roche prep
Van Poppel et al., 1992a, 1992b, 1995 Holland	143 male smokers, average age 39 y; randomly assigned to placebo or treatment	40 mg/d first 2 wk 20 mg/d next 12 wk
Allard et al., 1994 Canada	38 male nonsmokers, 25 male smokers, aged 20–75 y; randomly assigned to placebo or treatment	20 mg/d, Roche prep
Calzada et al., 1995 United States	12 healthy men and 7 women, aged 21–50 y; randomly assigned to placebo or treatment	15 mg/d, Roche prep
Gaziano et al., 1995 United States	4 healthy men and 12 women, aged 25–47 y; randomly assigned to either synthetic (BASF) or natural (Henkel) β-carotene	100 mg/d load dose; natural treatment, 66 or 100 mg/2d; synthetic treatment, 50 mg/2 d
Winklhofer-Roob et al., 1995 Switzerland	CF^m patients, 32 boys and girls; average age 10.8 y	0.5 mg/kg BW^n/d, 3M Medica, Ltd.
Clevidence et al., 1997 United States	5 healthy men and 7 women, aged 27–61 y	18 mg/d additional as foods; kale, tomato juice, sweet potato

Duration	Plasma β-Carotene (μmol/L)	Findings
6 wk	Baseline 0.50 (27 μg/dL) Trt[a]—2.06 (111 μg/dL)	No change in leukocyte sister chromatid exchange
2 wk 4 wk	Baseline—0.24 (13 μg/dL) Depletion—0.09 (5 μg/dL) 15 mg/d—3.32 (178 μg/dL) 120 mg/d—8.74 (469 μg/dL)	↓ Breath pentane on 120 mg/d only; ↓ Serum lipid peroxide levels, both repletion levels
2 wk 12 wk	Baseline—0.33 (18 μg/dL) Trt at 14 wk—4.36 (234 μg/dL)	↓ Sputum nuclei No change in lymphocyte sister chromatid exchange or urinary 8-oxodG[b]
4 wk	Placebo/NS[c]—0.38 (20 μg/dL) Placebo/S[d]—0.27 (14 μg/dL) Trt/NS—3.50 (188 μg/dL) Trt/S—3.38 (181 μg/dL)	↓ Breath pentane in smokers No change in breath pentane in nonsmokers No change in breath ethane, RBC[e], MDA[f] or plasma Se-GSHPx[g] in either group
14 d 56 d	Baseline—0.87 (47 μg/dL) Trt—3.07 (165 μg/dL)	No change in plasma Trolox equivalent antioxidant activity
6 d load; followed by 21 d treatment	Baseline—0.25 (13 μg/dL) Both Trts—1.39 (75 μg/dL)	↑ Cu^{2+}-induced LDL[k] oxidation No change in AAPH[L]-induced LDL oxidation
3 m	Baseline—0.09 (5 μg/dL) Trt—1.07 (57 μg/dL)	↓ Plasma MDA and Cu^{2+}-induced LDL oxidation
3 wk	Baseline—0.29 (15 μg/dL) Trt 0.76 (40.2 μg/dL)	No change in plasma ORAC[o], plasma hydroperoxides, LDL TBARS, or 8-oxodG

continued

TABLE 8-2 Continued

Reference, Country	Subjects	β-Carotene Dose
Hininger et al., 1997 France	11 healthy men and 11 females, aged 25–45 y; 11 smokers and 11 nonsmokers	10 mg/d additional as foods (primarily carrots)
Mosca et al., 1997 United States	Coronary artery disease patients; 39 men and 6 women, aged 39–80 y	12 mg/d + vit E and vit C; or 24 mg/d + vit E and vit C
Pool-Zobel et al., 1997 Germany	23 healthy men, aged 27–40 y	Low carotenoid depletion food diet; followed by 22 mg/d as carrot juice
Wang et al., 1997 Japan	192 healthy men; nonsmokers and smokers, aged 18–58 y	From foods; subjects grouped by plasma levels
Dixon et al., 1998; Lin et al., 1998 United States	9 healthy women, premenopausal, aged 18–45 y	≤ 0.58 mg/d as diet or diet + small supplement for depletion; repletion 3.3 mg/d, Roche prep
Rust et al., 1998 Austria	24 CF patients and 14 age-matched healthy children, average age 12.8 y	1 mg/kg BW/d to max of 50 mg/d
Steinberg and Chait, 1998 United States	8 men and 12 women who smoked were in Trt group; average age 29 y	Vegetable-based juice + 30 mg β-Carotene/d + vit C & vit E

SI Conversion factor used for β-carotene = $\mu mol/L \div 0.01863 = \mu g/dL$.

[a] Trt = treatment.
[b] 8-OxodG = 8-oxo-7,8-dihydro-2′-deoxyguanosine.
[c] NS = nonsmokers.
[d] S = smokers.
[e] RBC = red blood cell.
[f] MDA = malondialdehyde.
[g] Se-GSHPx = selenium glutathione peroxidase.
[h] TBARS = thiobarbituric acid reactive substances.

Duration	Plasma β-Carotene (μmol/L)	Findings
2 wk	Baseline/NS—0.95 (51 μg/dL) Baseline/S—0.58 (31 μg/dL) Trt/NS—1.13 (61 μg/dL) Trt/S—0.82 (44 μg/dL)	↑ RBC CuZn-SOD activity; No change in plasma MDA, GSH[p], GSSG, -SH groups, carbonyls, or Se-GSHPx activity
12 wk	Baseline—0.30 (16 μg/dL) 12 mg/d—1.99 (107 μg/dL) 24 mg/d—3.01 (162 μg/dL)	↓ Copper-induced LDL oxidation
2 wk depletion; 4 wk added food containing β-carotene	Not reported	↓ DNA strand breaks (COMET) and oxidized pyrimidine bases in lymphocytes
	0.56 (29.8 μg/dL) as criteria for establishing high/low intake	No difference in lymphocyte DNA adducts between high and low plasma β-carotene groups
100 d depletion; 20 d repletion	Baseline—0.76 (40.2 μg/dL) Depletion—0.33 (17.5 μg/dL) Repletion—1.73 (91.5 μg/dL)	Depletion ↑ plasma MDA and LDL oxidation rate (carbonyl production). Repletion ↓ LDL oxidation rate below baseline
12 wk	Baseline—0.08 (4.8 μg/dL) 12 wk—0.60 (31.7 μg/dL)	↓ Plasma MDA on high-dose βC
4 wk	Baseline—0.23 (12.3 μg/dL) Trt—1.21 (64.9 μg/dL)	↓ Breath pentane, LDL oxidation No change in plasma total peroxyl radical trapping

[i] SOD = superoxide dismutase.
[j] GSSG = erythrocyte oxidized glutathione.
[k] LDL = low-density lipoprotein.
[l] AAPH = 2,2′-azobis[2-amidinopropane]dihydrochloride.
[m] CF = cystic fibrosis.
[n] BW = body weight.
[o] ORAC = oxygen radical absorbance capacity.
[p] GSH = glutathione.

It is not known whether the parent carotenoids or their metabolites are the active factors (Hanusch et al., 1995), nor is it known whether carotenoids influence this communication process in vivo. More study is needed to ascertain whether carotenoids play a direct role in cell-cell communication and, if so, what health outcomes are influenced by this action.

Immune Function

There has been great interest in the potential role of carotenoids in enhancement of the immune response. Children with vitamin A deficiency suffer from compromised immunity and have difficulty protecting themselves from infections. It is important to remember, however, that studies conducted with provitamin A carotenoids may yield results that are attributable to the conversion of carotenoids to vitamin A or other retinoids, not to the effects of the intact carotenoid.

Santos et al. (1996) showed that long-term β-carotene supplementation enhanced natural killer cell activity in men 65 to 86 years of age, but not in men 51 to 64 years of age; enhancement by β-carotene in this age group was confirmed in a subsequent study (Santos et al., 1998). Hughes et al. (1997) evaluated mechanisms by which β-carotene might enable immune cells to act more efficiently. Subjects were supplemented for 26 days with either 15 mg of β-carotene or a placebo. Subjects receiving the β-carotene treatment had increases in expression of adhesion molecules by monocytes, in ex vivo secretion of tumor necrosis factor-α, and in the percentage of monocytes expressing major histocompatibility complex II, a cell surface molecule responsible for presenting antigen to T-helper cells.

Other immunological effects that carotenoids are reported to increase are lymphocyte response to mitogens (Kramer and Burri, 1997) and total white blood cells and helper T cells in human immunodeficiency virus-infected humans (Coodley et al., 1993). Whether these and the other effects noted are specific to carotenoids and are important in overall immunity is not confirmed. Therefore the usefulness of these as markers for disease has yet to be established.

Relationship of Carotenoid Intake to Chronic Disease

A vast number of observational studies, including both case-control and cohort studies, of carotenoids and chronic disease risk have been conducted. Many of the studies are based upon estimated intake of carotenoids in the diet, while many include biochemical evaluation of carotenoid concentrations in blood. Because the dietary intake data are generally obtained via food frequency questionnaires, they do not provide quantitative estimates of carotenoid intake, but rather allow for relative ranking of carotenoid intakes within a population. The blood concentration data, however, are more quantitative and generally more comparable across studies.

Prospective blood carotenoid concentration studies may be particularly informative because blood samples are generally obtained several years prior to the clinical detection of disease. Thus, for the purposes of evaluating the association between quantitative carotenoid exposure and risk of chronic disease, the prospective blood concentration studies are most useful and are given the greatest weight in the analysis that follows. The studies in which food intakes were the basis for evaluating risk of disease are less useful due to the inherent problems in adequately estimating carotenoid intake. These studies, however, may give support to the overall evaluation of the role of carotenoids in chronic disease. The following section briefly summarizes some key research findings from observational studies of the relationship between carotenoids and chronic disease risk.

Mortality

Greenberg et al. (1996) obtained blood samples from 1,188 men and 532 women enrolled in a skin cancer prevention trial and examined the relationship between plasma β-carotene concentrations at entry and subsequent mortality over a median follow-up period of 8.2 years (Table 8-3). Persons in the lowest quartile of plasma β-carotene had a significant increase in their risk of dying compared to those with higher plasma concentrations of β-carotene. The adjusted relative risk was lowest for persons with plasma β-carotene concentrations in the range of 0.34 to 0.53 μmol/L (18 to 28 μg/dL) (quartile 3), with a risk reduction (compared to the lowest quartile) of 43 percent for total deaths, 43 percent for cardiovascular disease deaths, and 51 percent for cancer deaths. The relative risk for overall mortality was 38 percent lower for persons who had plasma β-carotene concentrations in the highest quartile compared to the lowest quartile (relative risk [RR] = 0.62; 95 percent confidence interval [CI] = 0.44–0.87). Thus, these results suggest that plasma β-carotene concentrations in the range of 0.34 to 0.53 μmol/L (18 to 28 μg/dL) are associated with the lowest risk of all-cause

TABLE 8-3 Concentrations of β-Carotene and Total Carotenoids in Plasma or Serum Associated with a Lower Risk of Various Health Outcomes in Selected Studies

Author	Population
Nomura et al., 1985	Japanese men
Menkes et al., 1986	U.S. men and women
Connett et al., 1989	MRFIT[b] cohort men
Greenberg et al., 1996	U.S. men and women, 24–84 y
Jacques and Chylack, 1991	U.S. men and women, 40–70 y
Riemersma et al., 1991	British men
Stahelin et al., 1991	Swiss men
Batieha et al., 1993	U.S. women
EDCCSG, 1993	U.S. men and women
Eichholzer et al., 1992; Gey et al., 1993b	Swiss men
Zheng et al., 1993	U.S. men and women
Morris et al., 1994	U.S. men
West et al., 1994	U.S. men and women, ≥40 y
Sahyoun et al., 1996	U.S. men and women, >60 y
Bonithon-Kopp et al., 1997	French men, >58 y French women, >58 y

[a] Concentration in the quartile/quantile where the risk reduction was of the greatest magnitude. For studies that only report mean or median concentrations in the diseased and disease-free groups, the concentration is the level in the group that remained free of disease. SI Conversion factor used for β-carotene and total carotenoids = 0.01863 µg/dL to µmol/L, with the exception of Greenberg et al., 1996.

mortality in U.S. adults. Note that these blood concentrations reflect levels in the absence of supplementation with β-carotene. Thus, this prospective study emphasizes the inverse association between β-carotene-rich foods and the risk of all-cause mortality.

Another cohort study of carotenoids and mortality examined both dietary intake of total carotenoids and plasma concentrations of

Endpoint	β-Carotene Concentration (μmol/L)[a]	Total Carotenoid Concentration (μmol/L)[a]
Lung cancer	≥0.54 (29 μg/dL)	
Lung cancer	≥0.54 (29 μg/dL)	
Lung cancer	≥0.22 (12 μg/dL)[c]	≥1.84 (99 μg/dL)[c]
All-cause mortality	0.34–0.53 (18–28 μg/dL)	
Cataract		>3.3 (177 μg/dL)
Angina	>0.54 (29 μg/dL)[d]	
Total cancers	≥0.34 (18 μg/dL)[d]	
Lung cancer	≥0.34 (18 μg/dL)[d]	
Cervical cancer	≥0.26 (14 μg/dL)	≥1.73 (93 μg/dL)
Macular degeneration	≥0.74 (40 μg/dL)	≥2.39 (128 μg/dL)
Ischemic heart disease	≥0.18 (10 μg/dL)[d]	
Oropharyngeal cancers	≥0.28 (15 μg/dL)	≥1.75 (94 μg/dL)
CHD[e]		>3.16 (170 μg/dL)
Macular degeneration	>0.88 (47 μg/dL)	
Cancer mortality		>3.13 (168 μg/dL)
CHD mortality		1.73–3.13 (93–168 μg/dL)
All other causes, mortality		>3.13 (168 μg/dL)
Intima-media thickness		>2.1 (113 μg/dL)
Intima media thickness		>3.7 (199 μg/dL)

[b] MRFIT = Multiple Risk Factor Intervention Trial.

[c] Samples were stored at –50°C.

[d] Assumes value given for carotene is 80% β-carotene.

[e] CHD = coronary heart disease.

total carotenoids as predictors of mortality (Sahyoun et al., 1996). Results indicated that mortality from cancer and all causes other than coronary heart disease (CHD) was lowest at a plasma concentration of 3.13 μmol/L (168 μg/dL) total carotenoids or greater; mortality from CHD was lowest at plasma concentrations of 1.73 to 3.13 μmol/L (93 to 168 μg/dL). Overall mortality was lowest at dietary carotenoid intake levels of 8.6 mg/day (RR = 0.68 compared to those consuming 1.1 mg/day of carotenoids).

In the Western Electric cohort study, all-cause mortality was lowest for men who consumed the highest tertile of dietary β-carotene (RR = 0.80 for more than 4.1 mg/day of β-carotene versus less than 2.9 mg/day of β-carotene; p for trend = 0.01) (Pandey et al., 1995).

Cancer

Because there are literally hundreds of studies of carotenoids and cancer risk, this section emphasizes the results of epidemiological studies of all cancers combined, studies of carotenoids and lung cancer, and a few other selected tumor sites for which an inverse association with carotenoids is commonly seen.

Observational Epidemiological Studies. The Basel Prospective Study evaluated the relationship between plasma carotene concentrations in blood samples obtained in 1971–1973 and subsequent cancer mortality up to 1985 (Stahelin et al., 1991). Results showed that persons who went on to develop any cancer had significantly lower prediagnostic carotene concentrations than persons who remained alive and free of cancer in 1985 (mean plasma total carotenoid concentration 0.34 μmol/L [18 μg/dL] in those with cancer versus 0.43 μmol/L [23 μg/dL] in those free of cancer). The authors state that the reported carotene values represent approximately 80 percent β-carotene and 20 percent α-carotene; thus, plasma β-carotene concentrations of approximately 0.34 μmol/L (0.43 μmol/L × 0.8) (18 μg/dL [23 μg/dL × 0.8]) were typical for the survivors of this cohort. This concentration is within the range associated with lower risk elsewhere as shown in Table 8-3.

Numerous epidemiological studies have shown that individuals who consume a relatively large quantity of carotenoid-rich fruits and vegetables have a lower risk of cancer at several tumor sites (Block et al., 1992). The consistency of the results from observational studies is particularly striking for lung cancer, where carotenoid and fruit and vegetable intake has been associated with lower lung cancer risk in 8 of 8 prospective studies and 18 of 20 retrospective studies reviewed (Ziegler et al., 1996b).

Focusing on prospective blood analyses studies, the study with the largest number of cases (n = 99) was reported by Menkes et al. (1986) as part of the Washington County, Maryland, cohort. The risk of lung cancer increased in a linear fashion with decreasing serum concentrations of β-carotene, with the greatest risk at the lowest quintile (cutpoint not stated). The mean concentration of serum β-carotene in persons who subsequently developed lung cancer was 0.47 µmol/L (25 µg/dL), compared to 0.54 µmol/L (29 µg/dL) in persons who remained free of disease.

Nomura et al. (1985) conducted a prospective study of 6,860 men of Japanese ancestry in Hawaii; 74 men subsequently developed lung cancer. Men who later developed lung cancer had lower serum β-carotene concentrations (0.37 µmol/L [20 µg/dL]) than control subjects (0.54 µmol/L [29 µg/dL]). Similar results were reported in the Basel Prospective Study. Men who later developed lung cancer ($n = 68$) had α- plus β-carotene serum concentrations of 0.30 µmol/L (16 µg/dL) versus 0.43 µmol/L (23 µg/dL) in survivors (Stahelin et al., 1991). The Multiple Risk Factor Intervention Trial (MRFIT) cohort study had prediagnostic serologic data on 66 lung cancer cases and 131 control subjects (Connett et al., 1989). Lung cancer cases had lower serum β-carotene concentrations (mean of 0.17 µmol/L [9 µg/dL]) and total carotenoid concentrations (1.62 µmol/L [87 µg/dL]) compared to the control subjects (0.22 µmol/ L [12 µg/dL] and 1.84 µmol/L [99 µg/dL]), respectively. The absolute carotenoid concentrations in this study are lower than those in the previous studies, which may be a consequence of long-term storage of the samples at –50°C, rather than at –70°C or colder as is recommended for carotenoids.

As for dietary studies, the majority of the studies of carotenoids and lung cancer risk have relied upon the U.S. Department of Agriculture (USDA) Nutrient Database for Standard Reference, Release 13, which does not contain estimates of the amount of carotenoids in various food items, but simply contains estimates of provitamin A activity. With the release of a new carotenoid database in 1993 (Mangels et al., 1993), quantitative studies relating consumption of individual carotenoids to lung cancer risk are now available. Le Marchand et al. (1993) found that higher dietary intake of α-carotene, β-carotene, and lutein was significantly associated with lower lung cancer risk in both men and women. Optimal levels of intake for each of these three carotenoids were as follows: β-carotene more than 4.0 mg/day for men and more than 4.4 mg/day for women; α-carotene more than 0.6 mg/day for men and more than 0.7 mg/day for women; and lutein more than 3.3 mg/day for both males and females. Ziegler et al. (1996a) also found significant inverse trends for dietary α- and β-carotene and a marginally significant effect for lutein and zeaxanthin with risk of lung cancer. Optimal levels in this study were as follows: β-carotene 2.5–5.9 mg/day; α-carotene more than 1.5 mg/day; and lutein and zeaxanthin more than 4.2 mg/day.

As reviewed elsewhere, retrospective and prospective epidemiological studies of diet and serum carotenoids strongly indicate that greater consumption of fruits, vegetables, and carotenoids is inversely associated with risk of cancers of the oral cavity, pharynx, and larynx (Mayne, 1996; Mayne and Goodwin, 1993). In a review (Block et al., 1992), 13 of 13 studies indicated that fruit and vegetable intake was associated with reduced risk of cancers of the oral cavity, pharynx, and larynx. As for prospective serologic studies, Zheng et al. (1993) conducted a nested case-control study of serum micronutrients and subsequent risk of oral and pharyngeal cancer. Blood samples were collected and stored in 1974 from a cohort of 25,802 adults in Maryland. Over the next 15 years, 28 individuals developed oral or pharyngeal cancer. Serum analyses indicated that prediagnostic serum concentrations of all the major individual carotenoids, particularly β-carotene, were lower among the case group than among control subjects selected from the same cohort. β-Carotene concentrations in persons who later developed these cancers were 0.21 μmol/L (11 μg/dL) versus 0.28 μmol/L (15 μg/dL) in control subjects (mean; $p = 0.03$). Adjustment for smoking, which is known to be associated with lower serum carotenoid concentrations, attenuated the protective association slightly. The unadjusted and adjusted relative odds of oral or pharyngeal cancer, comparing the upper tertile of serum β-carotene concentrations (cutpoints not given) versus the lower tertile, were 0.50 and 0.69, respectively.

One recent prospective cohort study (Giovannucci et al., 1995) evaluated 47,894 participants in the Health Professionals Follow-up Study, 812 of whom were diagnosed with prostate cancer during the 6-year follow-up. Intake of tomato-based foods (tomato sauce, tomatoes, and pizza—but not tomato juice) and lycopene, which is found predominantly in tomato products, was associated with significantly lower prostate cancer risk. Risk was lowest for those who were estimated to consume more than 6.46 mg/day of lycopene. The lack of association for tomato juice may reflect the fact that lycopene is more bioavailable from processed tomato products than from fresh tomatoes (Gartner et al., 1997).

A prospective study of serum micronutrients and prostate cancer in Japanese men in Hawaii, however, found no difference in prediagnostic serum lycopene concentrations in 142 cases versus 142 matched control subjects (Nomura et al., 1997). The lack of effect seen in this study could possibly relate to the fact that serum lycopene concentrations were relatively low in this population (median 0.25 μmol/L [13 μg/dL]). This is likely a consequence of the fact that tomato products are not widely consumed in the Asian diet (thus the range of exposure may have been limited). Comprehensive reviews of the relationship between lycopene and prostate cancer have been published elsewhere (Clinton, 1998; Giovannucci, 1999).

Consumption of fruits and vegetables also has been reported to be inversely associated with cervical cancer risk in a number of studies. Batieha et al. (1993) conducted a nested case-control study, analyzing a variety of carotenoids in sera stored from 50 women who had developed either invasive cervical cancer or carcinoma in situ during a 15-year follow-up and in 99 control women pair-matched to the cases. The risk of cervical cancer was significantly higher among women with the lowest prediagnostic serum concentrations of total carotenoids (odds ratio [OR] = 2.7; 95 percent CI = 1.1–6.4), α-carotene (OR = 3.1; 95 percent CI = 1.3–7.6), and β-carotene (OR = 3.1; 95 percent CI = 1.2–8.1) compared to women in the upper tertiles. Mean serum concentrations of β-cryptoxanthin were also lower among cases relative to control subjects (p = 0.03). Optimal concentrations of these carotenoids for reducing the risk of cervical cancer were as follows: total carotenoids greater than 1.88 μmol/L (101 μg/dL); α-carotene greater than 0.05 μmol/L (2.7 μg/dL); β-carotene greater than 0.26 μmol/L (14 μg/dL); and cryptoxanthin greater than 0.17 μmol/L (9 μg/dL).

Intervention Trials. Three major double-blind, randomized intervention trials have been conducted using high-dose β-carotene supplements, either alone or in combination with other agents, in an attempt to evaluate any protective role in the development of lung or total cancers. In none of these studies was there any evidence of a protective role for supplementary β-carotene.

In current smokers participating in the Alpha-Tocopherol, Beta-Carotene (ATBC) Cancer Prevention Study, supplementation with 20 mg/day of β-carotene (with or without 50 mg of α-tocopherol) for 5 to 8 years led to a higher incidence in lung cancer but had no effect on the incidence of other major cancers occurring in this population (prostate, bladder, colon or rectum, or stomach) (ATBC Cancer Prevention Study Group, 1994). In addition, the Carotene and Retinol Efficacy Trial (CARET) used a nutrient combination of β-carotene (30 mg/day) plus retinyl palmitate (25,000 international units [IU]/day) versus placebo in asbestos workers and smokers (Omenn et al., 1996a, 1996b). This study reported more lung cancer cases in the supplemented group. The Physicians' Health Study (PHS) of supplemental β-carotene versus placebo in 22,071 male

U.S. physicians reported no significant effect of 12 years of supplementation of β-carotene (50 mg every other day) on cancer or total mortality (Hennekens et al., 1996).

Summary. Higher consumption of carotenoid-containing fruits and vegetables and higher plasma concentrations of several carotenoids, including β-carotene, are associated with a lower risk of many different cancers, especially lung, oral cavity, pharyngeal, laryngeal, and cervical cancers. These prospective blood concentration studies show that β-carotene concentrations in the range of 0.28 μmol/L (15 μg/dL) or less are associated with higher risk of many cancers (Table 8-3), whereas concentrations greater than 0.28 to 0.37 μmol/L (15 to 20 μg/dL) are associated with reduced risk of many cancers. This approximate threshold for cancer risk reduction is concordant with that for the prevention of all-cause mortality, given above. Furthermore, these studies show that increased consumption of foods containing these carotenoids, including carotenoids lacking vitamin A activity, is associated with risk reduction. However, in three large randomized clinical trials using high-dose β-carotene supplements (20 or 30 mg/day or 50 mg given every other day) for 4 to 12 years, no protection was reported with respect to lung cancer, or any other cancer.

Cardiovascular Disease

Epidemiological studies, including descriptive, cohort, and case-control studies, suggest that carotenoid- and β-carotene-rich diets are associated with a reduced risk of cardiovascular disease (Gaziano and Hennekens, 1993; Kohlmeier and Hastings, 1995; Manson et al., 1993). Beginning with biochemical epidemiological studies of plasma carotenoids, Gey et al. (1993a) reported data from the Vitamin Substudy of the World Health Organization's Monitoring Cardiovascular (WHO/MONICA) Project, in which plasma was obtained from approximately 100 apparently healthy men from each of 16 study sites within Europe. A comparison between median plasma β-carotene concentrations and ischemic heart disease mortality revealed no association when all 16 study sites were considered ($r^2 = 0.04$). However, a reasonably strong inverse association was evident ($r^2 = 0.50$) when three study sites, all apparent outliers (and all Finnish sites), were excluded from the analysis.

Men in the Basel Prospective Study, who had low blood concentrations of β-carotene and vitamin C initially and who were followed for 12 years, had a significantly higher risk of subsequent ischemic heart disease (RR = 1.96; p = 0.022) and stroke (RR = 4.17; p = 0.002) (Eichholzer et al., 1992; Gey et al., 1993b). Based upon these and other data, Gey et al. (1993a) proposed that more than 0.4 to 0.5 μmol/L (21 to 27 μg/dL) α-plus β-carotene or 0.3 to 0.4 μmol/L (16 to 21 μg/dL) β-carotene is needed to reduce the risk of ischemic heart disease.

Total serum carotenoids, measured at baseline in the placebo group of the Lipid Research Clinics Coronary Primary Prevention Trial, were inversely related to subsequent coronary heart disease events (Morris et al., 1994). Men in the highest quartile of total serum carotenoids (more than 3.16 μmol/L [172 μg/dL]) had an adjusted relative risk of 0.64 (95 percent CI = 0.44–0.92); among those who never smoked, the relative risk was 0.28 (95 percent CI = 0.11–0.73). Riemersma et al. (1991) reported that persons with plasma carotene concentrations in the lowest quintile (less than 0.26 μmol/L [14 μg/dL]) had 2.64 times the risk of angina pectoris. Adjustment for smoking reduced the magnitude of risk. However, because smoking may be part of the causal path, adjustment may not be appropriate.

The U.S. Health Professionals Follow-up Study of over 39,000 men reported a relative risk for coronary heart disease of 0.71 (95 percent CI = 0.55–0.92) for those at the top quintile of total carotene intake relative to the lowest quintile of intake (Rimm et al., 1993). The effect of β-carotene varied by smoking status: among current smokers, the relative risk was 0.30 (95 percent CI = 0.11–0.82); among former smokers, the risk was 0.60 (95 percent CI = 0.38–0.94), and among nonsmokers, the risk was 1.09 (95 percent CI = 0.66–1.79). A prospective cohort study of postmenopausal women found that the lowest risk of coronary heart disease was found for dietary carotenoid intakes greater than 8,857 IU/day (RR = 0.77; p = NS) (Kushi et al., 1996). A case-control study in 10 European countries found that lycopene concentrations, but not other carotenoid concentrations, in adipose tissue were inversely associated with the risk of myocardial infarction (Kohlmeier et al., 1997).

Cardiovascular epidemiology studies are now pursuing the use of intermediate endpoints, such as intima-media thickness, which can be estimated via ultrasonography as a measure of atherosclerosis. Bonithon-Kopp et al. (1997) reported a decrease in the intima-media thickness of the common carotid arteries with increasing concentrations of total plasma carotenoids in both men and women. Plasma carotenoid concentrations in excess of 2.07 μmol/L (111 μg/dL) were optimal for men; concentrations in excess of 3.73 μmol/L (200 μg/dL) were optimal for women. Salonen et al. (1993)

evaluated the change in the intima-media thickness as a measure of atherosclerotic progression and reported that progression was 92 percent greater in the lowest (less than or equal to 0.27 µmol/L [14 µg/dL]) versus the highest (more than or equal to 0.64 µmol/L [34 µg/dL]) quartile of plasma β-carotene.

Age-Related Macular Degeneration

Dietary carotenoids have been suggested to decrease the risk of age-related macular degeneration (AMD), the most common cause of irreversible blindness in people over age 65 in the United States, Canada, and Europe (Seddon et al., 1994; Snodderly, 1995). The macula lutea (macula) is a bright yellow spot in the center of the retina and is specialized and functions to maintain acute central vision. Of all the carotenoids circulating in the body, only two polar species, lutein and zeaxanthin, are contained in the macula (Bone et al., 1985; Handelman et al., 1988). Two groups of investigators have suggested pathways by which these two carotenoids are biochemically interchanged in the macula (Bone et al., 1993; Khachik et al., 1997a).

The potential role of carotenoids in the prevention of AMD has been comprehensively reviewed (Snodderly, 1995). Seddon et al. (1994) analyzed the association between carotenoid intake and advanced AMD in a large, multicenter, case-control study involving 356 cases and 520 control subjects with other ocular conditions. Those in the highest quintile of dietary carotenoid intake had a 43 percent lower risk for macular degeneration compared with those in the lowest (OR = 0.57; 95 percent CI = 0.35–0.92). Among the specific carotenoids, intake of lutein and zeaxanthin (grouped in the carotenoid food composition database) was most strongly associated with decreased risk. Those in the highest quintile of intake had a 60 percent lower risk compared to the lowest quintile of intake.

Some, but not all, studies using blood carotenoid concentrations also suggest protective effects against risk of AMD. The Eye Disease Case-Control Study (EDCCSG, 1993) measured serum carotenoids in 391 cases with neovascular AMD and 577 control subjects. The study reported protective effects of total carotenoids, α-carotene, β-carotene, β-cryptoxanthin, and lutein and zeaxanthin, with odds ratios ranging from 0.3 to 0.5 for the high group (more than the eightieth percentile) versus the low group (less than the twentieth percentile). Carotenoid concentrations associated with the lowest risk are shown in Table 8-4.

TABLE 8-4 Example of Plasma Carotenoid Concentrations Associated with Lowest Risk of Age-Related Macular Degeneration

Carotenoids	Concentrations (μmol/L)[a]
Total carotenoids	≥2.39 (128 μg/dL)
α-Carotene	≥0.19 (10 μg/dL)
β-Carotene	≥0.74 (40 μg/dL)
β-Cryptoxanthin	≥0.32 (18 μg/dL)
Lutein and zeaxanthin	≥0.67 (38 μg/dL)
Lycopene	≥0.61 (33 μg/dL)

[a] SI conversion factor used for total carotenoids, α- and β-carotene, and lycopene = 0.01863 μg/dL to μmol/L; for β-cryptoxanthin = 0.01809; and for lutein and zeaxanthin = 0.01758.
SOURCE: EDCCSG (1993).

Mares-Perlman et al. (1994) examined the association between serum carotenoid concentrations and age-related maculopathy in 167 case-control pairs and reported no association for any of the carotenoids, except lycopene, with persons in the lowest quintile of lycopene having a doubling in risk of maculopathy (cutpoint not stated). West et al. (1994) examined the relationship between plasma β-carotene concentration and AMD in 226 subjects and found the risk was lowest for the highest quartile of plasma β-carotene (more than 0.88 μmol/L [47 μg/dL]) (OR high quartile versus low = 0.62). Plasma lutein and zeaxanthin were not measured in this study.

Hammond and Fuld (1992) developed an optical system that, in situ, measures the intensity of the unique yellow color of the macula and presumably estimates the levels of lutein and zeaxanthin. This measure is known as Macular Pigment Optical Density (MPOD). Dietary intake of carotenoids, fat, and iron, as well as plasma concentrations of lutein and zeaxanthin, were positively related with MPOD in men, but only plasma concentrations of lutein and zeaxanthin were associated with MPOD values for women (Hammond et al., 1996). In the same studies, men had significantly higher MPOD readings than women despite similar plasma carotenoid concentrations and similar dietary intake, except for fat. These investigators also demonstrated that the MPOD of most subjects could be substantially increased by the addition of relatively small amounts of foods to the diet that are high in lutein ($^1/_2$ cup spinach per day) or lutein and zeaxanthin (1 cup of corn per day) (Hammond et al., 1997). Interestingly, when MPOD was enhanced following dietary modification, it was maintained at that level for several months despite resumption of an unmodified diet.

In summary, results of studies that have investigated MPOD as a biological indicator of carotenoid adequacy suggest that it has substantial potential as an indicator for estimating the requirements for lutein and zeaxanthin. Because of the unique metabolism of carotenoids in the macula, this technique will be useful in associating dietary intakes of lutein and zeaxanthin with the health of the macula. However, insufficient MPOD studies have been conducted to date to make recommendations relative to the dietary intakes of lutein and zeaxanthin.

Cataracts

Cataracts are also problematic, with cataract extraction being the most frequently performed surgical procedure in the elderly (Taylor, 1993). Although the etiology of this condition is not known, oxidative processes may play a role. Cataracts are thought to result from photo-oxidation of lens proteins, resulting in protein damage, accumulation, aggregation, and precipitation in the lens (Taylor, 1993). The cornea and lens filter out ultraviolet light, but visible blue light reaches the retina and may contribute to photic damage or other oxidative insults (Seddon et al., 1994).

Higher dietary intake of carotenoids or higher blood concentrations of carotenoids have been found to be inversely associated with the risk of various forms of cataract in some, but not all, studies. Jacques and Chylack (1991) reported that subjects with low plasma carotenoid concentrations (those with concentrations less than the twentieth percentile: less than 1.7 µmol/L [90 µg/dL]) had a 5.6-fold increased risk of any senile cataract and a 7.2-fold increased risk of cortical cataract, compared with subjects with high plasma total carotenoid concentrations (greater than the eightieth percentile; more than 3.3 µmol/L [177 µg/dL]). Mares-Perlman et al. (1995) performed a cross-sectional analysis of serum α-carotene, β-carotene, β-cryptoxanthin, lutein and zeaxanthin, and lycopene versus the severity of nuclear and cortical opacities, and found that higher concentrations of individual or total carotenoids were not associated with the severity of nuclear or cortical opacities overall. However, higher serum β-carotene (highest quintile median concentration 0.32 µmol/L [17 µg/dL]) was associated with less opacity in men, and higher concentrations of α-carotene (highest quintile median 0.14 μmol/L [7.5 μg/dL]), β-cryptoxanthin (highest quintile median 0.31 μmol/L [17 μg/dL]), and lutein (highest quintile median 0.44 μmol/L [25 μg/dL]) were associated with less nuclear sclerosis in men who smoked. In women, however, higher concentrations of some carotenoids (highest quintile median 2.19 μmol/L [118 μg/dL]) were associated with an increased severity of nuclear sclerosis.

Recently, the U.S. Health Professionals Follow-up Study reported a relative risk for cataract extraction in men of 0.81 (95 percent CI = 0.65–1.01) for those at the top quintile of lutein and zeaxanthin intake (median intake of 6.87 mg/day) relative to the lowest quintile of intake (Brown et al., 1999). Similar inverse associations for dietary lutein and zeaxanthin were seen in the Nurses' Health Study cohort, with a relative risk of 0.78 (95 percent CI = 0.63–0.95) for those at the top quintile of total lutein and zeaxanthin intake (median intake of 11.68 mg/day) relative to the lowest quintile of intake (Chasan-Taber et al., 1999). This decreased risk of cataracts (severe enough to require extraction) with higher intakes of lutein and zeaxanthin was not found with higher intakes of other carotenoids (α-carotene, β-carotene, lycopene, and β-cryptoxanthin) in either of these studies.

Plasma and Tissue Concentrations

As just detailed, plasma and tissue concentrations of carotenoids have been associated with a variety of health outcomes; that is, higher concentrations are associated with a lower risk of cancer, coronary heart disease, and all-cause mortality. This could be used as a possible indicator for establishing requirements for carotenoids. However, the limitation of this approach is that it is not clear whether observed health benefits are due to carotenoids per se or to other substances found in carotenoid-rich foods.

Thus, these data are suggestive of prudent intake levels, not required levels of intake. Recommendations have been made by a number of federal agencies and other organizations with regard to fruit and vegetable intake. Nutrient analysis of menus adhering to the U.S. Dietary Guidelines and the National Cancer Institute's Five-a-Day for Better Health Program, for example, indicates that persons following these diets would be consuming approximately 5.2 to 6.0 mg/day provitamin A carotenes on average if a variety of fruits and vegetables were consumed (Lachance, 1997). Similar levels would be obtained by following Canada's Food Guide for

Healthy Eating which specifies a minimum of five servings of vegetables and fruit (Health Canada, 1997). Other food-based dietary patterns recommended for the prevention of cancer and other chronic diseases would provide approximately 9 to 18 mg/day of carotenoids (WCRF/AICR, 1997).

The current U.S. and international guidelines encourage plant-based dietary patterns with less emphasis on foods of animal origin. With this type of dietary pattern, approximately 90 percent of the total ingested vitamin A would be in the form of provitamin A carotenoids (Lachance, 1997). This pattern is in stark contrast to current intake patterns in the United States, where less than 40 percent of vitamin A in the diet is derived from provitamin A carotenoids in fruits and vegetables (Figure 8-2), or to the intake patterns found in native Americans in some arctic regions of the United States and Canada (Kuhnlein et al., 1996).

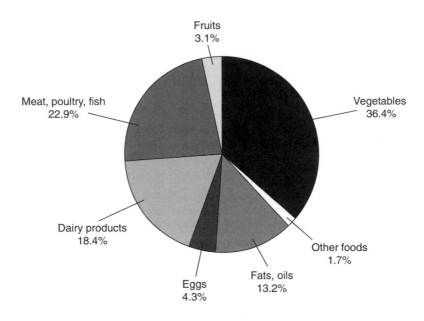

FIGURE 8-2 Contributors to Vitamin A intake in the U.S. food supply. The "other foods" category includes grain products (0.5 percent) and miscellaneous foods (1.2 percent).
SOURCE: LSRO/FASEB (1995).

An examination of human studies using dietary interventions with carotenoid-containing foods is necessary to determine the plasma carotene concentrations that an optimal diet would be expected to produce. In a controlled diet study (Micozzi et al., 1992), plasma β-carotene concentrations in the men who received the low carotenoid diet (less than 2 mg/day) to which broccoli had been added to provide 6 mg/day of carotenoids (3 mg of β-carotene, 3 mg of lutein) were raised significantly from 0.30 μmol/L (16 μg/dL) at baseline to 0.49 μmol/L (26 μg/dL) after six weeks, as were plasma lutein concentrations (from 0.38 μmol/L [22 μg/dL] to 0.63 μmol/L [36 μg/dL]). Plasma lycopene declined with this intervention because the baseline diet as well as broccoli was low in the content of lycopene and other carotenoids.

The Minnesota Cancer Prevention Research Unit feeding studies evaluated three experimental diets (two of which included carotenoids) and one control diet given for 9 days each to 23 young nonsmoking men and women. Persons on the control diet had a plasma β-carotene concentration of 0.26 μmol/L (14 μg/dL); 5 mg/day β-carotene from food increased plasma β-carotene to 0.37 μmol/L (19.5 μg/dL). When β-carotene from food was increased to 42 mg/day, plasma β-carotene increased further to 0.83 μmol/L (44 μg/dL) (Martini et al., 1995). Yong et al. (1994) studied dietary carotenoid intake and plasma carotenoids cross-sectionally in premenopausal nonsmoking women; the population had a geometric mean β-carotene intake of approximately 3 mg/day and a geometric mean plasma β-carotene concentration of 0.30 μmol/L (15.8 μg/dL). For total carotenoids, the geometric mean level of intake was 6.6 to 8.1 mg/day, with a total carotenoid concentration in plasma of approximately 1.51 μmol/L (80 μg/dL). A randomized, controlled trial on the effect of increasing fruit and vegetable intake for 8 weeks on plasma micronutrient concentrations was conducted with 87 subjects in New Zealand (Zino et al., 1997). β-Carotene intake increased from about 2.0 mg/day at baseline to 4.7 mg/day at week 4. This resulted in a mean plasma β-carotene increase from 0.34 μmol/L (18 μg/dL) at baseline to 0.48 μmol/L (25 μg/dL) at 4 weeks.

These data, although in varying populations, suggest that 3 to 6 mg/day of β-carotene from food sources is prudent to maintain plasma β-carotene concentrations in the range associated with a lower risk of various chronic disease outcomes (see Table 8-3).

FACTORS AFFECTING CAROTENOID BIOAVAILABILITY

Bioavailability

Bioavailability of carotenoids from food, concentrated extracts, or synthetic products is quite variable (Figure 8-3) because a complex set of factors affects carotenoid bioavailability. Erdman et al. (1993) and Castenmiller and West (1998) described the events necessary for adequate absorption of carotenoids from the diet: (1) digestion of the food matrix, (2) formation of lipid micelles in the gastrointes-

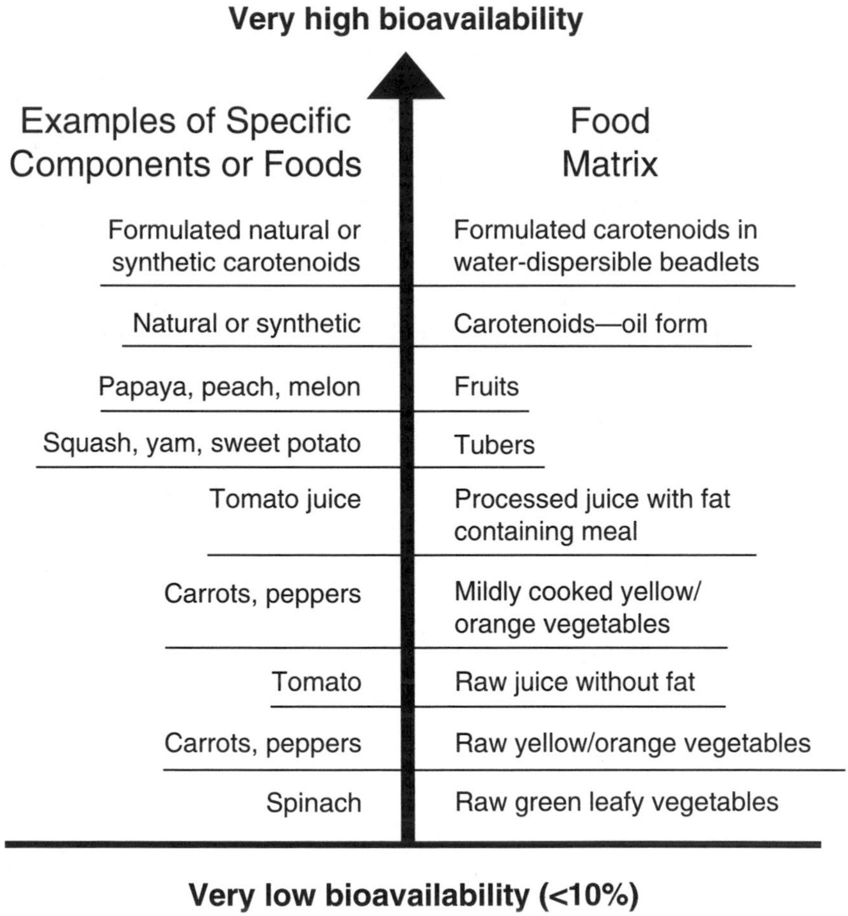

Very high bioavailability

Examples of Specific Components or Foods	Food Matrix
Formulated natural or synthetic carotenoids	Formulated carotenoids in water-dispersible beadlets
Natural or synthetic	Carotenoids—oil form
Papaya, peach, melon	Fruits
Squash, yam, sweet potato	Tubers
Tomato juice	Processed juice with fat containing meal
Carrots, peppers	Mildly cooked yellow/ orange vegetables
Tomato	Raw juice without fat
Carrots, peppers	Raw yellow/orange vegetables
Spinach	Raw green leafy vegetables

Very low bioavailability (<10%)

FIGURE 8-3 Effect of food matrix and processing on bioavailability of carotenoids. SOURCE: Adapted from Boileau et al (1999).

tinal tract, (3) uptake of carotenoids by intestinal mucosal cells, and (4) transport of carotenoids and their metabolic products to the lymph or portal circulation.

Food Matrix

Of the factors that affect carotenoid bioavailability, the food matrix effects on carotenoid absorption are generally the most critical. The absorption of β-carotene supplements that are solubilized with emulsifiers and protected by antioxidants can be 70 percent or more. In contrast, less than 5 percent bioavailability of carotenes has been reported from raw foods such as carrots (Rodriguez and Irwin, 1972). Recently, van het Hof et al. (1999) reported substantial differences between the relative bioavailabilities of β-carotene (14 percent) compared to lutein (67 percent) when feeding a high-vegetable diet (490 g of vegetables without supplements) and comparing it to a low-vegetable diet (130 g of vegetables) supplemented with β-carotene (6 mg/day) or lutein (9 mg/day), both of which were assumed to be 100 percent bioavailable. These differences were based on changes in plasma concentration of β-carotene or lutein.

Daily supplementation of dark-green leafy vegetables rich in carotenoids to lactating Indonesian women with low vitamin A status did not increase vitamin A status, whereas a similar amount of β-carotene given in a wafer supplement led to a significant increase in plasma retinol (de Pee et al., 1995). More recently, the same group (de Pee et al., 1998) studied anemic school children in Indonesia and calculated the relative vitamin A equivalency of β-carotene from different food sources. The calculated equivalencies were as follows: 26 μg of β-carotene from leafy vegetables and carrots corresponded to 12 μg of β-carotene from fruit, and equaled 1 μg of preformed vitamin A in vitamin A-rich foods. In contrast, Mahapatra and Manorama (1997), in a small study with vitamin A-deficient school children in India, concluded that β-carotene from red palm oil was as bioavailable as preformed vitamin A.

β-Carotene in the form of supplements has a much higher bioavailablity than β-carotene from foods. Micozzi et al. (1992) demonstrated that 30 mg/day of supplemental all-trans β-carotene produced more than a fivefold increase in plasma β-carotene compared to 29 mg/day of β-carotene from carrots. The relatively low bioavailability of plant carotenoids may be due to the fact that they can be bound in carotenoproteins and are often associated with the plant matrix. Typically in green leafy vegetables, carotenoids are found bound in chloroplasts where they play roles in photosynthesis. In carrot root, α- and β-carotene are largely in crystal forms. In both cases, the carotenoids are not easily solubilized out of these tissues by the digestive process.

Cooking

The hypothesis that cooking may improve the bioavailability of carotenoids has been tested. The bioavailability of lycopene from tomato juice is vastly improved by heat treatment in the presence of oil (Gartner et al., 1997; Stahl and Sies, 1992). When subjects consumed tomato juice (equivalent to a single lycopene dose of 2.5 μmol/kg body weight) that had been heated at 100°C for 1 hour with oil, they experienced a serum lycopene peak at 24 to 48 hours. In contrast, equivalent doses that were not heat treated did not result in an increase in serum lycopene. Steaming has also been shown to increase the amount of extractable carotenoids in spinach and carrots (Dietz et al., 1988). In contrast to steaming, more prolonged exposure to high temperatures (boiling) can reduce the carotenoid availability of vegetables by increasing the production of isomers or oxidation products. For example, canned carrots contain 73 percent all-trans β-carotene, 19 percent 13-cis-β-carotene, and 8 percent 9-cis-β-carotene, while fresh carrots contain 100 percent of the β-carotene in the all-trans configuration (Chandler and Schwartz, 1987). The relative vitamin A values of cis isomers of β-carotene compared to all-trans β-carotene is an active area of research.

Dietary Fat

Many research groups have shown that to optimize carotenoid absorption, dietary fat must be consumed during the same eating period as the carotenoid. Roels et al. (1958) demonstrated that in boys with vitamin A deficiency in an African village, supplementation of their carotene-sufficient but low-fat diets with 18 g/day of olive oil improved carotene absorption from 5 to 25 percent. More recently, Jalal et al. (1998) studied the roles of β-carotene-rich meals (mostly red sweet potatoes), extra dietary fat (15 g/day), and deworming on serum retinol concentrations of children in Sumatra. Prior to the intervention, these children all had intestinal infestations and were consuming diets with about 7 percent of calories from fat. A 3-week intervention of β-carotene-rich meals alone improved vitamin A status without added fat or deworming, but the combination of all three measures—β-carotene meals, added fat, and deworming—provided the greatest increase in serum retinol.

Other Factors

Lipid-lowering drugs have been shown to decrease serum carotenoids dramatically (Elinder et al., 1995). In a double-blind, randomized trial, treatment with cholestyramine (a lipid-lowering resin) for 4 months and probucol (antioxidant and lipid-lowering drug) for 2 months resulted in a 65 percent reduction in serum β-carotene and a 51 percent reduction in lycopene. The reductions were attributed to reduced intestinal absorption of lipids by cholestyramine and reduced lipoprotein particle number and size by probucol. Sucrose polyester (olestra), the nonabsorbable fat substitute, lowered carotenoid absorption when consumed at the same time as carotenoids (Koonsvitsky et al., 1997; Weststrate and van het Hof, 1995). Plant sterol-enriched margarines (Weststrate and Meijer, 1998) and dietary pectin supplementation also decreased β-carotene absorption (Rock and Swendseid, 1992).

Nutrient-Nutrient Interactions

Competitive interactions among different carotenoids during the absorptive process have been studied. Recipients of daily β-carotene supplements in either 12-mg or 30-mg capsules for 6 weeks had significantly lower plasma lutein concentrations than subjects who consumed both β-carotene and lutein from food sources (Micozzi et al., 1992). In addition, plasma β-carotene was higher in the subjects receiving β-carotene as supplements rather than as food, demonstrating the greater bioavailability of this source. Interactions between β-carotene and lutein have also been described by other investigators. When subjects were given purified crystalline β-carotene and crystalline lutein in a combined dose, β-carotene significantly reduced the serum area under the curve (AUC) value (a measure of total absorption) for lutein (Kostic et al., 1995). Lutein in a combined dose with β-carotene significantly enhanced β-carotene AUC in those subjects whose AUC for β-carotene (when dosed alone) was the lowest.

These studies (White et al., 1994) indicate that two carotenoids administered concurrently in controlled settings can affect the absorption of each other. Several investigators have examined the effect of daily supplementation with high-dose β-carotene on plasma concentrations of other carotenoids in participants in multiyear cancer prevention intervention trials (Albanes et al., 1997; Mayne et al., 1998; Nierenberg et al., 1997; Wahlqvist et al., 1994). These studies suggest no overall adverse effect on other carotenoids with high-dose supplementation of β-carotene daily for several years. This finding is not inconsistent with the results of the metabolic studies, because the trials were done in free-living individuals taking a supplement of β-carotene each day, which most likely is not consumed concurrently with an entire day's intake of other carotenoids from food.

FINDINGS BY LIFE STAGE AND GENDER GROUP

As discussed elsewhere in this document, this report does not establish a requirement for β-carotene or other carotenoids for any gender or life stage group. This issue will be considered in a subsequent report when addressing vitamin A. However, the following summarizes findings regarding carotenoid status, as measured by serum carotenoid concentrations, in different groups of the population.

Special Populations

If plasma carotenoid concentrations are considered as an indicator of adequacy with regard to reducing risk of chronic disease, it becomes apparent that certain subgroups of the population are known to have notably lower circulating concentrations of carotenoids. Thus, consumption of carotenoid-containing foods may have to be greater in these groups in order to achieve plasma carotenoid concentrations that are associated with a reduced risk of chronic disease (Table 8-3).

Adolescents

Serum carotenoid concentrations were measured in the Third National Health and Nutrition Examination Survey (NHANES III). As shown in Appendix Table F-4, serum β-carotene concentrations were lower during the period of adolescence and early adulthood in this U.S. population survey. The average concentration in children was approximately 0.34 μmol/L (18 μg/dL), which dropped to 0.28 μmol/L (15 μg/dL) or less in teenagers and did not return to childhood concentrations until the fourth decade (the thirties) for women, and the fifth decade (the forties) for men. This lower level during adolescence is also evident for α-carotene (Appendix Table F-5), β-cryptoxanthin (Appendix Table F-6), and lutein/zeaxanthin (Appendix Table F-7), but not lycopene (Appendix Table F-8). This may reflect relatively greater consumption of tomato products compared to other vegetables by adolescents in the United States.

Smoking

Many investigators have reported that those who smoke, on average, have lower plasma carotenoid concentrations compared to individuals that don't smoke (Brady et al., 1996; Chow et al., 1986; Comstock et al., 1988; Fukao et al., 1996; Herbeth et al., 1990; Margetts and Jackson, 1996, Pamuk et al., 1994; Stryker et al., 1988; Witter et al., 1982). The greater the intensity of smoking (cigarettes per day), the greater is the decrease in serum carotenoid concentrations. Fukao et al. (1996) studied 1,902 Japanese men in a cohort study and showed a dose-dependent decline in geometric mean serum β-carotene with greater smoking intensity (Table 8-5).

While smokers ingest less β-carotene than nonsmokers, it is unclear at present whether or not the lower serum concentrations seen can be fully explained by the reduced β-carotene intakes of smokers, as discussed recently by Brady et al. (1996). Many studies find differences in serum carotenoid concentrations even after adjusting for intake. However, because dietary intake is necessarily measured with some error, it is unclear whether full adjustment is possible. Tobacco smoke is known to be highly oxidative, and the gas phase of tobacco smoke has been shown to destroy β-carotene and other carotenoids in in vitro studies of human plasma (Handelman et al., 1996). As demonstrated recently by Baker et al. (1999), both smoke and gas-phase smoke oxidize β-carotene to carbonyls, epoxides, and nitro derivatives. Thus, it is possible that the smoke oxidatively degrades β-carotene in vivo and thus contributes to the reduction in circulating levels.

TABLE 8-5 Serum β-Carotene in Men in Relation to Smoking

	Mean[a] Serum β-Carotene (μmol/L)
Nonsmokers	0.39 (20.7 μg/dL)
Ex-smokers	0.31 (16.6 μg/dL)
Smokers	
1–10 cigarettes/d	0.25 (13.6 μg/dL)
11–20 cigarettes/d	0.23 (12.1 μg/dL)
21–100 cigarettes/d	0.20 (10.5 μg/dL)

[a] Geometric mean.
SOURCE: Fukao et al. (1996).

A first report in the area of putative mechanisms to explain the increase in lung cancer risk observed in heavy smokers taking high-dose supplements indicates that ferrets exposed to cigarette smoke and supplemented with β-carotene developed squamous metaplasia in their lungs as well as altered retinoid signaling (Wang et al., 1999). Another report suggests that oxidation products of β-carotene stimulate the binding of metabolites of benzo[a]pyrene to deoxyribonucleic acid (Salgo et al., 1999). These very new data await confirmation and further development.

Although smoking may result in a need for higher intakes of dietary carotenoids to achieve optimal plasma carotenoid concentrations, caution is warranted because β-carotene supplements, but not β-carotene-rich foods, have been suggested as causing adverse effects in smokers (see "Tolerable Upper Intake Levels"). Thus, any recommendations need to state clearly that those who smoke, in particular, may benefit from even higher average intakes of carotenoids *from foods.*

Alcohol Consumption

Alcohol intake, like tobacco, is inversely associated with serum β-carotene and carotenoid concentrations (Brady et al., 1996; Fukao et al., 1996; Herbeth et al., 1988, 1990; Stryker et al., 1988). Brady et al. (1996) reported that higher ethanol intake was associated with a decrease in all serum carotenoids measured, with the exception of lycopene. The inverse association appears to be dose dependent as shown by the cohort study in men of Fukao et al. (1996) in Table 8-6. It should be noted that in this study, the effects of smoking and alcohol consumption independently affected serum β-carotene concentrations in men.

Persons who consume large quantities of ethanol typically consume diets that are micronutrient deficient. Therefore, as is the case for smoking, it is not clear whether the observed decrements are fully attributable to reduced intakes or also reflect metabolic consequences of chronic ethanol ingestion.

INTAKE OF CAROTENOIDS

Food Sources

A database of values for α-carotene, β-carotene, β-cryptoxanthin, lutein plus zeaxanthin, and lycopene for 120 foods has been assembled (Mangels et al., 1993) and was recently updated and released

TABLE 8-6 Serum β-Carotene in Men in Relation to Alcohol Consumption

	Mean[a] Serum β-carotene (μmol/L)
Nondrinkers	0.38 (20.1 μg/dL)
Ex-drinkers	0.32 (16.9 μg/dL)
Drinkers	
1–15 g ethanol/d	0.33 (17.9 μg/dL)
15–28 g ethanol/d	0.30 (16.2 μg/dL)
29–56 g ethanol/d	0.19 (10.0 μg/dL)
56–140 g ethanol/d	0.15 (8.2 μg/dL)

[a] Geometric mean.
SOURCE: Fukao et al. (1996).

(Holden et al., 1999). Using an expansion of the earlier database and based on the 1986 U.S. Department of Agriculture Continuing Survey of Food Intake by Individuals (CSFII), Chug-Ahuja et al. (1993) reported that carrots were the major contributor of β-carotene to the diet of women of reproductive age (25 percent) with lesser contributions from the following food categories: cantaloupe, broccoli, vegetable beef or chicken soup, and spinach or collard greens. Similarly, the major contributors for α-carotene, β-cryptoxanthin, lycopene, and lutein and zeaxanthin were, respectively, carrots, followed by the categories of orange juice and its blends, tomatoes and tomato products, and spinach or collard greens.

A summary of the carotenoid content of human milk is shown in Table 8-7. It should be noted that the β-carotene content and the concentrations of other carotenoids in human milk are highly variable and appear to be altered easily by manipulation of the carotenoid content of the mother's diet. Most infant formulas, either milk or soy based, do not have carotenoids added to them and, as a result, would be expected to contain very low levels of β-carotene and other carotenoids.

Dietary Intake

Data for intakes of carotenoids (β-carotene, α-carotene, β-cryptoxanthin, lutein and zeaxanthin, and lycopene) from the 1988–1992 Third National Health and Nutrition Examination Survey (NHANES III) based on an expanded food composition database

TABLE 8-7 Carotenoid Content in Human Milk[a]

Author, Year	Country	Number of Subjects	Stage of Lactation[b]	Maternal Carotenoid Intake
Gebre-Medhin et al., 1976	Sweden	66	0.5–1.5 mo 1.5–3.5 mo 3.5–6.5 mo	Not reported
Butte and Calloway, 1981	U.S.[d]	23	19–62 d	Suboptimal
Chappell et al., 1985	Canada	24[f]	1 d 4 d 37 d	Not reported
Ostrea et al., 1986	U.S.	19[f]	1–5 d	Not reported
Patton et al., 1990	U.S.	11	Colostrum	Not reported
Giuliano et al., 1992	U.S.	3	1 mo	Not reported
Giuliano et al., 1994	U.S.	18	>1 mo	Not reported
Canfield et al., 1997	U.S.	12	≤6 mo	Dietary intake: β-carotene: 5.08 ± 2.5 mg/d α-carotene: 13.0 ± 0.8 mg/d Lycopene: 2.8 ± 2.6 mg/d β-Carotene supplements: Group 1: 60 mg/wk × 10 wk Group 2: 210 mg/wk × 3 wk

Carotenoid Content in Milk (μg/dL) [c]	Methods
β-Carotene: 16.3 ± 7.5 β-Carotene: 17.1 ± 7.5 β-Carotene: 20.8 ± 10.2	Spectrophotometric
Carotene: 19.7 ± 6.3 [e]	Spectrophotometric
Carotene: 200 ± 12 Carotene: 100 ± 4 Carotene: 23 ± 5	HPLC [g]
β-Carotene: day 1: 213 ± 167 day 2: 117 ± 112 day 3: 120 ± 63 day 4: 50 ± 20 day 5: 39 ± 35	Spectrophotometric
α-Carotene: 16 ± 17 β-Carotene: 66 ± 76 β-Cryptoxanthin: 71 ± 61 Lycopene: 96 ± 85	TLC [h], HPLC, and spectrophotometric
α-Carotene: 0.32 ± 0.02 β-Carotene: 1.01 ± 0.02 Lutein: 1.06 ± 0.03 Lycopene: 2.73 ± 0.13	HPLC
α-Carotene: 0.6 ± 0.4 β-Carotene: 2.5 ± 1.6 [i] β-Cryptoxanthin: 1.1 ± 0.4 Lycopene: 1.7 ± 0.9	HPLC

Initial β-carotene:
    1.9 ± 0.3 (group 1)
    2.7 ± 0.9 (group 2)
 	
Postsupplementation:
    β-carotene milk concentrations were
    4 times the initial for both groups.
    No significant increases in α-carotene,
    β-cryptoxanthin, lutein/zeaxanthin,
    or lycopene noted
	HPLC

continued

TABLE 8-7 Carotenoid Content in Human Milk[a]

Author, Year	Country	Number of Subjects	Stage of Lactation[b]	Maternal Carotenoid Intake
Johnson et al., 1997	U.S.	12	1–8 mo	Supplement: 64 mg all-trans-β-carotene + 69 mg 9-cis-β-carotene (1 dose/d × 7 d) Fed a low-carotenoid diet
Canfield et al., 1998	U.S.	5	>1 mo	Mean dietary intake of β-carotene at baseline = 4.0 ± 3.5 mg/d (measured by three 24-h dietary intake records) Supplemented with 30 mg β-carotene for 28 d

NOTE: For Guiliano et al. (1994), Canfield et al. (1997, 1998), and Johnson et al. (1997), milk carotenoid values were converted from nmol/L or μmol/L to μg/dL. The conversion factor used for β-carotene, α-carotene, lutein/zeaxanthin: μg/dL × 0.01863 = μmol/L. The conversion factor used for β-cryptoxanthin: μg/dL × 0.01809 = μmol/L.

[a] Unless noted otherwise, milk content was based on studies of healthy women with full-term pregnancies.
[b] pp = Postpartum.
[c] Mean ± standard deviation.
[d] U.S. = United States.
[e] Mean milk volume was reported as 634 ± 113 mL/d.

for carotenoids are presently being analyzed and are not available to be included in this report. Thus, they will be included in the appendix of the next DRI report that will include vitamin A.

However, dietary recall data from 1,102 adult women participating in the 1986 Continuing Survey of Food Intake by Individuals indicate mean intakes of β-carotene, α-carotene, lutein, and lycopene of 1.8, 0.4, 1.3, and 2.6 mg/day, respectively, with total carotenoid intake from β-carotene, α-carotene, β-cryptoxanthin, lutein, zeaxanthin, and lycopene of approximately 6 mg/day (Chug-Ahuja et al., 1993). Later food frequency data from the 8,341 adults participating in the 1992 National Health Interview Survey indicate that mean intakes of β-carotene, lutein, and lycopene for men were 2.9,

Carotenoid Content in Milk (µg/dL) [c]	Methods

all-trans-β-Carotene[j]
  prestudy: ≈ 42.9
  d 8: ≈ 225.4
9-*cis*-β-Carotene
  prestudy: ≈ 1.3
  d 8: ≈ 3.2
	HPLC

Initial[i,k]:
  α-carotene: 0.7 ± 0.2
  β-carotene: 3.6 ± 1.0
  β-cryptoxanthin : 1.4 ± 0.2
  Lutein/zeaxanthin: 1.2 ± 0.2
  Lycopene: 2.6 ± 0.3
Postsupplementation:
  β-carotene concentrations increased,
  on average, 6.4-fold over initial and
  remained elevated (≈ 2-fold over
  initial) 1 mo after supplementation
	HPLC

f Milk samples were obtained from both preterm and full-term pregnancies.

g HPLC = high-performance liquid chromatography.

h TLC = thin-layer chromatography.

i Large intra- and interindividual variability in milk carotenoid concentration.

j One month after the study, milk concentrations remained higher than baseline in the supplemented women. No changes in milk concentrations were seen in the placebo group.

k Mean milk volume was reported as 62.9 mL per human-feeding episode (Canfield et al., 1998).

2.2, and 2.3 mg/day, respectively, and for women 2.5, 1.9, and 2.1 mg/day, respectively (Nebeling et al., 1997). Another survey, the Nutritional Factors in Eye Disease Study, with 2,152 adults responding to a food frequency questionnaire, reported median dietary carotenoid intakes or ranges of 1.3 mg/day of β-carotene, 0.2 mg/day of α-carotene, 0.02–0.07 mg/day of β-cryptoxanthin, 0.7–0.8 mg/day of lutein and zeaxanthin, and 0.6–1.6 mg/day of lycopene (VandenLangenberg et al., 1996).

Intake levels of β-carotene for infants can be estimated using data on human milk concentrations of β-carotene (Table 8-7). Human milk β-carotene concentrations obtained at more than 1 month postpartum varied from 1 to 21 µg/dL. Assuming that infants receiving human milk consume 0.78 L/day on average in the first 6 months (Chapter 2); this would result in β-carotene intake levels of 8 to 163 µg/day.

Intake from Supplements

β-Carotene, α-carotene, lutein and zeaxanthin, and lycopene are available as dietary supplements. There are no reliable estimates of the amount of these dietary supplements consumed by individuals in the United States or Canada.

TOLERABLE UPPER INTAKE LEVELS

Hazard Identification

Adverse Effects

No adverse effects other than carotenodermia have been reported from the consumption of β-carotene or other carotenoids in food. Carotenodermia is a harmless but clearly documented biological effect of high carotenoid intake. It is characterized by a yellowish discoloration of the skin that results from an elevation of carotene concentrations.

β-Carotene is used therapeutically, at extremely high doses (approximately 180 mg/day), for the treatment of erythropoietic protoporphyria, a photosensitivity disorder. No toxic side effects have been observed at these doses. There is no evidence that β-carotene or other carotenoids are teratogenic, mutagenic, or carcinogenic in long-term bioassays in experimental animals (Heywood et al., 1985). In addition, long-term supplementation with β-carotene to persons with adequate vitamin A status does not increase the concentration of serum retinol (Nierenberg et al., 1997). However, two recent clinical trials reported an increase in lung cancer associated with supplemental β-carotene in current smokers (ATBC Cancer Prevention Study Group, 1994; Omenn et al., 1996a,b). These effects are discussed below.

Lung Cancer. The Alpha-Tocopherol, Beta-Carotene (ATBC) Cancer Prevention Study showed a significantly higher incidence of lung cancer (relative risk [RR] = 1.18; 95 percent confidence interval [CI] = 1.03–1.36) and total mortality (RR = 1.08; 95 percent CI = 1.01–1.16) in current smokers supplemented with 20 mg/day β-carotene (with or without 50 mg of α-tocopherol) for 5 to 8 years compared to the placebo group (ATBC Cancer Prevention Study Group, 1994). Supplemental β-carotene had no significant effect on the incidence of other major cancers occurring in this population (prostate, bladder, colon or rectum, stomach). In addition, the Carotene and Retinol Efficacy Trial (CARET), a multicenter lung cancer prevention trial of a nutrient combination versus placebo in asbestos workers and smokers (Omenn et al., 1996a,b) reported more lung cancer cases in the supplemented group. The nutrient combination used in CARET included supplemental β-carotene (30 mg/day) plus retinol (25,000 international units [IU]/day). Both CARET and ATBC included β-carotene in the intervention and reported similar effects on lung cancer. However, it should be noted that CARET used a nutrient combination, without a factorial design, and it is not clear whether the reported effects were attributable to β-carotene, retinol, or both acting in concert.

In contrast, the Physicians' Health Study of supplemental β-carotene versus placebo in 22,071 male U.S. physicians reported no significant effect of 12 years of supplementation with β-carotene (50 mg every other day) on cancer or total mortality (Hennekens et al., 1996). With regard to lung cancer, there was no indication of excess lung cancer in the β-carotene-supplemented individuals, even among smokers who took the supplements for up to 12 years.

One additional trial, which was not designed as a lung cancer prevention trial, nonetheless produced results that are of relevance to the topic of lung cancer prevention. The trial tested the efficacy of four different nutrient combinations in inhibiting the development of esophageal and gastric cancers in 30,000 men and women aged 40 to 69 years living in Linxian County, China (Blot et al., 1993). One of the nutrient supplements was a combination of β-carotene, selenium, and vitamin E. After a 5-year intervention period, those who were given this combination had a 13 percent reduction in cancer deaths (RR = 0.87; 95 percent CI = 0.75–1.00), a 9 percent reduction in total deaths (RR = 0.91; 95 percent CI = 0.84–0.99), a 4 percent reduction in esophageal cancer deaths (RR = 0.96; 95 percent CI = 0.78–1.18), and a 21 percent reduction in gastric cancer deaths (RR = 0.79; 95 percent CI = 0.64–0.99). For lung cancer, this trial had limited statistical power, with only 31 total lung cancer deaths (Blot et al., 1994). However, the relative risk of death from lung cancer was 0.55 (95 percent CI = 0.26–1.14) among those receiving the combination of β-carotene, α-tocopherol, and selenium. The smoking prevalence, including individuals who had ever smoked cigarettes for 6 or more months, was 30 percent.

At the present time, the data pertaining to a possible adverse effect of β-carotene in smokers are somewhat conflicting. The results of ongoing studies may help resolve this issue. There also appears to be a relationship between the adverse effects of β-carotene and both smoking and alcohol consumption in the ATBC and CARET trials. In the ATBC trial, only those men who consumed more than 11 g/day of alcohol (approximately one drink per day) showed an adverse response to β-carotene supplementation (Albanes et al., 1996). In the CARET study, adverse effects were associated with the individuals in the highest quartile of alcohol intake (Omenn et al., 1996a).

Carotenodermia. Carotenodermia is characterized by yellowish discoloration of the skin that results from an elevation of plasma carotene concentrations. This condition has been reported in adults taking supplements containing 30 mg/day or more of β-carotene for long periods of time or consuming high levels of carotenoid-rich foods such as carrots (Bendich, 1988) and is the primary effect of excess carotenoid intake noted in infants, toddlers, and young children (Lascari, 1981). Carotenodermia is distinguished from jaundice in that the ocular sclera are yellowed in jaundiced subjects but not in those with carotenodermia. Carotenodermia is considered harmless and is readily reversible when carotene ingestion is discontinued.

Lycopenodermia. Lycopenodermia results from high intakes of lycopene-rich foods such as tomatoes and is characterized by a deep orange discoloration of the skin. Lycopene is a more intensely colored pigment than carotene and may cause discoloration at lower concentrations than other carotenoids (Lascari, 1981).

Other Adverse Effects. Allergic reactions, increased incidence of prostate cancer, retinopathy, leukopenia, and reproductive disorders have been associated anecdotally with high carotene consumption (Bendich, 1988; Kobza et al., 1973; Shoenfeld et al., 1982). None of these effects has been confirmed by clinical trials. There is no evidence of hypervitaminosis A in individuals consuming high levels of β-carotene or other carotenoids (up to 180 mg/day) (Lewis, 1972; Mathews-Roth, 1986; Mathews-Roth et al., 1972, 1974).

Dose-Response Assessment

The data on the potential for β-carotene to produce increased lung cancer rates in smokers are conflicting and not sufficient for a dose-response assessment and derivation of a Tolerable Upper Intake Level (UL) for this endpoint. Supplements of 30 mg/day or more of β-carotene for long periods of time may be associated with carotenodermia, but this effect is more cosmetic than adverse and can be considered harmless and readily reversible. Because of the inconsistent data on adverse effects of β-carotene, a UL cannot be established at this time. ULs are not established for other carotenoids due to a lack of suitable data.

Intake Assessment

Data for intakes of carotenoids (β-carotene, α-carotene, β-cryptoxanthin, lutein and zeaxanthin, and lycopene) from the 1988–1992 Third National Health and Nutrition Examination Survey (NHANES III) based on an expanded food composition database for carotenoids are presently being analyzed and are not available to be included in this report. Thus, they will be included in the appendix of the next DRI report that will include vitamin A.

Risk Characterization

A possible increase in lung cancer incidence has been noted only in smokers taking high-dose supplements of β-carotene (20 mg/day or greater). As discussed earlier, supplemental forms of β-carotene have markedly greater bioavailability than β-carotene from foods. The bioavailability of β-carotene from supplements can also be variable depending on the formulation, nutritional status of the person or population, and dietary intake pattern (e.g., fat intake). Given these substantial differences in bioavailability, it is perhaps logical to characterize the risk as a function of plasma β-carotene concentration (see Figure 8-4). Median serum β-carotene concentrations in the participants receiving 20 mg/day of β-carotene in the Finnish trial rose from 0.32 μmol/L (17 μg/dL) at baseline to 5.66 μmol/L (300 μg/dL) at 3 years; this blood concentration was associated with an adverse effect (ATBC Cancer Prevention Study Group, 1994). In CARET, the median postintervention plasma concentration of β-carotene was 3.96 μmol/L (210 μg/dL); this blood concentration also was reported to be associated with an adverse effect (Omenn et al., 1996a). The first to ninety-ninth percentile for plasma β-carotene from NHANES III is also indicated in Appendix Table F-4. These data suggest that the concentrations associated with possible adverse effects on lung cancer are well beyond the concentrations achieved via dietary intake.

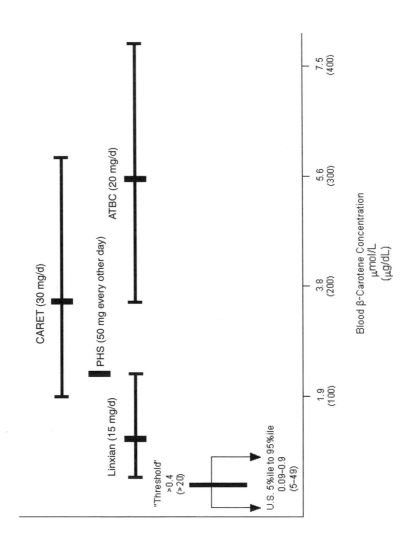

FIGURE 8-4 Risk characterization as a function of plasma β-carotene concentration in large population studies.
SOURCE: Mayne (1998).

Thus, while 20 mg/day of β-carotene in the form of a supplement is sufficient to raise blood concentrations to a range reported to be associated with an increase in lung cancer risk, the same amount of β-carotene in foods is not. Micozzi et al. (1992) demonstrated that 30 mg/day of supplemental β-carotene produced more than a five-fold increase in plasma β-carotene compared to 29 mg/day of β-carotene from carrots.

Based on these considerations, the existing recommendation for consumption of five or more servings of fruits and vegetables per day is supported because this would provide 3 to 6 mg/day of β-carotene. A UL has not been set for β-carotene or carotenoids. Instead, it is concluded that β carotene supplements are not advisable for the general population. This conclusion is based on a totality of evidence that includes several large-scale randomized trials of supplemental β-carotene. These trials indicate a lack of evidence of overall benefit on total cancer or cardiovascular disease and possible harm in certain subgroups such as current smokers or asbestos-exposed subjects. This advisement does not pertain to the possible use of supplemental β-carotene as a provitamin A source or for the prevention of vitamin A deficiency in populations with inadequate vitamin A nutriture or in patients suffering from erythropoietic protoporphyria.

RESEARCH RECOMMENDATIONS FOR β-CAROTENE AND OTHER CAROTENOIDS

• As described earlier, β-carotene and other carotenoids have been shown to modulate a variety of intermediate endpoints. However, studies validating that changes in an intermediate endpoint are predictive of changes in a health outcome are critically needed. As an example, macular pigment optical density (MPOD) is a promising intermediate marker for age-related macular degeneration (AMD), but human studies validating this endpoint prospectively are needed, as are studies demonstrating that changes in MPOD are predictive of changes in risk of macular degeneration.

• As a corollary, studies are needed on the effects of long-term depletion of β-carotene and subsequent repletion, with an evaluation of validated intermediate endpoints.

• Significantly more research is needed on health effects of dietary carotenoids other than β-carotene. Possible associations between lycopene and decreased prostate cancer risk, between lutein and zeaxanthin and lowered risk of AMD, and between α-carotene or lutein and various cancers have to be evaluated in additional observational studies, in animal models, and in human intervention trials, if justified. Studies should consider not only the other carotenoids, but also the *cis-* versus *trans*-configuration of the carotenoid.

• Since the data from the human intervention trials of β-carotene are contradictory, additional data are needed from intervention trials involving β-carotene, several of which are ongoing. An examination is needed of health effects in populations with varying baseline risk profiles and, in particular, of studies evaluating interventions in populations with poor baseline nutritional status. Posttrial follow-up of completed β-carotene trials is also needed.

• Studies aimed at the identification of correlates of higher β-carotene intake and plasma concentrations, which might help to explain the lower risks of cancer associated with carotene-rich diets, are needed.

• Additional research is needed that targets putative mechanisms to explain a possible increase in lung cancer risk in heavy smokers taking high-dose β-carotene supplements (animal studies, biochemical studies, and molecular studies). In particular, confirmation and extension of findings such as those of recent reports regarding lung metaplasia (Wang et al., 1999) and carotenoid oxidation products (Salgo et al., 1999), and their relevance to cancer development in humans, are needed.

• Surveys are needed that routinely assess and report dietary intakes of individual food carotenoids from large, representative population samples. Intakes from both foods and dietary supplements must be considered.

• Efforts should be directed toward evaluating equivalency and demonstrating efficacy of carotenoids in foods to meet vitamin A needs in vitamin A-deficient populations, in order to develop sustainable strategies to eradicate this worldwide public health problem.

REFERENCES

Albanes D, Heinonen OP, Taylor PR, Virtamo J, Edwards BK, Rautalahti M, Hartman AM, Palmgren J, Freedman LS, Haapakoski J, Barrett MJ, Pietinen P, Malila N, Tala E, Liippo K, Salomaa ER, Tangrea JA, Teppo L, Askin FB, Taskinen E, Erozan Y, Greenwald P, Huttunen JK. 1996. α-Tocopherol and ß-carotene supplements and lung cancer incidence in the Alpha-Tocopherol Beta-Carotene Prevention Study: Effects of base-line characteristics and study compliance. *J Natl Cancer Inst* 88:1560–1570.

Albanes D, Virtamo J, Taylor PR, Rautalahti M, Pietinen P, Heinonen OP. 1997. Effects of supplemental beta-carotene, cigarette smoking, and alcohol consumption on serum carotenoids in the Alpha-Tocopherol, Beta-Carotene Cancer Prevention Study. *Am J Clin Nutr* 66:366–372.

Allard JP, Royall D, Kurian R, Muggli R, Jeejeebhoy KN. 1994. Effects of beta-carotene supplementation on lipid peroxidation in humans. *Am J Clin Nutr* 59:884–890.

ATBC (Alpha-Tocopherol, Beta Carotene) Cancer Prevention Study Group. 1994. The effect of vitamin E and beta carotene on the incidence of lung cancer and other cancers in male smokers. *N Engl J Med* 330:1029–1035.

Baker DL, Krol ES, Jacobsen N, Liebler DC. 1999. Reactions of beta-carotene with cigarette smoke oxidants. Identification of carotenoid oxidation products and evaluation of the prooxidant/antioxidant effect. *Chem Res Toxicol* 12:535–543.

Batieha AM, Armenian HK, Norkus EP, Morris JS, Spate VE, Comstock GW. 1993. Serum micronutrients and the subsequent risk of cervical cancer in a population-based nested case-control study. *Cancer Epidemiol Biomarkers Prev* 2:335–339.

Bendich A. 1988. The safety of beta-carotene. *Nutr Cancer* 11:207–214.

Block G, Patterson B, Subar A. 1992. Fruit, vegetables, and cancer prevention: A review of the epidemiological evidence. *Nutr Cancer* 18:1–29.

Blot WJ, Li J-Y, Taylor PR, Guo W, Dawsey S, Wang G-Q, Yang CS, Zheng S-F, Gail M, Li G-Y, Yu Y, Liu B-Q, Tangrea J, Sun Y-H, Liu F, Fraumeni JF Jr, Zhang Y-H, Li B. 1993. Nutrition intervention trials in Linxian, China: Supplementation with specific vitamin/mineral combinations, cancer incidence, and disease-specific mortality in the general population. *J Natl Cancer Inst* 85:1483–1492.

Blot WJ, Li J-Y, Taylor PR, Li B. 1994. Lung cancer and vitamin supplementation. *N Engl J Med* 331:614.

Boileau TW, Moore AC, Erdman JW Jr. 1999. Carotenoids and vitamin A. In: Papas AM, ed. *Antioxidant Status, Diet, Nutrition, and Health.* Boca Raton, FL: CRC Press. Pp. 133–158.

Bone RA, Landrum JT, Tarsis SL. 1985. Preliminary identification of the human macular pigment. *Vision Res* 25:1531–1535.

Bone RA, Landrum JT, Hime GW, Cains A, Zamor J. 1993. Stereochemistry of the human macular carotenoids. *Invest Ophthalmol Vis Sci* 34:2033–2040.

Bonithon-Kopp C, Coudray C, Berr C, Touboul P-J, Feve JM, Favier A, Ducimetiere P. 1997. Combined effects of lipid peroxidation and antioxidant status on carotid atherosclerosis in a population aged 59–71 y: The EVA Study. *Am J Clin Nutr* 65:121–127.

Brady WE, Mares-Perlman JA, Bowen P, Stacewicz-Sapuntzakis M. 1996. Human serum carotenoid concentrations are related to physiologic and lifestyle factors. *J Nutr* 126:129–137.

Brown L, Rimm EB, Seddon JM, Giovannucci EL, Chasan-Taber L, Spiegelman D, Willett WC, Hankinson SE. 1999. A prospective study of carotenoid intake and risk of cataract extraction in US men. *Am J Clin Nutr* 70:517–524.

Burri BJ, Dixon ZR, Fong AK, Kretsch MJ, Clifford AJ, Erdman JW Jr. 1993. Possible association of skin lesions with a low-carotene diet in premenopausal women. *Ann NY Acad Sci* 691:279–280.

Butte NF, Calloway DH. 1981. Evaluation of lactational performance of Navajo women. *Am J Clin Nutr* 34:2210–2215.

Calzada C, Bizzotto M, Paganga G, Miller NJ, Bruckdorfer KR, Diplock AT, Rice-Evans CA. 1995. Levels of antioxidant nutrients in plasma and low density lipoproteins: A human volunteer supplementation study. *Free Radic Res* 23:489–503.

Canfield LM, Giuliano AR, Neilson EM, Yap HH, Graver EJ, Cui HA, Blashill BM. 1997. Beta-carotene in breast milk and serum is increased after a single beta-carotene dose. *Am J Clin Nutr* 66:52–61.

Canfield LM, Giuliano AR, Neilson EM, Blashil BM, Graver EJ, Yap HH. 1998. Kinetics of the response of milk and serum beta-carotene to daily beta-carotene supplementation in healthy, lactating women. *Am J Clin Nutr* 67: 276–283.

Castenmiller JJ, West CE. 1998. Bioavailability and bioconversion of carotenoids. *Annu Rev Nutr* 18:19–38.

Chandler LA, Schwartz SJ. 1987. HPLC separation of *cis-trans* carotene isomers in fresh and processed fruits and vegetables. *J Food Sci* 52:669–672.

Chappell JE, Francis T, Clandinin MT. 1985. Vitamin A and E content of human milk at early stages of lactation. *Early Hum Devel* 11:157–167.

Chasan-Taber L, Willett WC, Seddon JM, Stampfer M, Rosner B, Colditz GA, Speizer FE, Hankinson SE. 1999. A prospective study of carotenoid and vitamin A intakes and risk of cataract extraction in US women. *Am J Clin Nutr* 70:509–516.

Chow CK, Thacker RR, Changchit C, Bridges RB, Rehm SR, Humble J, Turbek J. 1986. Lower levels of vitamin C and carotenes in plasma of cigarette smokers. *J Am Coll Nutr* 5:305–312.

Chug-Ahuja JK, Holden JM, Forman MR, Mangels AR, Beecher GR, Lanza E. 1993. The development and application of a carotenoid database for fruits, vegetables, and selected multicomponent foods. *J Am Diet Assoc* 93:318–323.

Clevidence BA, Khachik F, Brown ED, Nair PP, Wiley ER, Prior RL, Cao G, Morel DW, Stone W, Gross M, Kramer TR. 1997. Human consumption of carotenoid-rich vegetables. In: Aruoma OI, Cuppett SL, eds. *Antioxidant Methodology: In Vivo and In Vitro Concepts*. Champaign, IL: AOCS Press. Pp 53–63.

Clinton SK. 1998. Lycopene: Chemistry, biology, and implications for human health and disease. *Nutr Rev* 56:35–51.

Clinton SK, Emenhiser C, Schwartz S, Bostwick DG, Williams AW, Moore BJ, Erdman JW Jr. 1996. *Cis-trans* lycopene isomers, carotenoids, and retinol in the human prostate. *Cancer Epidemiol Biomarkers Prev* 5:823–833.

Comstock GW, Menkes MS, Schober SE, Vuilleumier J-P, Helsing KJ. 1988. Serum levels of retinol, beta-carotene, and alpha-tocopherol in older adults. *Am J Epidemiol* 127:114–123.

Connett JE, Kuller LH, Kjelsberg MO, Polk BF, Collins G, Rider A, Hulley SB. 1989. Relationship between carotenoids and cancer. The Multiple Risk Factor Intervention Trial (MRFIT) Study. *Cancer* 64:126–134.

Coodley GO, Nelson HD, Loveless MO, Folk C. 1993. Beta-carotene in HIV infection. *J Acquir Immune Defic Syndr* 6:272–276.

de Pee S, West CE, Muhilal, Karyadi D, Hautvast J. 1995. Lack of improvement in vitamin A status with increased consumption of dark-green leafy vegetables. *Lancet* 346:75–81.

de Pee S, West CE, Permaesih D, Martuti S, Muhilal, Hautvast J. 1998. Orange fruit is more effective than are dark-green, leafy vegetables in increasing serum concentrations of retinol and beta-carotene in schoolchildren in Indonesia. *Am J Clin Nutr* 68:1058–1067.

Dietz JM, Kantha SS, Erdman JW Jr. 1988. Reversed phase HPLC analysis of alpha- and beta-carotene from selected raw and cooked vegetables. *Plant Food Hum Nutr* 38:333–341.

Dixon ZR, Burri BJ, Clifford A, Frankel EN, Schneeman BO, Parks E, Keim NL, Barbieri T, Wu M-M, Fong AK, Kretsch MJ, Sowell AL, Erdman JW Jr. 1994. Effects of a carotene-deficient diet on measures of oxidative susceptibility and superoxide dismutase activity in adult women. *Free Radic Biol Med* 17:537–544.

Dixon ZR, Shie F-S, Warden BA, Burri BJ, Neidlinger TR. 1998. The effect of a low carotenoid diet on malondialdehyde-thiobarbituric acid (MDA-TBA) concentrations in women: A placebo-controlled double-blind study. *J Am Coll Nutr* 17:54–58.

EDCCSG (Eye Disease Case-Control Study Group). 1993. Antioxidant status and neovascular age-related macular degeneration. *Arch Ophthalmol* 111:104–109.

Eichholzer M, Stahelin HB, Gey KF. 1992. Inverse correlation between essential antioxidants in plasma and subsequent risk to develop cancer, ischemic heart disease and stroke respectively: 12-year follow-up of the Prospective Basel Study. *Exp Suppl* 62:398–410.

Elinder LS, Hadell K, Johansson J, Molgaard J, Holme I, Olsson AG, Walldius G. 1995. Probucol treatment decreases serum concentrations of diet-derived antioxidants. *Arterioscler Thromb Vasc Biol* 15:1057–1063.

Erdman JW Jr, Bierer TL, Gugger ET. 1993. Absorption and transport of carotenoids. *Ann NY Acad Sci* 691:76–85.

Fukao A, Tsubono Y, Kawamura M, Ido T, Akazawa N, Tsuji I, Komatsu S, Minami Y, Hisamichi S. 1996. The independent association of smoking and drinking with serum beta-carotene levels among males in Miyagi, Japan. *Int J Epidemiol* 25:300–306.

Gartner C, Stahl W, Sies H. 1997. Lycopene is more bioavailable from tomato paste than from fresh tomatoes. *Am J Clin Nutr* 66:116–122.

Gaziano JM, Hennekens CH. 1993. The role of beta-carotene in the prevention of cardiovascular disease. *Ann NY Acad Sci* 691:148–155.

Gaziano JM, Hatta A, Flynn M, Johnson EJ, Krinsky NI, Ridker PM, Hennekens CH, Frei B. 1995. Supplementation with beta-carotene in vivo and in vitro does not inhibit low density lipoprotein oxidation. *Atherosclerosis* 112:187–195.

Gebre-Medhin M, Vahlquist A, Hofvander Y, Uppsall L, Vahlquist B. 1976. Breast milk composition in Ethiopian and Swedish mothers. I. Vitamin A and beta-carotene. *Am J Clin Nutr* 29:441–451.

Gey KF, Moser UK, Jordan P, Stahelin HB, Eichholzer M, Ludin E. 1993a. Increased risk of cardiovascular disease at suboptimal plasma concentrations of essential antioxidants: An epidemiological update with special attention to carotene and vitamin C. *Am J Clin Nutr* 57:787S–797S.

Gey KF, Stähelin HB, Eichholzer M. 1993b. Poor plasma status of carotene and vitamin C is associated with higher morbidity from ischemic heart disease and stroke: Basel Prospective Study. *Clin Invest* 71:3–6.

Giovannucci E. 1999. Tomatoes, tomato-based products, lycopene, and cancer: Review of the epidemiologic literature. *J Natl Cancer Inst* 91:317–331.

Giovannucci E, Ascherio A, Rimm EB, Stampfer MJ, Colditz GA, Willett WC. 1995. Intake of carotenoids and retinol in relation to risk of prostate cancer. *J Natl Cancer Inst* 87:1767–1776.

Giuliano AR, Neilson EM, Kelly BE, Canfield LM. 1992. Simultaneous quantitation and separation of carotenoids and retinol in human milk by high-performance liquid chromatography. *Methods Enzymol* 213:391–399.

Giuliano AR, Neilson SM, Yap H-H, Baier M, Canfield LM. 1994. Quantitation of and inter/intra-individual variability in major carotenoids of mature human milk. *J Nutr Biochem* 5:551–556.

Goodman DS, Blomstrand R, Werner B, Huang HS, Shiratori T. 1966. The intestinal absorption and metabolism of vitamin A and beta-carotene in man. *J Clin Invest* 45:1615–1623.

Gottlieb K, Zarling EJ, Mobarhan S, Bowen P, Sugerman S. 1993. Beta-carotene decreases markers of lipid peroxidation in healthy volunteers. *Nutr Cancer* 19:207–212.

Greenberg ER, Baron JA, Karagas MR, Stukel TA, Nierenberg DW, Stevens MM, Mandel JS, Haile RW. 1996. Mortality associated with low plasma concentration of beta carotene and the effect of oral supplementation. *J Am Med Assoc* 275:699–703.

Hammond BR Jr, Fuld K. 1992. Interocular differences in macular pigment density. *Invest Ophthalmol Vis Sci* 33:350–355.

Hammond BR Jr, Curran-Celentano J, Judd S, Fuld K, Krinsky NI, Wooten BR, Snodderly DM. 1996. Sex differences in macular pigment optical density: Relation to plasma carotenoid concentrations and dietary patterns. *Vision Res* 36:2001–2012.

Hammond BR Jr, Johnson EJ, Russell RM, Krinsky NI, Yeum K-J, Edwards RB, Snodderly DM. 1997. Dietary modification of human macular pigment density. *Invest Ophthalmol Vis Sci* 38:1795–1801.

Handelman GJ, Dratz EA, Reay CC, Van Kuijk JG. 1988. Carotenoids in the human macula and whole retina. *Invest Ophthalmol Vis Sci* 29:850–855.

Handelman GJ, Packer L, Cross CE. 1996. Destruction of tocopherols, carotenoids, and retinol in human plasma by cigarette smoke. *Am J Clin Nutr* 63:559–565.

Hanusch M, Stahl W, Schulz WA, Sies H. 1995. Induction of gap junctional communication by 4-oxoretinoic acid generated from its precursor canthaxanthin. *Arch Biochem Biophys* 317:423–428.

Health Canada. 1997. *Canada's Food Guide to Healthy Eating.* Minister of Public Works and Government Services Canada.

Hennekens CH, Buring JE, Manson JE, Stampfer M, Rosner B, Cook NR, Belanger C, LaMotte F, Gaziano JM, Ridker PM, Willett W, Peto R. 1996. Lack of effect of long-term supplementation with beta carotene on the incidence of malignant neoplasms and cardiovascular disease. *N Engl J Med* 334:1145–1149.

Herbeth B, Didelot-Barthelemy L, Lemoine A, Le Devehat C. 1988. Plasma fat-soluble vitamins and alcohol consumption. *Am J Clin Nutr* 47:343–344.

Herbeth B, Chavance M, Musse N, Mejean L, Vernhes G. 1990. Determinants of plasma retinol, beta-carotene, and alpha-tocopherol. *Am J Epidemiol* 132:394–396.

Heywood R, Palmer AK, Gregson RL, Hummler H. 1985. The toxicity of beta-carotene. *Toxicology* 36:91–100.

Hininger I, Chopra M, Thurnham DI, Laporte F, Richard M-J, Favier A, Roussel A-M. 1997. Effect of increased fruit and vegetable intake on the susceptibility of lipoprotein to oxidation in smokers. *Eur J Clin Nutr* 51:601–606.

Holden JM, Eldridge AL, Beecher GR, Buzzard M, Bhagwat S, Davis CS, Douglass LW, Gebhardt S, Haytowitz D, Schakel S. 1999. Carotenoid content of U.S. foods: an update of the database. *Food Comp Anal* 12:169–196.

Hollander D, Ruble RE. 1978. Beta-carotene intestinal absorption: bile, fatty acid, pH, and flow rate effects on transport. Am J Physiology. 235: e686–e691.

Hughes DA, Wright AJ, Finglas PM, Peerless AC, Bailey AL, Astley SB, Pinder AC, Southon S. 1997. The effect of beta-carotene supplementation on the immune function of blood monocytes from healthy male nonsmokers. *J Lab Clin Med* 129:309–317.

Jacques PF, Chylack LT Jr. 1991. Epidemiologic evidence of a role for the antioxidant vitamins and carotenoids in cataract prevention. *Am J Clin Nutr* 53:352S–355S.

Jalal F, Nesheim MC, Agus Z, Sanjur D, Habicht JP. 1998. Serum retinol concentrations in children are affected by food sources of beta-carotene, fat intake, and anthelmintic drug treatment. *Am J Clin Nutr* 68:623–629.

Johnson EJ, Russell RM. 1992. Distribution of orally administered beta-carotene among lipoproteins in healthy men. *Am J Clin Nutr* 56:128–135.

Johnson EJ, Qin J, Krinsky NI, Russell RM. 1997. Beta-carotene isomers in human serum, breast milk and buccal mucosa cells after continuous oral doses of *all-trans* and 9-*cis* beta-carotene. *J Nutr* 127:1993–1999.

Kaplan LA, Lau JM, Stein EA. 1990. Carotenoid composition, concentrations, and relationships in various human organs. *Clin Physiol Biochem* 8:1–10.

Khachik F, Bernstein PS, Garland DL. 1997a. Identification of lutein and zeaxanthin oxidation products in human and monkey retinas. *Invest Ophthalmol Vis Sci* 38:1802–1811.

Khachik F, Spangler CJ, Smith JC, Canfield LM, Steck A, Pfander H. 1997b. Identification, quantification, and relative concentrations of carotenoids and their metabolites in human milk and serum. *Anal Chem* 69:1873–1881.

Kobza A, Ramsay CA, Magnus IA. 1973. Oral carotene therapy in actinic reticuloid and solar urticaria. Failure to demonstrate a photoprotective effect against long wave ultraviolet and visible radiation. *Br J Dermatol* 88:157–166.

Kohlmeier L, Hastings SB. 1995. Epidemiologic evidence of a role of carotenoids in cardiovascular disease prevention. *Am J Clin Nutr* 62:1370S–1376S.

Kohlmeier L, Kark JD, Gomez-Gracia E, Martin BC, Steck SE, Kardinaal AF, Ringstad J, Thamm M, Masaev V, Riemersma R, Martin-Moreno JM, Huttunen JK, Kok FJ. 1997. Lycopene and myocardial infarction risk in the EURAMIC Study. *Am J Epidemiol* 146:618–626.

Koonsvitsky BP, Berry DA, Jones MB, Lin PY, Cooper DA, Jones DY, Jackson JE. 1997. Olestra affects serum concentrations of alpha-tocopherol and carotenoids but not vitamin D or vitamin K status in free-living subjects. *J Nutr* 127:1636S–1645S.

Kostic D, White WS, Olson JA. 1995. Intestinal absorption, serum clearance, and interactions between lutein and beta-carotene when administered to human adults in separate or combined oral doses. *Am J Clin Nutr* 62:604–610.

Kramer TR, Burri BJ. 1997. Modulated mitogenic proliferative responsiveness of lymphocytes in whole-blood cultures after a low-carotene diet and mixed-carotenoid supplementation in women. *Am J Clin Nutr* 65:871–875.

Krinsky NI. 1993. Actions of carotenoids in biological systems. *Annu Rev Nutr* 13:561–587.

Kuhnlein HV, Soueida R, Receveur O. 1996. Dietary nutrient profiles of Canadian Baffin Island Inuit differ by food source, season, and age. *J Am Diet Assoc* 96:155-162.

Kushi LH, Folsom AR, Prineas RJ, Mink PJ, Wu Y, Bostick RM. 1996. Dietary antioxidant vitamins and death from coronary heart disease in postmenopausal women. *N Engl J Med* 334:1156–1162.

Lachance PA. 1997. Nutrient addition to foods: The public health impact in countries with rapidly westernizing diets. In: Bendich A, Deckelbaum RJ, eds. *Preventive Nutrition: The Comprehensive Guide for Health Professionals.* Totowa, NJ: Humana Press. Pp. 441–454.

Lascari AD. 1981. Carotenemia. A review. *Clin Pediatr* 20:25–29.

Le Marchand L, Hankin JH, Kolonel LN, Beecher GR, Wilkens LR, Zhao LP. 1993. Intake of specific carotenoids and lung cancer risk. *Cancer Epidemiol Biomarkers Prev* 2:183–187.

Lewis MB. 1972. The effect of beta-carotene on serum vitamin A levels in erythropoietic protoporphyria. *Australas J Dermatol* 13:75–78.

Lin Y, Burri BJ, Neidlinger TR, Muller HG, Dueker SR, Clifford A. 1998. Estimating the concentration of beta-carotene required for maximal protection of low-density lipoproteins in women. *Am J Clin Nutr* 67:837–845.

LSRO/FASEB (Life Sciences Research Office/Federation of American Societies for Experimental Biology). 1995. *Third Report on Nutrition Monitoring in the United States*. Washington, DC: US Government Printing Office.

Mahapatra S, Manorama R. 1997. The protective effect of red palm oil in comparison with massive vitamin A dose in combating vitamin A deficiency in Orissa, India. *Asia Pacific J Clin Nutr* 6:246–250.

Mangels AR, Holden JM, Beecher GR, Forman MR, Lanza E. 1993. Carotenoid content of fruits and vegetables: An evaluation of analytic data. *J Am Diet Assoc* 93:284–296.

Manson JE, Gaziano JM, Jonas MA, Hennekens CH. 1993. Antioxidants and cardiovascular disease: A review. *J Am Coll Nutr* 12:426–432.

Mares-Perlman JA, Brady WE, Klein R, Klein BE, Palta M, Bowen P, Stacewicz-Sapuntzakis M. 1994. Serum levels of carotenoids and tocopherols in people with age-related maculopathy. *Invest Ophthalmol Vis Sci* 35:2004.

Mares-Perlman JA, Brady WE, Klein BE, Klein R, Palta M, Bowen P, Stacewicz-Sapuntzakis M. 1995. Serum carotenoids and tocopherols and severity of nuclear and cortical opacities. *Invest Ophthalmol Vis Sci* 36:276–288.

Margetts BM, Jackson AA. 1996. The determinants of plasma beta-carotene: Interaction between smoking and other lifestyle factors. *Eur J Clin Nutr* 50:236–238.

Martini MC, Campbell DR, Gross MD, Grandits GA, Potter JD, Slavin JL. 1995. Plasma carotenoids as biomarkers of vegetable intake: The University of Minnesota Cancer Prevention Research Unit Feeding Studies. *Cancer Epidemiol Biomarkers Prev* 4:491–496.

Mathews-Roth MM. 1986. Beta-carotene therapy for erythropoietic protoporphyria and other photosensitivity diseases. *Biochimie* 68:875–884.

Mathews-Roth MM, Pathak MA, Parrish J, Fitzpatrick TB, Kass EH, Toda K, Clemens W. 1972. A clinical trial of the effects of oral beta-carotene on the responses of human skin to solar radiation. *J Invest Dermatol* 59:349–353.

Mathews-Roth MM, Pathak MA, Fitzpatrick TB, Harber LC, Kass EH. 1974. Beta-carotene as an oral photoprotective agent in erythropoietic protoporphyria. *J Am Med Assoc* 228:1004–1008.

Mayne ST. 1996. Beta-carotene, carotenoids, and disease prevention in humans. *FASEB J* 10:690–701.

Mayne ST. 1998. Beta-carotene, Carotenoids and Cancer Prevention. In: DeVita VT Jr, Hellman S, Rosenberg SA, eds. *Principles and Practice of Oncology (PPO)*, 5th Edition Updates. Philadelphia, PA: Lippincott-Raven Publishers. Pp. 12:1–15.

Mayne ST, Goodwin WJ Jr. 1993. Chemoprevention of head and neck cancer. *Current Opinion Otolaryn Head Neck Surg* 1:126–132.

Mayne ST, Cartmel B, Silva F, Kim CS, Fallon BG, Briskin K, Zheng T, Baum M, Shor-Posner G, Goodwin WJ Jr. 1998. Effect of supplemental beta-carotene on plasma concentrations of carotenoids, retinol, and alpha-tocopherol in humans. *Am J Clin Nutr* 68:642–647.

Menkes MS, Comstock GW, Vuilleumier JP, Helsing KJ, Rider AA, Brookmeyer R. 1986. Serum beta-carotene, vitamins A and E, selenium, and the risk of lung cancer. N Engl J Med 315:1250–1254.

Micozzi MS, Brown ED, Edwards BK, Bieri JG, Taylor PR, Khachik F, Beecher GR, Smith JC. 1992. Plasma carotenoid response to chronic intake of selected foods and beta-carotene supplements in men. Am J Clin Nutr 55:1120–1125.

Mobarhan S, Bowen P, Andersen B, Evans M, Stacewicz-Sapuntzakis M, Sugerman S, Simms P, Lucchesi D, Friedman H. 1990. Effects of beta-carotene repletion on beta-carotene absorption, lipid peroxidation, and neutrophil superoxide formation in young men. Nutr Cancer 14:195–206.

Morris DL, Kritchevsky SB, Davis CE. 1994. Serum carotenoids and coronary heart disease: The Lipid Research Clinics Coronary Primary Prevention Trial and Follow-up Study. J Am Med Assoc 272:1439–1441.

Mosca L, Rubenfire M, Mandel C, Rock C, Tarshis T, Tsai A, Pearson T. 1997. Antioxidant nutrient supplementation reduces the susceptibility of low density lipoprotein to oxidation in patients with coronary artery disease. J Am Coll Cardiol 30:392–399.

Nebeling LC, Forman MR, Graubard BI, Snyder RA. 1997. Changes in carotenoid intake in the United States: The 1987 and 1992 National Health Interview Surveys. J Am Diet Assoc 97:991–996.

Nierenberg DW, Dain BJ, Mott LA, Baron JA, Greenberg ER. 1997. Effects of 4 y of oral supplementation with beta-carotene on serum concentrations of retinol, tocopherol, and five carotenoids. Am J Clin Nutr 66:315–319.

Nomura AM, Stemmermann GN, Heilbrun LK, Salkeld RM, Vuilleumier JP. 1985. Serum vitamin levels and the risk of cancer of specific sites in men of Japanese ancestry in Hawaii. Cancer Res 45:2369–2372.

Nomura AM, Stemmermann GN, Lee J, Craft NE. 1997. Serum micronutrients and prostate cancer in Japanese Americans in Hawaii. Cancer Epidemiol Biomarkers Prev 6:487–491.

Olson JA. 1989. Biological actions of carotenoids. J Nutr 119:94–95.

Olson JA. 1994. Absorption, transport, and metabolism of carotenoids in humans. Pure Appl Chem 66:1011–1016.

Olson JA. 1999. Carotenoids. In: Shils ME, Olson JA, Shike M, Ross AC, eds. Modern Nutrition in Health and Disease, 9th edition. Baltimore, MD: Williams & Wilkins. Pp. 525–541.

Omenn GS, Goodman GE, Thornquist MD, Balmes J, Cullen MR, Glass A, Keogh JP, Meyskens FL Jr, Valanis B, Williams JH Jr, Barnhart S, Cherniack MG, Brodkin CA, Hammar S. 1996a. Risk factors for lung cancer and for intervention effects in CARET, the Beta-Carotene and Retinol Efficacy Trial. J Natl Cancer Inst 88:1550–1559.

Omenn GS, Goodman GE, Thornquist MD, Balmes J, Cullen MR, Glass A, Keogh JP, Meyskens FL Jr, Valanis B, Williams JH Jr, Barnhart S, Hammar S. 1996b. Effects of a combination of beta carotene and vitamin A on lung cancer and cardiovascular disease. N Engl J Med 334:1150–1155.

Ostrea EM Jr, Balun JE, Winkler R, Porter T. 1986. Influence of breast-feeding on the restoration of the low serum concentration of vitamin E and beta-carotene in the newborn infant. Am J Obstet Gynecol 154:1014–1017.

Pamuk ER, Byers T, Coates RJ, Vann JW, Sowell AL, Gunter EW, Glass D. 1994. Effect of smoking on serum nutrient concentrations in African-American women. Am J Clin Nutr 59:891–895.

Pandey DK, Shekelle R, Selwyn BJ, Tangney C, Stamler J. 1995. Dietary vitamin C and beta-carotene and risk of death in middle-aged men. The Western Electric Study. *Am J Epidemiol* 142:1269–1278.

Parker RS. 1988. Carotenoid and tocopherol composition of human adipose tissue. *Am J Clin Nutr* 47:33–36.

Parker RS. 1996. Absorption, metabolism, and transport of carotenoids. *FASEB J* 10:542–551.

Patton S, Canfield LM, Huston GE, Ferris AM, Jensen RG. 1990. Carotenoids of human colostrum. *Lipids* 25:159–165.

Pool-Zobel BL, Bub A, Muller H, Wollowski I, Rechkemmer G. 1997. Consumption of vegetables reduces genetic damage in humans: First results of a human intervention trial with carotenoid-rich foods. *Carcinogenesis* 18:1847–1850.

Richards GA, Theron AJ, Van Rensburg CE, Van Rensburg AJ, Van der Merwe CA, Kuyl JM, Anderson R. 1990. Investigation of the effects of oral administration of vitamin E and beta-carotene on the chemiluminescence responses and the frequency of sister chromatid exchanges in circulating leukocytes from cigarette smokers. *Am Rev Respir Dis* 142:648–654.

Riemersma RA, Wood DA, Macintyre CC, Elton RA, Gey KF, Oliver MF. 1991. Risk of angina pectoris and plasma concentrations of vitamins A, C, and E and carotene. *Lancet* 337:1–5.

Rimm EB, Stampfer MJ, Ascherio A, Giovannucci E, Colditz GA, Willett WC. 1993. Vitamin E consumption and the risk of coronary heart disease in men. *N Engl J Med* 328:1450–1456.

Rock CL, Swendseid ME. 1992. Plasma beta-carotene response in humans after meals supplemented with dietary pectin. *Am J Clin Nutr* 55:96–99.

Rodriguez MS, Irwin MI. 1972. A conspectus of research on vitamin A requirements of man. *J Nutr* 102:909–968.

Roels OA, Trout M, Dujacquier R. 1958. Carotene balances on boys in Ruanda where vitamin A deficiency is prevalent. *J Nutr* 65:115–127.

Rust P, Eichler I, Renner S, Elmadfa I. 1998. Effects of long-term oral beta-carotene supplementation on lipid peroxidation in patients with cystic fibrosis. *Int J Vitam Nutr Res* 68:83–87.

Sahyoun NR, Jacques PF, Russell RM. 1996. Carotenoids, vitamins C and E, and mortality in an elderly population. *Am J Epidemiol* 144:501–511.

Salgo MG, Cueto R, Winston GW, Pryor WA. 1999. Beta carotene and its oxidation products have different effects on microsome mediated binding of benzo-[a]pyrene to DNA. *Free Radic Biol Med* 26:162–173.

Salonen JT, Nyyssonen K, Parviainen M, Kantola M, Korpela H, Salonen R. 1993. Low plasma beta-carotene, vitamin E and selenium levels associate with accelerated carotid atherogenesis in hypercholesterolemic eastern Finnish men. *Circulation* 87:678.

Santos MS, Meydani SN, Leka L, Wu D, Fotouhi N, Meydani M, Hennekens CH, Gaziano JM. 1996. Natural killer cell activity in elderly men is enhanced by beta-carotene supplementation. *Am J Clin Nutr* 64:772–777.

Santos MS, Gaziano JM, Leka LS, Beharka AA, Hennekens CH, Meydani SN. 1998. Beta-carotene-induced enhancement of natural killer cell activity in elderly men: An investigation of the role of cytokines. *Am J Clin Nutr* 68:164–170.

Schmitz HH, Poor CL, Wellman RB, Erdman JW Jr. 1991. Concentrations of selected carotenoids and vitamin A in human liver, kidney and lung tissue. *J Nutr* 121:1613–1621.

Seddon JM, Ajani UA, Sperduto RD, Hiller R, Blair N, Burton TC, Farber MD, Gragoudas ES, Haller J, Miller DT, Yannuzzi LA, Willett W. 1994. Dietary carotenoids, vitamins A, C, and E, and advanced age related macular degeneration. *J Am Med Assoc* 272:1413–1420.

Shoenfeld Y, Shaklai M, Ben-Baruch N, Hirschorn M, Pinkhaus J. 1982. Neutropenia induced by hypercarotenaemia. *Lancet* 1:1245.

Sies H, Stahl W. 1997. Carotenoids and intercellular communication via gap junctions. *Int J Vitam Nutr Res* 67:364–367.

Snodderly DM. 1995. Evidence for protection against age-related macular degeneration by carotenoids and antioxidant vitamins. *Am J Clin Nutr* 62:1448S–1461S.

Stahelin HB, Gey KF, Eichholzer M, Ludin E, Bernasconi F, Thurneysen J, Brubacher G. 1991. Plasma antioxidant vitamins and subsequent cancer mortality in the 12-year follow-up of the Prospective Basel Study. *Am J Epidemiol* 133:766–775.

Stahl W, Sies H. 1992. Uptake of lycopene and its geometrical isomers is greater from heat-processed than from unprocessed tomato juice in humans. *J Nutr* 122:2161–2166.

Stahl W, Schwarz W, Sundquist AR, Sies H. 1992. *Cis-trans* isomers of lycopene and beta-carotene in human serum and tissues. *Arch Biochem Biophys* 294:173–177.

Steinberg FM, Chait A. 1998. Antioxidant vitamin supplementation and lipid peroxidation in smokers. *Am J Clin Nutr* 68:319–327.

Stryker WS, Kaplan LA, Stein EA, Stampfer MJ, Sober A, Willett WC. 1988. The relation of diet, cigarette smoking, and alcohol consumption to plasma beta-carotene and alpha-tocopherol levels. *Am J Epidemiol* 127:283–296.

Taylor A. 1993. Cataract: Relationship between nutrition and oxidation. *J Am Coll Nutr* 12:138–146.

Taylor A, Jacques PF, Epstein EM. 1995. Relations among aging, antioxidant status, and cataract. *Am J Clin Nutr* 62:1439S–1447S.

Traber MG, Diamond SR, Lane JC, Brody RI, Kayden HJ. 1994. Beta-carotene transport in human lipoproteins. Comparisons with alpha-tocopherol. *Lipids* 29:665–669.

VandenLangenberg GM, Brady WE, Nebeling LC, Block G, Forman M, Bowen PE, Stacewicz-Sapuntzakis M, Mares-Perlman JA. 1996. Influence of using different sources of carotenoid data in epidemiologic studies. *J Am Diet Assoc* 96:1271–1275.

van het Hof KH, Brouwer IA, West CE, Haddeman E, Steegers-Theunissen RP, van Dusseldorp M, Weststrate JA, Eskes TK, Hautvast JG. 1999. Bioavailability of lutein from vegetables is 5 times higher than that of beta-carotene. *Am J Clin Nutr* 70:261–268.

van Poppel G, Kok FJ, Duijzings P, de Vogel N. 1992a. No influence of beta-carotene on smoking-induced DNA damage as reflected by sister chromatid exchanges. *Int J Cancer* 51:355–358.

van Poppel G, Kok FJ, Hermus RJ. 1992b. Beta-carotene supplementation in smokers reduces the frequency of micronuclei in sputum. *Br J Cancer* 66:1164–1168.

van Poppel G, Poulsen H, Loft S, Verhagen H. 1995. No influence of beta carotene on oxidative DNA damage in male smokers. *J Natl Cancer Inst* 87:310–311.

van Vliet T, Schreurs WH, van Den Berg H. 1995. Intestinal beta-carotene absorption and cleavage in men: Response of beta-carotene and retinyl esters in the triglyceride-rich lipoprotein fraction after a single oral dose of beta-carotene. *Am J Clin Nutr* 62:110–116.

Wahlqvist ML, Wattanapenpaiboon N, Macrae FA, Lambert JR, MacLennan R, Hsu-Hage BH. 1994. Changes in serum carotenoids in subjects with colorectal adenomas after 24 mo of beta-carotene supplementation. Australian Polyp Prevention Project Investigators. *Am J Clin Nutr* 60:936–943.

Wang X-D. 1994. Absorption and metabolism of beta-carotene. *J Am Coll Nutr* 13:314–325.

Wang X-D, Liu C, Bronson RT, Smith DE, Krinsky NI, Russell RM. 1999. Retinoid signaling and activator protein-1 expression in ferrets given beta-carotene supplements and exposed to tobacco smoke. *J Natl Cancer Inst* 91:60–66.

Wang Y, Ichiba M, Oishi H, Iyadomi M, Shono N, Tomokuni K. 1997. Relationship between plasma concentrations of beta-carotene and alpha-tocopherol and life-style factors and levels of DNA adducts in lymphocytes. *Nutr Cancer* 27:69–73.

West S, Vitale S, Hallfrisch J, Munoz B, Muller D, Bressler S, Bressler NM. 1994. Are antioxidants or supplements protective for age-related macular degeneration? *Arch Ophthalmol* 112:222–227.

Weststrate JA, Meijer GW. 1998. Plant sterol-enriched margarines and reduction of plasma total- and LDL-cholesterol concentrations in normocholesterolaemic and mildly hypercholesterolaemic subjects. *Eur J Clin Nutr* 52:334–343.

Weststrate JA, van het Hof KH. 1995. Sucrose polyester and plasma carotenoid concentrations in healthy subjects. *Am J Clin Nutr* 62:591–597.

White WS, Stacewicz-Sapuntzakis M, Erdman JW Jr, Bowen PE. 1994. Pharmacokinetics of beta-carotene and canthaxanthin after ingestion of individual and combined doses by human subjects. *J Am Coll Nutr* 13:665–671.

Winklhofer-Roob BM, Puhl H, Khoschsorur G, van't Hof MA, Esterbauer H, Shmerling DH. 1995. Enhanced resistance to oxidation of low density lipoproteins and decreased lipid peroxide formation during beta-carotene supplementation in cystic fibrosis. *Free Radic Biol Med* 18:849–859.

Witter FR, Blake DA, Baumgardner R, Mellits ED, Niebyl JR. 1982. Folate, carotene, and smoking. *Am J Obstet Gynecol* 144:857.

WCRF/AICR (World Cancer Research Fund/American Institute for Cancer Research). 1997. *Food, Nutrition and the Prevention of Cancer: A Global Perspective.* Menasha, WI: BANTA Book Group.

Yong LC, Forman MR, Beecher GR, Graubard BI, Campbell WS, Reichman ME, Taylor PR, Lanza E, Holden JM, Judd JT. 1994. Relationship between dietary intake and plasma concentrations of carotenoids in premenopausal women: Application of the USDA-NCI carotenoid food-composition database. *Am J Clin Nutr* 60:223–230.

Zhang L-X, Cooney RV, Bertram JS. 1991. Carotenoids enhance gap junctional communication and inhibit lipid peroxidation in C3H/10T1/2 cells: Relationship to their cancer chemopreventive action. *Carcinogenesis* 12:2109–2114.

Zheng W, Blot WJ, Diamond EL, Norkus EP, Spate V, Morris JS, Comstock GW. 1993. Serum micronutrients and the subsequent risk of oral and pharyngeal cancer. *Cancer Res* 53:795–798.

Ziegler RG, Colavito EA, Hartge P, McAdams MJ, Schoenberg JB, Mason TJ, Fraumeni JF Jr. 1996a. Importance of alpha-carotene, beta-carotene, and other phytochemicals in the etiology of lung cancer. *J Natl Cancer Inst* 88:612–615.

Ziegler RG, Mayne ST, Swanson CA. 1996b. Nutrition and lung cancer. *Cancer Causes Control* 7:157–177.

Zino S, Skeaff M, Williams S, Mann J. 1997. Randomised controlled trial of effect of fruit and vegetable consumption on plasma concentrations of lipids and antioxidants. *Br Med J* 314:1787–1791.

9

Uses of
Dietary Reference Intakes

OVERVIEW

The Dietary Reference Intakes (DRIs) may be used for many purposes. These fall into two broad categories: assessing nutrient intakes and planning for nutrient intakes. Each category may be further subdivided into uses for individual diets and uses for diets of groups (Figure 9-1).

For example, the Estimated Average Requirement (EAR) and Tolerable Upper Intake Level (UL) may be used as components of a dietary assessment of an individual client in a health care clinic; the Recommended Dietary Allowance (RDA) and Adequate Intake (AI) may be used as components to plan an improved diet for the same client. Likewise, the EARs and ULs may be used to assess the nutrient quality of a group of individuals participating in a dietary survey (such as those regularly conducted as part of the National Nutrition Monitoring System) or to plan nutritionally adequate diets for groups of people receiving meals in nursing homes, schools, and other group-feeding settings.

In the past, RDAs in the United States and Recommended Nutrient Intakes (RNIs) in Canada were the primary values available to health professionals for planning and assessing the diets of individuals and of groups and as a basis for making judgments about inadequate or excessive intake. However, these former RDAs and RNIs were not ideally suited for many of these purposes (IOM, 1994). The DRIs provide a more complete set of reference values. The transition from using RDAs or RNIs alone to using each different

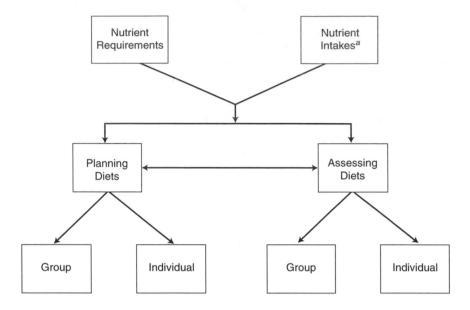

FIGURE 9-1 Conceptual framework—uses of Dietary Reference Intakes.
a Food plus supplements.

DRI appropriately will require time and effort by health profession-als and others.

Appropriate uses of each of the new DRIs are described briefly in this chapter and in more detail in upcoming reports on the uses and applications of the DRIs. Also included in this chapter are specific applications to the nutrients discussed in this report. Details on how the DRIs are set with reference to specific life stages and genders and the primary criteria used to define adequacy or adverse effects for each of these groups are given in Chapters 5 through 8 of this report.

ASSESSING NUTRIENT INTAKES OF INDIVIDUALS

Using the Estimated Average Requirement for Individuals

The Dietary Reference Intakes (DRIs) were not designed to be used alone in assessing the adequacy of the diet of a specific individ-ual because there is a wide range of requirements among individuals. The Estimated Average Requirement (EAR) estimates the median requirement of a distribution of requirements for a life stage or gender group, but it is not possible to know where an individual falls on this distribution without further physiological or biochemical measures. Thus, from dietary data alone, it is only possible to estimate the *likelihood* of nutrient adequacy. Furthermore, it is rare to have precise and representative data on usual intake of an individual, which adds additional uncertainty to the evaluation of an individual's dietary adequacy. Thus, true nutrient status can usually be determined only by obtaining physiological and biochemical data for the individual, and not from dietary assessment alone.

There are a number of inherent inaccuracies in dietary assessment methods. One is that individuals often underreport their intakes (Briefel et al., 1997; Mertz et al., 1991), and it appears that obese individuals do so to a greater extent than normal-weight individuals (Heitmann and Lissner, 1995). Furthermore, large day-to-day variations in intake, which occur for almost all individuals, necessitate many days of measurement to approximate usual intake. As a result, substantial caution must be used when interpreting nutrient assessments based on self-reported dietary data covering relatively few days of intake. Given the difficulties in accurately estimating usual intake, as well as the variance in requirements, a qualitative interpretation is recommended as described below:

- If usual intake of an individual is greater than or equal to the Recommended Dietary Allowance (RDA), there is *little likelihood* that intake is inadequate. Intake at this level is expected to be inadequate for fewer than 2 to 3 percent of individuals (IOM, 1997, 1998).
- If usual intake is between the RDA and the EAR, there is a great deal of uncertainty about whether that intake is inadequate and additional information about the individual may be needed. Usual intake between the RDA and the EAR is inadequate for about 3 to 50 percent of the individuals in the life stage group. If these individuals maintained intakes at this level over a prolonged time period, they might demonstrate the signs of inadequacy used to establish the EAR. For example, inadequate intake of vitamin C would lead to low ascorbate saturation of neutrophils.
- If usual intake is less than the EAR, there is a *high likelihood* that intake is inadequate. Usual intake at the EAR is expected to be inadequate for at least 50 percent of individuals.
- Because usual intakes are so difficult to measure, and because an individual's actual requirement is usually unknown, evaluation

based on dietary assessment should be confirmed by other measures, especially when a high likelihood of inadequacy is suspected.

For example, a 30-year-old woman who consumes an average of 55 mg/day of vitamin C from her food and takes a multiple vitamin four times a week containing 60 mg of vitamin C would average 89 mg/day (55 mg + [60 mg × 4/7]). Thus, her diet alone would put her at high likelihood of inadequacy, since it is below the EAR of 60 mg/day. Addition of the supplement, however, would add up to a sum on average above the RDA of 75 mg/day for adult women, thus suggesting little likelihood that intake is inadequate if the dietary assessment represents her true usual intake.

Using the Adequate Intake for Individuals

For vitamin C, vitamin E, and selenium, Adequate Intakes (AIs), rather than EARs or RDAs, have been set only for infants. By definition and observation, healthy infants who are exclusively fed human milk for the first 6 months of life by apparently healthy mothers are consuming an adequate amount of these nutrients. Infants who are consuming formulas with a nutrient profile similar to human milk (after adjustment for differences in bioavailability) for these three nutrients are also consuming adequate levels. In the case where an infant formula contains a lower level of these nutrients than human milk, the likelihood of nutrient adequacy for infants consuming this formula cannot be determined as data on infants at lower concentrations of intake are not available for review.

Using the Tolerable Upper Intake Level for Individuals

The Tolerable Upper Intake Level (UL) is used to determine the possibility of overconsumption of a nutrient. If an individual's usual nutrient intake remains below the UL, there is little risk of adverse effects from excessive intake. At intakes above the UL, the risk of adverse effects increases. However, the intake at which a given individual will develop adverse effects as a result of taking large amounts of a nutrient is not known with certainty. For example, an individual consuming supplements of vitamin C that exceed 2,000 mg/day may be at increased risk of adverse effects. In the case of vitamin C, the first adverse effects are osmotic diarrhea and gastrointestinal disturbances. It should be noted that there is no established benefit for presumably healthy individuals in consuming amounts of nutrients that exceed the RDA or AI.

ASSESSING NUTRIENT INTAKES OF GROUPS

Using the Estimated Average Requirement for Groups

The prevalence of nutrient inadequacy for a group of individuals may be estimated by comparing the distribution of usual intakes with the distribution of requirements. The Estimated Average Requirement (EAR) is the appropriate Dietary Reference Intake (DRI) to use for this purpose. In most situations, a cutpoint approach may be used to estimate the prevalence of inadequate intakes within the population group under study; this approach is a simplification of the full probability method of calculating the prevalence of inadequacy described by the National Research Council (NRC, 1986). The cutpoint approach allows the prevalence of inadequate nutrient intakes in a population to be approximated by determining the percentage of the individuals in the group whose usual intakes are less than the EAR for the nutrient of interest. This approach assumes that the intake and requirement distributions are independent, that the variability of intakes among individuals within the group under study is greater than the variability of their requirements, and that the requirement distributions are symmetrical.[1]

Before determining the percentage of the group whose intake is below the EAR, the intake distribution should be adjusted to remove the effect of day-to-day variation in intake (Nusser et al., 1996). This can be accomplished by collecting dietary data for each individual over many days or by statistical adjustments to the distribution that are based on information or assumptions about the day-to-day variation (Nusser et al., 1996). When this adjustment is performed (and intakes are thus more representative of the usual diet), the intake distribution narrows and gives a more precise estimate of the proportion of the group with usual intakes below the EAR. An explanation of an adjustment procedure was presented by the National Research Council (NRC, 1986) and is also described in the upcoming report on using DRIs for dietary assessment.

Figures 9-2 and 9-3 are a graphical representation of this approach for vitamin C. They compare the adjusted distribution of intakes of vitamin C for men and women 19 years of age and older from the Third National Health and Nutrition Examination Survey

---

[1]For free-living populations, it is reasonable to assume that the variability in requirements is smaller than the variability in intakes. For vitamin C, vitamin E, and selenium, requirement distributions are assumed to be symmetrical, and the intake and requirement distributions are thought to be independent.

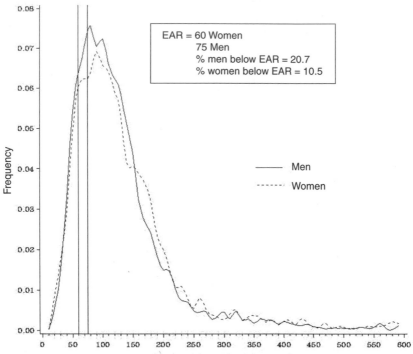

Vitamin C Intake (mg/day) for Men and Women Who Don't Smoke (Food and Supplements)

FIGURE 9-2 Distribution of reported vitamin C intake from all sources for men and women aged 19 years and older who don't smoke, from the Third National Health and Nutrition Examination Survey (NHANES III), 1988–1994. The area under the curve represents almost 100 percent of that population (the right tail of the distributions are not shown here). Approximately 21 percent of men and 11 percent of women who don't smoke have reported total vitamin C intakes (food plus supplements) below the Estimated Average Requirement (EAR) of 75 mg/day for men and 60 mg/day for women. Data have been adjusted for within-person variability (see note below).

NOTE: Nutrient intake from supplements in NHANES III is collected via an instrument similar to a food frequency questionnaire. Thus, the correct method for combining nutrient intake from food (collected with a 24-hour recall) and nutrient intake from supplements to assess total intake is uncertain. For the specific examples shown above, the following process was followed: (1) usual intakes from food were estimated for each individual using the Nusser et al. (1996) approach; (2) self-reported usual intake from supplements were added to obtain an estimate of the individual's total usual intake; and (3) these total usual intakes were compared to the EAR to obtain an estimate of the prevalence of inadequate intakes. This approach may not be optimal because it assumes that the self-reported usual supplement intake has no day-to-day variability. Therefore, the examples may not provide the best estimate of the prevalence of inadequacy of a nutrient, but they still serve to illustrate the use of the EARs when assessing intakes of groups.

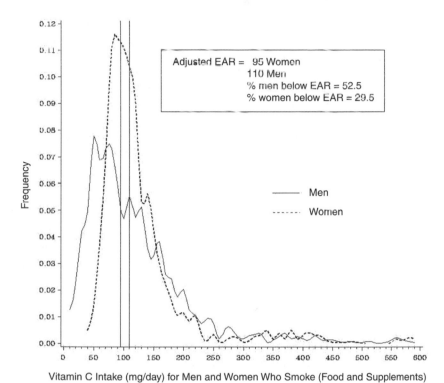

Vitamin C Intake (mg/day) for Men and Women Who Smoke (Food and Supplements)

FIGURE 9-3 Distribution of reported vitamin C intake from all sources for men and women who smoke aged 19 years and older, from the Third National Health and Nutrition Examination Survey (NHANES III), 1988–1994. The area under the curve represents almost 100 percent of that population (the right tail of the distributions are not shown). Approximately 53 percent of men who smoke and 30 percent of women who smoke have reported total vitamin C intakes (food plus supplements) below the Estimated Average Requirement (EAR) adjusted for the effect of smoking to 110 mg/day for men and 95 mg/day for women. Data have been adjusted for within-person variability (see note below).

NOTE: Nutrient intake from supplements in NHANES III is collected via an instrument similar to a food frequency questionnaire. Thus, the correct method for combining nutrient intake from food (collected with a 24-hour recall) and nutrient intake from supplements to assess total intake is uncertain. For the specific examples shown above, the following process was followed: (1) usual intakes from food were estimated for each individual using the Nusser et al. (1996) approach; (2) self-reported usual intake from supplements were added to obtain an estimate of the individual's total usual intake; and (3) these total usual intakes were compared to the EAR to obtain an estimate of the prevalence of inadequate intakes. This approach may not be optimal because it assumes that the self-reported usual supplement intake has no day-to-day variability. Therefore, the examples may not provide the best estimate of the prevalence of inadequacy of a nutrient, but they still serve to illustrate the use of the EARs when assessing intakes of groups.

(NHANES III) with the EARs for vitamin C. These data include intake from both food and supplements. Although the NHANES food intake data are based on a single 24-hour recall for all individuals, replicate 24-hour recalls were conducted on a subset of the participants, and these estimates of day-to-day variation derived from this subset have been used to adjust the intake distributions (see Appendix Tables C-1 and C-2).

The EARs for vitamin C are 60 mg/day for women and 75 mg/day for men. Based on the U.S. population that doesn't smoke, approximately 11 percent of women and 21 percent of men did not consume adequate amounts of vitamin C (from food sources and supplements) (Figure 9-2).

Those who smoke require an additional 35 mg/day of vitamin C, which would result in an adjusted average requirement of 95 mg/day for females and 110 mg/day for males. This is shown in Figure 9-3, in which a higher prevalence of inadequacy is estimated for smokers compared to nonsmokers. Even when vitamin C supplements are included, 53 percent of men and 30 percent of women who smoke were below the requirement. These prevalences indicate that a substantial percentage of Americans who smoke may have inadequate intakes of vitamin C and thus would be expected to have less than optimal ascorbate saturation of neutrophils.

The assessment of nutrient adequacy for groups of people requires unbiased, quantitative information on the intake of the nutrient of interest by individuals in the group. Care must be taken to ensure the quality of the information on which assessments are based, so they are not underestimates or overestimates of total nutrient intake. Estimates of total nutrient intake, including amounts obtained from supplements, should be acquired. It is also important to use appropriate food composition data with valid nutrient values for the foods consumed. In the example for vitamin C intakes, a database of vitamin C values for all foods that contribute substantially to the intakes of this nutrient, as well as a database with the vitamin C composition of the supplements consumed by the population under study, are required.

Overestimates of the prevalence of inadequate intakes could result if the data used are based on intakes that are systematically underreported or if foods rich in vitamin C are underreported. Conversely, underestimates of the prevalence of inadequacy would result if vitamin C-rich foods were overreported. A more extensive discussion of potential sources of error in self-reported dietary data can be found in the upcoming report on using DRIs in dietary assessment.

Using the Recommended Dietary Allowances for Groups

The Recommended Dietary Allowances (RDAs) are not useful in estimating the prevalence of inadequate intakes for groups. As described above, the EAR should be used for this purpose.

Using the Adequate Intake for Groups

In this report, Adequate Intakes (AIs) are assigned only for infants and reflect the average intake of the nutrient from human milk. Human milk and, in the case of nutrients reviewed in this report, infant formulas with the same nutrient composition as human milk (after adjustment for bioavailability) provide the appropriate levels of nutrients for infants of presumably healthy well-nourished mothers. Groups of infants consuming formulas with lower levels of nutrients than human milk may be at some risk of inadequacy, but the prevalence of inadequacy cannot be quantified.

Using the Tolerable Upper Intake Level for Groups

The proportion of the population with usual intakes below the Tolerable Upper Intake Level (UL) is likely to be at no risk of adverse effects due to overconsumption, while the proportion above the UL may be at some risk. In the case of vitamin C, the UL is 2,000 mg/day for adults; the NHANES III data in Figures 9-2 and 9-3, which include reported intake from supplements, illustrate that the U.S. adult population did not exceed this UL at the time of the survey.

In typical food-based diets, ULs for vitamin C, vitamin E, and selenium can rarely be exceeded. Supplement use would be the primary way to exceed these ULs.

The mean intake of a population cannot be used to evaluate the prevalence of intakes above the UL. A distribution of usual intakes, including intakes from supplements, is required in order to assess the proportion of the population that may be at risk of overconsumption.

PLANNING NUTRIENT INTAKES OF INDIVIDUALS

Using the Recommended Dietary Allowance for Individuals

Individuals should use the Recommended Dietary Allowance (RDA) as the target for their daily nutrient intakes. For example, to increase their vitamin C consumption to the RDA level (75 mg/day for women and 90 mg/day for men), adults can increase their intake of foods that provide ascorbate, such as citrus fruits, broccoli, or tomatoes. An 8-ounce glass of orange juice (from frozen concentrate) supplies about 100 mg of vitamin C (USDA, 1991).

Using the Adequate Intake for Individuals

For the nutrients in this report, vitamin C, vitamin E, and selenium, Adequate Intakes (AIs) are set only for infants. Human milk content for these nutrients should supply the AI, so it is not necessary to plan additional sources of intakes for infants exclusively fed human milk. Likewise, for these nutrients, an infant formula with a nutrient profile similar to human milk (after adjustment for any differences in bioavailability) should supply adequate nutrients for an infant.

PLANNING NUTRIENT INTAKES OF GROUPS

The Estimated Average Requirement (EAR) may be used as a basis for planning or making recommendations for the nutrient intakes of groups. The mean intake of a group should be high enough so that only a small percentage of the group would have intakes below the EAR, thus indicating a low prevalence of dietary inadequacy.

Using the EAR and Tolerable Upper Intake Level (UL) in planning intakes of groups involves a number of key decisions and the analysis of issues such as the following:

• determination of the current nutrient intake distribution of the group of interest;
• an evaluation of interventions to shift the current distribution, if necessary, so there is an acceptably low prevalence of intakes below the EAR, as well as an acceptably low prevalence of intakes above the UL (some interventions may increase the intake of those most at risk of inadequacy—usually by individual intervention—whereas others may increase the intake of the entire group [e.g., fortification of the food supply]); and

- the selection of the degree of risk that can be tolerated when planning for the group (e.g., a 2 to 3 percent prevalence versus a higher or lower prevalence).

NUTRIENT-SPECIFIC CONSIDERATIONS

Vitamin C

The effect of cigarette smoking on vitamin C status has led to recommending an increase to cover the higher vitamin C requirements for those who smoke. Thus, smoking status has to be considered in assessing and planning ascorbate intakes. Another consideration in evaluating vitamin C intake is the variability in the food supply and the loss during cooking of this water-soluble and heat-labile vitamin. Destruction of vitamin C in processing and cooking (Williams and Erdman, 1999) may be different than assumed by the values in the food composition tables resulting in an over- or underestimation of the population at risk, while underreporting of dietary intakes in general may lead to an overestimate of the population at risk.

The Tolerable Upper Intake Level (UL) for vitamin C for adults is 2,000 mg/day. Sensitive individuals who regularly consume more than 2,000 mg/day may be at risk of osmotic diarrhea and gastrointestinal disturbances.

Vitamin E

The Estimated Average Requirements (EARs), Recommended Dietary Allowances (RDAs), and Adequate Intakes (AIs) for vitamin E are based on α-tocopherol only and do not include amounts obtained from the other seven naturally occurring forms of vitamin E (β-, γ-, δ- tocopherol and the four tocotrienols). Although absorbed, these forms do not contribute to meeting the vitamin E requirement because they are not converted to α-tocopherol. Only the 2R-stereoisomeric forms of α tocopherol are preferentially secreted by the liver into the plasma for transport to tissues. Since the 2S-stereoisomeric forms of α-tocopherol are not maintained in human plasma or tissues, vitamin E is defined in this report as limited to the 2R-stereoisomeric forms of α-tocopherol to establish recommended intakes. However, all eight stereoisomers of supplemental α-tocopherol are used as the basis for establishing the Tolerable Upper Intake Level (UL) for vitamin E.

Currently, most nutrient databases, as well as nutrition labels, do not distinguish among all the different forms of vitamin E (Figure 6-1) in food. These databases often present the data as α-tocopherol equivalents (α-TE) and thus include the contribution of all eight naturally occurring forms of vitamin E, after adjustment for bioavailability using previously determined equivalencies (e.g., γ-tocopherol has been usually assumed to have only 10 percent of the availability of α-tocopherol) based on fetal resorption assays. This report (see Chapter 6) recommends that the use of α-TE be abandoned due to the lack of evidence of bioavailability via transport in plasma or tissues. Because these other forms of vitamin E occur in foods (e.g., γ-tocopherol is present in widely consumed oils such as soybean and corn oils), the intake of α-TE is greater than the intake of α-tocopherol alone.

All α-tocopherol in foods is *RRR*-α-tocopherol, but the *all rac*-α-tocopherol in fortified foods and supplements is an equal mix of the 2*R*- and 2*S*-stereoisomers. The EARs, RDAs, and AIs given in Chapter 6 apply only to the intake of the *RRR*-α-tocopherol from food and the 2*R*-stereoisomeric forms of α-tocopherol (*RRR*-, *RSR*-, *RRS*-, and *RSS*-α-tocopherol) that occur in fortified foods and supplements (see Chapter 6, Figure 6-2). The UL applies to all eight stereoisomeric forms of α-tocopherol that occur in fortified foods and supplements.

Conversion Factor for Vitamin E in Food and Supplements

The reported median vitamin E intake in the United States of all individuals surveyed in the Third National Health and Nutrition Examination Survey (NHANES III) was 9 mg (21 μmol)/day of α-TE (see Appendix Table C-3). Additional data from the NHANES III database indicate that α-tocopherol contributed 7 mg/day of the 9 mg/day median intake of total α-TE from food (see Appendix Table C-4). Thus, based on NHANES III, approximately 80 percent of the α-TE from foods in the survey are reported to be contributed by α-tocopherol. So to estimate the α-tocopherol intake from food surveys in the United States in which food intake data are presented as α-TE, the α-TE should be multiplied by 0.8.

$$\text{mg of } \alpha\text{-tocopherol in a meal} =$$
$$\text{mg of } \alpha\text{-tocopherol equivalents in a meal} \times 0.8.$$

In addition, the amount of chemically synthesized *all rac*-α-tocopherol compounds added to foods and multivitamin supplements in milligrams should be estimated at 50 percent to calculate the intake of the 2R-stereoisomers of α-tocopherol when assessing intakes to meet requirements.

If vitamin E in foods, fortified foods, and multivitamin supplements is reported in international units (IUs), the activity in milligrams of α-tocopherol may be calculated by multiplying the number of IUs by 0.67 if the form of vitamin E is RRR-α-tocopherol (natural vitamin E) (historically and incorrectly labeled d-α-tocopherol) (Horwitt, 1976), and by 0.45 if the form is all rac-α-tocopherol (synthetic vitamin E) (historically and incorrectly labeled dl-α-tocopherol compounds) (Horwitt, 1976)[2] (see Chapter 6, Table 6-1).

mg of α-tocopherol in food, fortified food, or multivitamin

= IU of the RRR-α-tocopherol compound × 0.67.

or

= IU of the all rac-α-tocopherol compound × 0.45.

For example, a person with intake from food of 15 mg/day of α-TE would have consumed approximately 12 mg/day of α-tocopherol (15 × 0.8 = 12). If this person took a daily multivitamin supplement with 30 IU of RRR-α-tocopheryl acetate, an additional 20 mg/day of α-tocopherol would have been consumed (30 × 0.67 = 20). Thus, this person would have an effective total intake of 32 mg/day of α-tocopherol (12 + 20). If the daily multivitamin supplement contained 30 IU of all rac-α-tocopherol, it would be equivalent to 13.5 mg/day of α-tocopherol (30 × 0.45 = 13.5), and the person's total intake of α-tocopherol would be 25.5 mg/day (12 + 13.5).

Vitamin E Intake from Food

Estimation of vitamin E intake is difficult. There is a propensity to

---

[2]The original international standard for vitamin E, dl-α-tocopheryl acetate (one asymmetric carbon atom in the 2 position on the chromal ring, ambo-α-tocopheryl acetate) is no longer commercially available. It was synthesized from natural phytol and was a mixture of two stereoisomers of α-tocopherols, RRR-α-tocopheryl acetate and SRR-α-tocopheryl acetate (Horwitt, 1976). For practical purposes at the time, the activity of 1 mg of dl-α-tocopheryl acetate was defined as equivalent to one IU of vitamin E. The dl-α-tocopheryl acetate of commerce currently available is synthesized from synthetic isophytol, has eight stereoisomers, and is labeled as dl-α-tocopheryl acetate. However, it is more accurately called all rac-α-tocopheryl acetate (AIN, 1990; IUPAC, 1974) because it contains three asymmetric carbon atoms in the 2, 4', and 8' positions (2RS, 4'RS, 8'RS-α-tocopherol). The all rac and ambo-α-tocopheryl acetates were shown to have the same biological activity in rats (Weiser et al., 1986).

underreport energy intake in national surveys, and fat intake is more underreported than energy intake in the NHANES III survey (Briefel et al., 1997). Since vitamin E is associated with fat in the food matrix, underreporting of the total intake of fat also results in the underreporting of vitamin E intake. Furthermore, there are uncertainties in the amount of α-tocopherol in fats and oils consumed, particularly when food labels do not provide the specific fat or oil used (e.g., "this product may contain partially hydrogenated soybean and/or cottonseed oil or vegetable oil"); in addition, because of the small number of samples, the vitamin E content of the foods in the Continuing Survey of Food Intake of Individuals (CSFII) and NHANES III databases are very variable (J. Holden, Agricultural Research Service, U.S. Department of Agriculture, personal communication, April 13, 1999). Finally, the amounts of fats and oils added during food preparation (and absorbed into the cooked product) is difficult to assess using diet recall methodologies, yet may contribute substantially to vitamin E intake.

UL for Vitamin E

The UL for α-tocopherol for adults is 1,000 mg/day of all eight stereoisomers of α-tocopherol. This UL is based on the intake of α-tocopherol from supplements only, because there is no evidence of adverse effects from the consumption of vitamin E naturally occurring in foods. In addition, the UL was based on animal studies feeding either *RRR*-α-tocopherol (natural vitamin E) or *all rac*-α-tocopherol (synthetic vitamin E), both of which had equivalent adverse effects. Although adults should not exceed the UL of 1,000 mg/day of any form of supplemental α-tocopherol, intakes above this amount may be appropriate for investigation in well-controlled clinical trials.

Sources of vitamin E available as supplements are usually labeled as international units (IUs) of natural vitamin E and its esters or as synthetic vitamin E and its esters. Table 9-1 shows the IUs of various sources of supplemental vitamin E that are equivalent to the UL for adults of 1,000 mg/day of any form of supplemental α-tocopherol.

Recommendation

Because the various forms of vitamin E are not interconvertible in humans, it is recommended that nutrient databases be specific enough to identify and report α-tocopherol intake separately from intake of other tocopherols. However, until this is done, it is possi-

TABLE 9-1 Amounts in International Units (IU) of Any Forms of α-Tocopherol[a] Contained in Vitamin E[b] Supplements Equivalent to the UL for Adults[c]

Sources of Vitamin E Available as Supplements	UL for Adults Total α-Tocopherol (mg/day)	IU from Source Providing Adult UL
Synthetic Vitamin E and Esters		
dl-α-Tocopheryl acetate	1,000	1,100
dl-α-Tocopheryl succinate	1,000	1,100
dl-α-Tocopherol	1.000	1,100
Natural Vitamin E and Esters		
d-α-Tocopheryl acetate	1,000	1,500
d-α-Tocopheryl succinate	1,000	1,500
d-α-Tocopherol	1,000	1,500

[a] All forms of supplemental α-tocopherol include all eight stereoisomers of α-tocopherol. The UL was based on animal studies feeding either *all racemic-* or *RRR-α-*tocopherol, both of which resulted in equivalent adverse effects.

[b] Vitamin E supplements have historically although incorrectly been labeled *d-* or *dl-*α-tocopherol (Horwitt, 1976). Sources of vitamin E include the *all racemic-* (*dl-α-*tocopherol [*RRR-, RRS-, RSR-, RSS-, SSS-, SRS-, SSR-,* and *SRR-*] or synthetic) form and its esters and the *RRR-α-*tocopherol (*d-α-*tocopherol or natural) form and its esters. All of these forms of vitamin E may be present in supplements.

[c] Conversion factors given in Table 6-1 to determine equivalency for meeting requirements are not directly applicable as they take into account lack of documented biological activity of 2S-forms of α-tocopherol in meeting requirements. The conversion factors used in this table are based on 2S-forms contributing to the adverse effects identified.

ble to estimate α-tocopherol intakes by multiplying the total α-TE in food (obtained from food composition tables) by 0.8. Also, the form of chemically synthesized α-tocopherol in fortified foods, multivitamin supplements, and vitamin E supplements has to be identified so that appropriate adjustments for activity can be made before calculating total intake of α-tocopherol.

Selenium

Dietary intakes of selenium depend on the selenium content of the soil where the plant was grown or the animal was raised. Food animals in the United States and Canada usually have controlled diets to which selenium is added, and thus, the amounts found in muscle meats, milk, and eggs are more consistent than for plant foods.

While the food distribution system in the United States and Canada ensures a mix of plant and animal foods from the broad range of soil selenium conditions (see Chapter 7), local foods (e.g., from farmers' markets) may vary considerably from the mean values in food composition databases. However, the variation in selenium content of food sources does not appear to exceed that for many other nutrients. For example, the variation in β-carotene content of

---

Box 9-1 Uses of Dietary Reference Intakes for Healthy Individuals and Groups

Type of Use	For the Individual	For a Group
Assessment	**EAR**[a]: use to examine the possibility of inadequacy of reported intake.	**EAR**[b]: use to estimate the prevalence of inadequate intakes within a group.
	AI[a]: intakes at this level have a low probability of inadequacy.	**AI**[b]: mean intake at this level implies a low prevalence of inadequate intakes.
	UL[a]: intake above this level has a risk of adverse effects.	**UL**[b]: use to estimate the prevalence of intakes that may be at risk of adverse effects.
Planning	**RDA**: aim for this intake.	**EAR**: use in conjunction with a measure of variability of the group's intake to set goals for the median intake of a specific population.
	AI: aim for this intake.	
	UL: use as a guide to limit intake; chronic intake of higher amounts may increase risk of adverse effects.	

EAR = Estimated Average Requirement
RDA = Recommended Dietary Allowance
AI = Adequate Intake
UL = Tolerable Upper Intake Level

[a] Requires accurate measure of usual intake. Evaluation of true status requires clinical, biochemical, and anthropometric data.
[b] Requires statistically valid approximation of usual intake.

food sources is similar to that of selenium (J. Holden, Agricultural Research Service, U.S. Department of Agriculture, personal communication, April 13, 1999).

Infant formulas are often fortified with selenium, and selenium supplements for adults (usually inorganic selenium salts) are becoming more common. The bioavailability of selenate and selenite, the two inorganic forms of selenium commonly used for supplementation, is roughly equivalent and generally exceeds 50 percent (Thomson and Robinson, 1986). Selenium found naturally in foods is primarily in the forms of selenomethionine and selenocysteine, which are organic selenium compounds. The bioavailability of selenium in the form of selenomethionine is greater than 90 percent (Thomson and Robinson, 1986). The selenium in selenocysteine is also highly bioavailable (Swanson et al., 1991). Thus selenium supplements with yeast as the selenium source have higher bioavailability than inorganic supplements. In general, food composition tables do not distinguish these sources. Estimated intakes through self-selected diets are shown in Appendix Table C-6, and total intakes (food and supplements) according to NHANES III are shown in Appendix Table C-7.

The contribution of water to selenium intakes is generally trivial in comparison to food selenium (NRC, 1980) and does not have to be added to intake assessments, unless water from an area known to be high in selenium is consumed.

The UL for adults for selenium is 400 µg/day. Individuals who regularly consume more than 400 µg/day may be at risk of adverse effects that include brittle nails and hair loss.

SUMMARY

With careful consideration to the points mentioned above, the various Dietary Reference Intakes (DRIs) may be used to assess as well as to plan nutrient intakes. Box 9-1 summarizes the appropriate uses of the DRIs for individuals and groups.

REFERENCES

AIN (American Institute of Nutrition). 1990. Nomenclature policy: Generic descriptors and trivial names for vitamins and related compounds. *J Nutr* 120:12–19.

Briefel RR, Sempos CT, McDowell MA, Chien S, Alaimo K. 1997. Dietary methods research in the third National Health and Nutrition Examination Survey: Underreporting of energy intake. *Am J Clin Nutr* 65:1203S–1209S.

Heitmann BL, Lissner L. 1995. Dietary underreporting by obese individuals—Is it specific or non-specific? *Br Med J* 311:986–989.

Horwitt MK. 1976. Vitamin E: A reexamination. *Am J Clin Nutr* 29:569–578.

IOM (Institute of Medicine). 1994. *How Should the Recommended Dietary Allowances be Revised?* Washington, DC: National Academy Press.

IOM (Institute of Medicine). 1997. *Dietary Reference Intakes for Calcium, Phosphorus, Magnesium, Vitamin D, and Fluoride.* Washington, DC: National Academy Press.

IOM (Institute of Medicine). 1998. *Dietary Reference Intakes for Thiamin, Riboflavin, Niacin, Vitamin B$_6$, Folate, Vitamin B$_{12}$, Pantothenic Acid, Biotin, and Choline.* Washington, DC: National Academy Press.

IUPAC-IUB Commission on Biochemical Nomenclature. 1974. Nomenclature of tocopherols and related compounds. Recommendations 1973. *Eur J Biochem* 46:217–219.

Mertz W, Tsui JC, Judd JT, Reiser S, Hallfrisch J, Morris ER, Steele PD, Lashley E. 1991. What are people really eating? The relation between energy intake derived from estimated diet records and intake determined to maintain body weight. *Am J Clin Nutr* 54:291–295.

NRC (National Research Council). 1980. *Drinking Water and Health,* Volume 3. Washington, DC: National Academy Press.

NRC (National Research Council). 1986. *Nutrient Adequacy. Assessment Using Food Consumption Surveys.* Washington, DC: National Academy Press.

Nusser SM, Carriquiry AL, Dodd KW, Fuller WA. 1996. A semiparametric transformation approach to estimating usual daily intake distributions. *J Am Stat Assoc* 91:1440–1449.

Swanson CA, Patterson BH, Levander OA, Veillon C, Taylor PR, Helzlsouer K, McAdam PA, Zech LA. 1991. Human [^{74}Se]selenomethionine metabolism: A kinetic model. *Am J Clin Nutr* 54:917–926.

Thomson CD, Robinson MF. 1986. Urinary and fecal excretions and absorption of a large supplement of selenium: Superiority of selenate over selenite. *Am J Clin Nutr* 44:659–663.

USDA (U.S. Department of Agriculture). 1999. USDA Nutrient Database for Standard Reference, Release, [Online]. Available: http://www.nal.usda.gov/fnic/foodcomp.

Weiser H, Vecchi M, Schlachter M. 1986. Stereoisomers of alpha-tocopherol acetate. IV. USP units and alpha-tocopherol equivalents of all-rac-, 2-ambo- and RRR-alpha-tocopherol evaluated by simultaneous determination of resorption-gestation, myopath and liver storage capacity in rats. *Int J Vitam Nutr Res* 56:45–56.

Williams AW, Erdman JW Jr. 1999. In: Shils ME, Olson JA, Shike M, Ross AC, eds. *Modern Nutrition in Health and Disease.* Baltimore, MD: Williams and Wilkins. P. 181.

10

A Research Agenda

The Panel on Antioxidants and Related Compounds and the Standing Committee on the Scientific Evaluation of Dietary Reference Intakes (DRI Committee) and its subcommittees were charged with developing a research agenda to provide a basis for public policy decisions related to recommended intakes of vitamin C, vitamin E, selenium, and β-carotene and other carotenoids, and ways to achieve them. This chapter describes the approach used to develop the research agenda, briefly summarizes gaps in knowledge, and presents a prioritized research agenda. A section at the end of each nutrient chapter (Chapters 5 through 8) presents a prioritized list of research topics for each nutrient.

APPROACH

The following approach resulted in the research agenda identified in this chapter:

1. Identify gaps in knowledge;
2. Examine data to identify any major discrepancies between intake and the Estimated Average Requirements (EARs); consider possible reasons for such discrepancies;
3. Consider the need to protect individuals with extreme or distinct vulnerabilities due to genetic predisposition or disease conditions; and
4. Weigh alternatives and set priorities based on expert judgment.

401

As a result of this approach, the following four areas were identified:

- nutrient requirements,
- methodological problems related to the assessment of intake of these nutrients and to the assessment of adequacy of intake,
  - relationships of nutrient intake to public health, and
  - adverse effects of nutrients.

MAJOR KNOWLEDGE GAPS

Requirements

To derive an Estimated Average Requirement (EAR), the criterion must be known for a particular status indicator or combination of indicators that is consistent with impaired status as defined by some clinical consequence. For the nutrients considered in this report, there is a dearth of information on the biochemical values that reflect abnormal function. A priority should be the determination of the relationship of existing status indicators to clinical endpoints in the same subjects to determine if a correlation exists. For some nutrients, either new clinical endpoints or intermediate endpoints of impaired function have to be identified and related to status indicators.

The depletion-repletion research paradigms that are often used in studies of requirements, although not ideal, are still probably the best approach to determining nutrient requirements. However, these studies should be designed to meet three important criteria:

1. An indicator of nutrient status is needed for which a cutoff point has been identified, below which nutrient status is documented to be impaired. (In the case of vitamin E, values are based on induced vitamin E deficiency and the correlation with hydrogen peroxide-induced hemolysis and plasma α-tocopherol concentrations, because there is little information relating levels of status indicators to functional sufficiency or insufficiency. Also with vitamin C, there is little information relating levels of status indicators to functional sufficiency or insufficiency, because dose-dependent absorption and renal regulation of ascorbate allow body conservation during low intakes and limitation of plasma levels at high intakes.)

2. The depletion and repletion periods should be sufficiently long to allow a new steady state to be reached. This can be very problematic for vitamin C because biological half-life ranges from

8 to 40 days and is inversely related to ascorbate body pool. For β-carotene and other carotenoids, no long-term depletion-repletion studies with validated intermediate endpoints exist. Study design should allow examination of the effects of initial status on response to maintenance or depletion-repletion.

3. Repletion regimen intakes should bracket the expected EAR intake to assess the EAR more accurately and to allow for a measure of variance. In addition, an accurate assessment of variance requires a sufficient number of subjects.

A relatively new and increasingly popular approach to determining requirements is kinetic modeling of body pools, using steady-state compartmental analyses. Although this approach is unlikely to supplant depletion-repletion studies, it may be the only technique available to obtain this type of information, despite a number of drawbacks. A number of assumptions that cannot be tested experimentally are often needed, and the estimates obtained for body pool sizes are inherently imprecise. Even if accurate assessments of body pools were possible and were obtained, such information would be useful in setting a requirement only if one could establish the body pool size at which functional deficiency occurs. The amount needed for restoration of biochemical status indicators to baseline values is not necessarily equivalent to the requirement for the nutrient.

For vitamin C, vitamin E, selenium, and β-carotene and other carotenoids, useful data are seriously lacking for setting requirements for infants, children, adolescents, pregnant and lactating women, and the elderly. Studies should use graded levels of nutrient intake and a combination of response indices, and should consider other points raised above. For some of these nutrients, studies should examine whether or not the requirement varies substantially by trimester of pregnancy. In addition, more information is needed for groups at increased risk for oxidative stress, especially those who smoke or who are subjected to second-hand smoke, athletes, and individuals living at high altitudes.

Data are lacking about gender issues with respect to metabolism and requirements of these nutrients. For example, women and children with low intakes of selenium are at higher risk of Keshan disease than are men with similar intakes. Women are at higher risk of macular degeneration even at similar plasma concentrations of carotenoids.

The understanding of the health effects of carotenoids is rudimentary compared with that of the other nutrients in this report.

Little information is available on bioavailability, toxicity, and effects of these compounds, apart from β-carotene. Although the only known validated function for carotenoids in humans is to act as a source of vitamin A in the diet, little is known about the relative contribution of dietary provitamin A carotenoids to vitamin A status.

Research to date has indicated little cause for concern about the adequacy of vitamin E intake for apparently healthy people; deficiency states can be produced only as a result of genetic abnormalities in α-tocopherol transfer protein, as a result of various fat malabsorption syndromes, or as a result of protein-energy malnutrition. However, the prevalence of these genetic abnormalities is unknown.

A growing number of studies suggest that there are complex interrelationships among nutrients, particularly those involved in protecting against oxidation (e.g., vitamin C, vitamin E, and selenium), but these are not well understood in relation to the maintenance of normal nutritional status and to the prevention of chronic degenerative disease. These interactions may affect the intake level for one or more of the nutrients.

Methodology

For some nutrients, serious limitations exist in the methods available to analyze laboratory values indicative of nutrient status, to determine the nutrient content of foods, or both. These limitations have slowed progress in conducting or interpreting studies of nutrient requirements. Although the analytical methodology for serum carotenoid status is becoming more routine, methods for the analysis of the major dietary carotenoids remain as a limiting methodological factor. A related gap, which is not strictly methodological, is the bioavailability of the various isomers of vitamin E. Major needs include: (1) a comparison of the biological potencies of the various forms of food vitamin E from mixed diets; (2) validation of dietary intake instruments to assess intake of vitamin E and of the major carotenoids in food; and (3) an examination of the mechanisms by which bioavailability is altered by food matrices.

Relationships of Intake to Public Health

Although interest is high and numerous studies have been conducted, serious gaps still exist in knowledge of the relationship of intakes of vitamin C, vitamin E, selenium, and β-carotene and other carotenoids to the risk of coronary heart disease, cancer, and other chronic degenerative diseases. An imbalance in oxidant stress and defenses can lead to the formation and excretion of oxidized products of nucleic acids, lipids, and proteins, which may play a role in chronic disease.

Many of these studies have been conducted with supplemental intakes that are far above those that can be obtained from food, and some questions and controversy remain regarding the linkage of these antioxidant nutrients with increased risk of chronic disease. For example, some clinical intervention trials have shown that in male long-term smokers, high doses of β-carotene supplements did not decrease and may have increased their risk of lung cancer.

Multiple factors are probably involved in disease, but in some cases, one particular nutrient may contribute significantly. For example, vitamin E is known to protect ex vivo low-density lipoprotein oxidation, whereas β-carotene offers no protection. Questions that have to be answered include the following: (1) what are the tissue uptake and subcellular distributions of these nutrients in humans; (2) what is the mechanism by which these nutrients are taken up and regulated by the cells; (3) what is the turnover of these nutrients in the various tissues; (4) in which tissues are they degraded and how rapidly; and (5) what are the major metabolic intermediates during degradation and do they have biological function?

Additional randomized clinical trials are needed to test whether or not supplementation with vitamin C, vitamin E, selenium, and/or β-carotene and other carotenoids can reduce the risk of chronic disease. A number of clinical intervention trials involving more than 100,000 people are in progress. However, whether the results are positive or negative, additional studies will be necessary. For example, if the results are negative, the question will arise as to whether treatment was instituted early enough and whether even longer trials starting at an earlier age are needed to test the hypothesis properly. If the results are positive, the relative importance of vitamin C, vitamin E, selenium, and β-carotene will have to be sorted out, because they are being used in combination in several of the studies. Also, the issue of dose will arise. Most of these studies are using doses that may be unnecessarily high. The questions of who should be treated, at what dosage, and at what age will have to be addressed, along with the impact of treatment on various subgroups (older adults, those who smoke, those with other chronic diseases such as diabetes, etc.). Again, if the results are positive, indicating that antioxidants do indeed offer protection, it will be important to determine if combinations of antioxidants in various doses can further increase the beneficial effect.

Adverse Effects

Considering these nutrients as a group, only a few studies have been conducted that were explicitly designed to address adverse effects of chronically high intake. Thus, information on which to base Tolerable Upper Intake Levels (ULs) is extremely limited. Although an unexpected result of the Alpha-Tocopherol, Beta-Carotene Cancer Prevention Study was a non-prespecified 50 percent increase in mortality from hemorrhagic stroke in Finnish men who smoked and were supplemented with 50 mg/day of vitamin E, additional randomized trial evidence is needed for confirmation or refutation of this result. Because data on the potential for β-carotene to produce increased lung cancer rates in smokers are conflicting, ongoing studies are needed to help resolve this issue.

THE RESEARCH AGENDA

Reporting Data

Because the various forms of vitamin E are not interconvertible and because plasma concentrations of vitamin E depend on the affinity of hepatic α-tocopherol transfer protein for the various forms, it is recommended that the relative biological potencies of the different forms of vitamin E be reevaluated. Until this is done, the actual concentrations of each of the various vitamin E forms in food and biological samples should be reported separately whenever possible.

Research

Five major types of information gaps were noted: (1) a dearth of studies designed specifically to estimate average requirements in presumably healthy humans; (2) a nearly complete lack of usable data on the nutrient needs of infants, children, adolescents, and pregnant women; (3) a lack of definitive studies to determine the role of these nutrients in reducing the risk of certain chronic diseases; (4) a lack of validated biomarkers to evaluate oxidative stress and the relationship between antioxidant intake and health and disease; and (5) a lack of studies designed to detect adverse effects of chronic high intakes of these nutrients.

Highest priority is thus given to research that has the potential to prevent or retard human disease processes and to prevent deficiencies with functional consequences. The following six areas for research were assigned the highest priority (other research recommendations are found at the end of Chapters 5 through 8):

- Studies to provide the basic data for constructing risk curves and benefit curves across the exposures to dietary and supplemental intakes of vitamin C, vitamin E, selenium, β-carotene and other carotenoids. Studies should be designed to determine the relationship of nutrient intakes to validated biomarkers of oxidative stress. These studies should be followed by nested case-control studies to determine the relationship of the biomarkers of oxidative stress to chronic disease. Finally, full-scale intervention trials should be done to establish the preventive potential of a nutrient for chronic disease.
- Investigations of the gender specificity of the metabolism and requirements for vitamin C, vitamin E, selenium, and β-carotene and the other carotenoids.
- Studies to validate methods and possible models for determining Dietary Reference Intakes in the absence of data for some life stage groups, such as children, pregnant and lactating women, and older adults.
- Research to determine the interactions and possible synergisms of vitamin C, vitamin E, selenium, and β-carotene with each other, with other nutrients and other food components, and with endogenous antioxidants. Multifactorial studies are needed to demonstrate in vivo actions as well as synergisms that have been shown in vitro.
- Studies to develop economical, sensitive, and specific methods to assess the associations of vitamin C, vitamin E, selenium, and β-carotene and the other carotenoids with the causation, prevalence, prevention, and treatment of specific viral or other infections.
- Investigations of the magnitude and role of genetic polymorphisms in the mechanisms of actions of vitamin C, vitamin E, selenium, and β-carotene and the other carotenoids.

Because of inconsistent data, a Tolerable Upper Intake Level (UL) could not be established for β-carotene, and due to a lack of sufficient data, ULs could not be set for other carotenoids from food. Thus, research is needed concerning the ULs for the carotenoids. In addition, research would be helpful relative to the adverse effects of vitamin C, vitamin E, and selenium. However, it was concluded that higher priority should be given to the areas listed above because of the possibility of adverse effects at intakes consumed from food and supplements in the United States and Canada.

A

Origin and Framework of the Development of Dietary Reference Intakes

This report is the third in a series of publications resulting from the comprehensive effort being undertaken by the Food and Nutrition Board's (FNB's) Standing Committee on the Scientific Evaluation of Dietary Reference Intakes (DRI Committee) and its panels and subcommittees.

ORIGIN

This initiative began in June 1993, when the Food and Nutrition Board (FNB) organized a symposium and public hearing entitled "Should the Recommended Dietary Allowances Be Revised?" Shortly thereafter, to continue its collaboration with the larger nutrition community on the future of the Recommended Dietary Allowances (RDAs), the FNB took two major steps: (1) it prepared, published, and disseminated the paper "How Should the Recommended Dietary Allowances Be Revised?" (IOM, 1994), which invited comments regarding the proposed concept; and (2) it held several symposia at nutrition-focused professional meetings to discuss its tentative plans and receive responses to this initial concept. Many aspects of the conceptual framework of DRIs came from the report *Dietary Reference Values for Food Energy and Nutrients for the United Kingdom* (COMA, 1991).

The five general conclusions presented in the FNB's 1994 paper are as follows:

1. Sufficient new information has accumulated to support a re-assessment of the RDAs.

2. Where sufficient data for efficacy and safety exist, reduction in the risk of chronic degenerative disease is a concept that should be included in the formulation of future recommendations.

3. Upper levels of intake should be established where data exist regarding risk of toxicity.

4. Components of food of possible benefit to health, although not meeting the traditional concept of a nutrient, should be reviewed, and if adequate data exist, reference intakes should be established.

5. Serious consideration must be given to developing a new format for presenting future recommendations.

Subsequent to the symposium and the release of the paper, the FNB held workshops at which invited experts discussed many issues related to the development of nutrient-based reference values, and FNB members have continued to provide updates and engage in discussions at professional meetings. In addition, the FNB gave attention to the international uses of the earlier RDAs and the expectation that the scientific review of nutrient requirements should be similar for comparable populations.

Concurrently, Health Canada and Canadian scientists were reviewing the need for revision of the *Recommended Nutrient Intakes* (RNIs) (Health Canada, 1990). The consensus following a symposium for Canadian scientists cosponsored by the Canadian National Institute of Nutrition and Health Canada in April 1995 was that the Canadian government should pursue the extent to which involvement with the developing FNB process would be of benefit to both Canada and the United States in terms of leading toward harmonization.

Based on extensive input and deliberations, the FNB initiated action to provide a framework for the development and possible international harmonization of nutrient-based recommendations that would serve, where warranted, for all of North America. To this end, in December 1995, the FNB began a close collaboration with the government of Canada and took action to establish the Standing Committee on the Scientific Evaluation of Dietary Reference Intakes.

THE CHARGE TO THE COMMITTEE

In 1995, the Standing Committee on the Scientific Evaluation of Dietary Reference Intakes (DRI Committee) was appointed to oversee and conduct this project. To accomplish this task, the DRI Committee devised a plan involving the work of seven or more expert nutrient group panels and two overarching subcommittees (Figure

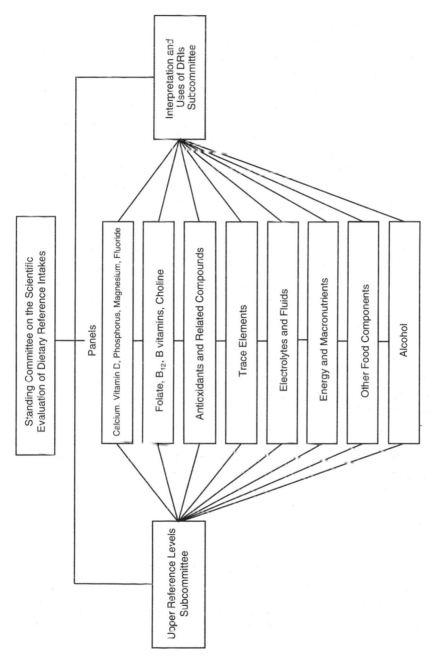

FIGURE A-1 Dietary Reference Intakes project structure.

A-1). The process described below is expected to be used for subsequent reports as well.

The Panel on Dietary Antioxidants and Related Compounds, composed of experts on these nutrients, has been responsible for the following: (1) propose a definition of a dietary antioxidant; (2) review the scientific literature concerning antioxidant nutrients and selected components of foods that may influence the bioavailability of these nutrients; (3) develop dietary reference levels of intake for the selected dietary antioxidants that are compatible with good nutrition throughout the life span and that may decrease the risk of developmental abnormalities and chronic disease; (4) address the safety of high intakes of these dietary antioxidants and, when appropriate, determine Tolerable Upper Intake Levels (ULs); and (5) identify a research agenda to provide a basis for public policy decisions related to recommended intakes and ways to achieve these intakes.

The panel was charged with analyzing the literature, evaluating possible criteria or indicators of adequacy, and providing substantive rationales for their choices of each criterion. Using the criterion chosen for each stage of the lifespan, the panel estimated the average requirement for each nutrient or food component reviewed, assuming that adequate data were available. As panel members reviewed data on ULs, they interacted with the Subcommittee on Upper Reference Levels of Nutrients, which assisted the panel in applying the risk assessment model to each selected nutrient. The panel also worked with the Subcommittee on Interpretation and Uses of Dietary Reference Intakes to determine appropriate examples for using the Recommended Dietary Allowances, Estimated Average Requirements, Adequate Intakes, and ULs. The Dietary Reference Intake values in this report are a product of the joint efforts of the DRI Committee, the Panel on Dietary Antioxidants and Related Compounds, the Subcommittee on Upper Reference Levels of Nutrients, and the Subcommittee on Interpretation and Uses of Dietary Reference Intakes, all under the oversight of the Food and Nutrition Board.

REFERENCES

COMA (Committee on Medical Aspects of Food Policy). 1991. *Dietary Reference Values for Food Energy and Nutrients for the United Kingdom.* Report on Health and Social Subjects, No. 41. London: Her Majesty's Stationery Office.

Health Canada. 1990. *Nutrition Recommendations. The Report of the Scientific Review Committee 1990.* Ottawa: Canadian Government Publishing Centre.

IOM (Institute of Medicine). 1994. *How Should the Recommended Dietary Allowances be Revised?* Washington, DC: National Academy Press.

B

Acknowledgments

The Panel on Dietary Antioxidants and Related Compounds, the Subcommittee on Upper Reference Levels of Nutrients, the Subcommittee on Interpretation and Uses of Dietary Reference Intakes, the Standing Committee on the Scientific Evaluation of Dietary Reference Intakes, and the Food and Nutrition Board (FNB) staff are grateful for the time and effort of the many contributors to this report and the workshops and meetings leading up to the report. Through openly sharing their considerable expertise and different outlooks, these individuals and organizations brought clarity and focus to the challenging task of defining dietary antioxidants and developing vitamin C, vitamin E, β-carotene, and selenium DRIs for humans. The list below mentions those individuals with whom we worked closely, but many others also deserve our heartfelt thanks. These individuals, whose names we do not know, made important contributions to the report by offering suggestions and opinions at the many professional meetings and workshops the committee members attended. The panel, subcommittee, and committee members, as well as FNB staff, thank the following named (as well as unnamed) individuals and organizations:

INDIVIDUALS

G. H. Anderson
Douglas Balentine
Adrianne Bendich
Bernice Berg

Hans Biesalski
Jeffrey Blumberg
Luke Bucci
Graham Burton

Mary Ellen Camire
Larry Clark
Steven Clinton
William Cohn

Paul Connett
John Cordaro
Michael Dourson
Gary Flamm
Balz Frei
Bernard Goldstein
Gary Goodman
E. Robert Greenberg
Roger Hammond
Suzanne Harris
John Hathcock
Harri Hemilä
Max Horwitt

Debra Jahner
Carol Johnston
John Landrum
Orville Levander
Mark Levine
Bernadette Marriott
Thomas McClure
Simin Meydani
Anna Moses
Alanna Moshfegh
Gilbert Omenn
Lester Packer
Sharon Ross

Robert Russell
Etta Saltos
Helmut Sies
Max Snodderly
Thressa Stadtman
Dan Steffen
Manfred Steiner
Roger Sunde
Thomas Tozer
Diane Tribble
George Truscott
Ron Walker

FEDERAL PROJECT STEERING COMMITTEE

Barbara Bowman
Elizabeth Castro
Margaret Cheney
Carolyn Clifford
Paul Coates
Rebecca Costello
Kathleen Ellwood
Nancy Ernst

Peter Fischer
Elizabeth Frazao
Karl Friedl
Nancy Gaston
Jay Hirschman
Van Hubbard
Clifford Johnson
Christine Lewis
Jean Lloyd

Melvin Mathias
Linda Meyers
Esther Myers
Cynthia Ogden
Susan Pilch
Pamela Starke-Reed
Jacqueline Wright
Elizabeth Yetley

DRI CORPORATE DONOR FUND REPRESENTATIVES

Rodney Ausich
Kati Chevaux
David Cook
Mark Dreher

Timothy Jacobson
Maureen Lennon
David Mastroianni
Debra Ponder

Vishwa Singh
Walter Whitehill
Cindy Yablonski

ORGANIZATIONS

American Academy of Neurology
American Academy of Pediatrics
American College of Obstetricians and Gynecologists
American Dietetic Association
American Society for Nutrition Sciences
American Medical Association
Canadian Paediatric Society
Canadian Society for Nutritional Sciences
Center for Science in the Public Interest
Council for Responsible Nutrition
The Dannon Institute
Federation of American Scientists for Experimental Biology
Health Canada
Institute of Food Technologists
Interagency Human Nutrition Research Council
International Life Sciences Institute
Life Sciences Research Organization
National Institute for Nutrition, Canada

C

Dietary Intake Data from the Third National Health and Nutrition Examination Survey (NHANES III), 1988–1994

TABLE C-1 Dietary Vitamin C Intake (mg): Mean and Selected Percentiles, United States, NHANES III, 1988–1994

Sex[a] and Age	Number of Persons Examined	Selected Percentiles		
		Mean	1st	5th
Both sexes, 0–6 mo	413	93.9	55.0	64.0
Standard error		6.5	2.5	4.0
Both sexes, 7–12 mo	579	110.2	56.0	69.0
Standard error		4.4	3.3	3.8
Both sexes, 1–3 y	3,623	91.5	50.0	60.0
Standard error		1.7	1.3	1.3
Both sexes, 4–8 y	4,663	104.6	57.0	68.0
Standard error		2.2	5.7	4.9
M, 9–13 y	1,262	109.9	42.0	56.0
Standard error		4.7	2.6	3.0
M, 14–18 y	938	128.0	41.0	57.0
Standard error		6.0	2.0	2.6
M, 19–30 y	1,960	122.2	39.0	55.0
Standard error		3.9	2.1	2.6
M, 31–50 y	2,611	115.1	37.0	52.0
Standard error		3.2	1.5	1.7
M, 51–70 y	2,029	110.6	33.0	47.0
Standard error		4.6	1.8	2.3
M, 71+ y	1,321	103.9	36.0	50.0
Standard error		3.3	1.3	1.6

10th	25th	50th	75th	90th	95th	99th
69.0	78.0	91.0	107.0	124.0	135.0	157.0
4.8	5.5	7.7	10.7	10.8	9.5	7.4
76.0	90.0	108.0	127.0	147.0	160.0	186.0
3.8	3.8	4.3	5.2	6.1	6.9	10.6
65.0	76.0	89.0	105.0	120.0	130.0	151.0
1.4	1.5	1.7	2.0	2.4	2.7	3.5
75.0	87.0	103.0	120.0	137.0	148.0	170.0
4.4	3.3	2.3	2.8	4.8	6.4	10.1
65.0	82.0	105.0	132.0	162.0	181.0	223.0
3.3	3.8	4.6	5.7	7.2	8.4	11.4
68.0	89.0	119.0	157.0	199.0	228.0	293.0
3.1	4.1	5.6	7.7	10.3	12.3	17.2
65.0	85.0	114.0	150.0	190.0	217.0	278.0
2.9	3.4	3.8	4.9	7.1	9.2	14.9
62.0	81.0	108.0	141.0	178.0	203.0	258.0
1.9	2.3	2.9	4.0	5.6	6.8	10.1
57.0	76.0	103.0	137.0	174.0	200.0	256.0
2.5	3.1	4.2	5.8	8.0	9.8	14.2
59.0	76.0	99.0	126.0	155.0	175.0	215.0
1.8	2.2	3.0	4.3	5.9	7.3	10.4

continued

TABLE C-1 Continued

Sex[a] and Age	Number of Persons Examined	Selected Percentiles		
		Mean	1st	5th
F, 9–13 y	1,279	103.2	47.0	60.0
Standard error		5.7	2.4	2.9
F, 14–18 y	707	94.4	32.0	44.0
Standard error		6.3	2.8	3.6
F, 19–30 y	1,106	84.1	31.0	42.0
Standard error		4.7	2.8	3.6
F, 31–50 y	2,644	90.0	32.0	43.0
Standard error		2.6	1.9	2.1
F, 51–70 y	2,143	102.4	35.0	49.0
Standard error		3.5	2.1	2.3
F, 71+ y	1,436	102.8	45.0	58.0
Standard error		2.6	1.8	1.9
Pregnant	214	124.0	49.0	65.0
Standard error		11.3	6.4	9.4
Lactating	100	136.8	50.0	65.0
Standard error		21.0	13.8	20.2
All individuals (+P/L)	29,022	105.5	46.0	58.0
Standard error		1.3	3.5	3.2
All individuals	28,714	105.3	45.0	58.0
Standard error		1.2	3.3	3.0

NOTE: Estimated mean and standard deviation, and selected percentiles of the usual intake distribution of vitamin C, computed using intake from food sources alone. Dietary intake data are from NHANES III, and the distribution was adjusted using C-SIDE and the method presented in Nusser SM, Carriquiry AL, Dodd KW, Fuller WA. 1996. A semiparametric transformation approach to estimating usual daily intake distributions. *J Am Stat Assoc* 91:1440–1449. Data corresponding to age groups 0–6 months,

10th	25th	50th	75th	90th	95th	99th
67.0	82.0	100.0	121.0	143.0	158.0	187.0
3.4	4.5	5.9	7.1	8.1	8.8	11.0
52.0	68.0	89.0	115.0	144.0	163.0	205.0
4.0	4.9	6.1	7.5	9.7	11.9	19.4
48.0	61.0	79.0	102.0	126.0	142.0	179.0
4.0	4.4	4.7	5.2	6.3	7.6	11.6
51.0	65.0	85.0	109.0	136.0	154.0	194.0
2.2	2.3	2.6	3.1	4.1	4.9	7.0
57.0	74.0	97.0	125.0	154.0	173.0	215.0
2.4	2.7	3.3	4.6	6.3	8.0	12.7
66.0	81.0	100.0	122.0	144.0	158.0	188.0
2.1	2.2	2.5	3.0	3.7	4.2	5.4
75.0	93.0	119.0	148.0	180.0	202.0	247.0
10.9	12.3	12.3	12.0	13.1	14.3	17.9
75.0	98.0	130.0	169.0	208.0	239.0	274.0
22.6	23.7	22.5	23.7	28.4	30.9	32.6
66.0	82.0	102.0	125.0	150.0	166.0	201.0
2.8	2.1	1.3	2.2	4.4	6.1	10.0
66.0	81.0	101.0	125.0	150.0	167.0	203.0
2.7	2.0	1.2	2.2	4.3	6.0	9.9

7–12 months, and 1–3 years of age were not adjusted because no replicate vitamin C intake data are available for children under 3 years.

[a] M = male, F = female.

SOURCE: Iowa State University Department of Statistics, 1999.

TABLE C-2 Total (Diet + Supplements) Vitamin C Intake (mg): Mean and Selected Percentiles, United States, NHANES III, 1988–1994

Sex[a] and Age	Number of Persons Examined	Selected Percentiles		
		Mean	1st	5th
Both sexes, 0–6 mo	413	100.3	54.9	65.5
Both sexes, 7–12 mo	579	122.5	62.8	70.9
Both sexes, 1–3 y	3,623	121.1	53.0	62.8
Both sexes, 4–8 y	4,663	136.2	58.7	70.9
M, 9–13 y	1,262	143.2	44.1	59.2
M, 14–18 y	938	156.7	37.3	60.8
M, 19–30 y	1,960	172.9	36.3	59.5
M, 31–50 y	2,611	187.1	36.4	55.8
M, 51–70 y	2,029	199.4	34.0	49.8
M, 71+ y	1,321	176.3	38.2	52.5
F, 9–13 y	1,279	129.8	44.2	63.5
F, 14–18 y	707	145.5	31.1	50.1
F, 19–30 y	1,106	121.9	31.1	44.4
F, 31–50 y	2,644	165.1	31.0	48.1
F, 51–70 y	2,143	202.4	37.7	52.3
F, 71+ y	1,436	192.3	46.8	62.2
Pregnant	214	192.7	68.9	77.7
Lactating	100	195.9	60.5	76.6
All individuals (+P/L)	29,022	167.2	45.5	61.9
All individuals	28,714	186.9	44.6	61.0

NOTE: Estimated mean and selected percentiles of the usual intake distribution of vitamin C, computed using intakes from food and supplement sources. Dietary intake data are from NHANES III. Intakes from food were adjusted using C-SIDE and the method presented by Nusser SM, Carriquiry AL, Dodd KW, Fuller WA. 1996. A semiparametric transformation approach to estimating usual daily intake distributions.

10th	25th	50th	75th	90th	95th	99th
73.0	79.4	95.5	113.6	137.1	145.5	194.0
77.6	94.9	114.1	139.4	165.3	177.7	423.9
70.1	83.7	104.4	137.6	168.2	190.7	378.7
79.3	95.3	117.7	151.0	185.3	256.8	395.1
65.9	85.6	119.3	158.3	216.6	334.6	598.3
72.1	91.9	126.3	182.3	254.8	358.8	617.0
68.6	91.1	127.1	177.7	264.0	400.4	1,176.1
66.6	88.7	121.3	175.9	293.3	503.2	1,237.8
62.9	84.3	123.5	186.9	372.9	629.5	1,301.6
64.1	82.5	118.0	169.4	349.1	605.8	1,131.6
70.2	87.5	111.7	141.3	188.9	232.7	621.3
55.0	68.9	94.2	130.7	179.6	226.4	723.0
52.9	67.0	90.1	129.2	176.6	233.8	721.6
55.4	72.8	102.3	151.4	311.6	552.2	1,132.9
63.5	86.0	123.7	185.9	422.1	655.7	1,236.1
70.8	89.7	119.2	175.0	386.0	607.9	1,178.6
96.7	129.4	185.0	237.1	266.7	359.6	540.0
103.9	137.2	181.9	236.4	287.8	296.7	418.6
70.6	88.1	116.3	158.8	246.3	427.6	1,131.0
69.6	87.4	115.9	158.1	246.7	430.3	1,131.2

J Am Stat Assoc 91:1440–1449. However, intakes from supplements are unadjusted, so the day-to-day variability in intakes may not have been totally removed from the data. Standard errors were not available for this data set.

[a] M = male, F = female.

SOURCE: Iowa State University Department of Statistics, 1999.

TABLE C-3 Dietary Vitamin E Intake (α-Tocopherol Equivalents, mg): Mean and Selected Percentiles, United States, NHANES III, 1988–1994

Sex[a] and Age	Number of Persons Examined	Mean	Selected Percentiles 1st	5th
Both sexes, 0–6 mo	414	12.3	7.5	8.8
Standard error		0.3	0.3	0.3
Both sexes, 7–12 mo	579	8.5	4.1	4.8
Standard error		0.3	0.2	0.3
Both sexes 1–3 y	3,624	5.5	3.4	3.9
Standard error		0.1	0.1	0.1
Both sexes, 4–8 y	4,664	7.2	4.7	5.3
Standard error		0.2	1.0	0.8
M, 9–13 y	1,262	9.1	5.1	6.0
Standard error		0.5	0.3	0.3
M, 14–18 y	938	12.0	5.9	6.8
Standard error		1.9	0.3	0.4
M, 19–30 y	1,960	11.6	6.8	7.9
Standard error		0.5	0.3	0.3
M, 31–50 y	2,611	12.1	6.3	7.6
Standard error		0.7	0.7	0.8
M, 51–70 y	2,029	10.6	5.3	6.3
Standard error		0.2	0.2	0.2
M, 71+ y	1,322	9.8	4.8	5.8
Standard error		0.4	0.2	0.2
F, 9–13 y	1,279	7.8	4.1	4.9
Standard error		0.2	0.1	0.2
F, 14–18 y	707	7.9	4.0	4.8
Standard error		0.5	0.2	0.3
F, 19–30 y	1,106	8.5	4.3	5.2
Standard error		0.4	0.3	0.4
F, 31–50 y	2,644	8.2	4.3	5.2
Standard error		0.3	0.3	0.3
F, 51–70 y	2,145	7.7	3.5	4.4
Standard error		0.3	0.3	0.3
F, 71+ y	1,436	8.0	4.1	4.9
Standard error		0.3	0.3	0.3
Pregnant	214	10.1	5.0	6.3
Standard error		1.2	0.5	0.7
Lactating	100	12.0	6.6	7.7
Standard error		1.5	0.6	0.8
All individuals (+P/L)	29,028	9.2	5.3	6.2
Standard error		0.1	0.7	0.6
All individuals	28,720	9.3	5.1	6.0
Standard error		0.1	0.7	0.6

NOTE: Estimated mean and standard deviation, and selected percentiles of the usual intake distribution of vitamin E, computed using intake from food sources alone. Dietary intake data are from NHANES III, and the distribution was adjusted using C-SIDE and the method presented in Nusser SM, Carriquiry AL, Dodd KW, Fuller WA. 1996. A semiparametric transformation approach to estimating usual daily intake distributions.

10th	25th	50th	75th	90th	95th	99th
9.5	10.7	12.2	13.7	15.2	16.1	17.8
0.3	0.3	0.4	0.4	0.4	0.5	0.6
5.3	6.4	8.2	10.3	12.1	13.1	14.8
0.4	0.5	0.4	0.6	0.8	0.7	0.6
4.1	4.7	5.3	6.1	6.9	7.4	8.5
0.1	0.1	0.1	0.1	0.2	0.2	0.3
5.7	6.3	7.1	8.1	9.0	9.6	10.9
0.7	0.5	0.3	0.3	0.6	0.9	1.5
6.5	7.5	8.8	10.4	12.0	13.2	15.7
0.3	0.3	0.4	0.6	0.7	0.8	1.1
7.6	9.2	11.3	13.8	17.2	19.7	25.4
0.5	0.8	1.2	2.3	4.2	6.0	11.4
8.5	9.8	11.4	13.2	15.0	16.1	18.4
0.3	0.4	0.5	0.7	0.7	0.8	1.0
8.4	9.9	11.7	13.9	16.3	17.8	21.3
0.8	0.8	0.8	0.8	0.9	1.0	1.3
7.0	8.4	10.1	12.4	14.9	16.6	20.7
0.2	0.2	0.2	0.3	0.4	0.6	1.0
6.4	7.6	9.3	11.4	13.9	15.7	20.0
0.3	0.2	0.3	0.5	0.9	1.1	1.9
5.4	6.4	7.5	9.0	10.5	11.5	13.9
0.3	0.2	0.3	0.3	0.3	0.3	0.5
5.4	6.3	7.6	9.2	10.9	12.1	14.7
0.3	0.3	0.4	0.6	0.8	1.0	1.5
5.8	6.9	8.2	9.9	11.6	12.8	15.6
0.4	0.4	0.4	0.6	0.7	0.7	2.1
5.7	6.7	8.0	9.5	11.1	12.1	14.3
0.3	0.3	0.3	0.3	0.5	0.6	0.9
4.9	6.0	7.4	9.1	11.0	12.3	15.1
0.3	0.3	0.3	0.3	0.5	0.7	1.1
5.4	6.4	7.7	9.3	11.0	12.2	14.7
0.3	0.2	0.3	0.4	0.6	0.8	1.2
7.0	8.3	9.8	11.6	13.5	14.9	18.1
0.9	1.1	1.2	1.4	1.7	1.9	2.5
8.4	9.8	11.6	13.8	16.1	17.7	21.2
0.9	1.1	1.4	1.8	2.3	2.7	3.5
6.7	7.7	9.0	10.4	11.5	12.9	14.9
0.5	0.4	0.2	0.3	0.7	1.0	1.6
6.6	7.8	8.9	10.5	12.0	13.1	15.3
0.5	0.4	0.2	0.3	0.7	0.9	1.6

J Am Stat Assoc 91:1440–1449. Data corresponding to age groups 0–6 months, 7–12 months, and 1–3 years of age were not adjusted because no replicate vitamin E intake data are available for children under 3 years.

[a] M = male, F = female.

SOURCE: Iowa State University Department of Statistics, 1999.

TABLE C-4 Dietary α-Tocopherol Intake (mg): Mean and Selected Percentiles, United States, NHANES III, 1988–1994

Sex[a] and Age	Number of Persons Examined	Selected Percentiles		
		Mean	1st	5th
Both sexes, 4–8 y	3,455	5.7	4.2	4.6
Standard error		0.1	2.2	1.8
M, 9–13 y	1,223	7.4	1.6	2.6
Standard error		0.3	0.1	0.1
M, 14–18 y	913	9.9	1.5	2.6
Standard error		1.6	0.1	0.2
M, 19–30 y	1,905	9.6	2.1	3.6
Standard error		0.3	0.1	0.2
M, 31–50 y	2,532	9.6	2.2	3.5
Standard error		0.2	0.1	0.1
M, 51–70 y	1,943	8.9	1.8	2.9
Standard error		0.2	0.1	0.2
M, 71+ y	1,256	8.2	1.6	2.5
Standard error		0.4	0.1	0.1
F, 9–13 y	1,241	6.3	1.5	2.3
Standard error		0.2	0.1	0.1
F, 14–18 y	1,029	6.9	1.2	2.4
Standard error		0.4	0.1	0.2
F, 19–30 y	2,204	7.1	1.4	2.4
Standard error		0.2	0.1	0.1
F, 31–50 y	3,060	7.4	1.7	2.8
Standard error		0.3	0.1	0.1
F, 51–70 y	2,080	6.6	1.4	2.4
Standard error		0.3	0.1	0.1
F, 71+ y	1,369	6.5	1.3	2.0
Standard error		0.3	0.1	0.1
All individuals	29,136	7.5	3.0	3.9
Standard error		0.1	0.3	0.3

NOTE: Estimated mean and standard deviation, and selected percentiles of the usual intake distribution of vitamin E, computed using intake from food sources alone. Dietary intake data are from NHANES III, and the distribution was adjusted using C-SIDE and the method presented in Nusser SM, Carriquiry AL, Dodd KW, Fuller WA. 1996. A

10th	25th	50th	75th	90th	95th	99th
4.8	5.2	5.6	6.1	6.6	6.9	7.5
1.5	1.0	0.3	0.7	1.7	2.4	4.0
3.3	4.4	6.4	9.2	12.4	15.5	24.9
0.2	0.2	0.2	0.3	0.7	1.2	3.3
3.5	5.3	7.7	11.4	16.2	22.0	51.9
0.2	0.2	0.4	0.9	2.8	5.6	28.2
4.4	5.9	8.5	11.9	15.6	19.2	29.3
0.2	0.2	0.3	0.4	0.7	1.1	2.4
4.4	5.9	8.4	11.9	15.9	19.8	30.7
0.1	0.1	0.2	0.2	0.4	0.7	1.9
3.7	5.1	7.5	10.8	15.1	19.5	33.3
0.2	0.3	0.2	0.5	0.6	1.0	2.7
3.2	4.3	6.5	9.8	14.3	19.2	35.6
0.2	0.2	0.2	0.4	0.9	1.6	4.3
2.9	3.9	5.6	7.7	10.1	12.6	20.0
0.1	0.1	0.2	0.3	0.4	0.6	1.5
2.9	3.8	5.6	8.6	11.9	15.1	27.8
0.2	0.1	0.3	0.5	0.7	1.6	4.7
3.0	4.2	6.1	8.7	11.9	15.2	24.9
0.1	0.1	0.1	0.3	0.5	0.8	2.1
3.3	4.4	6.4	9.2	12.5	14.8	24.0
0.1	0.1	0.3	0.5	1.0	1.0	2.6
2.9	3.9	5.6	8.1	11.0	14.0	24.8
0.1	0.1	0.2	0.3	0.6	1.1	3.4
2.6	3.7	5.2	7.6	11.6	15.4	26.9
0.1	0.1	0.1	0.3	0.7	1.1	3.0
4.5	5.6	7.1	9.0	11.1	12.6	16.1
0.2	0.2	0.1	0.1	0.4	0.6	1.1

semiparametric transformation approach to estimating usual daily intake distributions. *J Am Stat Assoc* 91:1440–1449.

[a] M = male, F = female.

SOURCE: Iowa State University Department of Statistics, 1999.

TABLE C-5 Total (Diet + Supplements) Vitamin E Intake (α-Tocopherol Equivalents, mg): Mean and Selected Percentiles, United States, NHANES III, 1988–1994

Sex[a] and Age	Number of Persons Examined	Selected Percentiles		
		Mean	1st	5th
Both sexes, 0–6 mo	414	12.6	7.4	8.6
Both sexes, 7–12 mo	579	9.3	3.9	4.9
Both sexes 1–3 y	3,624	11.5	3.4	4.2
Both sexes, 4–8 y	4,664	13.2	4.9	5.4
M, 9–13 y	1,262	13.6	5.0	6.4
M, 14–18 y	938	16.8	6.0	7.0
M, 19–30 y	1,960	22.8	6.7	8.1
M, 31–50 y	2,611	26.6	6.4	7.8
M, 51–70 y	2,029	35.3	5.3	6.5
M, 71+ y	1,322	39.9	5.1	6.2
F, 9–13 y	1,279	12.8	4.1	4.9
F, 14–18 y	707	12.2	4.3	4.9
F, 19–30 y	1,106	17.7	4.8	5.5
F, 31–50 y	2,644	30.1	4.4	5.5
F, 51–70 y	2,145	44.9	3.6	4.8
F, 71+ y	1,436	36.8	4.1	5.3
Pregnant	214	31.6	4.7	7.0
Lactating	100	29.2	7.5	8.3
All individuals (+P/L)	29,028	25.7	5.3	6.4
All individuals	28,720	25.7	5.0	6.2

NOTE: Estimated mean and selected percentiles of the usual intake distribution of vitamin E, computed using intakes from food and supplement sources. Dietary intake data are from NHANES III. Intakes from food were adjusted using C-SIDE and the method presented by Nusser SM, Carriquiry AL, Dodd KW, Fuller WA. 1996. A semiparametric transformation approach to estimating usual daily intake distributions.

10th	25th	50th	75th	90th	95th	99th
9.2	10.7	12.3	13.7	16.0	17.5	21.0
5.7	6.8	8.8	11.2	13.2	14.8	18.1
4.3	5.1	6.2	17.7	21.3	34.7	36.4
5.9	6.8	8.0	20.2	23.6	36.5	39.5
6.8	7.9	9.6	13.0	24.6	34.9	67.8
7.8	9.6	11.5	15.3	23.0	40.4	121.2
8.6	10.1	12.1	15.3	42.1	53.0	239.8
8.6	10.5	12.9	18.1	43.1	73.9	243.1
7.3	8.9	11.7	29.5	46.6	116.1	444.0
6.5	8.2	10.8	36.1	70.2	141.4	443.6
5.6	6.6	8.4	11.8	32.2	37.7	42.0
5.5	6.8	8.0	11.1	20.1	37.6	41.9
6.2	7.1	9.2	13.2	38.0	40.4	137.1
6.2	7.3	9.1	25.7	40.3	107.4	420.4
5.6	6.9	9.1	36.9	106.4	191.7	508.7
6.1	7.2	8.9	36.9	69.7	140.2	437.7
7.9	9.0	24.5	39.7	43.2	47.3	416.8
9.5	12.2	25.5	39.3	42.5	114.3	141.0
7.1	8.3	9.9	19.1	39.9	69.1	409.0
7.0	8.2	9.9	18.3	39.8	69.5	409.0

J Am Stat Assoc 91:1440–1449. However, intakes from supplements are unadjusted, so the day-to-day variability in intakes may not have been totally removed from the data. Standard errors were not available for this data set.

[a] M = male, F = female.

SOURCE: Iowa State University Department of Statistics, 1999.

TABLE C-6 Dietary Selenium Intake (µg): Mean and Selected Percentiles, United States, NHANES III, 1988–1994

Sex[a] and Age	Number of Persons Examined	Selected Percentiles		
		Mean	1st	5th
Both sexes, 0–6 mo	793	18.8	3.2	7.7
Both sexes, 7–12 mo	827	37.4	9.1	14.7
Both sexes, 1–3 y	3,309	65.5	15.5	27.0
Both sexes, 4–8 y	3,456	86.8	48.0	58.0
Standard error		1.5	8.4	6.9
M, 9–13 y	1,223	116.0	57.0	70.0
Standard error		5.2	2.5	3.7
M, 14–18 y	914	142.7	67.0	85.0
Standard error		4.2	3.0	4.4
M, 19–30 y	1,906	158.5	81.0	100.0
Standard error		3.5	2.9	3.5
M, 31–50 y	2,536	151.1	74.0	92.0
Standard error		3.3	3.0	3.2
M, 51–70 y	1,946	133.7	64.0	80.0
Standard error		2.6	1.9	1.9
M, 71+ y	1,257	112.0	57.0	69.0
Standard error		2.0	1.4	1.5
F, 9–13 y	1,241	91.9	53.0	63.0
Standard error		1.4	1.6	1.4
F, 14–18 y	697	87.9	44.0	54.0
Standard error		3.1	2.4	2.5
F, 19–30 y	1,084	103.3	52.0	62.0
Standard error		8.8	2.4	3.2
F, 31–50 y	2,587	100.5	55.0	66.0
Standard error		2.2	2.5	2.8
F, 51–70 y	2,080	93.7	51.0	61.0
Standard error		1.7	2.3	2.3
F, 71+ y	1,370	83.3	46.0	55.0
Standard error		1.7	1.0	1.0
Pregnant	211	115.9	60.0	73.0
Standard error		6.4	5.6	5.3
Lactating	96	139.2	86.0	99.0
Standard error		8.3	6.1	6.8
All individuals (+P/L)	27,528	113.7	43.0	57.0
Standard error		1.1	1.9	1.7
All individuals	27,226	113.5	43.0	57.0
Standard error		1.1	1.9	1.8

NOTE: Estimated mean and standard deviation, and selected percentiles of the usual intake distribution of selenium, computed using intake from food sources alone. Dietary intake data are from NHANES III, and the distribution was adjusted using C-SIDE and the method presented in Nusser SM, Carriquiry AL, Dodd KW, Fuller WA. 1996. A semiparametric transformation approach to estimating usual daily intake distributions. *J Am Stat Assoc* 91:1440–1449. Data corresponding to age groups 0–6 months, 7–12

10th	25th	50th	75th	90th	95th	99th
9.8	13.5	17.0	22.2	29.9	36.0	56.9
17.1	23.4	32.2	46.9	64.4	75.1	109.9
33.4	45.4	61.1	80.5	101.7	121.7	155.7
63.0	73.0	85.0	99.0	113.0	122.0	142.0
5.9	3.9	1.7	3.1	7.1	10.1	17.1
78.0	93.0	112.0	134.0	159.0	176.0	216.0
5.0	5.2	3.6	7.3	13.6	14.7	27.6
95.0	114.0	138.0	166.0	196.0	216.0	258.0
5.3	5.3	3.8	4.9	5.9	7.5	19.2
111.0	131.0	154.0	181.0	211.0	231.0	276.0
3.8	3.9	3.6	3.8	4.7	5.4	7.4
102.0	121.0	146.0	175.0	206.0	228.0	280.0
3.1	2.9	3.4	4.0	5.3	7.0	12.3
89.0	105.0	128.0	155.0	186.0	208.0	261.0
1.9	1.9	2.3	3.1	5.3	7.5	14.1
77.0	91.0	108.0	129.0	152.0	167.0	202.0
1.6	1.7	1.9	2.5	3.5	4.5	7.0
69.0	79.0	90.0	104.0	117.0	125.0	143.0
1.3	1.3	1.4	1.6	2.1	2.6	3.8
61.0	72.0	86.0	101.0	118.0	129.0	153.0
2.6	2.8	3.1	3.5	4.2	4.8	6.6
68.0	81.0	99.0	120.0	143.0	159.0	200.0
4.0	4.3	8.0	11.5	18.1	22.1	39.0
72.0	83.0	98.0	115.0	132.0	144.0	170.0
2.6	2.1	2.1	2.7	4.0	5.9	9.4
68.0	78.0	92.0	107.0	123.0	133.0	157.0
2.3	2.0	1.7	1.9	2.7	3.4	5.4
61.0	70.0	82.0	94.0	108.0	117.0	138.0
1.0	1.1	1.4	2.1	3.1	4.1	7.1
81.0	95.0	113.0	134.0	154.0	167.0	194.0
5.3	5.8	6.6	7.8	9.1	10.1	12.5
107.0	121.0	137.0	156.0	174.0	186.0	209.0
7.3	7.9	8.7	9.3	10.2	10.9	13.1
66.0	83.0	106.0	136.0	170.0	194.0	250.0
1.3	1.1	1.2	1.5	2.4	4.2	8.2
66.0	83.0	106.0	136.0	170.0	193.0	250.0
1.3	1.1	1.2	1.5	2.5	4.2	8.2

months, and 1–3 years of age were not adjusted because no replicate selenium intake data are available for children under 3 years.

[a] M – male, F – female.

SOURCE: Iowa State University Department of Statistics, 1999.

TABLE C-7 Total (Diet + Supplements) Selenium Intake (µg): Mean and Selected Percentiles, United States, NHANES III, 1988–1994

Sex[a] and Age	Number of Persons Examined	Selected Percentiles		
		Mean	1st	5th
Both sexes, 0–6 mo	793	35.3	17.2	24.0
Both sexes, 7–12 mo	827	49.7	25.7	31.8
Both sexes, 1–3 y	3,309	69.2	32.7	43.3
Both sexes, 4–8 y	3,456	87.0	49.4	58.2
M, 9–13 y	1,223	116.6	58.2	72.4
M, 14–18 y	914	143.8	68.7	87.9
M, 19–30 y	1,906	160.9	81.6	103.4
M, 31–50 y	2,536	154.1	74.2	94.3
M, 51–70 y	1,946	136.2	65.8	80.9
M, 71+ y	1,257	116.4	57.8	71.4
F, 9–13 y	1,241	92.5	53.6	65.3
F, 14–18 y	697	88.7	41.6	56.4
F, 19–30 y	1,084	105.1	53.9	63.9
F, 31–50 y	2,587	103.5	56.7	67.0
F, 51–70 y	2,080	98.4	53.6	63.3
F, 71+ y	1,370	87.7	47.0	56.5
Pregnant	211	123.9	52.0	82.5
Lactating	96	132.9	79.3	97.4
All individual (+P/L)	27,528	116.1	42.9	57.7
All individuals	27,226	116.0	43.1	57.8

NOTE: Estimated mean and standard deviation, and selected percentiles of the usual intake distribution of selenium, computed using intakes from food and supplement sources. Dietary intake data are from NHANES III. Intakes from food were adjusted using C-SIDE and the method presented by Nusser SM, Carriquiry AL, Dodd KW, Fuller WA. 1996. A semiparametric transformation approach to estimating usual daily intake

10th	25th	50th	75th	90th	95th	99th
26.4	30.7	34.2	39.3	45.2	49.1	66.9
34.3	40.5	46.9	56.0	68.5	77.1	99.7
47.5	55.1	66.4	80.4	93.4	107.0	126.5
63.3	73.0	84.8	98.8	113.3	122.2	139.7
79.1	92.8	111.1	136.2	160.6	172.5	203.1
98.7	115.0	139.3	167.0	195.6	219.0	263.1
114.8	131.7	156.1	184.3	213.4	233.6	291.1
103.0	123.2	147.8	178.5	209.4	235.9	286.4
89.9	106.3	129.9	156.6	189.8	215.9	256.9
79.2	92.3	112.1	134.1	157.5	173.2	222.2
69.9	78.2	91.2	105.0	116.7	124.1	150.9
62.3	71.9	87.3	103.4	119.0	130.2	159.3
68.0	81.7	101.0	122.7	150.3	159.5	184.9
72.5	84.6	100.2	119.0	136.9	147.9	178.4
68.7	80.6	95.8	112.5	128.7	142.5	174.8
61.7	71.0	84.6	100.2	115.1	128.2	160.1
86.8	97.4	118.0	146.8	180.5	186.1	199.1
101.4	110.5	131.6	154.4	168.4	169.8	203.5
67.3	84.6	108.6	139.5	175.4	197.8	250.3
67.4	84.6	108.5	139.1	175.0	197.6	250.4

distributions. *J Am Stat Assoc* 91:1440–1449. However, intakes from supplements are unadjusted, so the day-to-day variability in intakes may not have been totally removed from the data. Standard errors were not available for this data set.

[a] M = male, F = female.

SOURCE: Iowa State University Department of Statistics, 1999.

D

Dietary Intake Data from the Continuing Survey of Food Intakes by Individuals (CSFII), 1994–1996

TABLE D-1 Mean and Percentiles for Usual Intake of Vitamin C (mg), CSFII, 1994–1996

Sex[a] and Age	Number of Persons Examined	Selected Percentiles		
		Mean	1st	5th
0 to 6 mo	209	85.5	4.0	15.0
Standard error		4.6	1.5	4.4
7 to 12 mo	139	114.1	21.0	41.0
Standard error		5.2	7.4	7.9
1 to 3 y	1,908	98.0	23.0	35.0
Standard error		2.3	1.3	2.3
4 to 8 y	1,711	96.5	27.0	40.0
Standard error		2.0	1.8	1.9
M, 9 to 13 y	574	107.1	35.0	49.0
Standard error		5.0	4.1	4.3
M, 14 to 18 y	474	119.2	21.0	35.0
Standard error		7.2	2.1	2.7
M, 19 to 30 y	920	118.6	21.0	35.0
Standard error		5.7	2.0	2.6
M, 31 to 50 y	1,806	105.7	17.0	29.0
Standard error		3.7	3.5	4.2
M, 51 to 70 y	1,680	107.8	15.0	28.0
Standard error		2.2	1.2	1.5
M, 71+ y	722	101.9	10.0	21.0
Standard error		3.3	1.6	2.5

10th	25th	50th	75th	90th	95th	99th
25.0	46.0	75.0	112.0	158.0	192.0	273.0
3.4	7.0	4.9	7.4	16.7	24.5	31.2
54.0	77.0	106.0	141.0	183.0	215.0	293.0
v7.5	6.5	5.9	6.9	10.0	14.2	28.9
44.0	63.0	90.0	125.0	162.0	188.0	245.0
2.6	2.2	2.4	3.0	4.3	5.9	8.5
49.0	66.0	90.0	120.0	153.0	176.0	227.0
1.9	1.8	1.9	2.5	3.9	5.2	8.4
58.0	76.0	100.0	131.0	165.0	188.0	239.0
4.3	4.4	4.8	6.3	9.1	11.6	18.0
46.0	69.0	104.0	153.0	211.0	254.0	351.0
3.0	4.0	6.0	9.7	15.2	19.7	31.4
46.0	68.0	104.0	152.0	211.0	253.0	352.0
3.0	3.9	5.3	7.3	13.0	19.9	42.3
39.0	60.0	92.0	137.0	191.0	229.0	313.0
4.2	3.5	3.0	5.7	8.7	10.9	19.6
37.0	59.0	93.0	141.0	197.0	237.0	329.0
1.7	1.9	2.2	2.8	4.2	5.6	9.8
31.0	54.0	89.0	135.0	189.0	228.0	320.0
2.4	2.5	3.9	4.7	9.5	9.8	33.8

continued

TABLE D-1 Continued

Sex[a] and Age	Number of Persons Examined	Selected Percentiles		
		Mean	1st	5th
F, 9 to 13 y	586	93.8	20.0	32.0
Standard error		3.9	2.3	2.7
F, 14 to 18 y	449	91.2	21.0	32.0
Standard error		5.1	2.9	3.4
F, 19 to 30 y	808	85.1	22.0	33.0
Standard error		3.6	2.8	3.0
F, 31 to 50 y	1,690	86.0	15.0	26.0
Standard error		2.3	0.9	1.1
F, 51 to 70 y	1,605	97.1	17.0	28.0
Standard error		11.2	3.8	1.6
F, 71+ y	670	94.3	15.0	27.0
Standard error		5.7	2.9	4.7
F, Pregnant	80	132.9	27.0	44.0
Standard error		13.7	9.5	10.2
F, Lactating	43	134.2	14.0	29.0
Standard error		21.9	9.6	12.8
All Individuals	15,951	99.7	17.0	29.0
Standard error		1.3	0.6	1.6
All Individuals (+P/L)	16,075	100.1	17.0	29.0
Standard error		1.3	0.8	1.5

NOTE: Estimated mean and standard deviation, and selected percentiles of the usual intake distribution of vitamin C, computed using intake from food sources alone. Dietary intake data are from CSFII, and the distribution was adjusted using C-SIDE and the method presented in Nusser SM, Carriquiry AL, Dodd KW, Fuller WA. 1996. A semiparametric transformation approach to estimating usual daily intake distributions. *J Am Stat Assoc* 91:1440–1449. Data corresponding to age groups 0–6 months, 7–12

10th	25th	50th	75th	90th	95th	99th
41.0	58.0	85.0	119.0	158.0	187.0	250.0
2.9	3.1	3.6	5.2	8.3	11.0	18.5
40.0	57.0	82.0	115.0	154.0	181.0	243.0
3.5	3.8	4.6	6.7	10.7	14.2	23.6
40.0	56.0	78.0	107.0	139.0	161.0	211.0
3.0	3.0	3.3	4.9	7.8	10.3	16.7
33.0	50.0	76.0	111.0	152.0	181.0	248.0
1.2	1.5	2.1	3.1	4.7	6.1	9.8
36.0	55.0	86.0	127.0	173.0	203.0	270.0
1.7	2.4	6.8	22.3	32.9	33.6	26.3
36.0	57.0	86.0	122.0	162.0	189.0	252.0
4.2	3.5	8.8	8.5	6.6	8.1	22.7
56.0	81.0	119.0	169.0	228.0	269.0	365.0
10.4	10.7	12.6	19.3	30.8	40.6	66.1
40.0	66.0	111.0	176.0	258.0	320.0	467.0
14.5	17.3	21.1	30.4	50.8	70.8	128.0
38.0	57.0	87.0	128.0	177.0	212.0	299.0
1.4	1.1	2.3	2.1	5.9	6.5	6.7
38.0	57.0	88.0	129.0	178.0	214.0	301.0
1.4	1.2	2.4	2.0	5.6	6.1	7.4

months, and 1–3 years of age were not adjusted because no replicate vitamin C intake data are available for children under 3 years.

[a] M = male; F = female.

SOURCE: Iowa State University Department of Statistics, 1999.

TABLE D-2 Mean and Percentiles for Usual Intake of
Vitamin E (α-Tocopherol Equivalents, mg), CSFII, 1994–1996

Sex[a] and Age	Number of Persons Examined	Selected Percentiles		
		Mean	1st	5th
0 to 6 mo	209	10.7	0.4	1.5
Standard error		0.5	0.1	0.3
7 to 12 mo	139	10.3	1.0	2.8
Standard error		0.6	0.4	0.4
1 to 3 y	1,908	4.7	1.9	2.5
Standard error		0.1	0.1	0.1
4 to 8 y	1,711	5.8	3.1	3.7
Standard error		0.1	0.1	0.1
M, 9 to 13 y	574	8.1	3.4	4.4
Standard error		0.4	0.2	0.2
M, 14 to 18 y	474	9.3	3.9	5.1
Standard error		0.3	0.3	0.3
M, 19 to 30 y	920	10.3	3.9	5.1
Standard error		0.3	0.2	0.3
M, 31 to 50 y	1,806	10.2	3.7	4.9
Standard error		0.3	0.1	0.1
M, 51 to 70 y	1,680	9.6	3.1	4.4
Standard error		0.3	0.1	0.1
M, 71+ y	722	8.6	2.2	3.3
Standard error		0.3	0.1	0.1
F, 9 to 13 y	586	6.9	3.3	4.1
Standard error		0.2	0.2	0.2
F, 14 to 18 y	449	7.0	3.7	4.5
Standard error		0.3	0.6	0.5
F, 19 to 30 y	808	7.1	3.2	4.0
Standard error		0.2	0.2	0.2
F, 31 to 50 y	1,690	7.4	2.8	3.7
Standard error		0.2	0.1	0.1
F, 51 to 70 y	1,605	7.0	2.4	3.4
Standard error		0.1	0.1	0.1
F, 71+ y	670	6.4	2.1	2.9
Standard error		0.2	0.1	0.1
F, Pregnant	80	7.8	3.9	4.7
Standard error		0.7	1.1	0.9
F, Lactating	43	9.1	3.5	4.5
Standard error		1.1	1.0	1.0
All Individuals	15,951	8.1	2.4	3.5
Standard error		0.1	0.1	0.1
All Individuals (+P/L)	16,075	8.1	2.4	3.5
Standard error		0.1	0.1	0.1

NOTE: Estimated mean and standard deviation, and selected percentiles of the usual intake distribution of vitamin E, computed using intake from food sources alone. Dietary intake data are from CSFII, and the distribution was adjusted using C-SIDE and the method presented in Nusser SM, Carriquiry AL, Dodd KW, Fuller WA. 1996. A semiparametric transformation approach to estimating usual daily intake distributions. *J Am Stat Assoc* 91:1440–1449. Data corresponding to age groups 0–6 months, 7–12

10th	25th	50th	75th	90th	95th	99th
3.1	6.7	10.5	14.2	18.3	21.1	26.7
0.4	0.6	0.7	0.6	0.9	1.4	2.1
4.0	6.4	9.7	13.5	17.3	19.8	24.8
0.5	0.5	0.6	0.8	1.1	1.3	2.0
2.8	3.5	4.4	5.6	7.0	8.1	10.8
0.1	0.1	0.1	0.1	0.2	0.3	0.6
4.0	4.7	5.6	6.7	7.9	8.7	10.5
0.1	0.1	0.1	0.1	0.2	0.3	0.5
4.9	6.0	7.5	9.5	11.9	13.8	18.4
0.2	0.3	0.3	0.5	0.8	1.2	2.8
5.8	7.2	8.9	11.0	13.2	14.8	18.3
0.3	0.3	0.3	0.3	0.4	0.5	0.9
5.9	7.4	9.5	12.3	15.5	17.9	23.7
0.3	0.3	0.3	0.5	1.0	1.4	2.9
5.7	7.2	9.3	12.2	15.7	18.4	25.4
0.1	0.1	0.2	0.3	0.6	1.0	2.2
5.1	6.6	8.7	11.5	15.0	17.7	25.0
0.1	0.1	0.2	0.3	0.6	0.9	1.9
4.1	5.5	7.5	10.4	14.3	17.6	26.9
0.1	0.1	0.2	0.3	0.8	1.3	3.0
4.5	5.4	6.6	8.0	9.7	11.0	14.0
0.2	0.2	0.2	0.3	0.5	0.7	1.3
4.9	5.8	6.9	8.1	9.4	10.2	12.1
0.4	0.3	0.3	0.4	0.8	1.1	1.8
4.5	5.5	6.7	8.3	10.0	11.2	14.0
0.2	0.2	0.2	0.3	0.5	0.6	1.0
4.3	5.3	6.8	8.8	11.1	12.8	17.2
0.1	0.1	0.1	0.2	0.4	0.6	1.1
3.9	5.1	6.5	8.4	10.6	12.3	16.3
0.1	0.1	0.1	0.2	0.3	0.4	0.8
3.4	4.4	5.8	7.7	10.0	11.9	17.0
0.1	0.1	0.2	0.3	0.5	0.8	1.7
5.3	6.3	7.5	9.0	10.6	11.6	13.7
0.8	0.6	0.6	1.0	1.7	2.2	3.3
5.2	6.5	8.4	10.9	13.8	15.9	20.9
1.0	1.0	1.0	1.5	2.5	3.4	6.0
4.1	5.4	7.2	9.7	13.0	15.6	22.3
0.1	0.1	0.1	0.1	0.7	0.9	0.9
4.1	5.4	7.2	9.7	13.0	15.6	22.3
0.1	0.1	0.1	0.1	0.7	0.9	0.9

months, and 1–3 years of age were not adjusted because no replicate vitamin E intake data are available for children under 3 years.

[a] M = male; F = female.

SOURCE: Iowa State University Department of Statistics, 1999.

E

Canadian Dietary Intake Data, 1993, 1995

TABLE E-1 Dietary Vitamin C Intake (mg) of Adults Aged 19–74 Years: Mean and Selected Percentiles, Nova Scotia and Québec, Canada

| | | Selected Percentiles | |
Sex[a] and Age, y	Number of Respondents	Mean	5th
M, 19–30	536	123	32.0
Standard error			3.3
M, 31–50	724	96	25.0
Standard error			4.0
M, 51–70	663	88	23.0
Standard error			4.6
M, 71–74	149	97	18.0
Standard error			3.1
F, 19–30	548	105	18.0
Standard error			1.9
F, 31–50	826	88	16.0
Standard error			1.6
F, 51–70	657	105	20.0
Standard error			2.7
F, 71–74	148	83	19.0
Standard error			7.6

[a] M = male, F = female.

SOURCE: Nova Scotia Heart Health Program. 1993. *Report of the Nova Scotia Nutrition Survey.* Nova Scotia Department of Health, Health and Welfare Canada; Santé Québec.

10th	25th	50th	75th	90th	95th	99th
42.0	59.0	83.0	114.0	143.0	159.0	210.0
2.5	1.7	2.6	3.2	4.1	5.6	12.0
37.0	54.0	74.0	100.0	120.0	136.0	162.0
1.4	2.3	2.3	2.7	3.5	4.8	7.2
35.0	44.0	66.0	97.0	127.0	145.0	234.0
3.0	2.2	4.6	4.8	4.4	9.3	30.0
22.0	38.0	72.0	119.0	182.0	207.0	273.0
2.7	5.8	10.0	18.0	18.0	26.0	40.0
25.0	43.0	74.0	105.0	139.0	158.0	210.0
2.1	1.9	2.9	3.5	4.5	7.2	16.0
21.0	36.0	61.0	104.0	152.0	183.0	238.0
1.6	1.9	4.0	4.4	11.0	7.7	23.0
27.0	46.0	83.0	116.0	158.0	199.0	279.0
2.8	3.5	5.2	6.9	8.3	16.0	39.0
27.0	43.0	70.0	95.0	115.0	139.0	198.0
4.8	4.4	7.0	5.2	11.0	22.0	27.0

1995. *Les Québécoises et les Québécois Mangent-Ils Mieux? Rapport de l'Enquête Québécoise sur la Nutrition, 1990*. Montréal: Ministère de la Santé et des Services Sociaux, Gouvernement du Québec.

F

Serum Values from the Third National Health and Nutrition Examination Survey (NHANES III), 1988–1994

TABLE F-1 Serum Vitamin C (mg/dL) of Persons Aged 4 Years and Older: Mean and Selected Percentiles, United States, NHANES III, 1988–1994

| | Number of Persons Examined | Selected Percentiles | | |
Sex[a] and Age, y		Mean	1st	5th
Both sexes, 4–8	1,216	1.1	0.8	0.9
Standard error		0.02	0.17	0.12
M, 9–13	1,019	0.9	0.2	0.4
Standard error		0.03	0.03	0.03
M, 14–18	789	0.7	0.1	0.2
Standard error		0.03	0.03	0.04
M, 19–30	1,715	0.7	0.07	0.1
Standard error		0.02	0.007	0.01
M, 31–50	2,314	0.6	0.05	0.1
Standard error		0.02	0.006	0.01
M, 51–70	1,836	0.7	0.07	0.1
Standard error		0.02	0.007	0.01
M, 71+	1,150	0.8	0.06	0.2
Standard error		0.02	0.008	0.02

10th	25th	50th	75th	90th	95th	99th
0.9	1.0	1.1	1.2	1.3	1.4	1.5
0.09	0.05	0.02	0.05	0.10	0.13	0.21
0.5	0.7	0.9	1.2	1.4	1.5	2.0
0.03	0.03	0.03	0.03	0.04	0.06	0.14
0.3	0.5	0.7	0.9	1.2	1.3	1.6
0.03	0.03	0.04	0.03	0.03	0.04	0.20
0.2	0.4	0.6	0.9	1.1	1.3	1.8
0.01	0.02	0.02	0.02	0.03	0.07	0.19
0.2	0.3	0.6	0.9	1.1	1.3	1.7
0.01	0.02	0.02	0.02	0.04	0.07	0.11
0.2	0.4	0.7	1.0	1.2	1.4	2.0
0.01	0.02	0.02	0.02	0.04	0.05	0.10
0.2	0.5	0.7	1.0	1.3	1.5	2.1
0.02	0.03	0.02	0.03	0.04	0.06	0.18

continued

TABLE F-1 Continued

Sex[a] and Age, y	Number of Persons Examined	Selected Percentiles		
		Mean	1st	5th
F, 9–13	1,045	1.0	0.24	0.4
Standard error		0.03	0.03	0.03
F, 14–18	906	0.9	0.15	0.3
Standard error		0.04	0.03	0.03
F, 19–30	1,973	0.7	0.11	0.2
Standard error		0.02	0.01	0.03
F, 31–50	2,778	0.8	0.09	0.2
Standard error		0.02	0.009	0.01
F, 51–70	1,907	0.9	0.12	0.3
Standard error		0.03	0.01	0.02
F, 71+	1,251	1.0	0.14	0.3
Standard error		0.02	0.02	0.02
All individuals	19,899	0.8	0.09	0.2
Standard error		0.01	0.006	0.01

[a] M = male, F = female.

SOURCE: Iowa State University Department of Statistics, 1999.

10th	25th	50th	75th	90th	95th	99th
0.5	0.8	1.0	1.2	1.4	1.5	1.9
0.03	0.03	0.04	0.03	0.05	0.07	0.18
0.4	0.6	0.8	1.1	1.3	1.5	1.9
0.03	0.03	0.03	0.04	0.06	0.07	0.10
0.3	0.5	0.7	1.0	1.2	1.3	1.7
0.03	0.03	0.05	0.05	0.05	0.05	0.11
0.3	0.5	0.7	1.0	1.2	1.4	1.8
0.02	0.02	0.01	0.02	0.03	0.04	0.06
0.4	0.6	0.9	1.1	1.4	1.6	2.0
0.02	0.03	0.03	0.03	0.04	0.06	0.10
0.5	0.7	1.0	1.3	1.5	1.7	2.2
0.02	0.03	0.02	0.02	0.03	0.05	0.07
0.3	0.5	0.8	1.0	1.3	1.5	1.9
0.01	0.01	0.01	0.02	0.02	0.04	0.07

TABLE F-2 Serum Vitamin E (µg/dL) of Persons Aged 4 Years and Older: Mean and Selected Percentiles, United States, NHANES III, 1988–1994

Sex[a] and Age, y	Number of Persons Examined	Selected Percentiles		
		Mean	1st	5th
Both sexes, 4–8	2,835	814	542	611
Standard error		7.3	12.0	8.9
M, 9–13	1,072	790	507	571
Standard error		7.9	8.0	6.1
M, 14–18	816	739	459	522
Standard error		9.1	12.9	7.3
M, 19–30	1,782	894	498	594
Standard error		10.3	17.5	10.0
M, 31–50	2,391	1,128	563	675
Standard error		13.9	11.0	9.0
M, 51–70	1,895	1,294	567	739
Standard error		18.2	29.1	52.4
M, 71+	1,193	1,303	609	724
Standard error		30.9	20.6	10.7
F, 9–13	1,094	795	487	563
Standard error		11.3	10.3	8.0
F, 14–18	937	810	481	548
Standard error		10.5	20.8	15.0
F, 19–30	2,028	932	524	618
Standard error		9.5	11.4	7.9
F, 31–50	2,839	1,074	589	686
Standard error		10.3	8.14	6.4
F, 51–70	1,957	1,424	625	793
Standard error		25.7	32.3	24.6
F, 71+	1,290	1,489	640	834
Standard error		19.2	74.6	37.4
All individuals	22,129	1,071	534	618
Standard error		6.6	16.1	6.5

[a] M = male, F = female.

SOURCE: Iowa State University Department of Statistics, 1999.

10th	25th	50th	75th	90th	95th	99th
648	713	793	890	1,004	1,089	1,294
7.8	6.6	6.7	9.3	16.2	23.4	49.6
609	679	771	880	995	1,073	1,238
6.0	7.2	9.0	10.3	12.6	15.6	25.8
558	624	710	821	956	1,058	1,298
7.8	8.9	7.9	13.4	18.7	24.6	57.7
648	741	853	996	1,185	1,335	1,710
7.9	7.9	9.7	15.0	22.5	32.8	75.8
746	885	1,062	1,269	1,551	1,815	2,598
9.7	10.2	11.4	18.2	30.2	45.1	139.0
833	985	1,117	1,465	1,878	2,232	3,196
30.7	36.0	15.7	44.9	85.3	149.0	262.0
796	940	1,157	1,489	1,967	2,375	3,486
12.3	16.8	19.0	33.0	64.0	119.0	361.0
606	678	765	875	1,018	1,129	1,401
7.9	8.3	9.5	14.0	22.1	30.8	61.1
592	678	786	902	1,041	1,159	1,479
17.8	12.3	25.6	17.0	46.2	43.7	174.0
671	765	880	1,036	1,248	1,422	1,863
7.5	6.7	10.0	11.2	29.9	40.4	72.1
745	856	1,007	1,207	1,470	1,691	2,276
6.8	7.8	9.7	12.7	20.1	32.7	96.0
890	1,058	1,279	1,597	2,078	2,534	3,923
14.0	20.7	16.7	28.8	54.0	99.2	358.0
946	1,138	1,373	1,696	2,156	2,543	3,539
20.8	16.0	18.2	23.0	41.5	73.1	198.0
681	795	969	1,220	1,554	1,847	2,707
3.9	4.5	6.0	9.9	13.5	23.2	69.5

TABLE F-3 Serum Selenium (μg/dL) of Persons Aged 4 Years and Older: Mean and Selected Percentiles, United States, NHANES III, 1988–1994

Sex[a] and Age, y	Number of Persons Examined	Selected Percentiles		
		Mean	1st	5th
Both sexes, 4–8				
Standard error				
M, 9–13	344	11.81	9.19	9.99
Standard error		0.16	0.11	0.16
M, 14–18	799	12.28	9.92	10.51
Standard error		0.11	0.13	0.11
M, 19–30	1,751	12.55	9.84	10.62
Standard error		0.11	0.11	0.09
M, 31–50	2,365	12.73	9.78	10.68
Standard error		0.08	0.13	0.07
M, 51–70	1,869	12.69	9.69	10.53
Standard error		0.11	0.22	0.09
M, 71+	1,156	12.54	9.20	10.10
Standard error		0.11	0.13	0.11
F, 9–13	390	11.55	9.14	9.75
Standard error		0.13	0.17	0.14
F, 14–18	926	12.17	9.33	10.02
Standard error		0.10	0.11	0.09
F, 19–30	2,016	12.36	9.50	10.24
Standard error		0.11	0.19	0.06
F, 31–50	2,817	12.25	9.61	10.35
Standard error		0.07	0.08	0.07
F, 51–70	1,936	12.52	9.48	10.37
Standard error		0.09	0.22	0.09
F, 71+	1,261	12.45	9.12	10.15
Standard error		0.10	0.35	0.13
All individuals	17,630	12.45	9.51	10.36
Standard error		0.08	0.07	0.07

[a] M = male, F = female.

SOURCE: Iowa State University Department of Statistics, 1999.

10th	25th	50th	75th	90th	95th	99th
10.41	11.07	11.78	12.51	13.25	13.73	14.73
0.18	0.15	0.13	0.17	0.32	0.37	0.38
10.85	11.45	12.19	13.01	13.83	14.35	15.41
0.09	0.09	0.10	0.13	0.18	0.23	0.34
11.03	11.71	12.47	13.30	14.17	14.76	16.03
0.08	0.08	0.10	0.13	0.16	0.19	0.30
11.12	11.82	12.63	13.51	14.44	15.12	16.79
0.06	0.07	0.07	0.11	0.15	0.19	0.36
10.99	11.74	12.60	13.53	14.50	15.16	16.56
0.12	0.14	0.10	0.17	0.20	0.23	0.55
10.60	11.50	12.50	13.50	14.50	15.10	16.30
0.10	0.11	0.13	0.13	0.14	0.16	0.22
10.07	10.64	11.47	12.33	12.99	13.54	15.40
0.11	0.09	0.11	0.15	0.19	0.30	0.92
10.42	11.14	12.04	13.06	14.09	14.76	16.13
0.08	0.08	0.09	0.12	0.17	0.21	0.31
10.65	11.38	12.25	13.22	14.22	14.88	16.27
0.08	0.09	0.11	0.18	0.21	0.22	0.44
10.75	11.41	12.17	12.99	13.85	14.43	15.67
0.07	0.07	0.07	0.07	0.09	0.10	0.16
10.84	11.61	12.46	13.35	14.25	14.85	16.11
0.08	0.08	0.09	0.14	0.13	0.13	0.39
10.67	11.51	12.41	13.35	14.28	14.90	16.17
0.16	0.17	0.11	0.17	0.16	0.14	0.48
10.80	11.52	12.37	13.27	14.19	14.82	16.26
0.06	0.06	0.07	0.09	0.12	0.14	0.19

TABLE F-4 Serum β-Carotene (µg/dL) of Persons Aged 4 Years and Older: Mean and Selected Percentiles, United States, NHANES III, 1988–1994

Sex[a] and Age, y	Number of Persons Examined	Selected Percentiles		
		Mean	1st	5th
Both sexes, 4–8	2,834	18.7	6.0	8.2
Standard error		0.3	0.5	0.2
M, 9–13	1,072	16.7	4.5	6.3
Standard error		0.6	0.2	0.3
M, 14–18	816	12.4	3.8	5.1
Standard error		0.4	0.2	0.3
M, 19–30	1,782	12.9	2.4	4.0
Standard error		0.5	0.2	0.2
M, 31–50	2,388	16.2	2.2	4.1
Standard error		0.5	0.1	0.2
M, 51–70	1,892	19.5	2.3	4.7
Standard error		0.6	0.2	0.4
M, 71+	1,193	23.4	3.3	5.7
Standard error		0.9	0.5	0.2
F, 9–13	1,094	15.7	5.0	6.7
Standard error		0.4	0.2	0.2
F, 14–18	937	14.3	4.3	5.6
Standard error		0.6	0.2	0.2
F, 19–30	2,028	15.0	2.7	4.6
Standard error		0.4	0.2	0.1
F, 31–50	2,839	21.7	3.2	5.7
Standard error		0.5	0.2	0.2
F, 51–70	1,955	26.4	3.7	6.4
Standard error		0.8	0.4	0.3
F, 71+	1,289	31.1	5.4	8.4
Standard error		1.0	0.4	0.4
All individuals	22,119	18.9	3.0	5.2
Standard error		0.3	0.1	0.1

[a] M = male, F = female.

SOURCE: Iowa State University Department of Statistics, 1999.

10th	25th	50th	75th	90th	95th	99th
9.5	12.4	16.6	22.5	30.1	36.2	51.8
0.3	0.4	0.3	0.9	0.9	1.2	6.4
7.7	10.6	14.7	19.9	27.0	33.5	53.5
0.3	0.4	0.4	0.5	1.5	2.7	7.4
5.9	7.7	10.8	15.1	20.0	24.4	39.7
0.3	0.4	0.4	0.5	1.2	2.3	5.5
5.0	6.9	9.8	15.3	24.3	32.2	54.3
0.1	0.3	0.2	0.5	1.3	2.0	5.2
5.3	7.9	12.4	19.5	29.7	39.7	76.1
0.2	0.2	0.3	0.5	1.0	1.8	7.0
6.3	9.6	15.3	24.1	35.9	46.8	84.4
0.3	0.4	0.4	0.8	1.9	3.5	7.9
7.6	11.6	18.0	28.1	44.1	59.2	106.1
0.3	0.6	0.6	1.8	2.4	3.7	17.9
7.9	10.4	14.1	19.2	25.5	30.2	41.7
0.2	0.3	0.4	0.5	0.7	0.9	1.7
6.4	8.4	11.7	17.2	25.0	31.6	50.0
0.2	0.2	0.3	0.7	1.5	2.4	5.6
5.7	7.9	12.0	18.6	27.0	34.5	59.7
0.1	0.2	0.3	0.5	0.9	1.4	4.1
7.4	11.0	17.2	26.8	39.6	51.4	90.8
0.2	0.3	0.4	0.6	1.1	1.9	6.3
8.5	13.1	20.6	32.3	49.9	65.8	112.9
0.4	0.6	0.6	1.7	1.9	3.4	18.2
10.6	15.7	24.5	38.7	58.8	75.8	122.7
0.4	0.5	0.7	1.2	2.4	3.8	8.9
6.4	9.4	14.7	22.8	35.1	46.2	82.6
0.1	0.1	0.2	0.4	0.5	0.8	2.7

TABLE F-5 Serum α-Carotene (μg/dL) of Persons Aged 4
Years and Older: Mean and Selected Percentiles, United
States, NHANES III, 1988–1994

Sex[a] and Age, y	Number of Persons Examined	Selected Percentiles		
		Mean	1st	5th
Both sexes, 4–8	2,826	4.26	0.90	1.10
Standard error		0.12	0.03	0.07
M, 9–13	1,062	4.08	0.92	1.09
Standard error		0.34	0.03	0.06
M, 14–18	805	2.81	0.67	0.88
Standard error		0.17	0.02	0.01
M, 19–30	1,747	3.23	0.90	0.99
Standard error		0.14	0.01	0.06
M, 31–50	2,342	4.34	0.92	1.03
Standard error		0.18	0.01	0.04
M, 51–70	1,856	4.75	0.93	1.05
Standard error		0.14	0.01	0.04
M, 71+	1,175	4.79	0.96	1.12
Standard error		0.15	0.02	0.02
F, 9–13	1,087	3.66	0.60	1.00
Standard error		0.17	0.02	0.03
F, 14–18	626	3.12	0.90	0.99
Standard error		0.2	0.01	0.03
F, 19–30	996	3.44	0.65	0.89
Standard error		0.20	0.03	0.01
F, 31–50	2,375	5.37	0.70	1.10
Standard error		0.21	0.03	0.04
F, 51–70	1,938	6.01	1.00	1.20
Standard error		0.22	0.02	0.03
F, 71+	1,279	6.38	1.00	1.50
Standard error		0.20	0.02	0.08
Pregnant	186	4.47	0.57	1.09
Standard error		0.45	0.73	0.56
Lactating	90	5.99	0.90	1.70
Standard error		0.52	0.29	0.37
All individuals	20,114	4.59	0.60	1.00
Standard error		0.1	0.02	0.03
All individuals (+P/L)	20,386	4.59	0.60	1.00
Standard error		0.1	0.02	0.03

[a] M = male, F = female.

SOURCE: Iowa State University Department of Statistics, 1999.

10th	25th	50th	75th	90th	95th	99th
1.40	2.40	3.70	5.30	7.50	9.50	14.90
0.11	0.11	0.11	0.16	0.29	0.5	0.89
1.17	2.13	3.20	4.87	7.29	9.36	19.12
0.05	0.32	0.31	0.29	0.75	1.11	4.52
1.01	1.34	1.99	3.26	5.43	7.46	13.63
0.03	0.06	0.12	0.21	0.38	0.59	1.39
1.09	1.22	2.46	4.17	6.26	8.02	13.97
0.04	0.03	0.16	0.13	0.39	0.61	1.57
1.15	2.09	3.50	5.29	8.01	10.25	20.17
0.04	0.37	0.14	0.24	0.42	0.59	2.80
1.25	2.28	3.89	5.98	9.05	11.67	18.59
0.04	0.13	0.12	0.17	0.35	0.51	1.23
1.25	2.71	4.07	5.93	8.78	11.27	17.68
0.08	0.12	0.12	0.19	0.56	0.69	1.04
1.30	1.90	2.90	4.60	6.90	8.80	13.80
0.05	0.08	0.14	0.22	0.4	0.58	1.18
1.07	1.24	2.41	4.09	5.84	7.14	11.94
0.03	0.1	0.39	0.34	0.31	0.93	1.67
1.05	1.45	2.26	3.94	6.93	9.85	19.23
0.03	0.07	0.14	0.23	0.48	0.83	2.40
1.50	2.30	3.90	6.60	10.80	14.50	25.20
0.05	0.08	0.14	0.24	0.49	0.79	1.87
1.60	3.30	4.90	7.50	11.10	14.40	23.10
0.19	0.12	0.18	0.31	0.58	0.63	1.44
2.20	3.50	5.20	7.70	11.60	14.90	25.30
0.12	0.11	0.13	0.24	0.46	0.71	2.10
1.12	1.5	3.42	6.21	9	10.22	18.89
0.24	0.77	0.75	1.05	1.95	3.89	9.01
2.40	3.60	5.50	7.80	10.30	12.10	15.80
0.41	0.45	0.58	1.08	1.13	0.73	2.56
1.30	2.00	3.40	5.70	9.20	12.30	20.60
0.04	0.06	0.1	0.13	0.21	0.32	0.74
1.30	2.00	3.40	5.70	9.20	12.30	20.70
0.04	0.06	0.09	0.13	0.21	0.3	0.65

TABLE F-6 Serum β-Cryptoxanthin (µg/dL) of Persons Aged 4 Years and Older: Mean and Selected Percentiles, United States, NHANES III, 1988–1994

Sex[a] and Age, y	Number of Persons Examined	Selected Percentiles		
		Mean	1st	5th
Both sexes, 4–8	2,834	11.58	4.10	5.40
Standard error		0.17	0.26	0.31
M, 9–13	1,072	10.89	3.00	4.40
Standard error		0.31	0.57	0.24
M, 14–18	816	8.76	2.80	3.70
Standard error		0.25	0.2	0.17
M, 19–30	1,782	8.70	2.40	3.50
Standard error		0.24	0.19	0.10
M, 31–50	2,389	8.54	1.60	3.00
Standard error		0.17	0.14	0.17
M, 51–70	1,893	8.83	1.60	2.90
Standard error		0.21	0.14	0.14
M, 71+	1,193	8.58	1.40	2.60
Standard error		0.2	0.13	0.15
F, 9–13	1,094	10.51	3.80	4.90
Standard error		0.29	0.18	0.17
F, 14–18	632	9.12	3.40	4.20
Standard error		0.39	0.17	0.17
F, 19–30	1,019	7.33	2.11	3.41
Standard error		0.21	0.35	0.14
F, 31–50	2,407	8.84	2.10	3.30
Standard error		0.21	0.13	0.11
F, 51–70	1,954	10.25	2.20	3.30
Standard error		0.27	0.16	0.13
F, 71+	1,287	11.38	2.10	3.40
Standard error		0.45	0.20	0.19
Pregnant	188	10.67	2.80	3.80
Standard error		1.08	0.37	0.35
Lactating	90	9.74	3.90	4.90
Standard error		0.82	0.58	0.4
All individuals	20,372	9.35	2.20	3.30
Standard error		0.13	0.07	0.07
All individuals (+P/L)	20,646	9.36	2.30	3.30
Standard error		0.14	0.07	0.07

[a] M = male, F = female.

SOURCE: Iowa State University Department of Statistics, 1999.

10th	25th	50th	75th	90th	95th	99th
6.30	8.00	10.50	13.90	18.10	21.40	29.30
0.35	0.32	0.32	0.35	0.50	0.62	1.44
5.30	7.00	9.40	13.30	18.30	22.10	31.50
0.45	0.5	0.48	0.53	1.08	1.53	4.25
4.30	5.60	7.60	10.60	14.70	17.90	26.00
0.15	0.15	0.22	0.34	0.59	0.86	1.78
4.10	5.30	7.30	10.40	14.80	18.60	29.40
0.12	0.14	0.16	0.33	0.53	0.76	1.96
3.70	5.10	7.10	10.40	14.70	18.60	29.60
0.24	0.14	0.16	0.26	0.38	0.66	1.77
3.70	5.00	7.30	10.90	16.00	19.90	29.50
0.15	0.14	0.22	0.31	0.54	0.67	1.65
3.40	4.80	7.10	10.70	15.40	19.40	30.10
0.16	0.16	0.23	0.37	0.50	0.71	2.00
5.60	7.10	9.40	12.70	16.80	19.90	27.50
0.18	0.19	0.24	0.37	0.62	0.88	1.65
4.70	5.90	7.80	10.80	15.10	18.60	27.50
0.18	0.23	0.32	0.47	0.81	1.18	2.40
4.05	4.90	6.26	8.46	11.62	14.38	23.89
0.12	0.10	0.14	0.37	0.37	0.65	1.67
4.00	5.30	7.40	10.70	15.10	19.00	30.40
0.1	0.12	0.15	0.22	0.49	0.85	2.57
4.00	5.70	8.50	12.80	18.50	23.00	34.70
0.16	0.17	0.24	0.37	0.68	0.80	2.81
4.30	6.30	9.60	14.40	20.70	25.50	37.50
0.19	0.22	0.38	0.71	0.99	1.18	1.86
4.50	6.10	8.60	12.90	19.10	24.30	38.20
0.38	0.47	0.71	1.59	2.72	3.00	8.76
5.50	6.70	8.70	11.60	15.30	18.20	25.30
0.50	0.81	0.73	0.91	1.47	2.58	6.68
4.00	5.50	8.00	11.60	16.40	20.10	29.60
0.07	0.08	0.10	0.16	0.28	0.42	0.85
4.00	5.50	8.00	11.60	16.40	20.10	29.70
0.07	0.08	0.11	0.16	0.28	0.42	0.86

TABLE F-7 Serum Lutein and Zeaxanthin (µg/dL) of Persons Aged 4 Years and Older: Mean and Selected Percentiles, United States, NHANES III, 1988–1994

Sex[a] and Age, y	Number of Persons Examined	Selected Percentiles		
		Mean	1st	5th
Both sexes, 4–8	2,835	19.7	8.6	10.8
Standard error		0.3	0.3	0.3
M, 9–13	1,072	18.1	7.9	9.7
Standard error		0.3	0.4	0.3
M, 14–18	816	15.5	5.8	7.6
Standard error		0.4	0.4	0.4
M, 19–30	1,782	18.6	6.6	8.9
Standard error		0.4	0.3	0.2
M, 31–50	2,391	21.5	7.2	9.7
Standard error		0.4	0.3	0.2
M, 51–70	1,894	24.0	6.9	10.2
Standard error		0.5	0.4	0.3
M, 71+	1,193	23.5	7.4	10.1
Standard error		0.6	0.3	0.3
F, 9–13	1,094	18.1	8.0	9.9
Standard error		0.5	0.3	0.4
F, 14–18	937	16.2	6.6	8.4
Standard error		0.5	0.5	0.3
F, 19–30	2,028	18.6	7.3	9.3
Standard error		0.4	0.2	0.2
F, 31–50	2,839	21.4	7.2	9.8
Standard error		0.3	0.2	0.2
F, 51–70	1,956	24.4	7.2	10.2
Standard error		0.5	0.7	0.2
F, 71+	1,289	25.7	7.8	10.8
Standard error		0.7	0.3	0.4
All individuals	22,126	20.9	7.1	9.6
Standard error		0.3	0.1	0.1

[a] M = male, F = female.

SOURCE: Iowa State University Department of Statistics, 1999.

10th	25th	50th	75th	90th	95th	99th
12.2	15.0	18.7	23.4	28.5	32.2	40.3
0.3	0.3	0.3	0.4	0.5	0.6	1.0
10.9	13.3	16.7	21.5	27.2	31.4	41.5
0.3	0.3	0.5	0.4	1.1	1.1	3.2
8.8	11.1	14.4	18.6	23.5	27.0	35.1
0.3	0.3	0.3	0.5	0.7	1.0	1.9
10.4	13.2	17.0	22.2	28.7	33.8	46.9
0.2	0.3	0.3	0.5	0.7	0.9	1.8
11.3	14.7	19.7	26.3	34.1	39.8	53.4
0.2	0.3	0.4	0.5	0.7	1.0	1.9
12.4	16.4	21.7	28.7	37.9	45.5	65.8
0.3	0.3	0.4	0.6	1.0	1.7	4.6
11.9	15.6	21.2	28.8	37.9	44.7	61.1
0.3	0.3	0.5	0.7	1.4	2.0	4.0
11.2	13.8	17.3	21.4	25.9	29.3	38.0
0.5	0.5	0.5	0.6	0.9	1.1	1.6
9.5	11.8	15.1	19.3	24.2	27.7	35.8
0.4	0.5	0.5	0.7	0.8	1.1	3.7
10.5	13.2	17.0	22.2	28.6	33.3	44.7
0.2	0.3	0.3	0.4	0.7	0.9	1.7
11.5	14.8	19.4	25.7	33.7	40.0	56.0
0.2	0.2	0.3	0.4	0.7	1.1	2.4
12.2	16.2	21.7	29.4	39.6	47.9	69.8
0.5	0.7	0.4	1.4	1.4	1.7	9.5
12.9	17.2	23.4	31.6	41.1	48.1	64.2
0.4	0.5	0.7	0.9	1.3	1.8	3.3
11.1	14.3	18.9	25.0	33.0	38.9	55.4
0.1	0.2	0.3	0.4	0.6	0.6	1.9

TABLE F-8 Serum Lycopene (µg/dL) of Persons Aged 4 Years and Older: Mean and Selected Percentiles, United States, NHANES III, 1988–1994

Sex[a] and Age, y	Number of Persons Examined	Selected Percentiles		
		Mean	1st	5th
Both sexes, 4–8	2,835	23.3	7.1	10.7
Standard error		0.3	0.9	0.5
M, 9–13	1,072	25.0	8.2	12.3
Standard error		0.6	0.9	0.6
M, 14–18	816	25.3	10.2	13.5
Standard error		0.4	0.6	0.4
M, 19–30	1,782	26.8	9.2	13.3
Standard error		0.5	0.4	0.4
M, 31–50	2,388	26.0	6.9	11.3
Standard error		0.4	0.5	0.5
M, 51–70	1,893	22.0	4.2	7.7
Standard error		0.4	0.3	0.3
M, 71+	1,188	15.5	2.7	4.7
Standard error		0.4	0.3	0.2
F, 9–13	1,094	24.4	9.7	12.6
Standard error		0.5	0.4	0.4
F, 14–18	937	23.4	8.7	11.9
Standard error		0.4	0.9	0.7
F, 19–30	2,028	24.8	7.9	11.7
Standard error		0.4	0.5	0.3
F, 31–50	2,839	22.9	6.5	10.0
Standard error		0.3	0.3	0.3
F, 51–70	1,955	20.9	4.3	7.4
Standard error		0.4	0.3	0.3
F, 71+	1,282	17.0	2.9	5.2
Standard error		0.4	0.2	0.3
All individuals	22,109	23.4	5.6	9.4
Standard error		0.2	0.2	0.2

[a] M = male, F = female.

SOURCE: Iowa State University Department of Statistics, 1999.

10th	25th	50th	75th	90th	95th	99th
12.9	17.1	22.4	28.5	34.7	38.6	46.7
0.5	0.5	0.3	0.8	1.0	0.9	2.2
14.8	19.0	24.1	30.0	36.4	40.9	50.7
0.5	0.5	0.6	0.9	1.1	1.2	2.1
15.5	19.4	24.4	30.3	36.4	40.5	48.9
0.5	0.6	0.5	0.8	0.8	0.9	2.6
15.7	20.2	26.0	32.5	38.9	43.0	51.4
0.4	0.5	0.5	0.6	0.7	0.7	1.0
14.0	18.9	25.0	31.8	39.1	44.0	54.6
0.4	0.4	0.4	0.5	0.6	0.8	1.8
10.0	14.5	20.7	28.0	35.6	40.6	51.0
0.3	0.4	0.4	0.5	0.6	0.8	1.2
6.1	9.3	14.1	20.3	26.7	30.9	39.5
0.3	0.4	0.4	0.6	0.7	0.8	2.1
14.5	18.2	23.1	29.3	36.0	40.6	50.7
0.4	0.4	0.5	0.6	0.8	1.0	1.7
13.9	17.6	22.5	28.2	34.1	38.0	46.0
0.6	0.5	0.4	0.5	0.7	1.0	1.7
14.1	18.4	23.6	29.9	36.9	41.9	53.2
0.3	0.3	0.4	0.5	0.8	1.1	2.0
12.2	16.4	21.9	28.3	34.8	39.0	47.8
0.3	0.2	0.3	0.4	0.6	0.8	1.3
9.5	13.7	19.5	26.6	34.2	39.3	50.1
0.3	0.3	0.4	0.6	0.8	1.0	1.7
6.8	10.3	15.4	22.0	29.4	34.6	45.9
0.3	0.3	0.4	0.6	0.8	1.0	1.7
11.9	16.5	22.4	29.1	36.1	40.7	50.8
0.2	0.2	0.3	0.3	0.3	0.4	0.8

G
Options for Dealing with Uncertainties

Methods for dealing with uncertainties in scientific data are generally understood by working scientists and require no special discussion here except to point out that such uncertainties should be explicitly acknowledged and taken into account whenever a risk assessment is undertaken. More subtle and difficult problems are created by uncertainties associated with some of the inferences that must be made in the absence of directly applicable data; much confusion and inconsistency can result if they are not recognized and dealt with in advance of undertaking a risk assessment.

The most significant inference uncertainties arise in risk assessments whenever attempts are made to answer the following questions (NRC, 1994):

- What set or sets of hazard and dose-response data (for a given substance) should be used to characterize risk in the population of interest?
- If animal data are to be used for risk characterization, which endpoints for adverse effects should be considered?
- If animal data are to be used for risk characterization, what measure of dose (e.g., dose per unit body weight, body surface, or dietary intake) should be used for scaling between animals and humans?
- What is the expected variability in dose-response between animals and humans?
- If human data are to be used for risk characterization, which adverse effects should be used?

- What is the expected variability in dose-response among members of the human population?
- How should data from subchronic exposure studies be used to estimate chronic effects?
- How should problems of differences in route of exposure within and between species be dealt with?
- How should the threshold dose be estimated for the human population?
- If a threshold in the dose-response relationship seems unlikely, how should a low-dose risk be modeled?
- What model should be chosen to represent the distribution of exposures in the population of interest when data relating to exposures are limited?
- When interspecies extrapolations are required, what should be assumed about relative rates of absorption from the gastrointestinal tract of animals and of humans?
- For which percentiles on the distribution of population exposures should risks be characterized?

At least partial, empirically based answers to some of these questions may be available for some of the nutrients under review, but in no case is scientific information likely to be sufficient to provide a highly certain answer; in many cases there will be no relevant data for the nutrient in question.

It should be recognized that for several of these questions, certain inferences have been widespread for long periods of time; thus, it may seem unnecessary to raise these uncertainties anew. When several sets of animal toxicology data are available, for example, and data are not sufficient for identifying the set (i.e., species, strain, and adverse effects endpoint) that best predicts human response, it has become traditional to select that set in which toxic responses occur at lowest dose (the most sensitive set). In the absence of definitive empirical data applicable to a specific case, it is generally assumed that there will not be more than a ten-fold variation in response among members of the human population. In the absence of absorption data, it is generally assumed that humans will absorb the chemical at the same rate as the animal species used to model human risk. In the absence of complete understanding of biological mechanisms, it is generally assumed that, except possibly for certain carcinogens, a threshold dose must be exceeded before toxicity is expressed. These types of long-standing assumptions, which are necessary to complete a risk assessment, are recognized by risk assessors as attempts to deal with uncertainties in knowledge (NRC, 1994).

A past National Research Council (NRC) report (1983) recommended adoption of the concepts and definitions that have been discussed in this report. The NRC committee recognized that throughout a risk assessment, data and basic knowledge will be lacking and risk assessors will be faced with several scientifically plausible options (called inference options by the NRC) for dealing with questions such as those presented above. For example, several scientifically supportable options for dose scaling across species and for high- to low-dose extrapolation will exist, but there will be no ready means to identify those that are clearly best supported. The NRC committee recommended that regulatory agencies in the United States identify the needed inference options in risk assessment and specify, through written risk assessment guidelines, the specific options that will be used for all assessments. Agencies in the United States have identified the specific models to be used to fill gaps in data and knowledge; these have come to be called *default options* (EPA, 1986).

The use of defaults to fill knowledge and data gaps in risk assessment has the advantage of ensuring consistency in approach (the same defaults are used for each assessment) and minimizing or eliminating case-by-case manipulations in the conduct of risk assessment to meet predetermined risk management objectives. The major disadvantage of the use of defaults is the potential for displacement of scientific judgment by excessively rigid guidelines. A remedy for this disadvantage was also suggested by the NRC committee: risk assessors should be allowed to replace defaults with alternative factors in specific cases of chemicals for which relevant scientific data are available to support alternatives. The risk assessors' obligation in such cases is to provide explicit justification for any such departure. Guidelines for risk assessment issued by the U.S. Environmental Protection Agency (EPA, 1986), for example, specifically allow for such departures.

The use of preselected defaults is not the only way to deal with model uncertainties. Another option is to allow risk assessors complete freedom to pursue whatever approaches they judge applicable in specific cases. Because many of the uncertainties cannot be resolved scientifically, case-by-case judgments without some guidance on how to deal with them will lead to difficulties in achieving scientific consensus, and the results of the assessment may not be credible.

Another option for dealing with uncertainties is to allow risk assessors to develop a range of estimates based on application of both defaults and alternative inferences that, in specific cases, have some degree of scientific support. Indeed, appropriate analysis of uncertainties seems to require such a presentation of risk results. Although presenting a number of plausible risk estimates has the advantage that it would seem to more faithfully reflect the true state of scientific understanding, there are no well-established criteria for using such complex results in risk management.

The various approaches to dealing with uncertainties inherent in risk assessment are summarized in Table G-1.

As can be seen in the chapters on each nutrient, specific default assumptions for assessing nutrient risks have not been recommended. Rather, the approach calls for case-by-case judgments, with the recommendation that the basis for the choices made be explicitly stated. Some general guidelines for making these choices are, however, offered.

TABLE G-1 Approaches for Dealing with Uncertainties in a Risk Assessment Program

Program Model	Advantages	Disadvantages
Case-by-case judgments by experts	Flexibility; high potential to maximize use of most relevant scientific information bearing on specific issues	Potential for inconsistent treatment of different issues; difficulty in achieving consensus; need to agree on defaults
Written guidelines specifying defaults for data and model uncertainties (with allowance for departures in specific cases)	Consistent treatment of different issues; maximization of transparency of process; resolution of scientific disagreements possible by resort to defaults	Possible difficulty in justifying departure or achieving consensus among scientists that departures are justified in specific cases; danger that uncertainties will be overlooked
Presentation of full array of estimates from all scientifically plausible models by assessors	Maximization of use of scientific information; reasonably reliable portrayal of true state of scientific understanding	Highly complex characterization of risk, with no easy way to discriminate among estimates; size of required effort may not be commensurate with utility of the outcome

REFERENCES

EPA (U.S. Environmental Protection Agency). 1986. Proposed guidelines for carcinogen risk assessment. *Fed Regist* 51:33992–34003.

NRC (National Research Council). 1983. *Risk Assessment in the Federal Government: Managing the Process.* Washington, DC: National Academy Press.

NRC (National Research Council). 1994. *Science and Judgment in Risk Assessment.* Washington, DC: National Academy Press.

H
Glossary and Acronyms

AAP	American Academy of Pediatrics
ACE	Angiotensin-converting enzyme
Action	Demonstrated effects in various biological systems that may or may not have physiological significance
ADD	Attention deficit disorder
AGE	Advanced glycosylation end product
AI	Adequate Intake
AMD	Age-related macular degeneration
APTT	Activated partial thromboplastin times
Association	Potential interactions derived from epidemiological studies of the relationship between specific nutrients and chronic disease
ATBC	Alpha-Tocopherol, Beta-Carotene (Cancer Prevention Study)
AUC	Area under the curve
AVED	Ataxia and vitamin E deficiency
Bioavailability	Accessibility of a nutrient to participate in unspecified metabolic and/or physiological processes

BMI	Body mass index
CARET	Carotene and Retinol Efficacy Trial
Carotenodermia	Yellow discoloration of the skin with elevated plasma carotene concentrations
α-CEHC	2,5,7,8-tetramethyl-2-(2′-carboxyethyl)-6-hydroxychroman
γ-CEHC	2,7,8-trimethyl-2-(2′-carboxyethyl)-6-hydroxychroman
CHAOS	Cambridge Heart Antioxidant Study
CHD	Coronary heart disease
CLAS	Cholesterol Lowering Atherosclerosis Study
CSFII	Continuing Survey of Food Intakes by Individuals—a survey conducted by the Agricultural Research Service, U.S. Department of Agriculture
CV	Coefficient of variation: mean ÷ standard deviation
DDS	Delayed dermal sensitivity
DHA	Dehydroascorbic acid
DNA	Deoxyribonucleic acid
Dose-response assessment	Second step in a risk assessment, in which the relationship between nutrient intake and adverse effect (in terms of incidence or severity of the effect) is determined
DRI	Dietary Reference Intake
DTH	Delayed-type hypersensitivity
EAR	Estimated Average Requirement
F_2-isoprostane	Indicator of oxidative lipid damage and free-radical generation
FAO	Food and Agriculture Organization of the United Nations
Fore milk	Human milk collected at the beginning of an infant feeding

FOX	Ferrous oxidation/xylenol orange
FNB	Food and Nutrition Board
FT_3	Free triiodothyronine
Function	Role played by a nutrient in growth, development and maturation
GSH	Reduced glutathione
GSHPx	Selenium-dependent glutathione peroxidases
GSSG	Oxidized glutathione
Gun blue	Lubricant solution containing selenious acid, nitric acid, and copper nitrate
H_2O_2	Hydrogen peroxide
Hazard identification	First step in a risk assessment, which is concerned with the collection, organization, and evaluation of all information pertaining to the toxic properties of a nutrient
HDL	High-density lipoprotein
Hind milk	Human milk collected at the end of an infant feeding
HIV	Human immunodeficiency virus
HOCl	Hypochlorous acid
HOPE	Heart Outcomes Prevention Evaluation
HPLC	High-performance liquid chromatography
IAEA	International Atomic Energy Agency
ICAM-1	Intracellular cell adhesion molecule
IOM	Institute of Medicine
Kashin-Beck disease	Human cartilage disease found in some of the low-selenium intake areas in Asia
Keshan disease	Human cardiomyopathy that occurs only in selenium-deficient children
LDL	Low-density lipoprotein

LOAEL   Lowest-observed-adverse-effect level—lowest intake (or experimental dose) of a nutrient at which an adverse effect has been identified

LPL   Lipoprotein lipase

Lycopenodermia   Deep orange discoloration of the skin resulting from high intakes of lycopene-rich food

MHC   Major histocompatibility complex

MONICA Project   Monitoring Trends and Determinants in Cardiovascular Disease Project

MPOD   Macular pigment optical density

MUFA   Monounsaturated fatty acid

NADH   Nicotinamide adenine dinucleotide

NADPH   Nicotinamide adenine dinucleotide phosphate

NEC   Necrotizing enterocolitis

NHANES   National Health and Nutrition Examination Survey—survey conducted periodically by the National Center for Health Statistics of the Centers for Disease Control and Prevention

NHIS   National Health Interview Survey

NO   Nitric oxide

NOAEL   No-observed-adverse-effect level—highest intake (or experimental dose) of a nutrient at which no adverse effect has been observed

NRC   National Research Council

ORAC   Oxygen radical absorbance capacity

Oxidative stress   Imbalance between the production of various reactive species and the ability of the organism's natural protective mechanisms to cope with these reactive compounds and prevent adverse effects

OxLDL   Oxidized low-density lipoprotein

8-OxodG   8-Oxo-7,8-dihydro-2′-deoxyguanosine—a product of oxidative DNA damage

PHS	Physicians' Health Study
Provitamin A carotenoids	α-Carotene, β-carotene, and β-cryptoxanthin
PUFA	Polyunsaturated fatty acid
RBC	Red blood cell
RDA	Recommended Dietary Allowance
Risk assessment	Organized framework for evaluating scientific information, which has as its objective a characterization of the nature and likelihood of harm resulting from excess human exposure to an environmental agent (in this case, a nutrient); it includes the development of both qualitative and quantitative expressions of risk
Risk characterization	Final step in a risk assessment, which summarizes the conclusions from steps 1 through 3 of the risk assessment (hazard identification, dose-response, and estimates of exposure) and evaluates the risk; this step also includes a characterization of the degree of scientific confidence that can be placed in the UL
Risk management	Process by which risk assessment results are integrated with other information to make decisions about the need for, method of, and extent of risk reduction; in addition, risk management considers such issues as the public health significance of the risk, the technical feasibility of achieving various degrees of risk control, and the economic and social costs of this control
RNA	Ribonucleic acid
RNI	Recommended Nutrient Intake
RNS	Reactive nitrogen species
ROS	Reactive oxygen species
SD	Standard deviation
SE	Standard error

Selenite and selenate	Inorganic selenium, the forms found in many dietary supplements
Selenomethionine and selenocysteine	Major dietary forms of selenium
Selenosis	Selenium toxicity characterized by hair loss and nail sloughing
SEM	Standard error of the mean
SOD	Superoxide dismutase
TBARS	Thiobarbituric acid reactive substances, a nonspecific measure of lipid peroxidation
TD	Tardive dyskinesia
α-TE	α-Tocopherol equivalent
TEAC	Trolox equivalent antioxidant capacity
α-Tocopherol	The only form of vitamin E that is maintained in human plasma and thus it is the only form utilized to estimate the vitamin E requirement.
TRAP	Total radical-trapping antioxidant capability
α-TTP	α-Tocopherol transfer protein
UF	Uncertainty factor—number by which the NOAEL (or LOAEL) is divided to obtain the UL; the size of the UF varies depending on the confidence in the data and the nature of the adverse effect
UL	Tolerable Upper Intake Level
USDA	U.S. Department of Agriculture
USP	U.S. Pharmacopeia
VCAM-1	Vascular cell adhesion molecule
Vitamin E	The 2R-stereoisomeric forms of α-tocopherol (*RRR*-, *RSR*-, *RRS*-, and *RSS*-α-tocopherol)
VLDL	Very low density lipoproteins
WHO	World Health Organization

I

Biographical Sketches
of Panel and
Subcommittee Members

LENORE ARAB, Ph.D., is a professor of epidemiology and nutrition in the Departments of Epidemiology and Nutrition at the University of North Carolina at Chapel Hill, Schools of Medicine and Public Health. Dr. Arab's main research interests are anticarcinogens in foods, heterocyclic amines, breast cancer incidence and survival, the relationship of diet to athersclerosis, antioxidant nutrients in various diseases, iron nutriture, and multi-media approaches to dietary assessment. She has published over 140 original papers as well as numerous book chapters and monographs. Dr. Arab serves as a nutrition advisor to the World Health Organization (WHO) and is the founding director of the WHO Collaborating Center for Nutritional Epidemiology in Berlin. She is the North American Editor of the journal *Public Health Nutrition* and sits on the editorial boards of the *European Journal of Clinical Nutrition, Journal of Clinical Epidemiology, Nutrition in Clinical Care,* and *Nutrition and Cancer: An International Journal.* She is the program director for nutritional epidemiology and leader of a training program and NCI-sponsored training grant in that field. Dr. Arab received her M.Sc. from Harvard School of Public Health and her Ph.D. in nutrition from Justus Liebig University in Giessen, Germany.

SUSAN I. BARR, Ph.D., is a professor of nutrition at the University of British Columbia. She received a Ph.D. in human nutrition from the University of Minnesota and is a registered dietitian in Canada. Her research interests focus on the associations among nutrition, physical activity and bone health in women, and she has authored over 65 publications. Dr. Barr has served as vice president of the Canadian Dietetic Association (now Dietitians of Canada) and is a Fellow of both the Dietitians of Canada and the American College of Sports Medicine. She is currently a member of the Scientific Advisory Board of the Osteoporosis Society of Canada and the Medical Advisory Board of the Milk Processors Education Program.

GEORGE C. BECKING, Ph.D., is an associate with Phoenix OHC, Inc., Kingston, Canada, specializing in toxicology and risk assessment related to human health effects of chemicals. Previously, he was a scientist with the World Health Organization (WHO), Geneva, working in the International Programme on Chemical Safety, and a Research Scientist and Scientific Manager at Health Canada. At WHO, his responsibilities included the evaluation of human health risks from a wide range of chemicals including the essential metals copper and zinc. At Health Canada, Dr. Becking worked as a research scientist with a major focus on the effects of nutrition on the metabolism and toxicity of chemicals. Dr. Becking earned his Ph.D. in biochemistry from Queen's University in Kingston, Ontario. He has published over 60 papers and book chapters in the fields of biochemistry, toxicology, and risk assessment methodology.

GARY R. BEECHER, Ph.D., received his Ph.D. in biochemistry from the University of Wisconsin, Madison. Currently, Dr. Beecher is a research chemist in the Food Composition Laboratory at the U.S. Department of Agriculture Beltsville Human Nutrition Research Center. He has over 30 years of professional research experience in analytical chemistry of biological and food systems. Dr. Beecher's recent work has been on investigating the relationship of dietary and plasma carotenoids. He is involved in developing methods for the measurement of flavonoids and the analysis of foods for these constituents. Dr. Beecher was the co-chair of the Symposium on Healthy Diets and Food Trade: The Role of Food Composition Data at the International Congress of Nutrition in July 1997.

SUSAN T. BORRA, R.D., is Senior Vice-President and Director of Nutrition at the International Food Information Council. Ms. Borra is responsible for directing communications programs, executing public affairs strategies, and managing nutrition and food safety issues. Additionally, she oversees the development of consumer education materials and nutrition, food safety, and health programs. Ms. Borra is a member of the American Dietetic Association and is immediate past chair of the American Dietetic Association Foundation. In addition, she is active in the American Heart Association and the Society for Nutrition Education. She has a bachelor's degree in nutrition and dietetics from the University of Maryland and is a registered dietitian.

RAYMOND F. BURK, M.D., is Director of the Clinical Nutrition Research Unit and professor of medicine and pathology at Vanderbilt University. It was also at Vanderbilt that Dr. Burk received his M.D. Dr. Burk has been involved in research on the nutritional and metabolic significance of selenium for many years. He has participated in five workshops sponsored by the National Cancer Institute and has been a member of three World Health Organization task groups on selenium. He was awarded the Lederle Award in Human Nutrition in 1988 and the Osborne and Mendel Award in 1993. He sits on the editorial boards of *Hepatology* and the *American Journal of Clinical Nutrition*.

ALICIA L. CARRIQUIRY, Ph.D., is an associate professor in the Department of Statistics at Iowa State University. She has a Ph.D. in statistics and animal science from Iowa State. Since 1990, Dr. Carriquiry has been a consultant for the U.S. Department of Agriculture Human Nutrition Information Service. She has also done consulting for the U.S. Environmental Protection Agency, the National Pork Producers Council, and is an affiliate for the Law and Economics Consulting Group. At present, Dr. Carriquiry is investigating the statistical issues associated with the Third National Health and Nutrition Examination Survey (NHANES III) and she has recently completed reports on improving the USDA's food intake surveys and methods to estimate adjusted intake, and biochemical measurement distributions for NHANES III. Dr. Carriquiry is the President Elect of the International Society for Bayesian Analysis, a fellow of the American Statistical Association, and an elected member of the International Statistical Institute. She is editor of *Statistical Science*, and serves on the Executive Committee of the Board of Directors of the National Institute of Statistical Science and of the Institute of Mathematical Statistics. Her research interests include nutrition and dietary assessment, Bayesian methods and applications, mixed models and variance component estimation, environmental statistics, stochastic volatility, and linear and nonlinear filtering.

ALVIN C. CHAN, Ph.D., is a professor in the Department of Biochemistry, Microbiology and Immunology, Faculty of Medicine, at the University of Ottawa, Ontario, Canada. Dr. Chan received both his M.Sc. and Ph.D. in nutrition from the University of Minnesota. His primary research interest is to elucidate the function of vitamin E in the turnover of arachidonic acid and membrane phospholipids, the role of vitamin E in free radical formation during oxidative stress, and the relationship of antioxidants to atherogenesis. Dr. Chan has spoken at numerous national and international conferences and has authored four book chapters and over 40 recent publications relating to vitamin E function and interaction with other antioxidants. He served as consultant for Health and Welfare Canada in the review of Canada's Nutrition Recommendations in 1990. He has been on the editorial board of the *Journal of Nutrition* from 1995–present.

BARBARA L. DEVANEY, Ph.D., is a senior fellow at Mathematica Policy Research Inc. where she has specialized in designing and conducting program evaluations. She recently completed a study that produced a comprehensive and rigorous evaluation design for evaluating the impacts of a Universal-Free School Breakfast Program on dietary and educational outcomes of children. She currently is completing an evaluation of the effects of an infant mortality demonstration program, Healthy Start, and is involved in a study examining the impacts of child WIC participation on health care utilization and costs. She also is a co-investigator of a large national evaluation of abstinence education programs funded under the welfare reform legislation. Dr. Devaney was a member of the Institute of Medicine's Committee on Scientific Evaluation of WIC Nutrition Risk Criteria. She received her Ph.D. in economics from the University of Michigan.

JOHANNA T. DWYER, D.Sc., R.D., is director of the Frances Stern Nutrition Center at New England Medical Center and professor in the Departments of Medicine and of Community Health at the Tufts Medical School and School of Nutrition Science and Policy in Boston. She is also senior scientist at the Jean Mayer U.S. Department of Agriculture Human Nutrition Research Center on Aging at Tufts University. Dr. Dwyer's work centers on life-cycle related concerns such as the prevention of diet-related disease in children and adolescents and maximization of quality of life and health in the elderly. She also has a long-standing interest in vegetarian and other alternative lifestyles. Dr. Dwyer is currently the editor of *Nutrition Today* and on the editorial boards of *Family Economics* and *Nutrition Reviews*. She received her D.Sc. and M.Sc. from the Harvard School of Public Health, an M.S. from the University of Wisconsin, and completed her undergraduate degree with distinction from Cornell University. She is a member of the Food and Nutrition Board and its Standing Committee on Scientific Evaluation of Dietary Reference Intakes, and the Technical Advisory Committee of the Nutrition Screening Initiative, and is past president of the American Society for Nutrition Sciences, past secretary of the American Society for Clinical Nutrition, and a past president of the Society for Nutrition Education.

JOHN W. ERDMAN, JR., Ph.D., is a professor of nutrition in the Department of Food Science and Human Nutrition and in Internal Medicine at the University of Illinois at Urbana-Champaign. His research interests are the effects of food processing upon nutrient retention, the metabolic roles of vitamin A and carotenoids, and the bioavailability of minerals from foods. His research regarding soy protein has extended into studies on the impact of non-nutrient components of foods such as phytoestrogens on chronic disease. He is vice-chair of the Standing Committee on the Scientific Evaluation of Dietary Reference Intakes and a former member of the Food and Nutrition Board's Committee on Opportunities in the Nutrition and Food Sciences; the Committee on the Nutrition Components of Food Labeling; and the Subcommittee on Bioavailability of Nutrients of the Committee on Animal Nutrition, Board on Agriculture. Dr. Erdman presently serves on the Scientific Advisory Boards of the Mars Nutrition Research Council and the United Soybean Board.

JEAN-PIERRE HABICHT, M.D., Ph.D., is professor of nutritional epidemiology in the Division of Nutrition Sciences at Cornell University. His professional experience includes serving as special assistant to the director of the Division of Health Examination Statistics at the National Center for Health Statistics, World Health Organization (WHO) medical officer at the Instituto de Nutricion de Centro America y Panama, and professor of maternal and child health at the University of San Carlos in Guatemala. Currently, Dr. Habicht serves as an advisor to United Nations (UN) and government health and nutrition agencies. He is a member of the Expert Advisory Panel on Nutrition, WHO, and is past chairman of the United Nations' Advisory Group on Nutrition. He has consulted to the UN's World Food Program and is involved in research with the UN High Commission for Refugees about the adequacy of food rations in refugee camps. Dr. Habicht has served on numerous Institute of Medicine committees advising the U.S. Agency for International Development about issues in international nutrition. He served as a member of the IOM's Food and Nutrition Board (1981–1984) and as a member and past chair of the Committee on International Nutrition Programs. Dr. Habicht chaired the National Research Council's Coordinating Committee on Evaluation of Food Consumption Surveys, which produced the 1986 NRC report, *Nutrient Adequacy: Assessment Using Food Consumption Surveys.*

ROBERT A. JACOB, Ph.D., F.A.C.N., obtained a Ph.D. degree in 1970 in inorganic and analytical chemistry from Southern Illinois University, Carbondale. Currently, Dr. Jacob is a research chemist at the U.S. Department of Agriculture (USDA) Western Human Nutrition Research Center (WHNRC) in Davis, California. Dr. Jacob has been engaged in nutritional biochemistry research for 23 years, 20 years as a chemist or research chemist with the USDA Agricultural Research Service. His area of research has been the metabolism and nutritional requirements for vitamins and trace minerals, and biochemical assessment of nutritional status. At WHNRC, his primary focus has been on requirements for vitamin C, folic acid, and niacin and the role of diet in antioxidant protection. He has published over 110 related articles in scientific journals and textbooks.

ISHWARLAL JIALAL, M.D., Ph.D., is Professor of Internal Medicine and Pathology, Director of the Division of Clinical Biochemistry and Human Metabolism, Co-director of the Lipid Clinic, and Attending Physician, Division of Endocrinology and Metabolism at the University of Texas Southwestern Medical Center at Dallas. He also holds the C. Vincent Prothro Chair in Human Nutrition Research. To date Dr. Jialal has published over 216 original papers and invited reviews in the areas of nutrition, atherolsclerosis, metabolism, and endocrinology. He has received numerous awards for his work including the AHA Young Investigator Award; Fellow, Council of Arteriosclerosis, AHA; George Grannis Award, National Academy of Clinical Biochemistry; the VERIS Award for nutrition research; the Outstanding Clinical Chemist Award from the Texas Section, American Association of Clinical Chemistry and the International Hermes Prize for Vitamin Research, The Bennie Zak Award for Outstanding Research, Lipids and Lipoproteins Division, AACC. He received his M.D. and Ph.D. from the University of Natal Medical School, Natal, South Africa. Presently, his major research interests are atherosclerosis, antioxidants, hyperlipidemia, and diabetes.

RENATE D. KIMBROUGH, M.D., presently works as an independent consultant. From 1991 to 1999 she served as senior medical associate at the Institute for Evaluating Health Risks (IEHR). She earned her M.D. from the University of Goettingen in Germany. At the IEHR, Dr. Kimbrough conducted several studies and consulted on a variety of matters involving environmental contamination and human health effects. Dr. Kimbrough has served previously as the Director for Health and Risk Capabilities and as Advisor on Medical Toxicology and Risk Evaluation for the U.S. Environmental Protection Agency's Office of the Administrator and as medical toxicologist for the Centers for Disease Control and Prevention. She has over 130 scientific publications in the fields of toxicology and risk assessment. Dr. Kimbrough is certified as a diplomate for the American Board of Toxicology and an honorary fellow of the American Academy of Pediatrics. In 1991, she received the American Conference on Governmental Industrial Hygienists' Herbert E. Stokinger Award for outstanding achievement in industrial toxicology. She also has served on the Scientific Advisory Board, United States Air Force, and the American Board of Toxicology.

LAURENCE N. KOLONEL, M.D., Ph.D., M.P.H., is Deputy Center Director and Director of the Cancer Etiology Program at the Cancer Research Center of the University of Hawaii. Dr. Kolonel is a former member of the Food and Nutrition Board and has served on the Committee on Diet, Nutrition and Cancer; the Committee on Diet and Health; and the Committee on Comparative Toxicity of Naturally Occurring Carcinogens. Dr. Kolonel recently served on the National Cancer Institute Subcommittee on Prevention and Control, is on the advisory board of the Center for Communications, Health and the Environment, and is associate editor of *Cancer Epidemiology Biomarkers and Prevention* and *Cancer Research*. Recently, Dr. Kolonel has published on the relationship of dietary intake and racial variations to prostate and other types of cancer. Dr. Kolonel received his M.P.H. and Ph.D. in epidemiology from the University of California at Berkeley and his M.D. from Harvard Medical School.

NORMAN I. KRINSKY, Ph.D., received his Ph.D. in biochemistry from the University of Southern California. He is currently a professor in the Department of Biochemistry at Tufts University School of Medicine and a scientist at the Jean Mayer U.S. Department of Agriculture Human Nutrition Research Center on Aging, Tufts University. Dr. Krinsky is a member of the Advisory Committee of the International Antioxidant Research Centre at King's College in London. He is also the president of the New England Free Radical/ Oxygen Society. Currently, Dr. Krinsky's research is directed at examining the metabolism of carotenoids to retinoids and retinoic acid, the role of carotenoids in human vision, and the function of antioxidants.

HARRIET V. KUHNLEIN, Ph.D., R.D., is professor of human nutrition at McGill University and founding director of the Centre for Indigenous Peoples' Nutrition and Environment. She is a registered dietitian in Canada, and holds a Ph.D. in nutritional sciences from the University of California at Berkeley. The focus of Dr. Kuhnlein's research is on the nutrition, food patterns, and environment of indigenous peoples. Specifically, her work examines the traditional foods of indigenous peoples, nutrient and contaminant levels in indigenous food systems, and nutrition promotion programs for indigenous peoples. She has published numerous articles on these subjects. Dr. Kuhnlein is a member of both the American and Canadian Societies of Nutritional Sciences, the Society for International Nutrition Research, the Canadian Dietetic Association, and the Society for Nutrition Education. She serves on the Advisory Council of the Herb Research Foundation, and is a former co-chair of the Committee on Nutrition and Anthropology of the International Union of Nutritional Sciences. Dr. Kuhnlein is a member of the editorial boards of *Ecology of Food and Nutrition, Journal of Food Composition and Analysis, International Journal of Circumpolar Health*, and *Journal of Ethnobiology*.

JAMES R. MARSHALL, Ph.D., is a professor of public health and associate director of Cancer Prevention and Control at the Arizona Cancer Center. He received his Ph.D. in sociology from the University of California at Los Angeles. Dr. Marshall is currently involved in a colon cancer prevention program project and is principal investigator for a collaborative project to assemble a multi-state registry of familial colon cancer. Additionally, Dr. Marshall is involved in research focused on diet in the epidemiology of prostate cancer. His work on measurement error in epidemiology has emphasized the use of nutrient indices. He has been the invited speaker at the American Cancer Society Workshop on Nutrition and Cancer, the American Dietetic Association, and the Second International Conference on Dietary Assessment Methods.

SUSAN TAYLOR MAYNE, Ph.D., is an associate professor in chronic disease epidemiology at Yale University School of Medicine and associate director of the Yale Comprehensive Cancer Center for which she leads the Cancer Prevention and Control Research Program. The primary focus of Dr. Mayne's research is in the area of nutrition and cancer prevention. Currently, she directs a large cancer prevention clinical trial to determine whether supplemental β-carotene reduces the incidence of cancer. Additionally, she participated in the working group on carotenoids and cancer of the International Agency for Research on Cancer and the Steering Committee of the Carotenoid/Vitamin A Research Interaction Group. She was chair of the Carotenoid Research Interaction Group Annual Conference at Federation of American Societies for Experimental Biology in 1996. Dr. Mayne has a Ph.D. in nutritional biochemistry with minors in biochemistry and toxicology from Cornell University.

RITA B. MESSING, Ph.D., received her Ph.D. in physiological psychology from Princeton University and did postdoctoral research in the Department of Nutrition and Food Science at Massachusetts Institute of Technology in the Laboratory of Neuroendocrine Regulation. Dr. Messing has been in the Department of Pharmacology, University of Minnesota Medical School since 1981, and is currently an associate professor. Since 1990 her primary employment has been at the Minnesota Department of Health in Environmental Toxicology, where she supervises the Site Assessment and Consultation Unit, which conducts public health activities at hazardous waste sites and other sources of uncontrolled toxic releases. Dr. Messing has 70 publications in toxicology and risk assessment, neuropharmacology, psychobiology, and experimental psychology. She has taught at Rutgers University, Northeastern University, University of California at Irvine, and the University of Minnesota, and has had visiting appointments at Organon Pharmaceuticals in the Netherlands and the University of Paris.

SANFORD A. MILLER, Ph.D., is dean of the Graduate School of Biomedical Sciences and professor in the Departments of Biochemistry and Medicine at The University of Texas Health Science Center at San Antonio. He is the former director of the Center for Food Safety and Applied Nutrition at the Food and Drug Administration. Previously, he was professor of Nutritional Biochemistry at the Massachusetts Institute of Technology. Dr. Miller has served on many national and international government and professional society advisory committees, including the Federation of American Societies for Experimental Biology Expert Committee on GRAS Substances, the National Advisory Environmental Health Sciences Council of the National Institutes of Health, the Food and Nutrition Board and its Food Forum, the Joint World Health Organization (WHO)/

Food and Agriculture Organization (FAO) of the United Nations Expert Advisory Panel on Food Safety (chairman), and the Steering Committees of several WHO/FAO panels. He also served as chair of the Joint FAO/WHO Expert Consultation on the Application of Risk Analysis to Food Standards Issues. He is author or co-author of more than 200 original scientific publications. Dr. Miller received a B.S. in chemistry from the City College of New York, and an M.S. and Ph.D. from Rutgers University in physiology and biochemistry.

IAN C. MUNRO, Ph.D., is a consultant toxicologist and principal for CanTox, Inc., in Ontario, Canada. He is a leading authority on toxicology and has over 30 years experience in dealing with complex regulatory issues related to product safety. He has in excess of 150 scientific publications in the fields of toxicology and risk assessment. Dr. Munro formerly held senior positions at Health and Welfare Canada as director of the Bureau of Chemical Safety and director general of the Food Directorate, Health Protection Branch. He was responsible for research and standard setting activities related to microbial and chemical hazards in food and the nutritional quality of the Canadian food supply. He has contributed significantly to the development of risk assessment procedures in the field of public health, both nationally and internationally, through membership on various committees dealing with the regulatory aspects of risk assessment and risk management of public health hazards. Dr. Munro is a graduate of McGill University in biochemistry and nutrition and holds a Ph.D. from Queen's University in pharmacology and toxicology. He is a fellow of the Royal College of Pathologists, London, and a fellow of the Academy of Toxicological Sciences. He also was a former director of the Canadian Centre for Toxicology at Guelph, Ontario.

SUZANNE P. MURPHY, Ph.D., R.D., is a nutrition researcher (professor) at the Cancer Research Center of Hawaii at the University of Hawaii, Honolulu. She received her B.S. in mathematics from Temple University and her Ph.D. in nutrition from the University of California at Berkeley. Dr. Murphy's research interests include dietary assessment methodology, development of food composition databases, and nutritional epidemiology. She is a member of the National Nutrition Monitoring Advisory Council and the Year 2000 Dietary Guidelines Advisory Committee, and serves on editorial boards for the *Journal of Nutrition, Journal of Food Composition and Analysis, Family Economics and Nutrition Review,* and *Nutrition Today.* Dr. Murphy is a member of numerous professional organizations including the American Dietetic Association, American Society for Nutritional Sciences, American Public Health Association, American

Society for Clinical Nutrition, and Society for Nutrition Education. She has over 50 publications on dietary assessment methodology and has lectured nationally and internationally on this subject.

HARRIS PASTIDES, Ph.D., is dean of the University of South Carolina's School of Public Health and professor in the Department of Epidemiology and Biostatistics. Previously, he was chair and a professor of epidemiology in the Department of Biostatistics and Epidemiology at the School of Public Health and Health Sciences at the University of Massachusetts at Amherst. Dr. Pastides is a consultant to the World Health Organization's Program in Environmental Health and a fellow of the American College of Epidemiology. He has published widely and is the co-author of several books. He was a Fulbright Senior Research Fellow and visiting professor at the University of Athens Medical School in Greece from 1987–1988. Dr. Pastides earned his M.P.H. and his Ph.D. from Yale University; he has been a principal investigator or co-investigator on over 30 externally funded research grants, results of which have been published in numerous peer reviewed journals. He previously served on the National Academy of Sciences' Committee on Pediatric Respiratory Infections in Developing Nations.

ROSS L. PRENTICE, Ph.D., is director of the Division of Public Health Science of the Fred Hutchinson Cancer Research Center and professor of biostatistics, University of Washington. He has expertise in the areas of statistics, biostatistics, nutrition, health promotion and disease prevention, and epidemiology, and is principal investigator of the Women's Health Initiative Clinical Coordinating Center. Dr. Prentice received his Ph.D. in statistics from the University of Toronto. He currently serves as a member on the Food and Nutrition Board and is a member of the Institute of Medicine.

JOSEPH V. RODRICKS, Ph.D., is the managing director of The Life Sciences Consultancy LLC. He is one of the founding principals of the ENVIRON Corporation, with internationally recognized expertise in assessing the risks to human health of exposure to toxic substances. He received his B.S. from Massachusetts Institute of Technology and his Ph.D. in biochemistry from the University of Maryland. Dr. Rodricks is certified as a diplomate of the American Board of Toxicology. Before working as a consultant, he spent 15 years at the Food and Drug Administration (FDA). In his final 3 years at the FDA, he was Deputy Associate Commissioner for Science, with special responsibility for risk assessment. He was a member of the National Academy of Sciences (NAS) Board on Toxicology and

Environmental Health Hazards, and has also served on or chaired ten other NAS Committees. He has more than 100 scientific publications on food safety and risk assessment and has lectured nationally and internationally on these subjects. He is the author of *Calculated Risks,* a nontechnical introduction to toxicology and risk assessment.

IRWIN H. ROSENBERG, M.D., is an internationally recognized leader in nutrition science who serves as professor of physiology, medicine and nutrition at Tufts University School of Medicine and School of Nutrition, as well as director, Jean Mayer U.S. Department of Agriculture Human Nutrition Research Center on Aging at Tufts University and dean for nutrition sciences, Tufts University. He is the first holder of the Jean Mayer Chair in Nutrition at Tufts. Prior to joining Tufts, Dr. Rosenberg held faculty positions at Harvard Medical School and the University of Chicago where he served as the first director of the Clinical Nutrition Research Center. As a clinical nutrition investigator, he has helped develop a nutritional focus within the field of gastroenterology with his primary research interest being in the area of folate metabolism. His research for the past decade has focused on nutrition and the aging process. Among his many honors are the Josiah Macy Faculty Award, Grace Goldsmith Award of the American College of Nutrition, Robert H. Herman Memorial Award of the American Society of Clinical Nutrition, the Jonathan B. Rhoads Award of the American Society for Parenteral and Enteral Nutrition, and the 1994 W.O. Atwater Memorial Lectureship of the USDA. Dr. Rosenberg was elected to the Institute of Medicine in 1994 and he recently received the Bristol Myers Squibb/Mead Johnson Award for Distinguished Achievement in Nutrition Research, 1996.

KATHLEEN B. SCHWARZ, M.D., is director of the Pediatric Liver Center and chief of the Division of Pediatric Gastroenterology and Nutrition at Johns Hopkins University. She received her M.D. from Washington University School of Medicine and completed her residency in pediatrics at St. Louis Children's Hospital. She is a member of the editorial board of the *Journal of Pediatric Gastroenterology and Nutrition* and the Children's Liver Council of the American Liver Foundation. Dr. Schwarz has been involved in research on the effects of antioxidants in infants, children, and pregnant women.

DANIEL STEINBERG, M.D., Ph.D., is a biochemist and clinician with the Division of Endocrinology and Metabolism in the School of Medicine at the University of California, San Diego. His research interests are in the area of lipid and lipoprotein metabolism associated with disease, and his major focus in recent years has been the interaction of lipoproteins with cells and how this relates to atherogenesis. He holds an M.D. from Wayne University School of Medicine and a Ph.D. in biological chemistry from Harvard Medical School. He has served on numerous committees of the American Heart Association and is a member of the National Academy of Sciences' Section on Medical Physiology and Metabolism.

STEVE L. TAYLOR, Ph.D., serves as professor and head of the Department of Food Science and Technology and director of the Food Processing Center at the University of Nebraska. He also maintains an active research program in the area of food allergies through the Food Allergy Research & Resource Program at the University of Nebraska. He received his B.S. and M.S. in food science and technology from Oregon State University and his Ph.D. in biochemistry from the University of California at Davis. Dr. Taylor's primary research interests involve naturally occurring toxicants in foods, especially food allergens. His research involves the development of immunoassays for the detection of residues of allergenic foods contaminating other foods, the effect of processing on food allergens, and the assessment of the allergenicity of genetically engineered foods. Dr. Taylor has over 160 publications. He is a member of numerous professional associations including Institute of Food Technologists, American Chemical Society, American Academy of Allergy, Asthma, and Immunology, and Society of Toxicology.

JOHN A. THOMAS, Ph.D., received his undergraduate degree at the University of Wisconsin and his M.A. and Ph.D. degrees at the University of Iowa. He has held professorships in departments of pharmacology and toxicology in several medical schools including Iowa, Virginia, and West Virginia. From 1973 to 1982 he served as Associate Dean of the School of Medicine at West Virginia University. In 1982 Dr. Thomas became Vice President for Corporate Research at Baxter Healthcare. Dr. Thomas served as vice president at the University of Texas Health Science Center at San Antonio from 1988–1998. Professor Thomas serves on several editorial boards of biomedical journals and serves as chairman of the Society of Toxicology Education Committee, chairman of the Expert Advisory Committee of the Canadian Network of Toxicology Centers, and vice president of the Academy of Toxicology. He is a diplomate, fellow, and member of the Board of Trustees in the Academy of Toxicological Sciences, and serves on many scientific boards and committees in the chemical and the pharmaceutical industry. He has been named the 1999 recipient of the Distinguished Service

Award from the American College of Toxicology. He is the recipient of several national awards including the Merit Award from the Society of Toxicology, Certificate of Scientific Service (U.S. Environmental Protection Agency), Distinguished Lecturer in Medical Sciences (American Medical Association), Distinguished Service Award from the Texas Society for Biomedical Research. He is an elected foreign member of the Russian Academy of Medical Sciences. Dr. Thomas is the author of over a dozen textbooks and research monographs and has published over 350 scientific articles.

MARET G. TRABER, Ph.D., is principal investigator for the Linus Pauling Institute and an associate professor in the Department of Nutrition and Food Management at the Oregon State University in Corvallis as well as an associate research biochemist in the Department of Internal Medicine at the University of California School of Medicine at Davis. Formerly she was associate research biochemist in the Departments of Molecular and Cell Biology at the University of California at Berkeley. Dr. Traber received her Ph.D. in nutrition from the University of California at Berkeley. Her research is focused on lipid and lipoprotein metabolism and vitamin E deficiency in humans. Presently, Dr. Traber is principal investigator on a project examining the role of tocopherol transfer protein in vitamin E transport. She is the current chair of the Vitamin E Task Force of the Food and Nutrition Science Associations and is associate editor of *Lipids*. In 1993, Dr. Traber received the Henkel Vitamin E Research Information Award.

GARY M. WILLIAMS, M.D., is professor in the Department of Pathology and Director of Environmental Pathology and Toxicology at New York Medical College. He also serves as head of the Program on Medicine, Food and Chemical Safety. Previously, Dr. Williams served as director of the Naylor Dana Institute and chief of the Division of Pathology and Toxicology at the American Health Foundation. He earned his M.D. from the University of Pittsburgh. Dr. Williams received numerous honors including the Arnold J. Lehman Award of the Society of Toxicology and the Sheard-Sandford Award of the American Society of Clinical Pathologists. He has served on the editorial boards for many scientific reports and journals. He is the author or co-author of over 430 scientific publications. He previously served on the Committee on Research Opportunities and Priorities for the Environmental Protection Agency and the Committee on the Carcinogenecity of Cyclamates for the National Academy of Sciences.

Index

A

Abetalipoproteinemia, 202
Abnormal Involuntary Movements Scale
score, 223
Absorption of nutrients. *See also*
Bioavailability of nutrients;
Malabsorption syndromes
aging and, 31, 147 148, 238, 305
alpha-tocopherol, 196-198, 238, 251
carotenoids, 326, 328, 330, 354, 355,
356
food matrix and, 355
form of nutrient and, 191, 355
iron, 129, 158, 159, 161
selenium, 285-286, 306
vitamin C, 99-100, 103, 108, 128, 140,
147-148, 155, 157
vitamin E (all forms), 191, 193, 196,
243
Adequate intakes (AIs). *See also individual*
nutrients
defined, 3, 4, 7, 22, 25
extrapolation from other age groups,
26, 65-66, 138
methods used to set, 6-11, 22, 63-66
RDA compared, 4, 25-26
uses, 4, 15, 25, 383, 386, 391, 392,
398

Adolescents, ages 14 through 18 years. *See*
also Life-stage groups; Puberty,
pubertal development; *individual*
nutrients
EARs, 65-66
growth factors, 66
Kashin-Beck disease, 287
lactation, 151-152, 163-164, 240-241,
258-259, 307-308, 315
pregnancy, 149-150, 163-164, 239-240,
258-259, 306-307, 315
RDAs, 66
reference weights and heights, 32-33
special considerations, 358
ULs, 14
Adults, 19 through 50 years. *See also* Life-
stage groups; *individual nutrients*
circulating lipid levels, 234-235
depletion/repletion studies, 143-145,
233-234, 236
EARs, 31
peak bone mass, 30-31
PUFA intake, 235
reference weights and heights, 32
supplement use, 70
ULs, 14
Adults, 51+ years. *See also* Life-stage
groups; *individual nutrients*
absorption of nutrients, 31, 147-148

age-related macular degeneration, 49,
    348-350
asthma, 126
cardiovascular disease, 47-49, 121-122,
    211-217, 241-242, 346-348
cataracts, 49, 125-126, 221, 350
EARs, 31
immune function, 51, 117-119, 220-
    221, 338
institutionalized, 147
lean body mass, 148
oxidative stress in, 51, 148, 242
supplement use, 51, 70
ULs, 14
Advanced glycosylation end products, 50-51
Adverse effects, 3, 4-6
    alpha-tocopherol, 249, 251-255
    carotenoids, 366-368
    defined, 73
    evidence of, 85
    knowledge gaps, 406
    nutrient-nutrient interactions, 74
    selenium, 311-313
    vitamin C, 155-161
Age-related macular degeneration (AMD)
    carotenoids and, 18-19, 49, 348-350
    smoking and, 18, 49
Aging. See also Life-stage groups; individual
        life stages
    and absorption of nutrients, 31, 147-
        148, 238, 305
    alpha-tocopherol and, 51, 235
    carotenoids and, 330
    food consumption and, 51
    and immune function, 51, 220
    oxidative stress and, 44, 51
    and serum cholesterol, 235
Alcohol and drug abuse, 101, 150, 330,
    360, 368
Aldosterone, 99
Allergic response to nutrients, 160, 161, 368
Alpha-1-antiprotease, 108, 140
Alpha-carotene, 325, 329, 330, 332-333,
    342, 343, 347, 348, 349, 350-351,
    356, 358, 360-365, 366, 371, 450-451
Alpha-tocopherol, 186-283. See also
        Vitamin E
    absorption, 196-198, 238, 251
    adolescents, 230-231, 239-241, 258,
        259, 260-261
    adults (19-50 years), 228-229, 231-237,
        239-241, 255-257, 258, 259, 397

adults (51+ years), 220, 238-239, 241-
    242, 249, 259-260
adverse effects, 249, 251-255, 396
AIs, 8-9, 65, 226-230, 393, 394, 507
animal studies, 197, 203, 212, 216, 221,
    252, 254, 255
antioxidant activity, 195, 224-225
and ataxia, 199, 202-203, 204-209
bioavailability, 224, 238, 243, 251
body pool, 209-210, 225
body size and composition and, 242
and cancer, 196, 213-214, 218-220, 241
and cardiovascular disease, 36-41, 203,
    206-207, 211-217, 225, 238, 241-242,
    248, 252, 261
and cataracts, 221
and central nervous system disorders,
    221-223, 252
children, 202, 230-231, 258, 260-261
and cholestatic hepatobiliary disease,
    202, 203
and circulating lipoproteins, 193, 197,
    199, 216, 234-235, 261
critical endpoint, 254
deficiency, 186, 199, 202-203, 204-209,
    210-211, 220, 221, 231, 235, 239, 240
defined, 187, 192, 468
depletion/repletion studies, 203, 232,
    233-234, 236
and diabetes mellitus, 217-218
and DNA damage and repair, 208
dose-response assessment for ULs, 255-
    259
EARs, 2, 8-9, 10-11, 194, 230-237, 238,
    239, 240, 393, 394
excretion, 200, 208-209
exposure assessment, 259-260
factors affecting requirements, 224-226
fetal, 239, 243, 394
food sources, 224, 243, 244, 245, 248,
    250, 396
in fortified foods, 190-191, 194, 243,
    394
functions, 12, 43, 186, 195-196
gender and, 2, 231, 237, 245, 249
hazard identification, 249, 251-255
hemorrhagic toxicity, 13, 252, 253-254,
    255-256
in human milk, 226, 227, 228-229, 240
and hydrogen peroxide-induced
    hemolysis, 12, 43, 203, 210-211,
    231, 232-233, 234, 235, 402

and immune function, 51, 219, 220-221
indicators of adequacy, 8-9, 203, 208-224
infants, 65, 226-230, 239, 240, 253-254, 258, 259, 386, 392
intakes, 16, 230, 243-249, 250, 395-397, 424-425
interaction with drugs, 252, 259
interaction with other antioxidants, 195, 290
interaction with other nutrients, 36-41, 98-99, 102, 109, 128, 129, 213, 221, 222, 224-225, 232, 252, 254-255, 259
international comparisons, 204-209, 212-214, 216
international units converted to, 192, 244-245, 395, 396, 397
intervention trials, 2, 36-41, 213-217, 219-220, 221, 223-224, 226, 238, 241-242, 252, 254, 261-262, 367, 405
kinetic modeling, 209-210
laboratory values, 67
lactation and, 67, 228-229, 240-241, 258, 259
and LDLs, 211-212, 217, 226
by life-stage group, 8-9, 14, 226-243, 255-258, 422-427, 436-437, 444-445
and lipid peroxidation, 12, 43, 45, 195, 203, 211, 221, 222, 223, 225, 226, 243, 261
metabolism, 199-200, 208-210, 261
methodological considerations, 65, 67, 68-69
method used to set AIs, 226-230
and neuropathy, 202, 204-207, 218, 220, 221, 231, 232
NOAEL/LOAEL, 255-257
observational epidemiological studies, 212-213, 219, 221
and oxidative stress, 44-45, 51, 52, 203, 211, 217-218, 221, 222, 223, 242, 261
physical exercise and, 242
plasma concentrations, 197, 210, 232-237, 251, 444-445
platelet effects, 196, 211, 212, 218, 253
preferential secretion by liver, 197-199, 243
pregnancy and, 67, 239-240, 258, 259
and PUFAs, 195, 215, 225-226, 235, 248
RDAs, 2, 8-9, 12, 231, 237, 238-241, 248, 393, 394, 507
research recommendations, 20, 260-262

and retinopathy, 202, 208-209, 259
risk characterization, 260
serum concentrations, 236, 444-445
and skeletal myopathy, 202
smokers, 36-37, 213-214, 216, 219, 238, 242-243, 252
special considerations, 241-243, 259
storage, 201-202
supplement use, 70, 190-191, 194, 244-245, 249, 251, 258-260, 394-395, 396, 397
synthetic, 190-191, 192, 193, 244-245, 393-397
transport, 196-199
ULs, 13, 14, 249, 251-260, 396-397
uncertainty assessment, 91, 256-257
and vasodilation, 196, 210
vitamin C and, 98-99, 102, 109, 110-113, 128, 129, 213, 224-225
Alpha-Tocopherol, Beta-Carotene Cancer Prevention Study, 36-37, 49, 213-214, 216-217, 219, 221, 238, 241, 242, 252, 254, 345, 366-368, 369, 406
Alpha-tocopherol equivalents
conversion to alpha-tocopherol intakes, 16, 244, 394-395, 397
intakes, 230, 243, 244, 245-248, 422-423, 426-427, 436-437
usefulness of, 394
Alpha-tocopherol transfer protein (alpha-TTP)
form of vitamin E and affinity of, 193, 195, 197-198, 243, 262
function, 186, 197-198
genetic defects, 199, 202, 204-209
Alzheimer's disease, 19, 50, 222, 252
American Academy of Pediatrics, 28, 29, 65, 74, 259
Amino acids. See also individual amino acids
biosynthesis, 96
Aminotransferases, 163
Amyloid beta-peptide, 222
Amyotrophic lateral sclerosis, 19, 50
Anemia, hemolytic, 239, 259, 355
Angina, 47, 341, 347
Angiotensin-converting enzyme inhibitor, 38-39
Animal studies
alpha-tocopherol, 51, 59, 91, 197, 203, 212, 216, 251, 252, 254, 255, 396
of cardiovascular disease, 48-49, 212, 216
carotenoids, 59

extrapolation of data from, 91, 257, 301
for hazard identification, 84-85, 86
methodological considerations, 58-59
relevance of, 86
selenium, 287, 290
uncertainties in, 459
vitamin C, 103, 120, 131, 140
Anticoagulants, 252, 253, 259
Antioxidants. *See* Dietary antioxidants
Aquocobalamin, 158
Arachidonic acid cascade, 196
Asbestos workers, 36-37, 367, 371
Ascorbic acid. *See* Vitamin C
Aspirin, 150
Asthma, 126
Ataxia with vitamin E deficiency, 199, 202-203, 204-209
Atherogenesis, 47, 48, 50, 121-122, 212, 218, 225
Atherosclerosis, 18, 36-37, 48, 103, 109, 122, 203, 213, 340-341, 347-348
Atherosclerosis Risk in Communities Study, 122
Athletes, 117, 153, 242, 403
Attention-deficit disorder, 163

B

Balance studies, 59
Baltimore Longitudinal Study on Aging, 125
Basel Prospective Study, 121, 342, 343, 346-347
Benign breast disease, 219
Benzo[α]pyrene, 360
Beta-carotene, 325-382. *See also* Carotenoids
    absorption, 326-328, 355
    adolescents, 358
    adverse effects, 366-368, 405, 406
    and alcohol consumption, 360, 361, 368
    antioxidant activity, 36-37, 43-45, 98-99, 102, 109, 110-111, 325, 331-333, 334-337
    bioavailability, 328, 331, 354-355, 356, 357, 369-371
    blood concentrations, 330, 332-333, 353, 369, 372, 448-449
    body stores, 329-330

and cancer, 36-41, 213-214, 290, 330, 339, 343, 344, 345-346, 366-368, 369-371, 405, 406
and cardiovascular disease, 36-41, 336-337, 346-347
carotenodermia, 366, 368, 369
and cystic fibrosis, 331, 336-337
depletion/repletion studies, 331, 332, 334-337, 371, 403
and DNA damage and repair, 109, 110-111, 331-332
erythropoietic protoporphyria, 366, 371
excretion, 328-329
and eye diseases, 49, 348, 349, 350-351
food sources, 331, 332, 334, 353, 355-356, 360-363, 398-399
and immune function, 338
infants, 361, 362-365
intakes, 361, 364-366, 369
interaction with drugs, 357
interaction with other nutrients, 36-41, 102, 109, 110-111, 290, 357-358
international comparisons, 334-337
intervention trials, 36-41, 213-214, 216-217, 219, 221, 238, 241, 242, 252, 254, 345, 366-368, 369, 372, 405
by life-stage group and, 358-360, 448-449
and lipid peroxidation, 332, 334-337
and oxidative stress, 332
provitamin A activity, 12-14, 36-37, 325, 356, 366, 367
research recommendations, 2, 20, 371-372
smokers, 36-39, 330, 331, 334-337, 345, 347, 359, 366-368, 372, 405, 406
supplement use, 325-326, 355, 357, 366
transport, 329
ULs, 5-6, 13-14, 27, 368-369
vitamin C and, 102, 109, 110-111
Beta-Carotene and Retinol Efficacy Trial, 36-37
Beta-cryptoxanthin, 13, 44, 325, 330, 332-333, 345, 348, 349, 350-351, 358, 360-365, 366, 452-453
Beta-glucuronidase, 106-107, 116
Bioavailability of nutrients
    alpha-tocopherol, 224, 243, 251, 394
    carotenoids, 328, 331, 344, 354-357, 369-371, 403
    defined, 463
    dietary fat and, 68, 224, 248, 356

drug interactions and, 357
food matrix and, 354, 355-356, 404
form of intake and, 83, 251, 354
form of nutrient and, 193, 194-195,
    357, 369-371
in infant formulas, 29, 64
iron in, 129
nutrient-nutrient interactions and, 83,
    357-358
nutritional status of individuals and,
    83, 356
processing of foods and, 29, 354, 356
and risk assessment, 82-83
selenium, 291-292, 306, 307, 399
vitamin C, 99, 128
vitamin E (all forms), 16, 193, 194-195,
    224, 243
Biomarkers
of cancer, 113-116
of DNA damage, 45, 46-47, 109-111,
    116
of lipid peroxidation, 45, 104-105, 116,
    132, 151, 203, 211
Bladder cancer, 106-107, 113, 116
Bleomycin, 112, 114-115
Blood coagulation, 99, 101
Body Mass Index, 32, 33, 330
Body pools
alpha-tocopherol, 201-202, 225
carotenoids, 329-330, 351-353
kinetic modeling of, 209-210, 403
selenium, 286, 313
vitamin C, 100, 103, 132, 140, 142, 145,
    152-153, 166, 225, 403
vitamin E (all forms), 210
Body size considerations, 133, 146, 242
Body water considerations, 133, 138, 146
Body weight. See also Reference body
    weight ratio method
reference weights, 31-33
Bone formation and growth, 98, 101, 202
Boston Nutritional Status Survey of the
    Elderly, 154, 155, 242, 249
Breast cancer, 123, 219
Breast Cancer Serum Bank cohort study,
    219
Breastfeeding. See Human milk, Lactation
Breath ethane, 132, 150-151, 203, 211, 231
Breath pentane, 334-337

C

Cambridge Heart Antioxidant Study, 36-
    37, 214-215, 241
Canada
antioxidant intervention trials, 38-39
cancer, 124
cardiovascular disease, 38-39
dietary intakes, 16, 154, 284, 309, 438-
    439
Food Guide for Healthy Eating, 351-352
Recommended Nutrient Intakes, 28,
    383, 410
reference weights and heights, 32, 33
selenium, 284, 293
vitamin C, 69, 124, 154
Canadian Paediatric Society, 28, 29, 63-65
Cancer. See also individual sites
alpha-tocopherol and, 36-37, 196, 213-
    214, 218-220, 241, 290, 366, 367
antioxidant intervention trials, 36-41,
    218-219, 339, 357-358
biomarkers, 113-116
carotenoids, 14, 36-41, 213-214, 290,
    326, 330, 333, 339, 340-341, 342-
    346, 351, 352, 357, 360, 366-372,
    405, 406
DNA damage and, 218-219
gap junctional communication and,
    333, 338
mortality, 14, 339
oxidative stress and, 17, 46-47, 218-219
selenium and, 36-41, 290-291, 319, 367
vitamin C and, 36-37, 40-41, 106-107,
    113-116, 123-125, 127, 128, 160
Cardiomyopathy, 159, 206-207, 287, 288
Cardiovascular disease. See also Coronary
    artery disease; Coronary heart
    disease
alpha-tocopherol and, 18, 36-41, 48-49,
    187, 203, 206-207, 211-217, 225,
    238, 241-242, 248, 252, 261, 406
animal studies, 48-49, 212, 216
carotenoids and, 18, 36-41, 326, 331,
    336-337, 339, 340-341, 346-348, 351,
    371
diabetes mellitus and, 50
intervention trials, 48, 213-216
iron and, 159

LDLs and, 47-48, 50, 211-212
lipid peroxidation and, 225
mortality, 339
observational studies, 212-213
oxidative stress and, 18, 47-49, 50, 101-102, 225
RNA/ROS and, 216
selenium and, 40-41, 287, 288
smokers, 37-39, 48-49, 103, 106-107, 216, 238, 252, 347
vitamin C and, 18, 38-41, 101-102, 106-107, 109, 121-122, 127, 128, 346-347
women, 38-41, 121, 122, 212, 347
Carnitine biosynthesis
iron and, 120
vitamin C and, 95, 96, 99, 120, 153, 166
Carotene and Retinol Efficacy Trial (CARET), 36, 345, 367, 368, 369
Carotenodermia, 366, 368, 464
Carotenoids, 325-382. *See also* Beta-carotene; *other individual carotenoids*
absorption, 326, 328, 330, 354, 355, 356
adolescents, 355, 358
adults (19-50 years), 330-331, 334-337, 339-345, 364-365
adults (51+ years), 336-337, 338, 340-341, 347, 348-351
adverse effects, 366-368, 405, 406
and age-related macular degeneration, 18-19, 49, 326, 340-341, 348-350, 371, 403
aging and, 330
alcohol consumption and, 330, 360, 361, 368
allergic reactions, 368
antioxidant activity, 36-37, 43-45, 98-99, 102, 109, 110-111, 325, 326, 331-333, 334-337
bioavailability, 328, 331, 344, 354-357, 369-371
blood concentrations, 329-330, 332-333, 338, 346, 351-353, 358, 368, 448-457
body mass index and, 330
body stores, 329-330, 351-353
and cancer, 36-41, 213-214, 290, 326, 330, 333, 339, 340-341, 342-346, 351, 352, 357, 360, 366-372, 405, 406

and cardiovascular disease, 18, 36-41, 326, 331, 336-337, 340-341, 346-348, 351, 371
and cataracts, 18, 326, 340-341, 350-351
children, 338, 355, 356, 358, 368
cholesterol and, 330
and cystic fibrosis, 331, 336-337
depletion/repletion studies, 331, 332, 334-337, 371, 403
dietary fat and, 356
and DNA damage and repair, 109, 110-111, 331-332, 336-337
dose-response assessment for ULs, 368-369
DRIs, 12-13, 16, 325
excretion, 328-329
exposure assessment, 369
fat substitutes and, 357
food sources, 325, 331, 332, 334, 342, 344-345, 346, 349-350, 351-352, 353, 354, 355-356, 360-363, 368, 371, 398-399
functions, 12, 43, 325, 326
and gap junctional communication, 333, 338
gender and, 330, 351, 364-365
hazard identification, 366-368
health effects, 326, 338-351, 403-404
in human milk, 361, 362-366
and immune function, 326, 338
indicators of adequacy, 325, 331-353
infants, 361, 362-366, 368
intakes, 361, 364-366, 369
interactions with drugs, 357
interactions with other nutrients, 36-41, 102, 109, 110-111, 290, 325, 326, 327, 328, 330, 331, 332, 338, 343, 352, 355, 356, 357-358, 366, 367
international comparisons, 334-337
intervention trials, 2, 14, 36-41, 213-214, 216-217, 219, 221, 238, 241, 242, 252, 254, 345-346, 353, 366-368, 369, 372, 405
lactation, 355, 362, 363
by life-stage group and, 358-360, 448-457
and lipid peroxidation, 332, 334-337
lipoproteins and, 329, 330, 332, 334-337

metabolism, 328-329
methodological issues, 16, 68-69, 339, 359, 404
and mortality from chronic disease, 14, 339-342, 351
nonprovitamin A, 326, 327, 346, 351
observational epidemiological studies, 338-339, 342-345, 346 347
and oxidative stress, 332
provitamin A activity, 12-14, 36-37, 43-44, 325, 326, 327, 328, 330, 331, 338, 343, 352, 355, 356, 366, 367, 371, 372, 403, 467
research recommendations, 2, 20, 371-372, 403-404
risk characterization, 369-371
smokers, 18, 36-39, 49, 330, 331, 334-337, 344, 345, 347, 351, 359, 366-371, 372, 405, 406
special considerations, 358-360
structure, 326, 327
supplement use, 325-326, 355, 357, 366
transport, 329
ULs, 5-6, 13-14, 27, 366-371, 407
Catalase, 45
Cataracts, 18, 49, 340-341
alpha-tocopherol and, 18, 49, 221
carotenoids and, 18, 326, 340-341, 350-351
oxidative stress and, 18, 49, 350
smoking and, 351
vitamin C and, 18, 98, 125-126, 127
Catecholamines, 96, 127, 222-223
Central nervous system disorders, 19, 50, 127, 221-223
Ceruloplasmin oxidase activity, 129, 160
Cervical cancer, 17, 123, 340-341, 345, 346
Children, ages 1 through 13 years. *See also* Life-stage groups; *individual nutrients*
abetalipoproteinemia, 202
AIs, 65-66
anemia, 355
attention-deficit disorder, 163
cardiomyopathy, 287, 288, 292
cholestasis, 235
common colds, 163
cystic fibrosis, 202, 210-211, 336-337
EARs, 30, 33, 65-66
growth factors, 66
Keshan disease, 287, 288, 292, 299-300, 301-302
reference weights and heights, 31-32

supplement use, 163, 260
ULs, 14, 33
vitamin A deficiency, 338, 356
Cholestasis, 235
Cholestatic hepatobiliary disease, 202, 203
Cholesterol
aging and, 235
carotenoids and, 330
dietary, 99, 248
LDL, 47, 330
serum, 235
vitamin C and, 99
Cholesterol Lowering Atherosclerosis Study, 213
Cholestyramine, 357
Chromosomal damage and aberrations, 109, 110-111, 112, 114-115
Chronic cholestatic hepatobiliary disease, 202, 203
Chronic obstructive pulmonary disease, 126, 127
Chylomicron secretion, 196-197, 224, 330
Circulating lipid levels, 234-235
Cobalamins, vitamin C and, 158
Cognitive function, 19, 50, 127
Collagen metabolism
iron and, 118-119
vitamin C and, 95, 96, 98, 99, 101, 118-119, 166
Colorectal cancer, 36-37, 113, 116, 123-124
Colorectal polyps, 113, 114-115, 219-220
Common cold, 117, 126-127
Complementary DNA (cDNA), 197
Conjugated dienes, 104-105, 203
Connective tissue synthesis, 98, 101
Continuing Survey of Food Intakes by Individuals (CSFII)
alpha-tocopherol, 68, 240, 245, 247, 248, 396, 436-437
carotenoids, 361, 364
design, 69
vitamin C, 135, 138, 432-435
Copper
infants, 129, 159-160
and LDL oxidation, 211
metabolism, 129
and oxidative stress, 203
vitamin C and, 96, 97-98, 128, 129, 156, 159-160, 161
Coronary artery disease, 106-107, 121, 122, 241, 248, 336-337

Coronary heart disease, 18, 49, 121, 122, 212, 214-215, 238, 241, 261, 341, 347, 351
Corticosteroids, 99
Coxsackie B3 virus, 287
Cretinism, 287
Critical endpoints, identification of, 88-89, 254, 313
CSFII. See Continuing Survey of Food Intakes by Individuals
Cyclooxygenase-1, 196, 212, 223
Cystic fibrosis, 202, 210-211, 331, 336-337

D

Data and database issues
    alpha-tocopherol, 232, 243-248, 255, 393-396
    for dose-response assessment for ULs, 88-89, 161, 255, 313, 315
    food compostion data, 16, 19, 67-68, 309, 360-361, 393-394, 396-397, 398, 399
    nutrient intakes, 16, 68, 69-70, 194-195, 243, 309, 385
    quality and completeness of data, 8-9, 61-62, 67-68, 87, 309, 385, 390
    selenium, 309, 310, 398-399
    supplement use, 70
    types of data used, 58-63
    vitamin C, 139-140, 143, 161
    vitamin E. See Alpha-tocopherol
Dehydroascorbic acid (DHA)
    absorption and transport, 99
    chemical structure, 96, 97
    in smokers, 130
Delayed dermal sensitivity, 117, 118-119, 220
Dental enamel erosion, 156, 160, 161
Depletion/repletion studies
    alpha-tocopherol, 203, 232, 233-234, 236, 402
    carotenoids, 331, 332, 334-337, 371
    limitations of, 59, 402-403
    vitamin C, 108, 117, 140, 143-145, 402-403
Diabetes mellitus
    alpha-tocopherol and, 217-218
    cardiovascular complications, 50
    LDLs and, 50
    oxidative stress and, 19, 50-51, 217-218

and platelet hyperactivity, 218
    type I, 106-107
    type II, 50, 106-107
Diabetic neuropathy, 218
Diacylglycerol, 196
Diarrhea. See Osmotic diarrhea
Dietary antioxidants
    alpha-tocopherol activity, 43, 44-45, 98-99, 102, 109, 110-113, 186, 195, 224-225
    carotenoid activity, 36-37, 43-45, 98-99, 325, 326, 331-333, 334-337
    criteria for, 43-44
    defined, 17, 42
    and immune function, 407
    interaction among, 195, 224-225, 290, 332, 367, 404
    intervention trials, 36-41, 50, 219-220, 339, 348-350, 357-358
    mechanisms of action, 44-46
    selenoprotein activity, 43, 44-45, 284, 285
    supplement efficacy, 45, 48, 49
    vitamin C activity, 43, 44-45, 96, 98-99, 101-109, 116, 124-125, 139-143, 146, 154, 166
Dietary intakes. See also Canada; Food sources of nutrients; Nutrient intakes; Supplements; individual nutrients
    data and database issues, 16, 68, 69-70, 194-195, 243, 309, 385
    day-to-day variation, 69, 385
    infants, 28, 65, 135, 138, 230, 307
    measurement errors, 68, 69, 313, 359, 385-386
    research recommendations, 165-166, 406
    self-reported, 60, 68, 385, 396
    smokers, 130, 359, 360
    survey data, 245-247
    underreporting of, 16, 60, 68, 69, 186, 232, 240, 247-248, 385, 390, 393, 395-396
Dietary Reference Intakes (DRIs)
    applicable population, 22
    categories, 2, 3, 22-27; see also Adequate Intakes; Estimated Average Requirements; Recommended Dietary Allowances; Tolerable Upper Intake Levels
    criteria for, 6-11, 12-13, 42

defined, 2-6, 21-22, 33
extrapolation from other age groups,
    65-67, 91
framework, 384, 410-412
group applications, 14-16, 25, 387-391,
    392-393, 398
individual applications, 4, 15, 22, 384-
    386, 392, 398
nutrient-specific considerations, 393-399
origin, 409-410
parameters for, 27-33; *see also* Life stage
    groups; Reference weights and
    heights
precision of values, 8-11
risk of inadequacy, 15-16
sources of data, 6-7; *see also*
    Methodological considerations
uses, 4, 14-16, 383-399
DNA damage and repair
    adduct formation, 106-107, 116, 208
    alpha-tocopherol and, 109, 110-113, 208
    biomarkers of, 45, 46-47, 109-111, 116
    and cancer, 46-47, 113-116, 218-219
    carotenoids and, 109, 110-111, 331-
        332, 336-337, 360
    ex vivo, 112-113, 114-115, 116, 130
    in gastric mucosa, 106-107, 116
    glutathione and, 109-110
    ionizing radiation and, 46, 112, 130
    iron and, 109, 160
    lymphocytes, 110-111, 112, 114-115
    oxidative stress and, 46-47, 109
    repair enzymes, 106-107, 116
    RNS and, 116
    smoking and, 110-113, 130-131, 360
    vitamin A and, 112-113
    vitamin C and, 98, 109-115, 116, 130-
        131, 160
Dopamine, 222-223
Dopamine-β-hydroxylase, 96, 98
Dose-response assessment for ULs
    adolescents, 162-164, 258, 315-316
    adults (19-50 years), 161-162, 255-257,
        313-315
    alpha-tocopherol, 255-259
    carotenoids, 368-369
    children, 162-164, 258, 315-316
    components and process, 85, 88-92
    critical endpoints, 88-89, 161, 254, 313
    data selection, 88-89, 161, 255, 313, 315
    defined, 77-78, 464

infants, 162, 258, 315-316
lactation, 164, 258, 315
NOAEL/LOAEL identification, 89-90,
    161-162, 255-256, 314, 316
pregnancy, 163-164, 258, 315
selenium, 313-316
special considerations, 92, 164-165, 259
UL derivation from, 91-92, 162, 257,
    315, 316
uncertainty assessment, 90-91, 162,
    256-257, 315, 316
vitamin C, 161-165
vitamin E. *See* Alpha-tocopherol
Down's syndrome, 222
Drinking water, 309-310, 311, 317, 399
Drug abuse. *See* Alcohol and drug abuse
Drug interactions
    with alpha-tocopherol, 40-41, 252, 259
    with carotenoids, 357
    with vitamin C, 99, 150
Dyspepsia, 106-107, 116

E

Elastin, 98
Elderly people. *See* Adults, 51+ years
Embryogenesis, 285
Emotional stress, 153
Endothelial cells
    dysfunction, 103, 106-107, 131
    monocyte adhesion to, 103
Endothelium-dependent vasodilation, 106-
    107, 131
Endothelium-derived relaxing factor, 103
Energy expenditures, 24-25
Energy intakes, 60, 68, 69, 247, 396
Energy status
    and antioxidant interactions, 224-225
    and PUFA metabolism, 226
Epinephrine, 96
Erythrocyte
    glutathione, 128
    hydrogen peroxide-induced lysis, 210-
        211, 231
    vitamin C, 140
Erythropoietic protoporphyria, 366, 371
Esophageal cancer, 367
Established Populations for
    Epidemiological Studies of the
    Elderly, 122, 213

Estimated Average Requirements (EARs).
  See also individual nutrients
  children, 30, 33, 65-66
  coefficient of variation, 3, 24-25
  criteria used to derive, 6-7, 8-11
  defined, 3, 5, 23, 24
  evidence considered, 10-11, 25
  extrapolation to/from other age
    groups, 65-66
  group applications, 15, 387-390, 392
  knowledge gaps, 402-404
  methods used to set, 25, 43, 65-66, 402-
    404
  and RDA, 2-4, 23-25
  reference weight and height and, 31-
    33
  risk of inadequacy, 24
  standard deviation, 3, 23-24
  uses, 15, 23, 25, 383, 384-386, 387-390,
    392-393
Ethane, 132, 150-151, 203, 211, 231
Ethical considerations, 84
European Commission Concerted Action
    on Fundamental Food, 42
Exposure
  duration of, 86
  route of, 86, 256
Exposure assessment
  alpha-tocopherol, 259-260
  carotenoids, 369
  defined, 77, 78
  process, 92
  selenium, 317
  supplements, 92
  vitamin C, 165
Extrapolation of data
  from animal studies, 91, 257
  body weight basis, 65-66, 138-139, 163-
    164, 230-231, 258-259, 299-300, 315-
    316
  from one gender group to another,
    146-147, 235, 237
  from other age groups, 25, 26, 65-66,
    138-139, 163-164, 166, 230, 231,
    258-259, 299-300, 315-316
  NOAEL from LOAEL, 162, 256-257
  from subchronic to chronic intake, 257
Eye Disease Case-Control Study, 348
Eye diseases. *See also* Age-related macular
    degeneration; Cataracts
  alpha-tocopherol and, 18, 49, 221

antioxidant intervention trials, 40-41,
    348-350
  carotenoids and, 49, 348, 349, 350-351
  vitamin C and, 18, 125-126

F

Familial hypercholesterolemia, 47
Fat, dietary
  and alpha-tocopherol, 68, 225-226,
    235, 248, 396
  and carotenoid, 356
  intakes, 16, 68, 69, 232, 247, 248, 261,
    396
  malabsorption syndromes, 202, 404
  and MOPD, 349
Fat substitutes, 357
Fatty streak lesions, 47
F_2-isoprostanes, 45, 48, 203, 217-218, 464
Ferritin, 159
Ferrous oxidation/xylenol orange (FOX)
    assay, 46
Fetal nutrition. *See also* Pregnancy
  alpha-tocopherol, 67, 239, 243, 258, 394
  selenium, 67, 306, 315
  vitamin C, 67, 149, 150, 163
Fibrillin, 98
Fibronectin, 98
Flavonoids, 98-99, 102, 128, 129, 225
Foam cells, 47-48
Food and Agriculture Organization, 22,
    73-74, 79
Food and Drug Administration, 309
Food composition data
  analytical methods, 67
  carotenoids, 360-361, 364-365, 369
  quality and completeness of, 68-69,
    309, 390, 393-394, 399
  recommendations, 19, 396-397
  selenium, 309, 398-399
  vitamin C, 154, 390
  vitamin E, 19, 68-69, 244-248, 393-394
Food matrix and bioavailability of
    nutrients, 250, 354, 355-356, 404
Food sources. *See also* Fortified foods
  alpha-tocopherol, 224, 243, 244, 245,
    248, 250, 396
  carotenoids, 325, 331, 332, 334, 342,
    344-345, 346, 349-350, 351-352, 353,
    354, 355-356, 360-363, 368, 371,
    398-399

selenium, 286, 292, 298-299, 308, 309, 397
vitamin C, 101, 130, 154, 392
Formulas, infant
  AIs, 386, 391, 392
  alpha-tocopherol, 230
  bioavailability of nutrients, 29, 64
  carotenoids, 361
  DRIs, 28-29
  selenium, 310, 399
  vitamin C, 101, 135
Fortified foods. *See also* Formulas, infant
  alpha-tocopherol in, 12, 16, 190-191, 243, 394
  selenium in, 286
  ULs and, 5, 26, 74
Fruits and vegetables, 17, 18, 45, 47, 130, 133, 154, 245, 342, 344-345, 346, 351, 353, 355, 368, 371
Furunculosis, 117, 118-119

G

Gastric cancer, 36-37, 106-107, 113, 114-115, 116, 124-125, 196, 290, 367
Gastric mucosa
  DNA damage, 106-107, 116
  nitrotyrosine, 102, 106-107, 116
  oxidant scavengers, 95, 102, 116, 124
Gastritis, 102, 106-107, 113, 116, 124-125
Gastrointestinal effects
  of vitamin C, 95, 100, 102, 106-107, 124-125, 156, 161-162, 163, 166, 386, 393
Gender. *See also* Men; Women; *individual nutrients*
  and cataracts, 351
  dietary intakes, 15-16, 154, 165, 245-247, 259-260, 364-365
  extrapolation of data on basis of, 146-147, 235, 237
  and Keshan disease, 299, 304
  and lean body mass, 2, 65, 146-147
  and metabolism, 20, 133, 403, 407
  reference weights and heights, 32
  and relative body weight, 65-66, 138
  and supplement use, 70, 260
Genetic defects, in alpha-TTP, 199, 202, 204-209
Genetic markers of disease susceptibility, 60

Geographic differences in nutrient intakes, 309, 311-312, 315, 316, 317, 318-319
Gingivitis, 120
GISSI Prevention Trial, 38-39, 215, 216, 217, 238, 241, 242, 252
Glial cells, 98
Glucose-6-phosphate dehydrogenase deficiency, 160-161, 164
Glutathione
  and asthma, 126
  deficiency, 128
  and DNA damage, 109-110
  erythrocyte, 128
  and oxidative stress, 128, 129, 224
  reduced, 104-105, 128, 225
  vitamin C and, 43, 96, 98, 99, 103, 105, 109-110, 126, 128, 129
Glutathione peroxidase activity, 12, 45, 284, 285, 286, 289-290, 293, 299, 301-302, 303, 304, 318
Growth factors, 66
Growth velocity, 28, 64
Gulonolactone oxidase, 95-96
Gun blue, 312, 465

H

Hazard identification
  adverse effects, 85, 155-161, 249, 251-255, 311-313, 366-368
  alpha-tocopherol, 249, 251-255
  animal studies, 84-85, 86
  carotenoids, 366-368
  causality, 85-86
  components of, 85-88
  data quality and completeness and, 87
  data sources, 84-85
  defined, 77, 465
  experimental data on nutrient toxicity and, 86
  mechanisms of toxicity and, 87
  pharmacokinetic and metabolic data and, 86-87
  selenium, 311-313
  sensitive subpopulations, 87-88
  vitamin C, 155-161
Health Canada, 410, 438-439
Heart Outcomes Prevention Evaluation Study, 38-39, 216, 217, 241, 242, 252

Helicobacter pylori infection, 106-107, 113, 116, 124-125
Hemochromatosis, 158, 159, 160, 164
Hemolysis
    hydrogen peroxide-induced, 12, 43, 186, 203, 210-211, 231, 232-233, 234, 235, 402
    in infants, 162, 163-164, 166
Hemorrhagic toxicity, 13, 252, 253-254, 255-256
Hemostatic dysfunction, 131
High-altitude resistance, 160
High-density lipoproteins, 329
Human immunodeficiency virus (HIV), 338
Human milk. *See also* Lactation
    alpha-tocopherol in, 226, 227, 228-229, 240, 386
    analysis of nutrient content, 227
    carotenoids in, 361, 362-366
    colostrum, 227, 293, 294
    fore milk, 293, 464
    hind milk, 293, 465
    intakes, 28, 65, 135, 138, 151, 227, 230, 298, 307, 391
    interindividual variation in nutrients, 293, 295
    selenium in, 292-298, 307, 315, 316
    smokers, 132
    vitamin C in, 101, 132, 134-138, 151, 164, 386
    vitamin E (all forms), 227, 228-229
Human studies
    ethical considerations, 84
    for hazard identification, 84
    methodological considerations, 59
Hydrogen peroxide, 112, 130-131
Hydrogen peroxide-induced hemolysis, 12, 43, 186, 203, 210-211, 231, 232-233, 234, 235, 402
Hydroxynonenal, 104-105
4-Hydroxyphenylpyruvatedioxygenase, 96
8-Hydroxy-7,8-dihydro-2´-deoxyguanosine (8-oxoxdG), 109, 110-113, 131
Hypercholesterolemia, 47, 106-107, 226
Hypertension, 106-107
Hypertriglyceridemia, 50
Hypervitaminosis A, 368
Hypochlorous acid (HOCl), 108, 140
Hypovitaminosis C, 132, 153

I

Immune function
    aging and, 51, 220
    alpha-tocopherol, 51, 220-221
    assessment of antioxidant role, 407
    carotenoids and, 326, 338
    measures of, 118-119
    vitamin C and, 108, 117-119, 127
Indicators of nutrient adequacy. *See also specific indicators, life stages, and nutrients*
    defined, 27
    risk reduction-based, 3, 27, 42
Infants, premature, 129, 159-160, 227, 239, 253-254, 259
Infants, 0 to 12 months. *See also* Formulas, infant; Human milk
    ages 0 through 6 months, 29, 64, 66
    ages 7 through 12 months, 29, 64-65, 66
    AI derivation for, 4, 28-29, 63-65, 391, 392
    cretinism, 287
    dietary intakes, 28, 65, 135, 138, 227, 230, 298, 307, 391
    growth velocity, 28, 64
    hemolysis, 162, 163-164, 166
    methodological considerations, 63-65, 66
    oxidant damage, 162, 166
    recommended food sources, 28-29
    reference weight, 32
    scurvy, 135, 159, 161, 162, 163-164, 166
    solid foods, 29, 64, 151, 293, 298-299
    special considerations, 160, 259
    ULs, 14
Infectious and inflammatory stresses, 103, 108, 130
Intake assessment to derive ULs. *See* Exposure assessment
Interactions. *See* Nutrient-nutrient interactions
Intercellular cell adhesion molecule (ICAM-1), 196, 212, 223
International Atomic Energy Agency (IAEA), 22, 74
International comparisons
    alpha-tocopherol, 204-209, 212-214, 216
    antioxidant intervention trials, 36-41
    cardiovascular disease, 121
    carotenoids, 334-337
    vitamin C, 121, 123, 124, 127, 135, 153

Intervention trials
    alpha-tocopherol, 2, 36-41, 213-217,
        219-220, 221, 223-224, 226, 238,
        241-242, 252, 254, 261-262, 367,
        405
    antioxidants, 36-41, 50, 218-220, 339,
        357-358
    cancer, 36-41, 219-220, 345-346
    cardiovascular disease, 36-41, 213-217
    carotenoids, 2, 14, 36-41, 213-214, 216-
        217, 219, 221, 238, 241, 242, 252,
        254, 345-346, 353, 366-368, 369,
        372, 405
    eye diseases, 40-41, 348-350
    intakes above ULs, 13, 27, 74, 155, 165,
        249, 260
    methodological issues, 58, 61
    selenium, 36-41, 290, 303-304, 311,
        318, 319, 367, 405
    vitamin C, 38-39, 405
Intestinal parasites, 356
Intracellular glutathione peroxidase, 289
Intracellular recycling, 108
Iodothyronine deiodinases, 285
Iowa Women's Health Study, 122, 123
Iron
    absorption, 129, 158, 159, 161
    bioavailability, 129
    cardiovascular disease, 159
    and carnitine biosynthesis, 120
    and collagen metabolism, 118-119
    and DNA damage and repair, 109, 160
    infants, 159
    and lipid peroxidation, 159, 221
    metabolism, 129
    and MOPD, 349
    and neurodegenerative diseases, 221
    overload, 158, 166
    transfer and storage, 129
    and vitamin C, 96, 97-98, 99, 109, 118-
        119, 120, 128, 129, 158, 159, 160,
        161, 164, 166
Ischemic heart disease, 36-37, 214, 216,
        341, 346-347
Isoprostane excretion, 95, 102, 130

K

Kashin-Beck disease, 12, 43, 287, 465
Keshan disease, 12, 43, 287, 288, 292, 299-
        300, 301-302, 304, 465

Kidney stones, 156, 157, 160
Kinetic modeling of body pools, 209-210,
        403

L

Laboratory values
    analytical considerations, 62-63, 139-
        140, 143, 231-232
    estimates of, 67, 404
Lactation. See also Human milk; individual
        nutrients
    derivation of DRIs for, 31
    length of, 134-135, 151
    methodological considerations, 67
    preterm delivery and, 227
    stage of, 228-229, 293, 294-297
    ULs, 82
Laryngeal cancer, 17
Latinos, vitamin C, 132
Lean body mass, 133, 138, 146, 148
Leukocytes, vitamin C in, 43, 95, 103, 108-
        109, 110-111, 130, 133, 139, 140,
        141, 142, 144, 146, 147, 148, 150
Leukopenia, 368
Life-stage groups. See also Adolescents;
        Adults; Children; Infants; Lactation;
        Pregnancy; individual nutrients
    Body Mass Index by categories, 27-31
    and derivation of DRIs, 27-31
    intakes of nutrients by, 416-439
    serum nutrient values by, 440-457
    supplement use by, 70
    ULs by, 14
Linoleic acid, 235, 248
Linxian Cancer Prevention Study, 36-37
Lipid-lowering drugs, 357
Lipid peroxidation
    alpha-tocopherol and, 12, 43, 45, 186,
        195, 203, 211, 221, 222, 223, 225,
        226, 243, 261, 405
    biomarkers/measures of, 45, 104-105,
        116, 132, 151, 203, 211
    and cardiovascular disease, 225
    carotenoids and, 332, 334-337
    iron and, 159, 221
    and neurodegenerative diseases, 221-
        222
    in passive smokers, 153
    pregnancy and, 150-151
    selenium and, 287

in smokers, 104-105, 130, 131, 132,
150-151, 153
vitamin C and, 45, 95, 98, 102, 104-
105, 109, 116, 130, 131, 132, 146,
150-151, 153, 159
Lipid Research Clinics Coronary Primary
Prevention Trial, 347
Lipoprotein lipase, 330
Lipoproteins. *See also* High-denisty
lipoproteins; Low-density
lipoproteins
alpha-tocopherol and, 193, 197, 199,
216, 234-235, 261, 405
carotenoids and, 329, 330
Liver fluke infection, 106-107
Liver necrosis, 287
Low-density lipoproteins (LDLs)
alpha-tocopherols and, 211, 217, 226
and cardiovascular disease, 47-48, 50,
211-212
carotenoids and, 329, 332, 334-337
copper and, 211
defined, 79, 466
and diabetes mellitus, 50
oxidation, 18, 47-48, 50, 211, 226, 405
smoking and, 130, 132, 153
vitamin C and, 98, 101-102, 104-105,
109, 132, 153
Low-fat diets, 226, 248, 356
Lowest-Observed-Adverse-Effect Level
(LOAEL)
alpha-tocopherol, 255-257
extrapolation of NOAEL from, 162,
256-257
identification of, 89-90, 161-162, 255-
256, 314
instead of NOAEL, 91
selenium, 314, 318
sensitive subpopulations and, 92
vitamin C, 161-162, 163
Lung cancer
beta-carotene and, 13-14, 340-341, 342-
343, 345-346
smoking and, 36-39, 124, 213-214, 219,
360, 366-371, 372, 405, 406
Lung lesions, 254
oxidant scavengers, 95, 108
Lutein, 18, 44, 49, 329, 330, 332-333, 343,
348, 349, 350-351, 353, 355, 357,
358, 360-365, 366, 371, 454-455

Lycopene, 44, 329, 332-333, 344-345, 347,
349, 350, 353, 356, 357, 358, 360-
365, 366, 368, 371, 456-457
Lycopenodermia, 368, 466
Lymphatic leukemia, 196
Lymphocytes
DNA damage, 110-111, 112, 114-115
vitamin C in, 99-100
Lysine, 98, 118-119

M

Macular Pigment Optical Density
(MOPD), 349-350, 371
Major histocompatibility complex II, 338
Malabsorption syndromes, 202, 210-211,
404
Malnutrition, protein-energy, 202, 404
Malondialdehyde, 104-105, 116, 203, 334-
335
Marathon runners, 117, 118-119
Margarine, plant sterol-enriched, 357
Men. *See also* Gender
alcohol consumption, 361, 368
alpha-tocopherol, 49, 232-233, 235,
237, 245, 249, 260
carotenoids, 49, 338, 349, 351, 353,
359, 361, 368
cataracts, 49, 351
dietary intakes, 154, 165, 245
immune response, 338
Keshan disease, 301-302
kidney stone formation, 157
MOPD values, 349
smokers, 359
supplement use, 249, 260
vitamin C, 95, 117, 118-119, 121, 126,
133, 146, 148, 149, 154, 157, 165
Metabolism of nutrients
aerobic, 46
alpha-tocopherol, 195, 199-200, 208-
210, 261
basal rate considerations, 24-25
carotenoids, 328-329, 350
copper, 129
drug, 99
gender differences, 20, 133, 292, 403,
407
iron, 129

selenium, 285, 286, 299, 308
vitamin C, 12, 43, 95, 100, 108, 130,
    133, 148, 152-153, 157, 158
Metalloenzyme reduction, 96, 97-98
Methionine, 284
Methionine sulfoxide, 45
Methodological considerations. *See also*
    Data and database issues;
    Extrapolation of data; Indicators of
    nutrient adequacy; Uncertainty
AIs, 63 66
alpha-tocopherol, 59, 65, 67, 68-69
animal studies, 58-59, 459
carotenoids, 16, 68-69, 339, 359, 404
children, 65-66
data limitations, 62-63
depletion/repletion studies, 59, 402-403
dietary intakes, 68, 69, 313, 359, 385-
    386
EARs, 65-66, 402-404
epidemiological studies, 127-128
in extrapolation of data, 62, 65-66
human feeding studies, 59
infants, 63-65, 66
intervention trials, 58, 61
kinetic modeling of body pools, 209-
    210, 403
laboratory assays, 67, 160, 404
lactation, 67
measurement errors, 68, 69, 313, 359,
    385-386
nutrient intake estimates, 67-69, 247,
    339, 385, 404 405
observational studies, 59-61, 127-128
pathways to nutrient requirements, 63
pregnancy, 67
randomized clinical trials, 61
RDAs, 66
in risk assessment, 458-461
types of data used, 58-63
vitamin C, 67, 68-69, 127-128, 139-140
weighing the evidence, 61-62
Minnesota Cancer Prevention Research
    Unit, 353
Monocyte adhesion, 103
Monounsaturated fatty acids, 226
Mortality from chronic disease, 14, 339-
    342, 351
MRC/BHF Heart Protection Study, 38-39
Multiple Risk Factor Intervention Trial,
    343
Multiple sclerosis, 50

Myelin, 98
Myeloperoxidase, 108, 109, 140
Myocardial infarction, 36-41, 47, 159, 214-
    215, 216, 238, 241, 312, 347
Myocarditis, 287

N

National Cancer Institute, 154
Five-a-Day for Better Health Program,
    351
National Health and Nutrition
    Examination Survey I (NHANES I),
    Epidemiological Follow-up Study,
    122, 124, 126, 219
National Health and Nutrition
    Examination Survey II (NHANES
    II), 121, 152, 235, 248
National Health and Nutrition
    Examination Survey III (NHANES
    III)
anthropometric data, 31, 32-33
carotenoids, 330, 358, 361, 364, 369,
    448-457
defined, 466
design, 69
energy intakes, 68, 69
fat intakes, 68, 69, 247, 396
selenium, 16, 69-70, 309, 310, 399, 428-
    431, 446-447
serum values of nutrients, 440-457
supplement data, 70
total intakes, 388, 389, 420-421, 426-
    427, 430-431
vitamin C, 15-16, 69-70, 133, 155, 165,
    387-390, 391, 416-421, 440-443
vitamin E (all forms), 16, 68, 69-70,
    210, 230, 233, 244, 245-246, 247,
    248, 259-260, 394, 422-427, 444-445
National Health Interview Survey, 70, 249,
    260, 310-311, 364-365
National Health Interview Survey
    Epidemiological Supplement, 249
National Nutrition Monitoring System, 383
Necrotizing enterocolitis, 253
Nervous system, 19, 50, 96, 98, 131, 153, 202
Neurodegenerative diseases
alpha-tocopherol and, 19, 50, 186, 202,
    204-207, 218, 220, 221, 222, 231, 232
iron and, 221
lipid peroxidation and, 221-223

oxidative stress and, 19, 50, 221-222
ROS and, 222-223
Neuroleptic drugs, 222-223
Neurons, 98, 131, 202
Neuropeptide biosynthesis, 98
Neurotransmitters, 95, 98, 153, 222-223
Neutrophils
    vitamin C in, 12, 43, 95, 98, 99-100,
        139, 140, 141, 143, 144-146, 150, 385
New York State Cohort Study, 123, 124
Niacin, 225
Nicotinamide adenine dinucleotide
    (NADH), 43, 96, 98, 224-225
Nicotinamide adenine dinucleotide
    phosphate (NADPH), 43, 96, 98,
    224-225
Nitric oxide scavengers, 262
Nitric oxide synthesis, 103
Nitrosoproline, 106-107
Nitrotyrosine, 45, 102, 106-107, 116
No-Observed-Adverse-Effect Level
    (NOAEL)
    alpha-tocopherol, 255-257
    defined, 79, 466
    extrapolation from LOAEL, 162, 256-
        257
    identification of, 89-90, 255-256, 316
    LOAEL used instead of, 91
    selenium, 314, 316
    sensitive subpopulations and, 92
    subchronic to predict chronic, 91
    vitamin C, 163
Norepinephrine, 96, 98
Normative requirement, 22
Nurses Health Study, 123, 125-126, 212, 351
Nutrient intakes. *See also* Dietary intakes;
    Exposure assessment; *individual
    nutrients*
    Canadian, 69, 154, 309, 438-439
    cooking losses, 154, 356
    day-to-day variation adjustments, 69,
        385, 387, 390
    extrapolation from subchronic to
        chronic, 257
    form of, 83
    geographic differences in, 284, 288,
        309, 311-312, 315, 316, 317, 318-319
    interpretation of, 385-359
    methodological considerations, 67-69,
        247, 339, 385, 404-405
    public health implications, 404-405

quality of data, 385, 390
    from supplements, 70, 155, 244-245,
        249, 366
    total calculated, 388, 389
    U.S., 70, 416-431, 432-437
Nutrient-nutrient interactions. *See also
    specific entries under individual
    nutrients*
    adverse, 74
    and bioavailability of nutrients, 83,
        357-358
    energy status and, 224-225
    research recommendations, 20, 407
    risk assessment, 83
Nutrition Canada Survey, 32
Nutrition During Lactation report, 28, 29
Nutrition labels, 16, 68, 194, 243, 393-394,
    396
Nutritional Factors in Eye Disease Study,
    365
Nutritional Prevention of Cancer Study,
    38-39

O

O^6-alkyltransferase, 106-107, 116
Obese individuals, 60, 385
Observational studies
    alpha-tocopherol, 212-213, 219, 221
    cancer, 219
    of cardiovascular disease, 212-213
    carotenoids, 338-339, 342-345, 346-347
    hazard identification, 84
    methodological issues, 59-61, 127-128
Oils, edible, 16, 68, 245, 246, 250, 396
Olestra, 357
Ophthalmoplegia, 202
Oropharyngeal cancers, 17, 341, 344, 346
Osmotic diarrhea, 13, 95, 100, 154, 161-
    162, 163, 166, 386, 393
Oxalate excretion, 156
Oxidant damage, 44-51
Oxidant scavengers, 95, 102, 108, 116, 124
Oxidative stress
    in adults (51+ years), 51, 148, 242
    and age-related macular degeneration,
        18-19, 49
    aging and, 44, 51
    alpha-tocopherol and, 44-45, 51, 52,
        203, 211, 217-218, 221, 222, 223,
        242, 261

and asthma, 126
and cancer, 17, 46-47, 218-219
and cardiovascular disease, 18, 47-49, 50, 101-102, 225
carotenoids and, 332
and cataracts, 18, 49, 350
cholestatic liver disease and, 202, 203
copper and, 203
defined, 44, 466
and diabetes mellitus, 19, 50-51, 217-218
and DNA damage, 46-47, 109
glutathione and, 128, 129, 244
indicators of, 20, 45-52, 102, 103, 109, 126, 128, 203, 217, 223, 407
mechanisms in, 44-45, 46, 47, 50
and neurodegenerative disease, 19, 50, 221-222
physical exercise and, 242
protective enzymes, 45
selenium, 41, 43, 44-45, 52, 285
smoking and, 43, 48, 102, 130, 131, 132
vitamin C and, 12, 43, 95, 101-102, 109, 126, 128, 130, 131, 132, 148, 152, 162, 166
8-Oxy-7,8-dihydro-2′-deoxyguanosine (8-oxodG), 46, 110, 112, 466
Oxygen demand, 156, 161
Oxygen radical absorbance capacity (ORAC) assay, 46
Ozone, 108

P

Pancreatic cancer, 124
Parkinson's disease, 19, 50, 221-222
Passive smokers, 132, 146, 153
Pauling, Linus, 126-127
Pectin, 357
Pentane, 203, 231, 334-337
Peptide hormones, amidation of, 96, 98
Peptidyl-glycine monoxygenase, 96
Periodontal health, 120, 156, 160, 161, 166
Peripheral artery disease, 216
Peroxynitrate, 45
Phospholipase A_2, 196, 212, 223
Phospholipid transfer protein, 197
Photosensitivity disorders, 366
Physical exams, 164
Physical exercise, 153, 242
Physicians' Health Study I, 38-39, 345-346, 367

Physicians' Health Study II, 40-41, 252
Plant phenolic compounds, 225
Plasma concentration of nutrients. See individual nutrients
Platelet effects, 196, 211, 212, 218, 253
Polyp Prevention Study, 36-37
Polyunsaturated fatty acids (PUFAs)
alpha-tocopherol and, 38-39, 195, 215, 225-226, 233, 235, 248
metabolism, 226
Pregnancy. See also Lactation; individual nutrients
alcohol and drug abuse, 150
aspirin use, 150
derivation of DRIs for, 67
eclampsia, 149
lipid peroxidation and, 150-151
methodological considerations, 67
premature birth, 149
and smoking, 132, 149, 150-151
special considerations, 150-151
ULs, 82
Probucol, 357
Proline, 98, 99, 106-107, 118-119
Pro-oxidant effects of nutrients, 129, 156, 159-160, 161, 166
Prostacyclin, 196, 212, 223
Prostaglandin synthesis, 99
Prostate cancer, 213-214, 219, 220, 290-291, 344-345, 368, 371
Protein, dietary
oxidation, 222
requirements for growth, 66
Protein-energy malnutrition, 202, 404
Protein kinase C inhibitors, 196, 211, 223
Proteoglycans, 98
Puberty. See also Adolescents
pubertal development, 30, 33

Q

Quercetin, 129

R

Race/ethnicity
and puberty onset, 30
and smoking, 132
and vitamin C, 132
Radiation, ionizing, 46, 112, 130

Randomized clinical trials, 61
Reactive nitrogen species (RNS)
  and cardiovascular disease, 216
  and DNA damage, 116
  measure of activity, 102, 106-107, 116
  mechanism of action, 44
  myeloperoxidase-derived, 109, 140
  vitamin C and, 98, 102, 106-107, 109,
    124, 140
Reactive oxygen species (ROS)
  and cardiovascular disease, 216
  and gastric cancer, 106-107, 116, 124
  and infectious and inflammatory
    stresses, 103
  mechanism of action, 44
  and neurodegenerative diseases, 222-223
  smoking and, 131
  sources of, 46
  vitamin C and, 98, 102, 103, 106-107,
    116, 124, 131
Recommendations. See also Research
    recommendations
  food composition data, 19, 396-397
Recommended Dietary Allowances
    (RDAs). See also individual nutrients
  AI compared, 4, 25-26, 138
  children, 66
  coefficient of variation, 66
  criteria used to derive, 10-11
  defined, 3, 5, 7, 22, 23, 24
  EAR and, 2-4, 23-25
  indicators of nutrient adequacy, 6-13
  method used to set, 23-25, 66
  uses, 4, 15, 23, 383, 391, 392
Recommended Dietary Allowances (reports),
    21
Reference body weight ratio method, 65-66
  alpha-tocopherol, 231
  selenium, 299
  vitamin C, 138
Reference weights and heights, 31-32
Renal disease/failure, 31, 50, 312
  vitamin C and, 157, 160, 164
Reproductive disorders, 368
Requirement, defined, 21
Research recommendations
  adverse effects, 21, 406
  alpha-tocopherol, 2, 20, 260-262, 406-407
  approach to setting, 19-20, 401-402
  carotenoids, 2, 20, 371-372, 403-404,
    406-407

dietary intakes, 165-166, 406
  kinetic modeling of body pools, 403
  priorities, 20, 140, 406-407
  selenium, 2, 20, 318-319, 406-407
  vitamin C, 2, 20, 140, 165-166, 406-407
Respiratory burst, 108
Respiratory distress syndrome, 108, 312
Retinaldehyde binding protein, 197
Retinol/retinoic acid, 36-37, 328, 332,
    355, 356, 367
Retinopathy, 50, 202, 208-209, 259, 368
Rheumatoid arthritis, 108
Riboflavin, 225
Risk assessment, defined, 75, 467
Risk assessment models. See also Dose-
    response assessment; Exposure
    assessment; Hazard identification;
    Risk characterization
  application to nutrients, 80-83
  basic concepts, 13, 75-76
  bioavailability considerations, 82-83
  default options, 460
  defined, 75, 467
  and food safety, 75-80
  inference options, 460
  methodological considerations, 458-461
  nutrient interactions, 83
  process, 76-78
  sensitivity of individuals, 82
  special problems with nutrients, 80-81
  thresholds, 78-80
  uncertainties, 76, 79-80, 458-461
Risk characterization, 92-94
  alpha-tocopherol, 260
  carotenoids, 369-371
  defined, 75, 77, 78, 467
  process, 92-93
  selenium, 13, 317-318
  vitamin C, 165
Risk management, 76, 467

S

Scurvy
  infants, 135, 159, 161, 162, 163-164,
    166
  rebound, 156, 158-159, 162, 163, 166
  vitamin C deficiency and, 98, 100, 101,
    119, 120, 135, 139, 145, 150, 156,
    158-159, 162, 163, 166

Selenium, 284-324
　absorption, 285-286, 306
　adolescents, 287, 299-300, 306, 307,
　　308, 315-316
　adults (19-50 years), 284, 300-305, 306-
　　308, 313-315, 399
　adults (51+ years), 70, 305-306
　adverse effects, 284, 311-313, 399, 407
　AIs, 10-11, 65, 292-299, 507
　animal studies, 287, 290, 301, 302
　bioavailability, 284, 291-292, 306, 307,
　　399
　in blood, 288-289, 301-302, 310, 312,
　　313, 314, 318, 446-447
　body stores, 286, 313
　breath excretion, 313
　and cancer, 36-41, 290-291, 319, 367
　and cardiovascular disease, 40-41, 287,
　　288
　children, 25, 65, 287, 288, 292, 299-
　　300, 301-302, 315-316, 318, 403
　critical endpoint, 313
　deficiency, 43, 287, 298
　dose-response assessment, 313-316
　in drinking water, 309-310, 311, 317,
　　399
　EARs, 10-11, 25, 299-304, 305, 306, 307
　excretion, 285, 286-287, 291, 313
　exposure assessment, 317
　factors affecting requirements, 291-292
　fetal, 67, 306
　food sources, 286, 292, 298-299, 308,
　　309, 397
　forms of, 285-286, 308, 312, 314, 468
　in fortified foods, 286, 310, 399
　functions, 43, 284, 285, 302
　gender and, 292, 299, 403
　geographic differences, 284, 309, 311-
　　312, 315, 316, 317, 318-319
　in hair and nails, 288, 313, 399
　hazard identification, 311-313
　in human milk, 292-298, 307, 315, 316,
　　386
　indicators of adequacy, 10-11, 12, 43,
　　287-291, 301-302, 312-313, 318
　infants, 65, 287, 292-299, 307, 315-316,
　　386, 392, 399
　intakes, 16, 284, 308-311, 317, 397-399,
　　428-431
　interaction with other nutrients, 36-37,
　　40-41, 285, 290, 367

　intervention studies, 2, 36-41, 290, 303-
　　304, 311, 318, 319, 367, 405
　and Kashin-Beck disease, 12, 43, 287,
　　465
　and Keshan disease, 12, 43, 287, 288,
　　292, 299-300, 301-302, 304, 403,
　　465
　lactation, 67, 293, 294-297, 307-308,
　　315
　by life-stage group, 10-11, 14, 292-308,
　　313-316, 428-431, 446-447
　and lipid peroxidation, 287
　metabolism, 285, 286, 299, 308
　method used to set AI, 65, 292-298
　NOAEL/LOAEL, 314, 316, 318
　and oxidative stress, 41, 43, 44-45, 52,
　　285
　pregnancy, 67, 287, 306-307, 315
　radiolabeled, 291
　RDAs, 2, 10-11, 12, 284, 300, 304-307,
　　308, 318, 507
　research recommendations, 20, 318-
　　319
　smokers, 367
　soil content, 16, 293, 298, 308, 397
　supplements, 286, 292, 310-311, 312,
　　317, 399
　and thyroid disorders, 287
　ULs, 13, 14, 26-27, 284, 311-318, 391,
　　399
　uncertainty assessment, 314, 315, 316
Selenocysteine, 284, 285, 286, 289, 291-
　　292, 308, 399, 468
Selenomethionine, 284-285, 286, 289, 291,
　　303, 307, 308, 312, 313, 314, 399,
　　468
Selenophosphate synthetase, 285
Selenoprotein P, 289, 290, 301-302
Selenoproteins
　absorption, 285
　antioxidant role, 41, 44-45, 284, 285
　in blood, 288, 289-290, 303, 304, 310
　defined, 285
　functions, 12, 43, 285, 318
　as indices of selenium status, 12, 43,
　　301-302, 312-313
　sources, 284-285
　synthesis, 286, 289, 291, 301
Selenosis, 284
　acute, 312
　biochemical indicators of, 312-313, 315

chronic, 311-312
defined, 468
form of intake and, 312, 314
overt signs of, 315
risk characterization, 13, 317-318
Semen, 98
Sensitivity
delayed dermal, 117, 118-119, 220
interindividual variability, 91, 82, 257
Sepsis, 253
Serum
alpha-carotene, 450-451
alpha-tocopherol, 236, 444-445
beta-carotene, 448-449
beta-cryptoxanthin, 452-453
cholesterol, 235
lutein and zeaxanthin, 454-455
lycopene, 456-457
vitamin C, 121, 132, 133, 152, 153, 156,
440-443
vitamin E (all forms), 444-445
Sjögren's syndrome, 101
Skeletal myopathy, 202
Skin cancer, 36-39, 290, 339
Skin Cancer Prevention Study, 36-37
Smokers and smoking
and alpha-tocopherol, 36-37, 213-214,
216, 219, 238, 242-243, 252, 367, 406
AMD, 18, 49
cardiovascular disease, 37-39, 48-49,
103, 106-107, 131, 216, 238, 252,
347
and carotenoids, 18, 36-39, 49, 330,
331, 334-337, 344, 345, 347, 351,
359, 366-371, 372, 405, 406
cataracts, 351
dietary intakes, 130, 359, 360
DNA damage, 110-113, 130-131, 360
endothelium-dependent vasodilation,
106-107, 131
lactating, 132
LDLs, 130, 132, 153
lipid peroxidation, 104-105, 130, 131,
132, 150-151
lung cancer, 36-39, 124, 213-214, 219,
360, 366-371, 372, 405, 406
metabolism of nutrients, 43
organic free radicals per puff, 132
and oropharyngeal cancers, 344
oxidative stress, 43, 48, 102, 130, 131,
132

passive, 132, 146, 153
pregnant, 132, 149, 150-151
prostate cancer, 219
racial/ethnic differences, 132
research needs, 403
and ROS, 131
and selenium, 367
special considerations, 150-151, 152-
153, 160-161, 164-165
and vitamin C, 12, 43, 95, 102, 103,
104-105, 108, 110-113, 124, 130-132,
146, 149, 150-151, 152-153, 242,
390, 393
Socioeconomic status, and nutrient status,
101, 136-137
Special considerations
adolescents, 358
alcohol and drug abusers, 150, 360
alpha-tocopherol, 241-243, 259
body size and composition extremes,
242
cancer, 241
cardiovascular disease, 241-242
carotenoids, 358-360
drug interactions, 150, 259
emotional stress, 153
glucose-6-phosphate dehydrogenase
deficiency, 160-161, 164
hemochromatosis, 160, 164
identification of, 87-88
infants, 160, 259
and NOAEL/LOAEL, 92
passive smokers, 153
physical exercise, 153, 242
in pregnancy, 150
renal disorders, 160, 164
smokers, 150-151, 152-153, 242-243,
359-360
ULs, 87-88, 92, 164-165, 259
vitamin C, 150-151, 152-153, 160-161,
164-165
vitamin K deficiency, 259
Sperm, 8-oxodG, 109, 110-111
Spinocerebellar ataxia, 202
Steroid hormone biosynthesis, 96, 98, 99,
153
Stomach cancer. See Gastric cancer
Stroke, 36-41, 121, 214, 216, 252, 254, 346-
347, 406
Superoxide, 103, 140-141, 211, 223
Superoxide dismutase, 45, 222

Supplements, dietary. *See also individual nutrients*
  bioavailability of nutrients, 191, 224, 251, 355, 357, 399
  data sources on intake, 70
  form of nutrient in, 192, 251, 286, 292, 312, 399
  gender differences, 70, 246-247, 260
  intakes from, 70, 155, 244-245, 249, 310-311
  multivitamin, 244, 246-247, 310, 386, 395
  quality of, 317
  shelf life, 190-191
  ULs and, 5, 26, 74, 155, 165, 249, 259, 310, 317, 396, 397
  units, 191, 244-245, 394-397
  usage, 70
SUVIMAX, 40-41
Systemic conditioning, 156, 158-159, 161

T

Tardive dyskinesia (TD), 222-223
Teratogenicity of nutrients, 315
Thiobarbituric acid reactive substances (TBARS), 45, 103, 104-105, 131, 203, 217, 334-335, 468
Thioredoxin reductases, 285
Thrombin, 211, 223
Thrombophlebitis, 253
Thromboxane, 217
Thyroid disorders, 287, 315
Tocopherol. *See* Alpha-tocopherol; Vitamin E
Tocotrienols. *See* Vitamin E
Toddlers, 29-30
Tolerable, defined, 26, 73
Tolerable Upper Intake Levels. *See also* Dose-response assessment; Hazard identification; Risk assessment models; *individual nutrients*
  appropropriateness of intakes above, 13, 27, 74, 155, 165, 249, 260, 311, 317-318, 369-371
  children, 33
  critical endpoints, 88-89
  defined, 3, 4, 5, 7-8, 26, 73, 91-92, 468
  derivation of, 7-8, 13, 26, 75, 80-83, 91-92, 162, 257, 315, 316
  development steps, 84-92
  fortification of foods and, 5, 26, 74

by life-stage groups, 14
  supplement use and, 5, 26-27, 80-81
  uses, 5-6, 15, 74, 383, 386, 391, 392-393, 398
Total Antioxidant Capacity, 104-105
Total radical-trapping antioxidant capability (TRAP) assay, 45
Toxicity
  experimental data, 86
  mechanism of action, 87
Triiodothyronine, 315
Trolox equivalent antioxidant capacity (TEAC) assay, 46
Tropical sprue, 220
Tumor necrosis factor-alpha, 338
Tyrosine metabolism, 45, 96

U

Ubiquinols, 224
Uncertainty
  alpha-tocopherol, 91, 231-232, 256-257
  assessment, 90-91, 162, 256-257, 315, 316
  dose-response assessment for ULs, 88-92
  in dietary assessment methods, 68, 248, 385, 396
  extrapolation from experimental animals to humans, 76, 79, 91
  factor, 79, 89, 90-91, 162, 256-257, 315, 468
  in risk assessment, 76, 79-80, 458-461
  selenium, 315, 316
  sources of, 256, 314, 386
  vitamin C data, 139-140, 162
United States Pharmacopeia, 191
Uric acid excretion, 156, 157
U.S. Department of Agriculture, 69, 135, 154, 343, 361
U.S. Department of Health and Human Services, 69
U.S. Dietary Guidelines, 351
U.S. Health Professionals Follow-up Study, 122, 290, 344, 347, 351

V

Vascular cell adhesion molecule-1 (VCAM-1), 196, 212, 223

Vasodilation
    alpha-tocopherol and, 196, 210
    endothelium-dependent, 106-107, 131
    smoking and, 131
    vitamin C and, 103, 106-107, 131
Vegans/vegetarians, 247, 297, 309
Vegetables. *See* Fruits and vegetables
Very low density lipoproteins, 104-105,
    197
Vitamin A
    carotenoids and, 12-14, 36-37, 43-44,
        325, 326, 327, 328, 330, 331, 338,
        343, 352, 355, 356, 366, 367, 371,
        372, 403, 467
    children, 338, 356
    deficiency, 43, 325, 338, 356, 371
    and DNA damage and repair, 112-113
    intakes, 352
    and lactation, 355
    vitamin C and, 112-113
Vitamin B$_{12}$, 156, 158, 161
Vitamin C (ascorbic acid), 95-185. *See also*
        Dehydroascorbic acid
    absorption and transport, 99-100, 103,
        108, 128, 140, 147-148, 155, 157
    adolescents, 65, 138-139, 149-151, 162-
        163
    adults (19-50 years), 12, 95, 121-122,
        126, 139-147, 149-151, 154, 157,
        161-162, 386, 387-390, 391, 392,
        393, 438-439
    adults (55+ years), 101, 118-119, 121,
        133, 147-149, 154, 155, 157, 438-439
    adverse effects, 13, 95, 100, 155-161,
        386, 407
    AIs, 6-7, 134-138, 507
    and alcohol/drug abuse, 101, 150
    allergic response, 160, 161
    animal studies, 59, 103, 120, 131, 140
    antioxidant role, 43, 44-45, 52, 95, 96,
        98-99, 101-109, 116, 124-125, 139-
        143, 146, 154, 166
    and asthma, 126
    and attention-deficit disorder, 163
    and beta-carotene, 102, 109, 110-111
    bioavailability, 99, 128
    and blood coagulation, 99, 101
    body pool, 100, 103, 132, 140, 142,
        145, 152-153, 166, 225, 403
    and bone growth, 101

    and cancer, 36-37, 40-41, 106-107, 113-
        116, 123-125, 127, 128, 160
    and cardiovascular disease, 18, 38-41,
        101-102, 103, 106-107, 109, 121-122,
        127, 128, 131, 346-347
    and carnitine biosynthesis, 95, 96, 99,
        120, 153, 166
    and cataracts, 18, 98, 125-126, 127
    chemistry, 95-96, 97
    children, 25, 65, 138-139, 161, 162-163,
        166
    and cholesterol, 99
    and chronic obstructive pulmonary
        disease, 126, 127
    and cognitive function, 19, 50, 127
    and collagen metabolism, 95, 96, 98,
        99, 101, 118-119, 166
    and common cold, 117, 126-127, 163
    and connective tissue synthesis, 98, 101
    and copper, 96, 97-98, 128, 129, 156,
        159-160, 161
    data selection, 161
    deficiency effects, 98, 99, 101, 108,
        119, 120, 145, 148, 149
    and dental enamel erosion, 156, 160,
        161
    dependence, 156, 158-159, 162, 163,
        166
    depletion/repletion studies, 108, 117,
        140, 143-145, 148, 402-403
    and DNA damage and repair, 98, 106-
        107, 109-115, 116, 130-131, 160
    dose-response assessment for ULs, 161-
        165
    EARs, 6-7, 23, 45, 65, 139, 146-151, 390
    emotional stress and, 153
    and endothelial dysfunction, 103, 106-
        107, 131
    erythrocyte, 140
    excretion, 12, 43, 95, 100, 140, 142,
        144, 147, 148, 151, 157, 158, 164
    exposure assessment, 165
    and factors affecting requirement, 128-
        133
    fetal, 67, 149, 150, 163, 166
    and flavonoids, 98-99, 102, 128, 129
    food sources, 101, 130, 154, 392
    functions, 12, 43, 95, 96-99, 165-166
    gastrointestinal effects, 95, 100, 102,
        106-107, 124-125, 156, 161-162, 163,
        166, 386, 393

gender and, 2, 12, 65, 95, 101, 121, 122, 124, 126, 133, 146-147, 154, 387-390
and glucose-6-phosphate dehydrogenase deficiency, 160-161, 164
and glutathione, 43, 96, 98, 99, 103, 105, 109-110, 126, 128, 129
hazard identification, 155-161
and hemostatic dysfunction, 131
and high-altitude resistance, 160
in human milk, 101, 132, 134-138, 151, 164, 386
and immune function, 108, 117-119, 127
indicators of adequacy, 6-7, 11, 101-128
infants, 65, 101, 129, 134-138, 159-160, 161, 162, 163-164, 386, 392
and inflammatory stress, 103, 108, 130
intakes, 15-16, 95, 135, 138, 154-155, 165-166, 387-390, 393, 416-421, 432-435, 438-439
interaction with drugs, 99, 150
interaction with other nutrients, 38-41, 96, 97-99, 102, 109, 110-113, 118-119, 120, 128-129, 156, 158, 159, 160, 161, 164, 166, 224-225, 285, 332
international comparisons, 121, 123, 124, 127, 135, 153
intervention trials, 38-39, 405
intracellular recycling, 108
and iron, 96, 97-98, 99, 109, 118-119, 120, 128, 129, 158, 159, 160, 161, 164, 166
and kidney stone formation, 156, 157, 160, 161
laboratory values, 67
and lactation, 67, 134-135, 136-137, 151-152, 164
and LDLs, 98, 101-102, 104-105, 109, 132, 153
in leukocytes, 43, 95, 103, 108-109, 110-111, 130, 133, 139, 140, 141, 142, 144, 146, 147, 148, 150
by life-stage group, 6-7, 14, 134-153, 161-164, 416-421, 432-435, 440-443
and lipid peroxidation, 45, 95, 98, 102, 104-105, 109, 116, 130, 131, 132, 146, 150-151, 153, 159
in lymphocytes, 99-100
metabolism, 12, 43, 95, 100, 108, 130, 133, 148, 152-153, 157, 158

method used to set AIs, 134-138
method used to set EARs, 139-145, 147-148, 149-151
methodological issues, 67, 68-69, 127-128, 402-403
and nervous system, 19, 50, 96, 98, 131, 153
in neutrophils, 12, 43, 95, 98, 99-100, 139, 140, 141, 144, 145, 146, 150, 385
NOAEL/LOAEL, 161-162, 163
and osmotic diarrhea, 13, 95, 100, 154, 161-162, 163, 166, 386, 393
and oxalate excretion, 156
and oxidative stress, 12, 43, 95, 101-102, 109, 126, 128, 130, 131, 132, 148, 152, 162, 166
and oxygen demand, 156, 161
passive smokers, 132, 146, 153
and periodontal health, 120, 156, 160, 161, 166
and physical exams, 164
and physical exercise, 153
plasma concentrations, 100, 101, 121, 123, 126, 127, 128, 130, 132, 133, 134-135, 140, 141, 142, 144, 146, 147, 148, 155, 158
and pregnancy, 67, 82, 132, 149-151, 159, 161, 163-164, 166
pro-oxidant effects, 129, 156, 159-160, 161, 166
race/ethnicity and, 132
RDAs, 2, 6-7, 12, 43, 95, 138, 139, 147, 149, 150, 151-152, 386, 392, 507
and renal disease, 157, 160, 164
research recommendations, 2, 20, 140, 165-166
and respiratory distress syndrome, 108
and rheumatoid arthritis, 108
risk characterization, 165
RNS/ROS and, 98, 102, 103, 106-107, 109, 116, 124, 131, 140
and scurvy, 98, 100, 101, 119, 120, 135, 139, 145, 150, 156, 158-159, 162, 163, 166
serum concentrations, 121, 132, 133, 152, 153, 156, 440-443
smokers, 12, 43, 95, 102, 103, 104-105, 108, 110-113, 124, 130-132, 146, 149, 150 151, 152-153, 242, 390, 393

socioeconomic status and, 101, 136-137
special considerations, 150-151, 152-153, 160-161, 164-165
and steroid hormone biosynthesis, 96, 98, 99, 153
supplements, 70, 155
systemic conditioning, 156, 158-159, 161
turnover, 43, 95, 130-131, 152-153, 158
ULs, 13, 14, 26-27, 82, 95, 155-165, 391, 393
uncertainties in data, 140, 162
and uric acid excretion, 156, 157
and vitamin A, 112-113
vitamin E and, 98-99, 102, 109, 110-113, 128, 129, 213, 224-225
and vitamin B_{12}, 156, 158, 161
Vitamin E (all forms), 186-293. *See also* Alpha-tocopherol
absorption, 191, 193, 196, 243
affinity of alpha-TTP to forms of, 2, 12, 19, 193, 195, 197-198, 243, 262
bioavailability, 193, 194-195, 243, 404
body pools, 210
conversion factors, 244-245, 394-395
defined, 187, 393
food composition data, 68-69, 393-394
forms of, 2, 12, 16, 186, 187-190, 193, 194-195, 210, 243, 262, 393-394, 404, 406
in human milk, 227, 228-229
intakes, 68, 69-70, 186, 194, 232, 243, 393-394, 395-396, 404, 406, 422-423
interconversion of units, 191-192, 244, 246
serum values, 444-445
shelf life, 190-191
structure, 187-195
units of activity, 186, 190 n.1, 191-195
Vitamin K, 252, 254-255, 256, 259

W

Warfarin therapy, 252
Weight. *See* Body weight; Reference weights and heights

Western Electric cohort study, 121-122, 341
Women. *See also* Gender; Lactation; Pregnancy
alpha-tocopherol, 40-41, 212, 219, 226, 237, 245, 246-247, 249, 259-260
aspirin, 40-41
breast cancer, 123, 219
cardiovascular disease, 38-41, 121, 122, 212, 347
carotenoids, 38-41, 330-331, 349, 351
cataracts, 126, 351
cervical cancer, 17, 123, 340-341, 345, 346
dietary intakes, 154, 165, 245
fish oil supplements, 226
Keshan disease, 292, 304
kidney stone formation, 157
MOPD values, 349
postmenopausal, 122, 123, 212, 219, 226, 259-260, 330-331, 347
selenium, 292
supplement use, 249, 260
vitamin C, 40-41, 95, 118-119, 122, 123, 126, 133, 146-147, 149, 154, 157, 165, 386
Women's Antioxidant Cardiovascular Study, 40-41, 252
Women's Health Study, 40-41, 252
World Health Organization
definition of adverse effect, 73
Monitoring Cardiovascular Project, Vitamin Substudy, 346
uncertainty factors, 79

X

Xanthophylls, 329, 330

Z

Zeaxanthin, 18, 44, 49, 329, 330, 348, 349, 350, 351, 358, 360-361, 364, 366, 371, 454-455
Zinc, 40-41